The Maxillary Sinus

Medical and Surgical Management

Thieme

The Maxillary Sinus

Medical and Surgical Management

James A. Duncavage, MD, FACS
Professor and Vice-Chairman
Department of Otolaryngology
Vanderbilt University Medical Center
Nashville, Tennessee

Samuel S. Becker, MD
Director of Rhinology
Becker Nose and Sinus Center, LLC
Voorhees, New Jersey

Thieme
New York • Stuttgart

Thieme Medical Publishers, Inc.
333 Seventh Avenue
New York, NY 10001

Executive Director: Timothy Y. Hiscock
Managing Editor: J. Owen Zurhellen IV
Editorial Assistant: Emma Lassiter
Editorial Director: Michael Wachinger
Production Editor: Martha L. Wetherill, MPS Content Services
International Production Director: Andreas Schabert
Vice President, International Marketing and Sales: Cornelia Schulze
Chief Financial Officer: James Mitos
President: Brian D. Scanlan
Illustrator: Birck Cox
Compositor: MPS Content Services, A Macmillan Company
Printer: Leo Paper USA

Library of Congress Cataloging-in-Publication Data
The maxillary sinus : medical and surgical management / [edited by] James A. Duncavage, Samuel S. Becker.
p. ; cm.
Includes bibliographical references and index.
ISBN 978-1-60406-280-9
1. Maxillary sinus—Diseases. 2. Maxillary sinus—Surgery. I. Duncavage, James A. II. Becker, Samuel S.
[DNLM: 1. Maxillary Sinus—surgery. 2. Maxillary Sinusitis—therapy. WV 345 M464 2010]
RF421.M365 2010
616.2'12059—dc22

2010002162

Important note: Medical knowledge is ever-changing. As new research and clinical experience broaden our knowledge, changes in treatment and drug therapy may be required. The authors and editors of the material herein have consulted sources believed to be reliable in their efforts to provide information that is complete and in accord with the standards accepted at the time of publication. However, in view of the possibility of human error by the authors, editors, or publisher of the work herein or changes in medical knowledge, neither the authors, editors, nor publisher, nor any other party who has been involved in the preparation of this work, warrants that the information contained herein is in every respect accurate or complete, and they are not responsible for any errors or omissions or for the results obtained from use of such information. Readers are encouraged to confirm the information contained herein with other sources. For example, readers are advised to check the product information sheet included in the package of each drug they plan to administer to be certain that the information contained in this publication is accurate and that changes have not been made in the recommended dose or in the contraindications for administration. This recommendation is of particular importance in connection with new or infrequently used drugs.

Some of the product names, patents, and registered designs referred to in this book are in fact registered trademarks or proprietary names even though specific reference to this fact is not always made in the text. Therefore, the appearance of a name without designation as proprietary is not to be construed as a representation by the publisher that it is in the public domain.

Printed in China

5 4 3 2 1

ISBN 978-1-60406-280-9

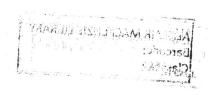

I dedicate this book to Lillian, my wife,
for all of her patience and understanding.

—JAD

I dedicate this book to my wife, Jennifer, and to our children, Emily and Katharine, as well as to my parents, Merle and William Becker, and to my brothers, Richard, Paul, and Daniel. Together they give my life the texture that makes each day different and lovely.

—SSB

Contents

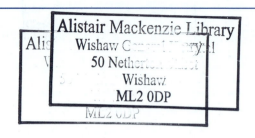

DVD-Video Contents

Disk 2

17.1. Caldwell–Luc Procedure
17.2. Endoscopic Caldwell–Luc Procedure

18.1. MIST
18.2. Balloon Sinuplasty
18.3. Maxillary Antrostomy
18.4. Resection of Juvenile Nasopharyngeal Angiofibroma

19.1. Anatomic Dissection of the Pterygopalatine Fossa

20.1. Endoscopic Orbital Decompression

21.1. FESS for Persistent Maxillary Sinusitis

[Chapter 22 no videos]

23.1. Identification of the Natural Ostium of the Maxillary Sinus: Two Cases
23.2. Identification of the Orifice of the Nasolacrimal Duct
23.3. Removing the Cyst Wall of a Dentigerous Cyst via the Middle Meatus and Inferior Meatus

24.1. Recurrent Maxillary Inverted Papilloma—Part I
24.2. Recurrent Maxillary Inverted Papilloma—Part II

25.1. Creating an Anterior Transseptal Approach for a Right Maxillary Inverted Papilloma
25.2. Trans-Septal Approach to Anterolateral Sinus Disease
25.3. Recurrent Left Inverted Papilloma—3 Weeks Postoperative
25.4. Endoscopic Anterior/Medial Buttress Excision of Left Maxillary Mass

26.1. Medial Maxillectomy for Inverted Papilloma

27.1. Surgical Challenges Involving the Maxillary Sinus—Part I
27.2. Surgical Challenges Involving the Maxillary Sinus—Part II

28.1. Six-Week Postoperative View after Revision Maxillary Sinus Surgery

Preface

Traditionally, the maxillary sinus has been seen as the easiest sinus to open surgically, with the frontal sinus being the most challenging. Over time, however, it has become clear that the maxillary sinus is, in fact, the sinus that most often requires revision surgery. This sinus is also the most difficult to keep consistently healthy after surgery. Consequently, the maxillary sinus presents the greatest challenge to those who treat patients with sinusitis. Now that endoscopic sinus surgery has been a staple of most otolaryngology practices over the past three decades, these practices are caring for increasing numbers of patients with refractory maxillary sinusitis. Meanwhile, there has been a variety of advancements regarding the efficacy of different surgical techniques to treat the maxillary sinus, as well as advances in our understanding of the pathophysiology and medical management of sinus disease. It is for this reason that we have found this single sinus deserving of the focus and detailed analysis allowed in this combined book and audiovisual format.

This book brings together authors from around the world—international experts on their respective topics—to discuss wide-ranging issues related to the medical and surgical management of maxillary sinus disease. For the surgeons and nonsurgeons alike, 73 carefully narrated videos representing more than 3 hours of detailed, step-by-step endoscopic procedures are included to complement and bring to life the ideas discussed in the text. Endoscopic photographs, illustrations, charts, and pearls are likewise provided to help increase understanding of the concepts presented.

By addressing the management of sinus disease from the perspective of a single sinus, we hope that this text and accompanying DVD-Videos will help otolaryngologists attain an increased understanding of the range of pathologic conditions that their patients bring to their offices, and ultimately, assist them in delivering improved care to their patients.

Acknowledgments

A project like this one is only possible through the hard work and support of many groups and individuals. We would first like to thank the contributors to this book and accompanying DVD-Videos, the rhinologists from around the world who have generously shared their experience with the readers. Special thanks go to Rashod Ezell, the Media Services specialist at Vanderbilt University whose tireless "behind the scenes" efforts allowed for the on time, high-quality production of this book and video project, and our thanks to artist Birck Cox, who has done a fabulous job with the illustrations. Our thanks also go to J. Owen Zurhellen, the managing editor at Thieme Publishers. Finally, we would like to thank Stryker Craniomaxillofacial for their financial support of this project.

Dr. Becker would like to acknowledge and to thank the outstanding mentors he has had over the years, who have encouraged him to maintain perseverance, creativity, and diligence in the face of obstacles. These mentors include Thom Haxo, Joel Upton, John Walker, Robert Jackler, Michael Merzenich, Charles Gross, and James Duncavage. They have selflessly shared the lessons of their own experiences, and have been teachers in the true sense of the word.

Dr. Duncavage would like to acknowledge Robert Toohill, his own mentor during residency at the Medical College of Wisconsin. In addition, he would like to thank all the staff at the Bill Wilkerson Center for Otolaryngology and Communication Sciences, Vanderbilt School of Medicine.

James A. Duncavage, MD, FACS
Samuel S. Becker, MD

Contributors

Adam M. Becker, MD
Assistant Professor of Otolaryngology
Section of Rhinology
Division of Otolaryngology–Head and Neck Surgery
Duke University
Durham, North Carolina

Samuel S. Becker, MD
Director of Rhinology
Becker Nose and Sinus Center, LLC
Voorhees, New Jersey

Jacquelyn M. Brewer, MD, MPH
Resident
Department of Otolaryngology–Head and Neck Surgery
University of Texas Southwestern Medical Center
University of Texas Southwestern
Dallas, Texas

Roy R. Casiano, MD
Professor and Vice Chairman
Department of Otolaryngology
University of Miami School of Medicine
University of Miami Hospital and Clinics
Miami, Florida

Peter J. Catalano, MD, FACS, FARS
Chief of Surgery
Department of Otolaryngology–Head and Neck Surgery
St. Elizabeth's Hospital
Boston, MA 02135

Rakesh K. Chandra, MD
Associate Professor
Northwestern Sinus and Allergy Center
Department of Otolaryngology–Head and Neck Surgery
Northwestern University Feinberg School of Medicine
Chicago, Illinois

Alexander G. Chiu, MD
Associate Professor
Director, Rhinology and Skull Base Surgery Fellowship Program
Department of Otorhinolaryngology
University of Pennsylvania Medical Center
Philadelphia, Pennsylvania

Venkatakarthikeyan Chokkalingam, MD
Assistant Professor
Department of Otolaryngology
All India Institute of Medical Sciences
New Delhi, India

Eugene A. Chu, MD
Clinical Instructor
Department of Otolaryngology–Head and Neck Surgery
Johns Hopkins University Hospital
Baltimore, Maryland

Nick I. Debnath, MD
Assistant Professor
Department of Otolaryngology–Head and Neck Surgery
Washington University in St. Louis School of Medicine
St. Louis, Missouri

Ramesh C. Deka, MD
Professor
Department of Otolaryngology
Director
All India Institute of Medical Sciences
New Delhi, India

Wolfgang Draf, Dr Med, Dr hc
Professor and Head
Department of Ear, Nose and Throat Diseases, Head and Neck Surgery
International Neuroscience Institute at the University of Magdeburg
Hannover, Germany

James A. Duncavage, MD
Professor and Vice-Chairman
Department of Otolaryngology
Vanderbilt University Medical Center
Nashville, Tennessee

Jean Anderson Eloy, MD
Director, Rhinology and Sinus Surgery
Assistant Professor of Surgery
Department of Surgery, Division of Otolaryngology–Head and Neck Surgery
University of Medicine and Dentistry of New Jersey–New Jersey Medical School
Newark, New Jersey

Berrylin J. Ferguson, MD
UPMC Mercy
Pittsburgh, Pennsylvania

Wytske J. Fokkens, MD, PhD
Department of Otorhinolaryngology
Academic Medical Center
Amsterdam, Netherlands

B. Forer, MD
Clinical Fellow
National University of Singapore
Singapore

Christos C. Georgalas, PhD, MRCS, DLO, FRCS (ORL-HNS)
Department of Otolaryngology
Academic Medical Center
Amsterdam, Netherlands

Richard J. Harvey, MD
Clinical Associate Professor
Rhinologist and Skull Base Surgeon
Department of Otolaryngology/Skull Base Surgery
St. Vincent's Hospital
Sydney, New South Wales
Australia

Peter H. Hwang, MD
Professor
Chief, Division of Rhinology
Department of Otolaryngology–Head and Neck Surgery
Stanford University School of Medicine
Stanford, California

Keiichi Ichimura, MD, PhD
Professor and Chairman
Department of Otolaryngology–Head and Neck Surgery
Jichi Medical University School of Medicine
Shimotsuke, Tochigi
Japan

Andrew P. Lane, MD
Director, Division of Rhinology and Sinus Surgery
Associate Professor
Department of Otolaryngology–Head and Neck Surgery
Johns Hopkins School of Medicine
Baltimore, Maryland

Theodore C. Larson III, MD
Director of Neurointervention and the Neurointerventional Fellowship Program
InterMountain Neurosurgery
St. Anthony Central Hospital
Denver, Colorado

John Lee, MD, FRCSC
Lecturer
Department of Otolaryngology–Head and Neck Surgery
University of Toronto
St. Michael's Hospital
Toronto, Ontario
Canada

Man-Kit Leung, MD
Pacific Ear, Nose, & Throat Associates, Inc.
San Francisco, California

Valerie J. Lund, CBE, MS, FRCS, FRCSEd
Professor of Rhinology
Honorary Consultant Otolaryngologist
Royal National Throat, Nose and Ear Hospital
Ear Institute
London, United Kingdom

Bradley F. Marple, MD
Department of Otolaryngology–Head and Neck Surgery
UT Southwestern Medical Center
Dallas, Texas

Ralph B. Metson, MD
Clinical Professor
Department of Otology and Laryngology
Harvard Medical School
Department of Otolaryngology
Massachusetts Eye and Ear Infirmary
Boston, Massachusetts

Amir Minovi, MD
Associate Professor
Department of Otorhinolaryngology, Head and Neck Surgery
Ruhr University Bochum
St. Elisabeth Hospital
Bochum, Germany

Abusaleh Muneif, MD
Otorhinolaryngology Hospital of the First Affiliated Hospital of Sun Yat-sen University
Otorhinolaryngology Institute of Sun Yat-sen University
Guangzhou, Guangdong
China

Jayakar V. Nayak, MD, PhD
Assistant Professor
Stanford Sinus and Skull Base Center
Department of Otolaryngology–Head and Neck Surgery
Stanford University
Stanford, California

João Flávio Nogueira, MD
Otolaryngologist
Director–Sinus Centro
Hospital Geral de Fortaleza
Fortaleza, Ceará
Brazil

Leslie A. Nurse, MD
Rhinology Fellow
Department of Otolaryngology
Vanderbilt University Medical Center
Nashville, Tennessee

Bradley A. Otto, MD
Assistant Professor
Department of Otolaryngology–Head and Neck Surgery
The Ohio State University
OSU Eye and Ear Institute
Columbus, Ohio

James N. Palmer, MD
Associate Professor
Director, Division of Rhinology
Department of Otorhinolaryngology–Head and Neck Surgery
University of Pennsylvania
Philadelphia, Pennsylvania

Shirley S. N. Pignatari, MD, PhD
Head
Division of Pediatric Otolaryngology
Department of Otolaryngology–Head and Neck Surgery
Federal University of São Paulo
São Paulo, Brazil

Simon Robinson, MBChB, FRACS
Director
Wakefield Sinus and Facial Plastic Centre
Wellington, New Zealand

Paul T. Russell, MD
Department of Otolaryngology–Head and Neck Surgery
Vanderbilt University Medical Center
Nashville, Tennessee

Hesham Saleh, FRCS (ORL-HNS)
Consultant Rhinologist and Facial Plastic Surgeon
Charing Cross and Royal Brompton Hospitals
Imperial College
London, United Kingdom

Zoukaa Sargi, MD
Assistant Professor of Clinical Otolaryngology
Department of Otolaryngology–Head and Neck Surgery
University of Miami Miller School of Medicine
Miami, Florida

Rodney J. Schlosser, MD
Department of Otolaryngology–Head and Neck Surgery
Medical University of South Carolina
Charleston, South Carolina

D. S. Sethi, FRCSEd
Clinical Associate
University of Singapore
Senior Consultant
Department of Otolaryngology
Singapore General Hospital
Singapore

Jianbo Shi, MD, PhD
Professor and Director of Rhinology
Department of Otorhinolaryngology
Otorhinolaryngology Institute of Sun Yat-sen University
The First Affiliated Hospital of Sun Yat-sen University
Guangzhou, Guangdong Province
China

Hwa J. Son, MD
Resident Physician
Department of Otolaryngology–Head and Neck Surgery
Feinberg School of Medicine
Northwestern Memorial Hospital
Chicago, Illinois

Aldo C. Stamm, MD, PhD
Director
São Paulo ENT Center
Hospital Professor
Hospital Edmundo Vasconcelos
São Paulo, Brazil

James A. Stankiewicz, MD
Professor and Chair
Department of Otolaryngology–Head and Neck Surgery
Loyola University Stritch School of Medicine
Senior Attending Physician
Loyola University Medical Center
Maywood, Illinois

Belachew Tessema, MD
Connecticut Sinus Institute
Assistant Clinical Professor
Department of Surgery, Division of Otolaryngology
University of Connecticut
Farmington, Connecticut

Marc A. Tewfik, MDCM, MSc, FRCSC
Assistant Professor
Department of Otolaryngology–Head and Neck Surgery
The Royal Victoria Hospital
McGill University
Montreal, Quebec
Canada

Roy F. Thomas, MD
Department of Otolaryngology
Brooke Army Medical Center
San Antonio, Texas

Ronaldo Nunes Toledo, MD, PhD
Department of Otolaryngology–Head and Neck Surgery
A.C. Camargo Cancer Hospital
São Paulo, Brazil

Winston C. Vaughan, MD
California Sinus Institute
East Palo Alto, California

Kevin C. Welch, MD
Assistant Professor
Department of Otolaryngology–Head and Neck Surgery
Loyola University Medical Center
Maywood, Illinois

Matthew Whitley, MD
Chief Resident
Department of Otolaryngology
University of Miami
Miami, Florida

Maria L. Wittkopf, MD
Resident, Otolaryngology and Head and Neck Surgery
Vanderbilt University Medical Center
Nashville, Tennessee

Peter-John Wormald, MD
Professor and Chairman
Department of Otorhinolaryngology and Head and Neck Surgery
University of Adelaide
Adelaide, South Australia
Australia

Guanxia Xiong, MD, PhD
Assistant Professor
Otorhinolaryngology Hospital of the First Affiliated Hospital of Sun Yat-sen University
Otorhinolaryngology Institute of Sun Yat-sen University
Guangzhou, Guangdong
China

Geng Xu, MD, PhD
Professor and Director
Otorhinolaryngology Hospital of the First Affiliated Hospital of Sun Yat-Sen University
Guangzhou, Guangdong
China

Ramzi T. Younis, MD
Professor and Chief
Division of Pediatric Otolaryngology
Department of Otolaryngology–Head and Neck Surgery
Leonard M. Miller School of Medicine
Holtz Children Hospital/Jackson Memorial Hospital
Bascom Palmer Eye Institute
Miami, Florida

Kejun Zuo, MD
Attending Doctor
Otorhinolaryngology Hospital of the First Affiliated Hospital of Sun Yat-sen University
Otorhinolaryngology Institute of Sun Yat-sen University
Guangzhou, Guangdong
China

Additional Video Contributors

Ross M. Germani, MD
Holzer Clinic
Proctorville, Ohio

Bjorn Herman, MD
Resident
Department of Otolaryngology
University of Miami
Miami, Florida

1 Surgical Anatomy and Embryology of the Maxillary Sinus and Surrounding Structures

Adam M. Becker and Peter H. Hwang

The maxillary sinus, the most accessible of the sinuses, is also one of the most commonly revised sites following primary functional endoscopic sinus surgery. A thorough understanding of maxillary sinus anatomy is critical to the optimal treatment of maxillary sinus disease.

Embryology

Although paranasal sinus development begins in utero, only the maxillary and ethmoid sinuses are present at birth. During the seventh to eighth week of development, a series of five to six ridges known as ethmoturbinals appear.[1] Via differential growth and development, only three to four ridges ultimately persist. The first ethmoturbinal undergoes partial regression during development; its ascending portion forms the agger nasi and its descending portion forms the uncinate process. The second ethmoturbinal forms the middle turbinate, the third forms the superior turbinate, and the fourth and fifth ethmoturbinals fuse to form the supreme turbinate. In addition to the ethmoturbinals, the maxilloturbinal is an inferiorly oriented ridge of maxillary origin that ultimately forms the inferior turbinate.

Ossification of the maxilla begins at approximately 6 weeks of life. Conflicting data exist regarding the exact process of osteogenesis. One theory is that bone formation begins in two initial foci, one in the maxilla proper and one in the premaxilla. Alternatively, Vacher and colleagues demonstrated maxillary ossification beginning on either side from a single layer of ossification situated cranially in relation to the dental lamina. Ossification then spreads medially to the entire palate, while respecting the median transverse mesenchymal septum, which separates the primary from the secondary palate.[2]

The primary furrows that lie between the ethmoturbinals form the various nasal meatus and recesses. The first of these, located between the first and second ethmoturbinals, has a descending portion that forms the ethmoid infundibulum, hiatus semilunaris, and middle meatus. The ascending aspect likely provides contributions to the frontal recess. The primordial maxillary sinus develops from the inferior aspect of the ethmoidal infundibulum at about 16 weeks.[3] The second primary furrow forms the superior meatus and the third primary furrow forms the supreme meatus. In addition to the ridge and furrow development, a cartilaginous capsule surrounds the developing nasal cavity and has an important role in sinonasal development.[4,5] Ultimately, the cartilaginous structures resorb or ossify as development progresses. Over the second and third trimesters the maxillary sinus continues to enlarge from the maxillary infundibulum.

At birth, the maxillary sinus measures ~7 millimeters (mm) in anteroposterior depth, 4.0 mm in height, and 2.7 mm in width.[6] The maxillary sinus continues to pneumatize most rapidly between ages 1 and 8, by which time the sinus extends laterally past the infraorbital canal, and inferiorly to the midinferior meatus. The floor of the maxillary sinus is initially oriented above the level of the nasal floor. Pneumatization reaches the level of the nasal floor following exfoliation and replacement of the primary dentition. In childhood, the roof of the maxillary sinus slopes inferolaterally, gradually assuming its more horizontal orientation seen in adulthood as pneumatization progresses. At 16 years of age, the maxillary sinus reaches its adult dimensions, measuring 39 mm in depth, 36 mm in height, and 27 mm in width. The final size of the maxillary sinus varies between individuals and can be influenced by several factors. Hypoplasia of the maxillary sinus is relatively rare: it has been related to conditions such as severe infection, trauma, tumor, irradiation, and syndromes affecting the first branchial arch.[7]

Anatomy

Maxillary Sinus

Osteology

The maxillary sinus usually consists of a single pyramidal chamber with an adult volume of 15 milliliters (mL) (**Fig. 1.1**). The medial wall of the maxillary sinus consists of a thin bony plate composed of the maxilla, the inferior turbinate, the uncinate process, the perpendicular plate of the palatine bone, and the lacrimal bone. The maxillary sinus ostium measures ~3 to 4 mm in diameter and lies in an anteromedial position. Its medial aspect is partially covered by the uncinate process (**see Video 1.1**). The lateral apex of the sinus extends into the zygomatic process of the maxillary bone or into the zygoma. The roof of the maxillary sinus is formed by the bony orbital floor. The infraorbital nerve can often be seen as a ridge or groove along the roof of the sinus as the nerve passes from a posterior to anterior direction. Occasionally, the infraorbital nerve may be dehiscent in the

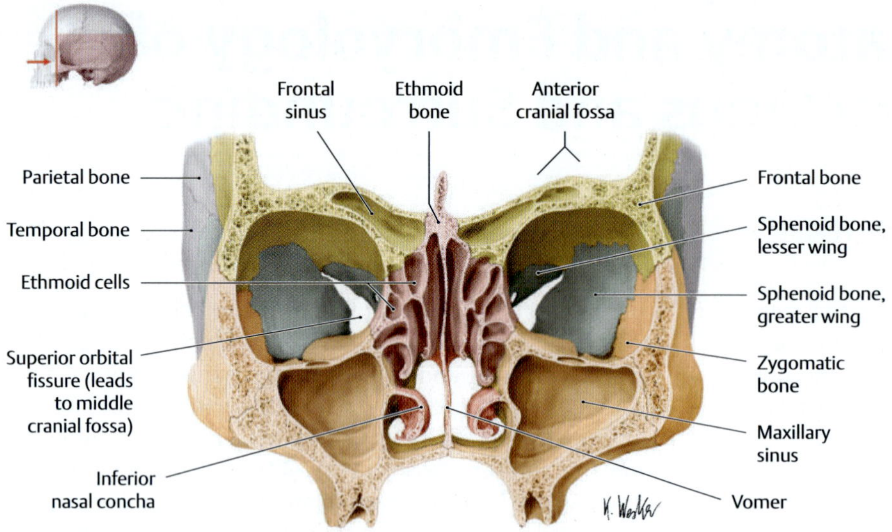

Fig. 1.1 The maxillary sinus and surrounding bony structures. From THIEME Atlas of Anatomy, Head and Neuroanatomy, © Thieme 2007, Illustration by Karl Wesker.

roof of the sinus, which some authors report to be a potential cause of facial pain and headache.[8]

The floor of the maxillary sinus is formed by the alveolar and palatine processes of the maxilla and generally lies 1.0 to 1.2 cm below the level of the floor of the nasal cavity. The maxillary sinus is usually separated from the molar dentition by a layer of compact bone. Occasionally, this layer of bone may be thin or absent, providing a direct route for odontogenic infections to spread into the sinus. The anterior wall of the maxillary sinus contains the infraorbital foramen located at the midsuperior portion. The canine fossa makes up the thinnest portion of the anterior wall and is located just above the canine tooth. The posterior wall of the sinus forms the anterior border of the pterygomaxillary fossa, which contains the internal maxillary artery, sphenopalatine ganglion, vidian nerve, greater palatine nerve, and the second branch of the trigeminal nerve.

Innervation

The posterior superior alveolar nerve supplies most of the sensation of the maxillary sinus. The anterior superior alveolar nerve innervates the anterior portion of the maxillary sinus and the middle superior alveolar nerve contributes secondary mucosal innervation. The maxillary ostium receives its innervation via the greater palatine nerve; the infundibulum is supplied by the anterior ethmoidal branch of V1.[9] Multiple branching patterns of the anterior superior and middle superior alveolar nerves exist along the anterior face of the maxilla.[10]

Secretomotor fibers from the facial nerve originate in the nervus intermedius, synapse at the pterygopalatine ganglion, and are carried to the sinus mucosa with the trigeminal sensory branches.[11] Vasoconstrictor branches originate from the sympathetic carotid plexus.

Vascular Supply

The infraorbital, lateral branches of the sphenopalatine, greater palatine, and the alveolar arteries supply the maxillary sinus. Venous drainage runs anteriorly into the facial vein and posteriorly into the maxillary vein as well as the jugular and dural sinus systems.

Lymphatic

The maxillary sinus mucosa has a superficial and deep longitudinal lymphatic capillary network oriented toward the natural maxillary sinus ostium. The density of lymphatics increases from cranial to caudal, and from dorsal to ventral, reaching its maximum density at the natural ostium.[12] At this point, the lymphatic network connects directly to the nasal vessels and travels to the nasopharynx. Besides the ostial route of lymphatic drainage, there are lymphatic connections over the pterygopalatine plexus to the eustachian tube and the nasopharynx. The primary lymphatic basins of the paranasal sinuses are the lateral cervical and retropharyngeal lymph nodes.[13]

The most common anatomic variation in the maxillary sinus region is the infraorbital ethmoid air cell (Haller cell). This is an ethmoid cell that pneumatizes along the medial roof of the maxillary sinus and inferomedial portion of the lamina papyracea. These cells, which are present in ~34% of patients, arise most commonly from the anterior ethmoid and frequently encroach on the infundibulum.[14] Bolger et al[15] investigated the role of the infraorbital air cell in sinusitis and found no statistically significant difference between its prevalence in patients presenting with recurrent maxillary sinusitis and that of asymptomatic patients.

Another rare anatomic variation is hypoplasia or atelectasis of the maxillary sinus.[16] Several investigators propose that the pathophysiology of this variation involves obstruction of the natural ostium by a lateralized uncinate process.[17–19] This, in turn, leads to a negative pressure environment with subsequent remodeling and involution of the bony maxillary walls. Although the atelectatic maxillary sinus is typically filled with thick mucus, the condition is often asymptomatic. In fact, the presenting clinical finding is often enophthalmos owing to descent of the orbital floor.

This clinical presentation is termed *silent sinus syndrome* or *silent maxillary sinus atelectasis with enophthalmos*.

Middle Turbinate

Of the three turbinates, the middle turbinate is the most influential in the development of the middle meatal anatomy. The middle turbinate has a complex series of attachments. Anteriorly, the middle turbinate assumes a sagittal orientation, fusing with the anterior uncinate process, the medial wall of the agger nasi, and the cribriform plate. More posteriorly, the middle turbinate basal lamella assumes a coronal orientation, attaching to the roof of the ethmoid sinus and the lamina papyracea. The basal lamella forms the boundary between the anterior and the posterior ethmoid sinuses. As the middle turbinate projects posteriorly, the body of the middle turbinate provides the medial border for the posterior aspect of the middle meatus.

Concha bullosa refers to a pneumatized middle turbinate (**see Video 1.2**). The actual prevalence of concha bullosa is unclear in the literature due to significant variation in the criteria used across studies; however, when present, conchae bullosa usually occur bilaterally.[20] Several authors have suggested that concha bullosa play a role in recurrent inflammatory sinus disease because of its tendency to compress the uncinate process and compromise or obstruct the middle meatus and infundibulum.[20,21] Others have suggested that the size of the concha bullosa, rather than its mere presence, was more significantly associated with inflammatory disease.[22]

Paradoxical middle turbinates occur when the normal convex curvature of the middle turbinate is reversed (**Fig. 1.2**). In the paradoxical middle turbinate, the inferior free edge of the turbinate orients toward the nasal septum, while the body of the turbinate is displaced laterally toward the middle meatus. Because of the potential to obscure drainage through the middle meatus, the presence of a paradoxical turbinate has been implicated as a contributing factor in chronic sinusitis. Lloyd, however, reported that this variation had no correlation with sinus disease in otherwise asymptomatic individuals.[20]

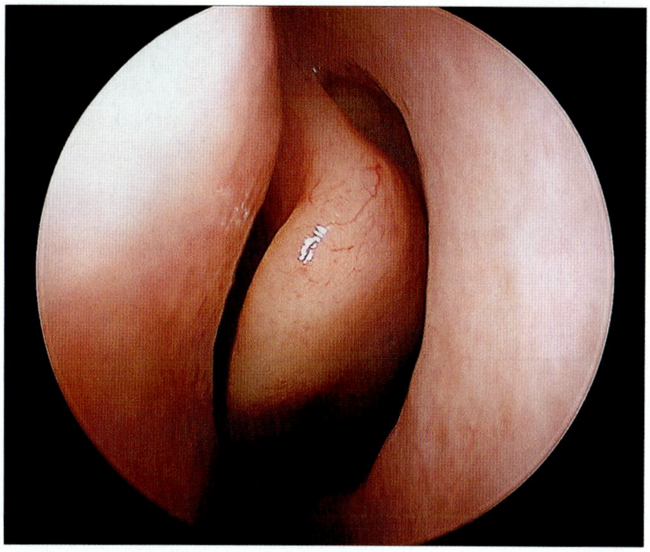

Fig. 1.2 Endoscopic view of a left middle meatus. The paradoxical middle turbinate has a convex lateral surface, which can result in narrowing of the maxillary sinus outflow tract.

Uncinate Process

The uncinate process is the most anterior of the classically described ethmoidal lamellae.[23] It is a sagittally oriented structure that forms the anteromedial boundary of the ethmoid infundibulum. The hiatus semilunaris lies directly between the posterior margin of the uncinate and the anterior wall of the bulla ethmoidalis. For most of its course, the uncinate has three layers: nasal or middle meatal mucosa on its medial aspect, infundibular mucosa on its lateral aspect, and ethmoid bone in between. Anteriorly and superiorly, the uncinate process attaches to the ethmoidal crest of the maxillae, just inferior to the attachments of the middle turbinate and agger nasi. Directly inferior to this, it fuses with the posterior aspect of the lacrimal bone. Posteriorly and inferiorly, the uncinate attaches to the ethmoidal process of the inferior turbinate bone. The superior aspect of the uncinate projects posteriorly and superiorly to the middle turbinate attachment. At this level, several patterns of attachment exist. The superior attachment of the uncinate most commonly bends laterally to insert on the lamina papyracea. In this configuration, the space inferior and lateral to this portion of the uncinate is the blind ending superior aspect of the infundibulum, an area referred to as the recessus terminalis. Superior and medial to this portion of the uncinate lies the floor of the frontal recess.

Alternatively, the uncinate can attach centrally to the skull base or medially to the superior aspect of the vertical lamella of the middle turbinate near the turbinate's insertion to the cribriform plate.[1] It can also fuse with an anterior ethmoid cell, such as the agger nasi. In these cases, the frontal sinus drains into the infundibulum. Rarely, the superior portion of the uncinate can divide to attach to the lamina papyracea, skull base, and middle turbinate.[1] Each leaflet can develop variably to produce partial or complete septations with accompanying inlets. The inlets vary as well, from shallow, blind pouches to small cells, which underscore the complexity and variability of this region.

The most common orientation of the uncinate process in relationship to the lateral nasal wall and lamina papyracea is ~140 degrees; however, there is a significant amount of variability.[3] There are two main primary variations of the uncinate process: deviation and pneumatization.[24] Lateral deviation of the uncinate may lead to narrowing of the infundibulum, whereas medial deviation may obstruct the middle meatus. The uncinate can be displaced laterally

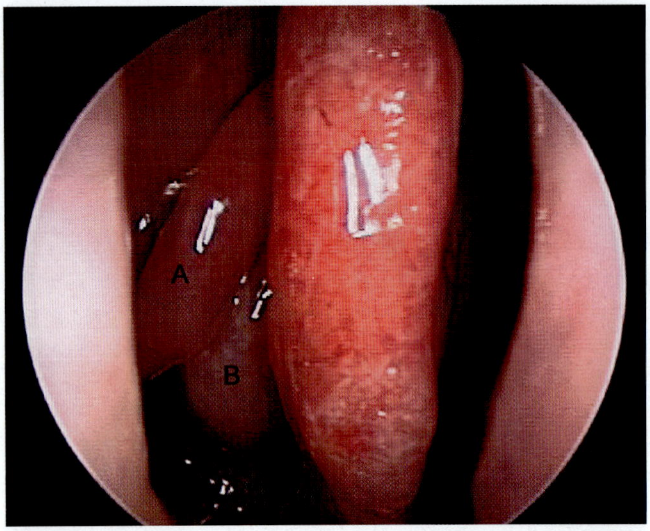

Fig. 1.3 Endoscopic view of a right middle meatus. A: Elongated uncinate process, which is everted anteriorly. B: Enlarged bulla ethmoidalis.

against the orbit, as commonly occurs in maxillary sinus hypoplasia. If atelectasis of the infundibulum is not appreciated during uncinectomy incision, inadvertent orbital injury can result. The uncinate may also be displaced medially, as commonly occurs in cases with extensive polypoid disease within the infundibulum. Occasionally, the uncinate is so medially displaced that it may evert and be misinterpreted as a duplication of the middle turbinate (**Fig. 1.3**).

Uncinate process pneumatization is rarely encountered, occurring in around 1% of people.[24,25] Pneumatization of the uncinate has been theorized to occur when an agger nasi cell extends into the most anterosuperior region of the uncinate process.[23]

Ethmoid Bulla

The ethmoid bulla is formed by pneumatization of the second ethmoid lamella or bulla lamella. In rare instances, this structure may remain unpneumatized, the resulting structure being referred to as the torus lateralis.[1] More often, the bulla ethmoidalis is one of the largest of the anterior ethmoid air cells. It is located within the middle meatus directly posterior to the uncinate process and anterior to the basal lamella of the middle turbinate. The bulla is relatively constant in location and is based on the lamina papyracea from which it projects into the middle meatus. Superiorly, the anterior wall of the ethmoid bulla usually extends to the skull base and forms the posterior limit of the frontal recess. Alternatively, there may be a suprabullar recess, a space above the bulla ethmoidalis that is in continuity with the middle meatus. There is typically a space behind the bulla known as the retrobullar recess; however, in ~25% of patients there is no retrobullar recess, and instead the posterior wall of the bulla ethmoidalis is fused with the basal lamella.[3] When highly pneumatized, the ethmoid bulla can lie in the lower aspect of the middle meatus and, in some cases, impair mucociliary transport and ventilation.

Excessive growth and pneumatization of the ethmoid bulla can encroach upon the infundibulum, potentially leading to obstruction and sinusitis (**Fig. 1.3**). Lloyd[20] reported that this variation was difficult to assess and suggested that it may be overdiagnosed. His study also found that, when compared with other variations, enlarged ethmoid bulla had a slightly lower incidence of correlation with sinus disease.

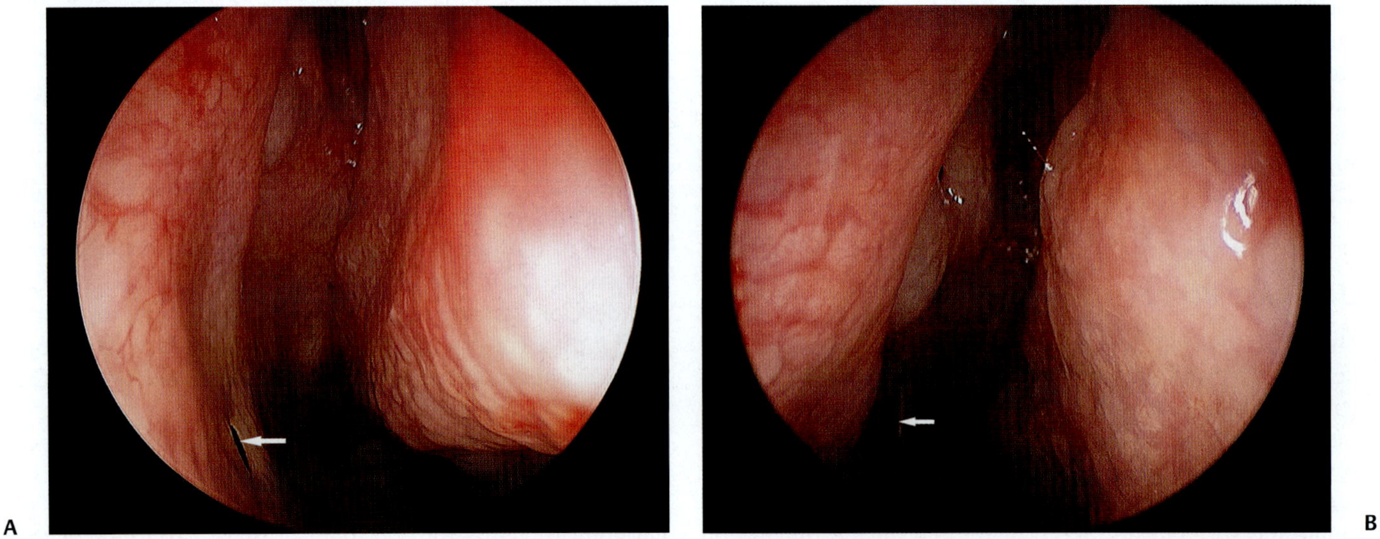

Fig. 1.4 **(A)** Endoscopic view of a right middle meatus. An anterior accessory ostium (*white arrow*) is seen at the anterior aspect of the uncinate process's inferior attachment. **(B)** Endoscopic view of a right middle meatus. A posterior accessory ostium (*white arrow*) is visualized at the posterior aspect of the uncinate process's inferior attachment.

Hiatus Semilunaris

The hiatus semilunaris is a crescent-shaped space between the posterior-free margin of the uncinate process and the anterior wall of the ethmoid bulla. The middle meatus communicates with the ethmoid infundibulum through this two-dimensional, sagittally oriented cleft.

Ethmoidal Infundibulum

The ethmoidal infundibulum is a three-dimensional space bordered medially by the uncinate process, laterally by the lamina papyracea, anterosuperiorly by the frontal process of the maxilla and lacrimal bone, and posteriorly by the anterior wall of the ethmoid bulla.[1] It forms a funnel-shaped passage through which the secretions from various anterior ethmoid cells, the maxillary sinus, and, in some cases, the frontal sinus are transported into the middle meatus. The ethmoidal infundibulum communicates with the middle meatus through the hiatus semilunaris. The maxillary ostium has been noted as a posterior, superoanterior, or medial opening, depending on the individual patient's anatomy (**see Video 1.3**). Understanding the superior aspect of the infundibulum is critical to understanding the drainage pathway of the frontal sinus, a relationship that is determined by the attachment of the uncinate process.

Fontanelles

The lateral nasal wall contains bony fontanelles composed of nasal mucosa, a small layer of intervening connective tissue, and sinus mucosa. The anterior and posterior fontanelles may perforate, creating accessory ostia that can be mistaken

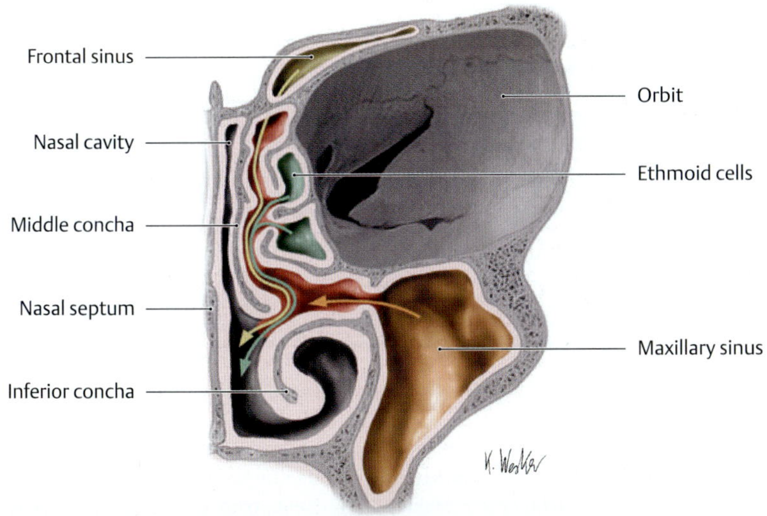

A

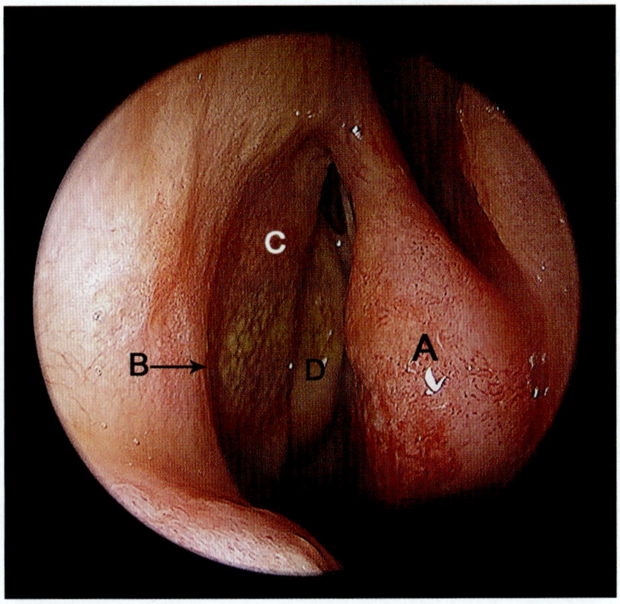

B

Fig. 1.5 **(A)** Osteomeatal unit of the left maxillary sinus. **(B)** Endoscopic view of a right middle meatus. A: Middle turbinate; B: maxillary line; C: uncinate process; D: bulla ethmoidalis. (**[A]** From THIEME Atlas of Anatomy, Head and Neuroanatomy, © Thieme 2007, Illustration by Karl Wesker.

for the natural maxillary sinus ostia. Posterior accessory ostia are more frequent and occur in ~20 to 25% of people (**Figs. 1.4A,B**).[26]

Ostiomeatal Unit

The ostiomeatal unit is a functional entity that represents a confluence of the drainage pathways of the maxillary, anterior ethmoid, and frontal sinuses. The ostiomeatal unit is composed of several structures within the middle meatus including the uncinate process, the ethmoid infundibulum, the anterior ethmoid air cells, maxillary, and frontal sinuses (**Figs. 1.5A,B**). The ostiomeatal unit is functionally important because a small amount of inflammation in this region can lead to disease upstream within the maxillary and/or frontal sinuses.[3]

Mucociliary Function

The cilia in the maxillary sinus propel the mucus stream in a starlike pattern from the floor of the maxillary sinus toward the ostium. From the primary ostium, mucus is swept superiorly through the ethmoid infundibulum. Posterior to the uncinate process mucus is propelled inferior to the ethmoidal bulla, through the middle meatus, and anterior to the torus tubarius into the nasopharynx, where it is swallowed. Recirculation of mucus may occur when discontinuity exists between the natural ostium and a secondary ostium. Secretions exiting the natural ostium may return to the sinus through a surgically created antrostomy or naturally occurring accessory ostium (**see Video 1.4**). This phenomenon may increase the risk of recurrent or persistent sinus infection.

Conclusion

A thorough understanding of the middle meatal anatomy is paramount to successful surgical treatment of the maxillary sinus and avoidance of complications. Anatomic variants are relatively common in the evaluation of patients with maxillary sinusitis and may also present in a significant number of persons without sinus disease.[27,28] The pathogenic role of each anatomic variation should be evaluated on an individual basis with considerations given to the size, position, and presence of inflammation.

Pearls

- The middle turbinate is a critical landmark in surgery of the middle meatus.
- Understanding the anatomy of the uncinate process and ethmoid infundibulum facilitates surgery of the maxillary sinus.
- It is important to understand anatomic variations, and critically assess their impact on the disease process.

References

1. Stammberger H. Functional Endoscopic Sinus Surgery: The Messerklinger Technique. Philadelphia, PA: BC Decker; 1991
2. Vacher C, Copin H, Sakka M. Maxillary ossification in a series of six human embryos and fetuses aged from 9 to 12 weeks of amenorrhea: clinical implications. Surg Radiol Anat 1999;21(4):261–266
3. Kennedy D, Bolger W, Zinreich S. Diseases of the Sinuses: Diagnosis and Management. London: BC Decker; 2001
4. Bingham B, Wang RG, Hawke M, Kwok P. The embryonic development of the lateral nasal wall from 8 to 24 weeks. Laryngoscope 1991;101(9):992–997
5. Wang RG, Jiang SC, Gu R. The cartilaginous nasal capsule and embryonic development of human paranasal sinuses. J Otolaryngol 1994;23(4):239–243
6. Barghouth G, Prior JO, Lepori D, Duvoisin B, Schnyder P, Gudinchet F. Paranasal sinuses in children: size evaluation of maxillary, sphenoid, and frontal sinuses by magnetic resonance imaging and proposal of volume index percentile curves. Eur Radiol 2002;12(6):1451–1458
7. Kapoor PK, Kumar BN, Watson SD. Maxillary sinus hypoplasia. J Laryngol Otol 2002;116(2):135–137
8. Whittet HB. Infraorbital nerve dehiscence: the anatomic cause of maxillary sinus "vacuum headache"? Otolaryngol Head Neck Surg 1992;107(1):21–28
9. Larrabee WF, Makielski KH, Henderson JL. Facial sensory innervation. In: Larrabee WF, Makielski KH, Henderson, eds. Surgical Anatomy of the Face. Philadelphia: Lippincott Williams & Wilkins;2003
10. Robinson S, Wormald PJ. Patterns of innervation of the anterior maxilla: a cadaver study with relevance to canine fossa puncture of the maxillary sinus. Laryngoscope 2005;115(10):1785–1788
11. Navarro JAC. Surgical anatomy of the nose, paranasal sinuses, and pterygopalatine fossa. In: Stamm A, Draf W, eds. Micro-Endoscopic Surgery of the Paranasal Sinuses and the Skull Base. Heidelberg, Germany: Springer; 2000
12. Hosemann W, Kühnel T, Burchard AK, Werner JA. Histochemical detection of lymphatic drainage pathways in the middle nasal meatus. Rhinology 1998;36(2):50–54
13. Chaboki H, Wanna GB, Westreich R, Kao J, Packer SH, Lawson W. Carcinomas of the nasal cavity and paranasal sinus. In: Genden EM., Varvares MA, eds. Head and Neck Cancer: An Evidence-Based Team Approach. New York: Thieme; 2008
14. Stackpole SA, Edelstein DR. The anatomic relevance of the Haller cell in sinusitis. Am J Rhinol 1997;11(3):219–223
15. Bolger WE, Butzin CA, Parsons DS. Paranasal sinus bony anatomic variations and mucosal abnormalities: CT analysis for endoscopic sinus surgery. Laryngoscope 1991;101(1 Pt 1):56–64
16. Bolger WE, Woodruff WW Jr, Morehead J, Parsons DS. Maxillary sinus hypoplasia: classification and description of associated uncinate

process hypoplasia. Otolaryngol Head Neck Surg 1990;103(5 (Pt 1)):759–765
17. Virgin F, Ling FT, Kountakis SE. Radiology and endoscopic findings of silent maxillary sinus atelectasis and enophthalmos. Am J Otolaryngol 2008;29(3):167–170
18. Wise SK, Wojno TH, DelGaudio JM. Silent sinus syndrome: lack of orbital findings in early presentation. Am J Rhinol 2007;21(4):489–494
19. Annino DJ Jr, Goguen LA. Silent sinus syndrome. Curr Opin Otolaryngol Head Neck Surg 2008;16(1):22–25
20. Lloyd GAS. CT of the paranasal sinuses: study of a control series in relation to endoscopic sinus surgery. J Laryngol Otol 1990;104(6):477–481
21. Bolger WE, Butzin CA, Parsons DS. Paranasal sinus bony anatomic variations and mucosal abnormalities: CT analysis for endoscopic sinus surgery. Laryngoscope 1991;101(1 Pt 1):56–64
22. Nadas S, Duvoisin B, Landry M, Schnyder P. Concha bullosa: frequency and appearances on CT and correlations with sinus disease in 308 patients with chronic sinusitis. Neuroradiology 1995;37(3):234–237
23. Kim SS, Lee JG, Kim KS, Kim HU, Chung IH, Yoon JH. Computed tomographic and anatomical analysis of the basal lamellas in the ethmoid sinus. Laryngoscope 2001;111(3):424–429
24. Bolger WE, Woodruff WW, Parsons DS. CT demonstration of uncinate process pneumatization: a rare paranasal sinus anomaly. AJNR Am J Neuroradiol 1990;11:552
25. Chao TK. Uncommon anatomic variations in patients with chronic paranasal sinusitis. Otolaryngol Head Neck Surg 2005;132(2):221–225
26. Stammberger H. Secretion transportation. In: Functional Endoscopic Sinus Surgery. Philadelphia, PA: BC Decker;1991: 17–47
27. Bolger WE, Butzin CA, Parsons DS. Paranasal sinus bony anatomic variations and mucosal abnormalities: CT analysis for endoscopic sinus surgery. Laryngoscope 1991;101(1 Pt 1):56–64
28. Calhoun KH, Waggenspack GA, Simpson CB, Hokanson JA, Bailey BJ. CT evaluation of the paranasal sinuses in symptomatic and asymptomatic populations. Otolaryngol Head Neck Surg 1991;104(4):480–483

2 Imaging of the Maxillary Sinus and Surrounding Structures

Samuel S. Becker and Theodore C. Larson III

Effective diagnosis of abnormalities of the maxillary sinus and surrounding structures is dependent on clinical and radiologic findings. The easy availability and minimal invasiveness of nasal endoscopy has dramatically increased the ability of the otolaryngologist to correctly characterize and diagnose sinonasal findings. In many cases, however, nasal endoscopy is insufficient for complete evaluation. In unoperated sinuses, for instance, the endoscope does not allow visualization within the maxillary sinus proper. Moreover, lesions on the anterior maxillary sinus wall are all but impossible to see directly with nasal endoscopy. Many lesions—even those that are visible on endoscopy—require further evaluation for complete understanding of their extent and impact on surrounding structures. It is in this context that high-resolution computed tomography (CT) scans of the paranasal sinuses have become indispensable for the complete evaluation of maxillary sinus lesions. The widespread availability of multislice CT technology has produced thin slices, small voxel sizes with submillimeter resolution, multiplanar and volumetric reconstruction, and improved patient comfort by examining the patient in a recumbent posture utilizing scanning times of less than 5 minutes. Many otolaryngology offices are now equipped with CT scan machines that allow for "point-of-service" imaging for patients directly within the confines of a clinic setting.

Inherent in all x-ray-based imaging is radiation exposure, with the typical CT examination of the paranasal sinuses producing 3.5 to 25 mGy (0.35–2.5 rad) to the lens of the eye depending on the imaging parameters.[1] A total lifetime cumulative radiation value from all sources of 0.5 to 2 Gy (50–200 rad) or more may be expected to produce cataracts.[2] Magnetic resonance imaging (MRI) utilizes static and varying gradient magnetic fields plus radiofrequency radiation. It has the potential to cause induced currents, heating, function deviation or motion in an implanted ferromagnetic device, and projectile hazards; effects that are stronger at higher magnetic fields.[3]

Multiple radiologic modalities exist to assist in the evaluation of the maxillary sinus and its surrounding structures. Although MRI, Panorex, computed radiography, traditional plain films, and angiography can each be contributory, the focus of this chapter will be on effective utilization of CT because this is the most common imaging modality used by otolaryngologists on a daily basis.

Maxillary Sinus Shape and Volume

Abnormalities of the maxillary sinus itself can be well visualized with CT. Typically pyramidal-shaped with a normal adult volume ranging from 5 to 20 mL, asymmetry is common, and variations in size and shape can be appreciated on a CT scan. Some abnormalities in particular warrant mention. Maxillary sinus hypoplasia has been classified into three types: mild, significant, and profound (**Fig. 2.1**).[4] Significant and profound hypoplasia are associated with uncinate process abnormalities; mild hypoplasia is not. It is recommended that any associated uncinate process variations be recognized on preoperative CT because failure to do so may lead to disorientation during sinus surgery. Although profound maxillary sinus hypoplasia and sinus aplasia are uncommon in the general population, there is an increased incidence in patients with cystic fibrosis,[5] secondary to chronic and repeated infections with poor aeration and consequent limited sinus expansion.

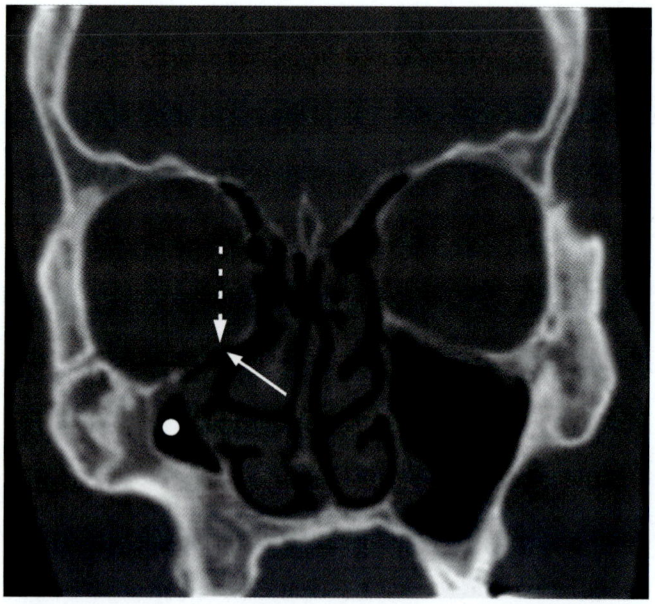

Fig. 2.1 Coronal computed tomography (CT) of a patient with a hypoplastic right maxillary sinus (*white circle*). Although the uncinate process (*solid white arrow*) is retracted laterally, the infundibulum (*dashed white arrow*) in this patient appears patent.

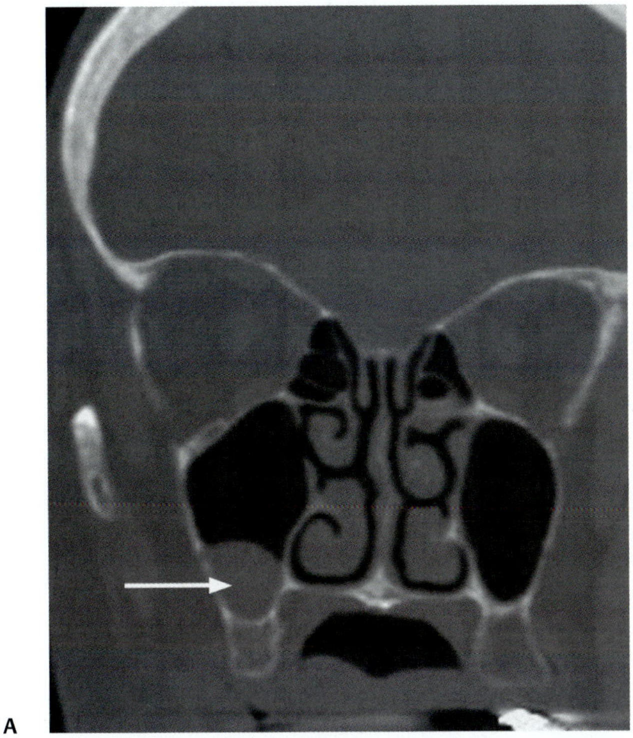

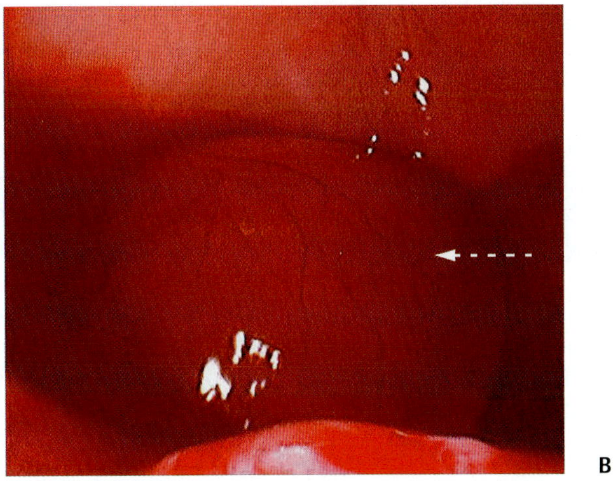

Fig. 2.2 **(A)** Coronal computed tomography (CT) with right maxillary retention cyst (*solid white arrow*). **(B)** The endoscopic view of another patient, seen in a transnasal view with a 70-degree endoscope reveals a maxillary retention cyst in this patient's left maxillary sinus (*dashed white arrow*).

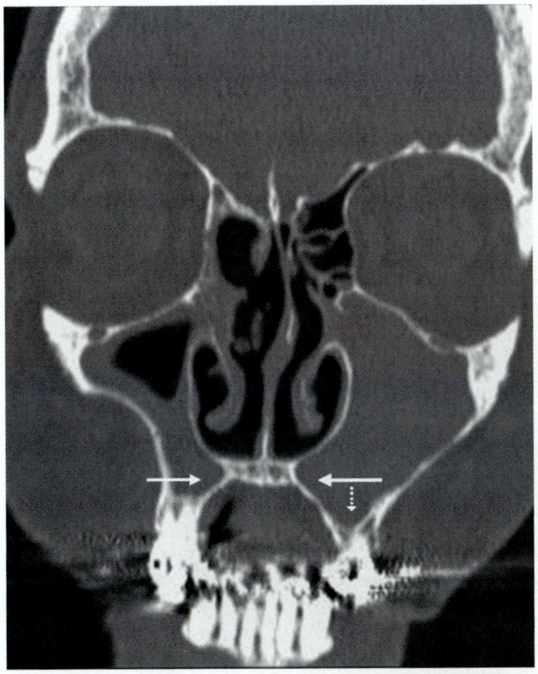

Fig. 2.3 Coronal computed tomography (CT) of a patient with partial right maxillary sinus opacification and total left maxillary sinus opacification. The maxillary sinuses also demonstrate bilateral palatine recesses (*solid white arrows*) and a left alveolar recess (*dotted white arrow*).

The shape and volume of the maxillary sinus may be affected by anatomic formations within the sinus. Bony septations may impact the natural flow of mucous within the sinus, which may lead to mucous retention cyst or localized mucocele formation (**Fig. 2.2**). Septations and irregular pneumatization patterns may also lead to the formation of

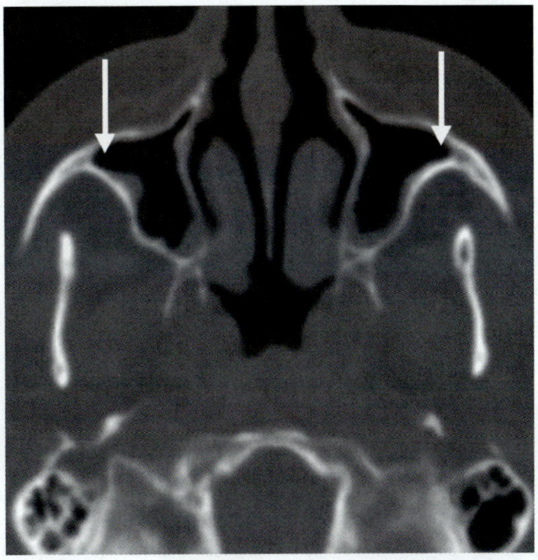

Fig. 2.4 Zygomatic recesses are anterolateral pneumatizations of the sinus in the direction of the infratemporal fossa. They are seen here on axial CT (*solid white arrows*).

recesses including the palatine, infraorbital, alveolar, and zygomatic recesses. Although the palatine recess represents an inferomedial pneumatization of the sinus into the hard palate (**Fig. 2.3**), the infraorbital recess represents an anterior pneumatization adjacent to the infraorbital canal in the maxillary sinus roof.[6] Alveolar recesses are pneumatizations inferiorly in the area of the molar and premolar dentition (**Fig. 2.3**). Zygomatic recesses are anterolateral pneumatizations of the sinus in the direction of the infratemporal fossa (**Fig. 2.4**). Although these pneumatizations are of unclear clinical significance, they do assist the otolaryngologist in appreciation of the unique character and details of each patient's sinus anatomy.

The Inferior Turbinate

The maxillary sinus is intimately associated with the inferior turbinate. Embryologically distinct from the other paranasal sinus structures, the inferior turbinate sits within the nasal cavity adjacent to, and just medial to the maxillary sinus proper where it is attached to the medial wall of the maxillary sinus. The cancellous turbinate bone is covered by highly vascularized mucosa with a respiratory epithelium and glandular lamina propria.[7] Functionally, the turbinate assists with thermoregulation, humidification, and filtration of inspired air.

Variations in inferior turbinate anatomy have been well documented. Absent and hypoplastic, as well as bifid, pneumatized, and paradoxically curved inferior turbinates have all been reported in the literature.[8] Hemangiomas, angiofibromas, polyps, pleomorphic adenomas, fibroosseous lesions, and schwannomas, as well as malignant lesions within the inferior turbinate have all been documented.[9–15] For most otolaryngologists, however, the inferior turbinate is pertinent in so far as it affects nasal airflow. Hypertrophy has been associated with allergic and nonallergic rhinitis and owes, in part, to the abundance of inflammatory cells that reside within the lamina propria. Because the turbinate sits at the anterior portion of the nasal cavity, hypertrophy

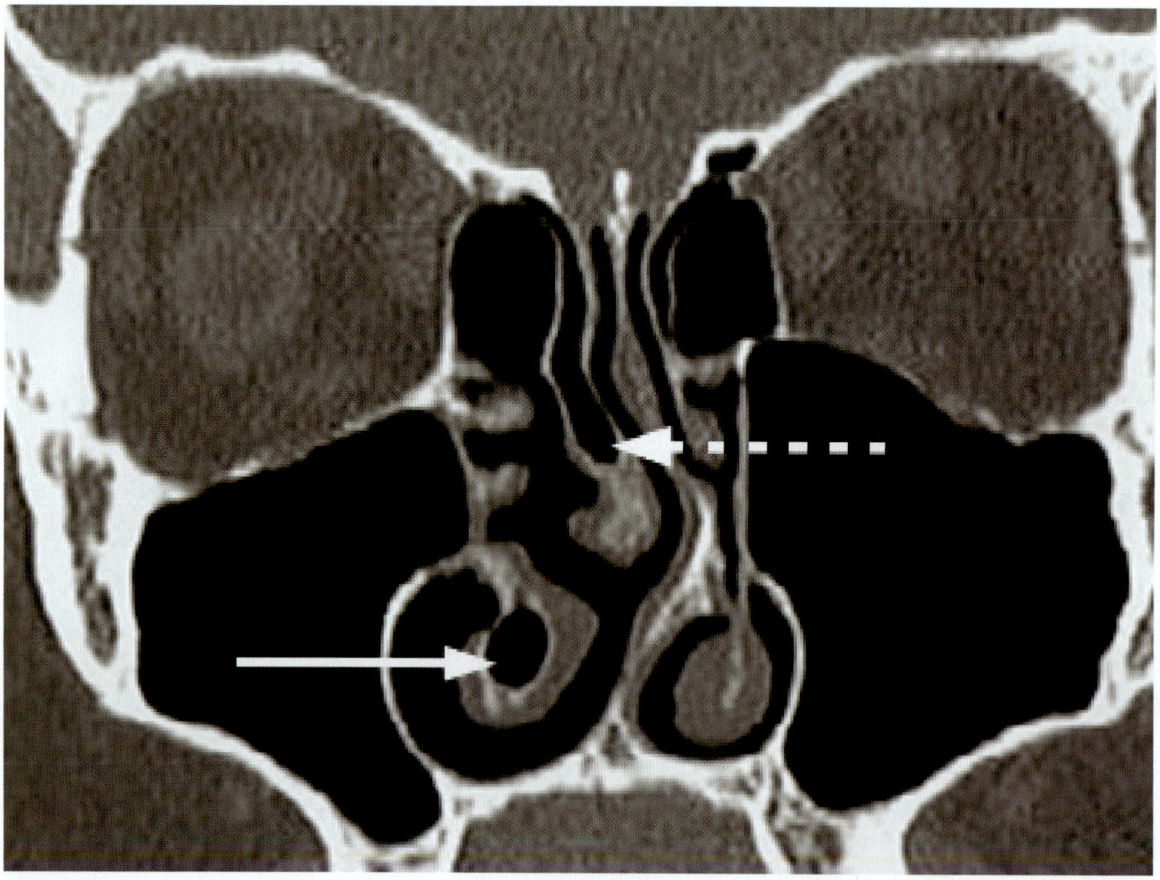

Fig. 2.5 Coronal computed tomography (CT) demonstrates a pneumatized right inferior turbinate (*solid white arrow*). Note that this patient also has a pneumatized right middle turbinate (concha bullosa) as well (*dotted white arrow*).

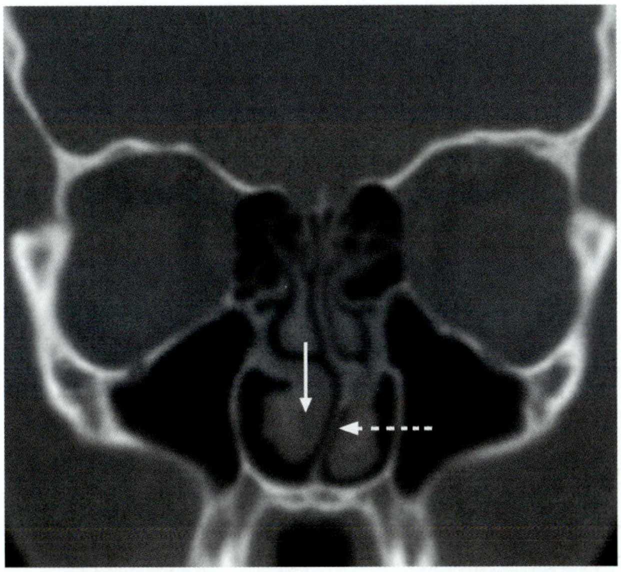

Fig. 2.6 Coronal sinus computed tomography (CT) demonstrates septal deviation to the patient's left side (*dotted white arrow*), with compensatory hypertrophy of the right inferior turbinate (*solid white arrow*).

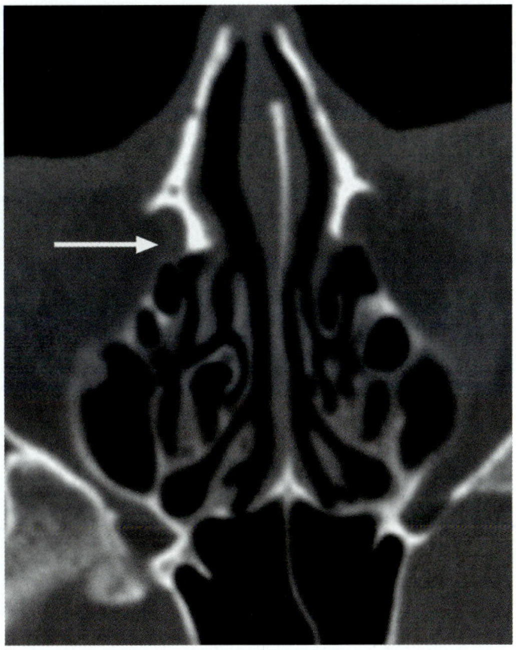

Fig. 2.7 The lacrimal sac (*solid white arrow*) is housed within the bony lacrimal fossa, seen on this axial CT view. The lacrimal fossa is formed by the frontal process of the maxilla anteriorly and medially, and the lacrimal bone posteriorly and laterally.

may lead to nasal obstruction. Although turbinate hypertrophy is usually a submucosal phenomenon, it may on occasion be secondary to an unusually large or pneumatized turbinate skeleton (**Fig. 2.5**). The bony skeleton is variable, and can be characterized as lamellar, compact, combined, or bullous.[16] Preoperative CT scans should be evaluated for these particulars so that the surgical intervention can be individualized to address the specific anatomic source of turbinate hypertrophy.

Interplay between hypertrophied turbinates and septal deviation should also be noted prior to surgical intervention. The presence of compensatory inferior turbinate hypertrophy in the context of septal deviation has been well-documented (**Fig. 2.6**),[17] and should be reviewed as part of the decision to treat turbinate hypertrophy concomitant with septoplasty. Often there exists a hypoplastic or paradoxical inferior turbinate on the side of the septal deviation, while the contralateral side (away from the septal deviation) has a hypertrophied inferior turbinate.

The Nasolacrimal Duct

Tear drainage occurs when tears that are collected by the lacrimal punctua enter the lacrimal canaliculi, pass through the valve of Rosenmüller, and enter the lacrimal sac. The lacrimal sac is housed within the bony lacrimal fossa, bounded anteriorly by the frontal process of the maxilla and posteriorly by the lacrimal bone (**Fig. 2.7**). From the lacrimal sac, tears drain into the nasolacrimal duct to pass through the Hasners valve and enter the inferior meatus of the nose ~1 cm posterior to the anterior tip of the inferior turbinate. The superior aspect of the duct is housed in the bony nasolacrimal canal, which directs the duct along a path just medial and anterior to the maxillary sinus. Obstruction along any portion of this tear duct pathway may present as epiphora. Cysts, tumors, mucoceles, dacryocystoceles, and polyps, among other lesions, have all been reported along this pathway.[18–20]

Although diagnosis of these lesions may fall to otolaryngologists, the tear duct is most pertinent insofar as it sits in the field during surgery on the maxillary sinus, and can be harmed inadvertently. The tear duct pathway can be appreciated on axial, coronal, and sagittal CT views (**Fig. 2.8**). In some cases, the bony covering over the duct may be thinned, or—in the case of revision surgery—violated. Preoperative CT evaluation should be performed so that the surgeon may be aware of these abnormalities and, subsequently, treat these areas cautiously if warranted. When epiphora does occur secondary to duct obstruction either from natural or iatrogenic causes, management via dacryocystorhinostomy has increasingly involved otolaryngologists.[21] In these situations, the CT scan may demonstrate both the site of obstruction and the location and bone thickness of the surrounding lacrimal fossa.

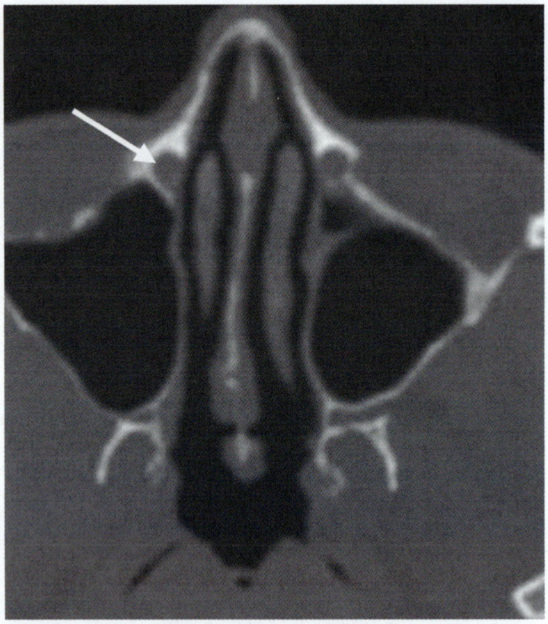

A

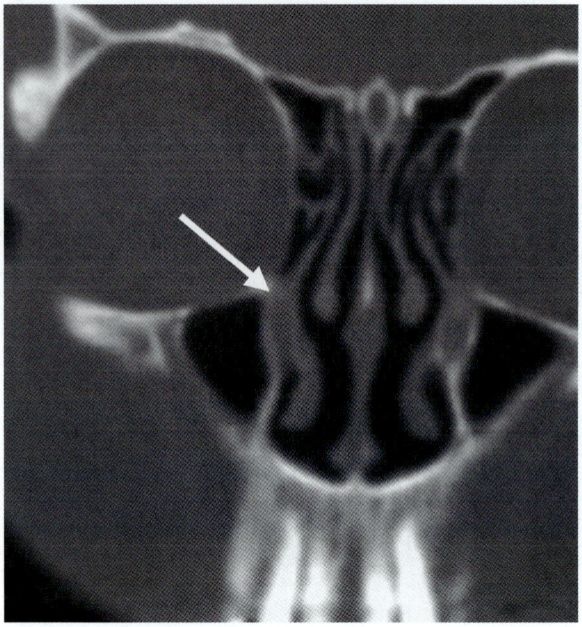

B

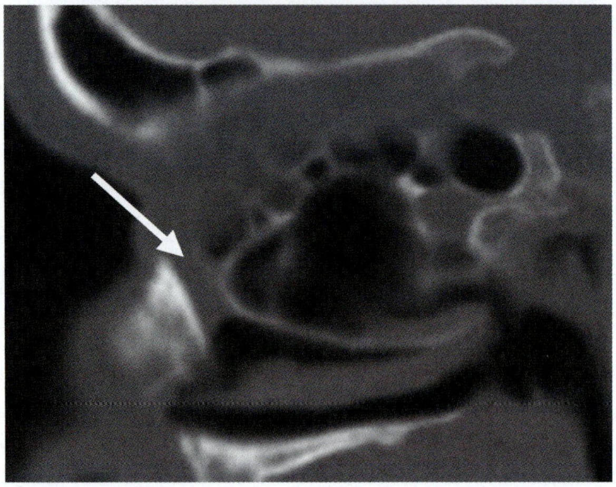

C

Fig. 2.8 **(A–C)** The lacrimal duct pathway can be appreciated in computed tomography (CT) on axial, coronal, and sagittal views (*solid white arrows*).

The Uncinate Process

The uncinate process is a thin, sagittally oriented sickle-shaped bone that lies along the superior aspect of the lateral nasal wall, above the inferior turbinate, projecting anterosuperiorly into the frontal recess where it has an anterior attachment. The uncinate forms the medial boundary of the ethmoidal infundibulum through which maxillary and ethmoid sinus drainage occurs. The two dimensional orifice of the superomedial infundibulum is the hiatus semilunaris inferior. Blockage in this area has a major impact on drainage of the surrounding sinuses, and is most easily evaluated on coronal imaging (**Fig. 2.9**).

Extensive cadaveric dissection has delineated the existence of at least eight variations of this posteroinferior attachment of the uncinate process.[22] In addition to its natural sinus ostia, the maxillary sinus may also have accessory ostia, or fontanelles, along its medial wall, the lateral nasal wall of the nasal cavity. The presence, location, and shape

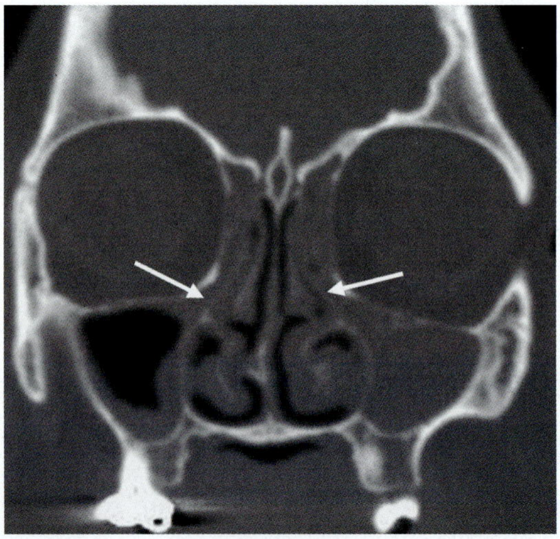

Fig. 2.9 Coronal sinus computed tomography (CT) demonstrates partial bilateral sinus opacification including opacification of the blocked infundibula bilaterally (*solid white arrows*).

A B C D

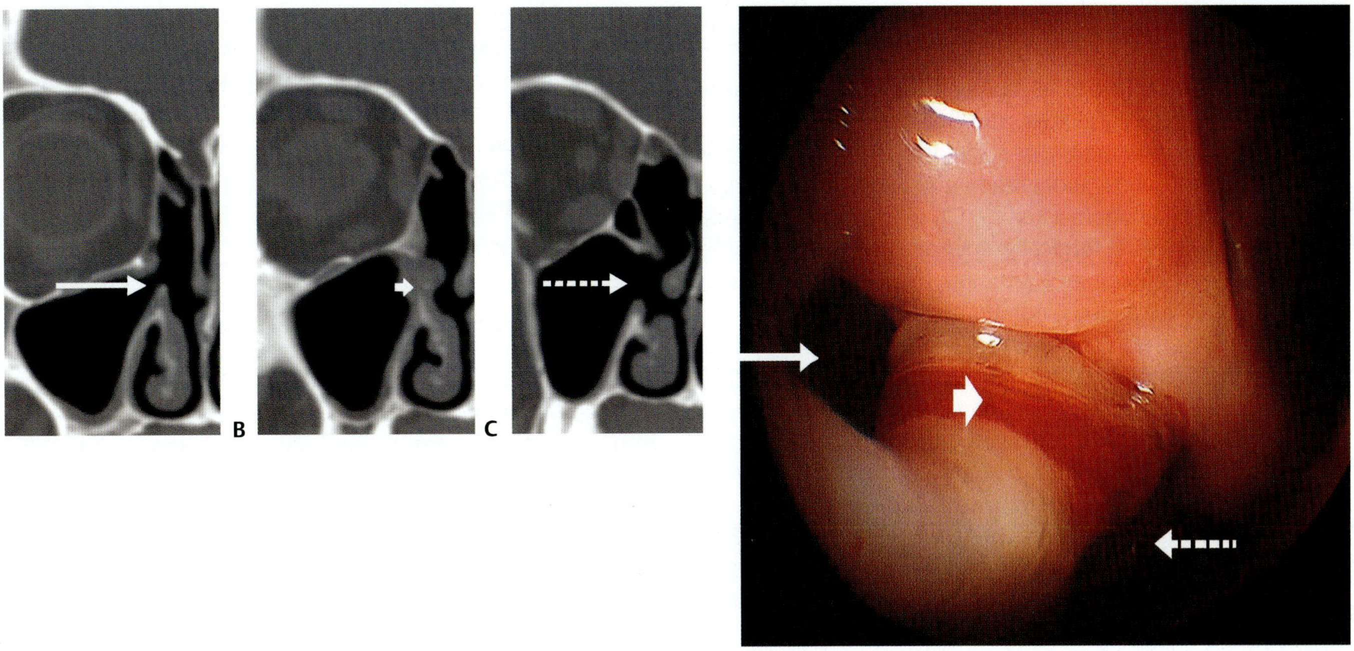

Fig. 2.10 Sequential coronal images of a missed ostium sequence. **(A)** The patient's right maxillary sinus natural ostium is seen (*solid white arrow*). **(B)** A coronal cut just posterior to **(A)**. Here scar tissue and retained uncinate can be appreciated (*short arrow*). **(C)** Just posterior to **(B)**, the surgical antrostomy (*dotted white arrow*) which is separate from the natural opening seen in **(D)**. An endoscopic picture of the findings seen in **A–C**.

of the fontanelles are dependent on the particular variation in the posteroinferior attachment of the uncinate process. Although it is debatable whether or not recirculation occurs between natural and accessory ostia in the absence of prior surgery, the presence of this phenomenon in the postsurgical patient is a common source of recurrent sinus disease, and can be recognized both endoscopically, and secondarily on CT (**Fig. 2.10**).

The uncinate process is usually located in a position medial to the lateral nasal wall; however, it may have a variation by which it is oriented superolaterally (lateral to the lamina papyracea). This malformation of "silent sinus syndrome" is addressed in detail in Chapter 10. Characterized by an atelectatic uncinate process and painless enophthalmos, the diagnosis is easily appreciated on CT scan (**Fig. 2.11**). A "silent sinus" represents an extreme on a continuum of atelectatic uncinates; in many circumstances the uncinate process may be retracted, although not as severely as in a silent sinus. These abnormalities can be recognized on CT. Other variations include aberrant inferior and superior attachments, pneumatization, and paradoxical curvature.

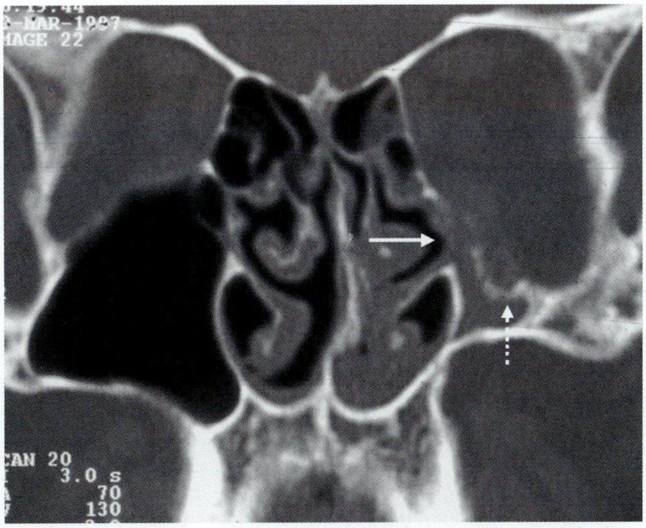

Fig. 2.11 This coronal computed tomography (CT) image demonstrates a left silent sinus. Note the retracted, atelectatic left uncinate process (*solid white arrow*) and the sunken orbit (*dotted white arrow*).

Infraorbital Nerve

The infraorbital nerve and its branches provide sensation to the upper lip, maxillary gingiva, and skin of the cheek over the maxilla. The nerve courses along the orbital floor within the infraorbital canal whose indentation into the roof of the maxillary sinus is easily appreciated on CT, as well as directly on nasal endoscopy (in a surgically opened sinus). The infraorbital canal may be examined radiographically for dehiscence, as well as for an anomalous course.

In most cases, the infraorbital canal courses anteriorly in the roof of the maxillary sinus, lateral to the midpoint of the roof, far away from the site of instrumentation in endonasal endoscopic maxillary sinus surgery. In some cases, however, the nerve and its canal take a more medial course toward the anterior maxillary sinus wall (**Fig. 2.12**). The frequency and prevalence of this irregular course has not been quantified, however, it is prudent to note the course of the nerve prior to surgical intervention in the maxillary sinus.[23] This is particularly applicable in cases that require instrumentation within the sinus itself, as is often the case in removal of allergic fungal mucin, inverted papilloma, and large mucous retention cysts, as well as during the Caldwell–Luc procedure and other anterior approaches. More unusual and uncommon is the presence of an infraorbital canal that courses through the sinus itself, separate from the orbital floor. Although such a variation is most uncommon, and usually due to developmental sinus enlargement or hyperpneumatization, it is easily recognized on CT and should be appreciated prior to surgical intervention (**Fig. 2.13**).[24]

The infraorbital canal has been noted to be dehiscent ~14% of the time.[25] Canal dehiscence may also be appreciated on CT scan in many cases. As with recognition of variations in the course of the nerve and canal, it would seem prudent to evaluate for canal dehiscence in any surgical case that might involve instrumentation within the maxillary sinus proper (**see Video 2.1**).

Haller (Infraorbital Ethmoid) Cells

Haller cells, also known as infraorbital ethmoid cells or ethmomaxillary cells were first described by the Swiss anatomist and poet Albrecht von Haller in 1765. Traditionally believed to represent an anomalous embryonic migration of ethmoid cells into the maxillary sinus, others have proposed that these cells are—in fact—superior maxillary septations that are distinct from the bulla ethmoidalis via continuance in the roof of the maxillary sinus laterally beyond the two-dimensional maxillary sinus ostium. Haller cells come in a range of sizes, and have been variously reported to have a prevalence ranging from 5 to 45%.[26–29] Their clinical import is similarly unclear. While reported to have a role in rhinogenic headache,[30] and orbital edema,[31] Haller cells are most clinically relevant in so far as they may impact maxillary sinus drainage via narrowing of the sinus infundibulum.[32] They may also be blocked themselves, which may then lead to secondary inflammatory obstruction of the maxillary sinus ostium.

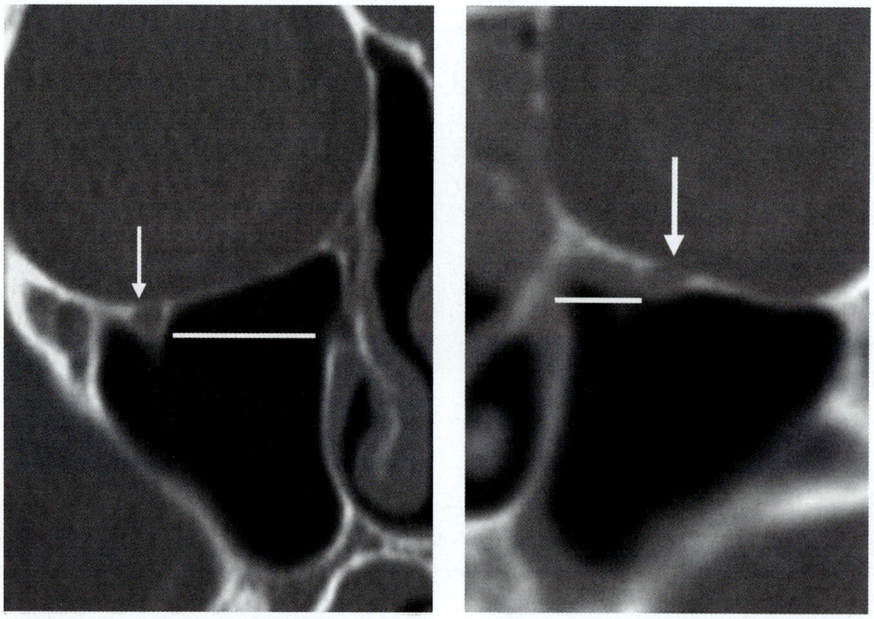

A,B

Fig. 2.12 **(A,B)** Coronal sinus computed tomography (CT) images through the maxillary sinuses of two different patients. Both images are roughly halfway between the posterior and the anterior walls of the maxillary sinus. **(A)** A patient's right maxillary sinus demonstrates the infraorbital nerve (*solid white arrow*) in a very lateral position, as indicated in the distance from the medial maxillary wall (*solid white line*). **(B)** A separate patient's left maxillary sinus demonstrates the infraorbital nerve (*solid white arrow*) in a very medial position, as indicated in the slight distance from the medial maxillary wall (*solid white line*).

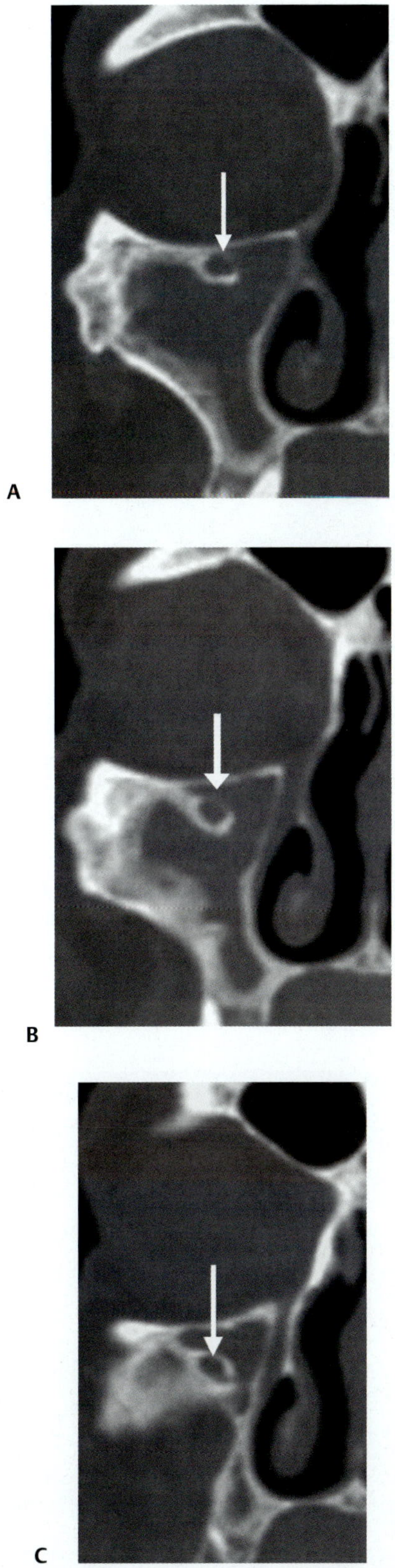

Fig. 2.13 (A–C) Sequential coronal computed tomography (CT) images, from posterior to anterior, follow the right infraorbital nerve coursing anteriorly through its canal (*solid white arrows*). Note that the bony canal is free and separate from the orbital floor/maxillary sinus roof. Surgery in the maxillary sinus could place this nerve at risk if this anomaly were unrecognized on preoperative CT.

Intraoperatively, Haller cells may obstruct identification of the natural sinus ostium leading to a surgical antrostomy separate from the natural ostium. Such a surgical error—the "missed ostium sequence"—is one source of the iatrogenic recirculation phenomenon, which occurs in patients with recurrent maxillary sinusitis despite surgical intervention.[33] In this situation, the Haller cell obscures the natural opening, which is left untouched and separate from the surgical antrostomy, in part, because of insufficient removal of the uncinate process. Fortunately, Haller cells are easily identifiable on preoperative CT scan, particularly on coronal view (**Fig. 2.14**). Awareness of the presence of a Haller cell should lead to increased vigilance on the part of the surgeon to identify the natural sinus opening with angled scopes if necessary to avoid iatrogenic sinusitis caused by recirculation from a missed ostium (**see Videos 2.2 and 2.3**).

Pterygopalatine Fossa

The pterygopalatine fossa (PPF), through which many vital structures pass, has communication to the middle cranial fossa, orbital apex, infratemporal fossa, foramen lacerum, and oral cavity. It is located just posterior to the maxillary sinus. Its borders and detailed anatomy are reviewed separately in Chapter 19. On axial and coronal CT views, the inferior orbital fissure, sphenopalatine foramen, and pterygoid plates are easily visualized (**Fig. 2.15**). On axial views, the greater palatine foramen and pterygomaxillary fissure, as well as the overall shape and size of the PPF contents are well illustrated (**Fig. 2.16**). The vidian canal, foramen

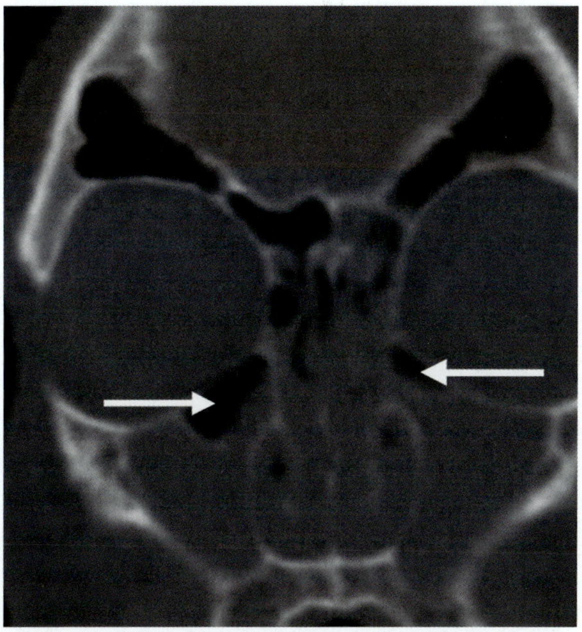

Fig. 2.14 Coronal computed tomography (CT) shows patient with bilateral maxillary and ethmoid sinus disease. There are large Haller (Infraorbital ethmoid) cells on both sides (*solid white arrows*).

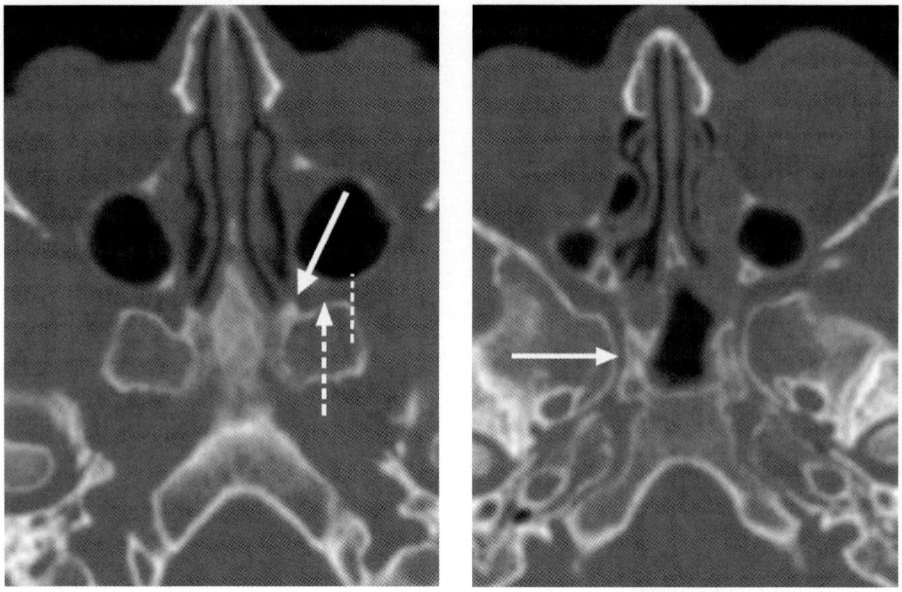

A B

Fig. 2.15 **(A)** Axial computed tomography (CT) scan demonstrates normal location of the pterygopalatine fossa (*dotted white arrow*), sphenopalatine foramen (*solid white arrow*), and pterygomaxillary fissure (*dotted white line*). **(B)** Axial CT also demonstrates location of the vidian canal (*solid white arrow*).

rotundum, and infraorbital canal may be appreciated best on coronal, and less readily on axial views as they course anteriorly (**Fig. 2.17**). The sagittal view is useful for viewing the profile and dimensions of the greater palatine canal (**Fig. 2.18**), and helpful for confirming many of the preceding landmarks. Although several studies have evaluated the length of the greater palatine canal[34–36]—useful to know prior to injection in this area for intraoperative hemostasis during sinus surgery—this measurement is variable and can easily be measured on CT prior to surgical intervention. Changes to the PPF from surgery, trauma, as well as from benign and malignant tumors may also be appreciated on CT. Widening of the sphenopalatine foramen is often noted in many tumors and expansile lesions (**Fig. 2.19**). Anterior bowing of the posterior wall of the maxillary sinus, the so-called Holman–Miller sign (**Fig. 2.20**), is considered

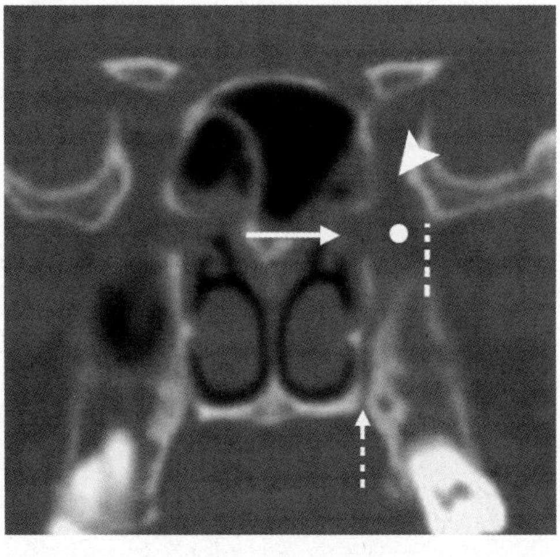

Fig. 2.16 Coronal computed tomography (CT) shows location of the pterygopalatine fossa (solid white dot), sphenopalatine foramen (*solid white arrow*), pterygomaxillary fissure (*dotted white line*), greater palatine foramen and canal (*dotted white arrow*), and infraorbital fissure (*solid white arrowhead*).

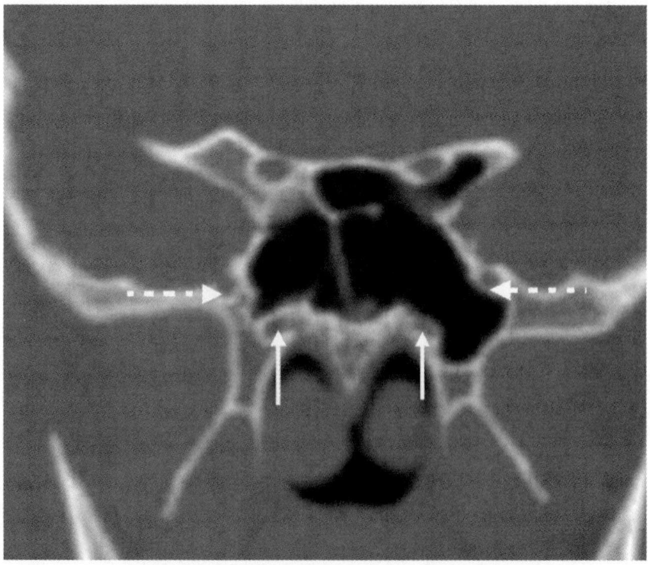

Fig. 2.17 Coronal computed tomography (CT) shows the locations of the vidian canal (*solid white arrows*) and foramen rotundum (*dotted white arrows*) brought into relief by a pneumatized pterygoid process.

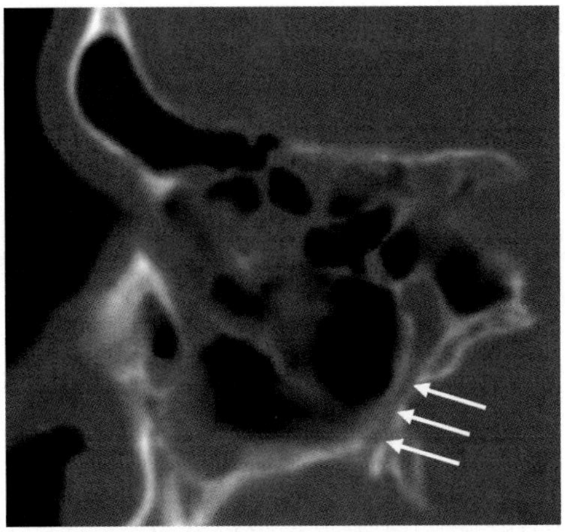

Fig. 2.18 Sagittal computed tomography (CT) demonstrates the greater palatine canal (*solid white arrows*) leading into the pterygopalatine fossa. Some surgeons will inject local anesthetic through this canal as a means of vasoconstricting the internal maxillary and sphenopalatine arteries, which pass through the pterygopalatine fossa before entering the sinonasal cavity.

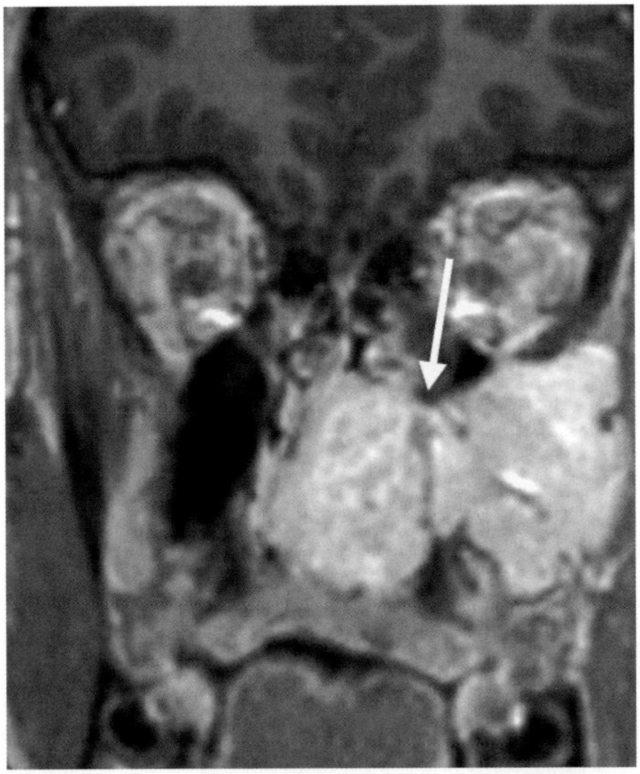

Fig. 2.19 Widening of the sphenopalatine foramen is often noted in many tumors and expansile lesions. This postcontrast T1-weighted coronal magnetic resonance image (MRI) shows a juvenile nasopharyngeal angiofibroma extending from the pterygopalatine fossa through the sphenopalatine foramen (*solid white arrow*), and into the nasal space. On computed tomography (CT), widening of this foramen can be appreciated.

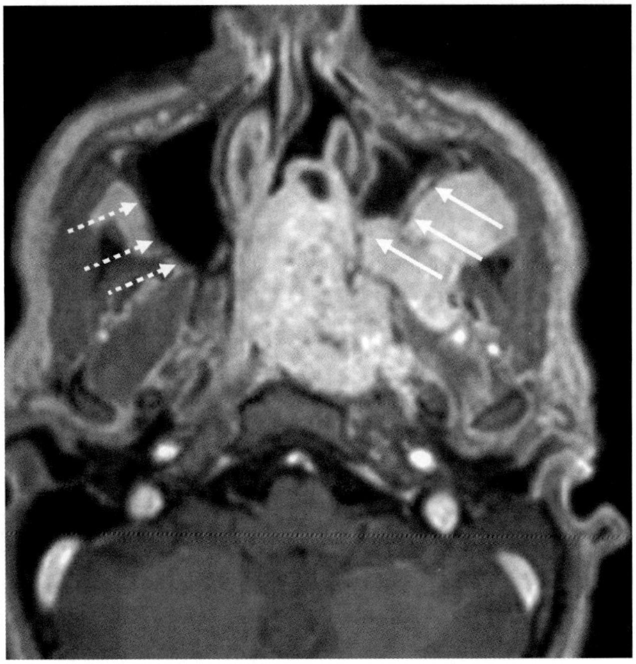

Fig. 2.20 Anterior bowing of the posterior wall of the maxillary sinus, the so-called Holman–Miller sign, can be appreciated on sinus computed tomography (CT), and here on postcontrast axial T1-weighted magnetic resonance image (MRI) of a patient with a juvenile nasopharyngeal angiofibroma. Note the impact on the left posterior maxillary sinus wall (*solid white arrows*) in comparison to the normal location of the right posterior maxillary sinus wall (*dotted white arrows*). This mass effect of the tumor is a telltale sign of a pterygopalatine fossa lesion, often a juvenile nasopharyngeal angiofibroma (JNA).

pathognomonic for the presence of juvenile nasopharyngeal angiofibroma (JNA), although other tumors such as a slowly growing, chronic schwannoma could also cause this appearance. Visualization and embolization of feeding vessels during catheter angiography confirms the diagnosis of a JNA and assists with hemostasis during surgical resection. Angiography and embolization are most commonly scheduled within 24 to 48 hours before surgical removal of the JNA to encourage tumor vessel thrombosis without recanalization. Although much can be learned about the extent and character of PPF masses from CT imaging, MRI continues to play an important role in the diagnosis of lesions within this area. Though beyond the scope of this chapter, many studies have suggested that patients with PPF lesions be evaluated with MRI as part of an optimal preoperative diagnostic algorithm.[37,38]

Radiology of Sinus Infection and Inflammation

CT is the primary tool in the diagnosis and staging of rhinosinusitis. Acute sinusitis is most commonly of infectious origin due to bacterial, viral, and/or fungal agents and associated with air–fluid levels and air bubbles (**Fig. 2.21**). In some cases, acute infections—particularly when unilateral—are associated with an odontogenic source, and an effort should be made to closely evaluate a patient's dentition. The radiologic appearance of mucosal thickening may also occur in patients with acute sinusitis; however, the chronically inflamed sinuses are more typically characterized by varying degrees of mucosal thickening that are less gravity dependent (**Fig. 2.22**). Persistent, chronic secretions may sometimes be characterized by increased density on CT due to elevated protein concentration or calcifications (**Fig. 2.23**). Of course, patients with chronic sinus inflammation may develop acute infections as well, and distinguishing these may require evaluating prior CT studies for a patient's baseline level of mucosal thickening.

Acute sinusitis fluid levels sometimes can be difficult to differentiate from mucosal thickening. Changing the patient's head position and repeating the CT scan will reveal an alternate orientation of the fluid level, confirming mobile fluid. The inflammatory character of this fluid, however, requires confirmation by sinus aspiration. Hyperplastic mucosa is a unique condition in which chronic mucosal inflammation results in mucosal enlargement and redundancy. Secretion stranding is the hallmark of subacute disease, but can also be identified in some patients with acute sinusitis. Chronic sinusitis is also associated with sinus wall chronic osteitis, a benign bony wall proliferation that is not true osteomyelitis. True osteomyelitis is most frequently seen in patients with an odontogenic source of infection.

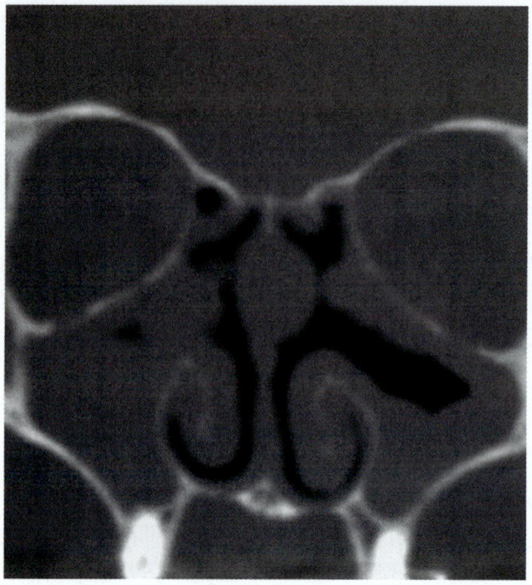

Fig. 2.22 This coronal computed tomography (CT) of a patient who has had prior sinus surgery demonstrates mucosal swelling and partial opacification in the maxillary sinuses consistent with a diagnosis of chronic rhinosinusitis. Notice that the mucosal lining is swollen throughout the sinus, and not simply in a gravity-dependent manner.

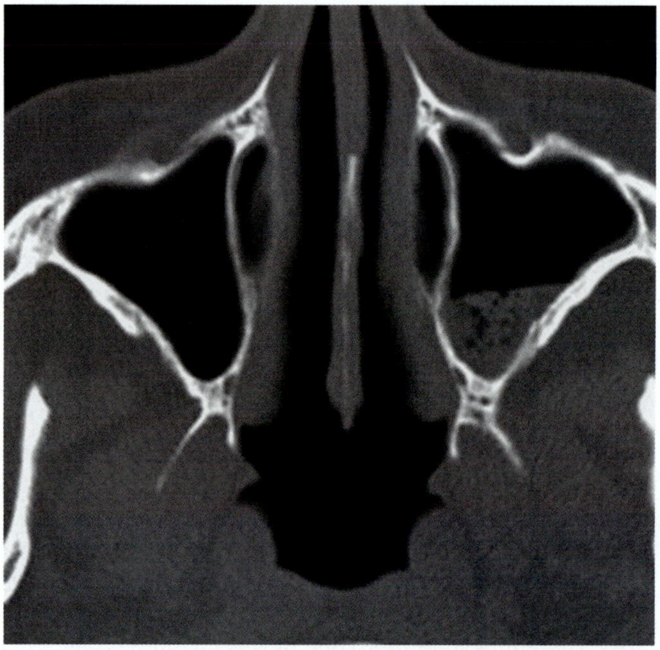

Fig. 2.21 Axial sinus computed tomography (CT) demonstrates an air–fluid level and air bubbles in the left maxillary sinus consistent with an acute sinus infection.

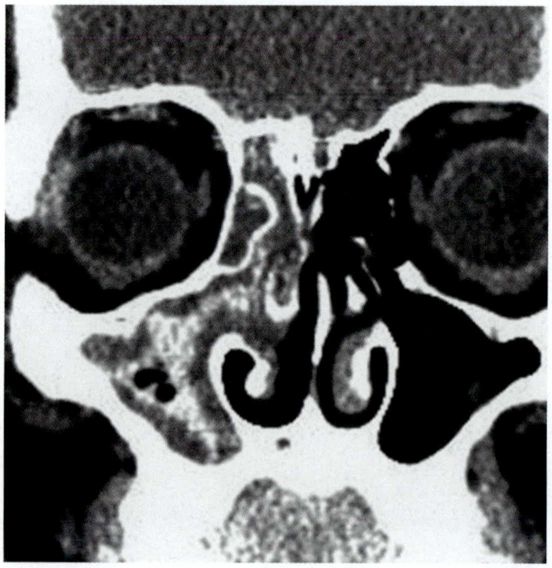

Fig. 2.23 This coronal computed tomography (CT), shown in a soft tissue window, demonstrates right-sided sinus opacification. Note the heterogeneity of the right maxillary sinus contents. The increased protein deposition of the chronically inflamed sinus contents lead to a heterogeneous density on CT scan.

Radiology of the Postsurgical Maxillary Sinus

There are many iatrogenic sources of chronic rhinosinusitis. Middle turbinate lateralization, maxillary sinus recirculation, retained uncinate processes, and oral-antral fistula are some of the iatrogenic abnormalities with distinctive radiologic appearances that can be appreciated and characterized on CT scans. Middle turbinate lateralization occurs when a middle turbinate, whose stability has been weakened by surgical manipulation, scars in a lateralized position. This occurrence has been noted to occur in over 75% of patients undergoing revision sinus surgery, and may block drainage patterns of the maxillary, ethmoid, and frontal sinuses.[39] Several techniques and spacers have been described to prevent lateralization; however, this iatrogenic abnormality continues to challenge sinus surgeons.[40–42] Fortunately, repair of this abnormality can be straightforward. It is imperative, however, to recognize its presence because repair will usually require some type of surgical intervention. Middle turbinate lateralization can be recognized on CT as well as during nasal endoscopy (**Fig. 2.24**) (**see Video 2.4**).

Retained uncinate processes and recirculation (also referred to as circular flow) often occur together. When an uncinate process is incompletely resected, the natural maxillary sinus ostium may be missed and, as a consequence, the surgical antrostomy is separate from the natural ostium. Mucous then flows in a circular pattern from the natural opening to the surgical opening and then back into the sinus. As mucociliary clearance is consequently impaired due to reentry of infected and inflammatory debris into the maxillary sinus, its ostium, and the ethmoidal infundibulum, patients with this iatrogenic complication often require a revision procedure to remove the uncinate remnant and create a single opening for mucous to flow from the maxillary sinus. Recognizing this defect on endoscopy may require angled scopes; however, it is clearly evident on coronal and axial CT images (**Fig. 2.10**) (**see Video 2.2**).

Oral-antral fistulas may occur after dental procedures and often present with unilateral maxillary sinusitis. Patients may present with drainage into their oral cavity, although edema and inflammation at the fistula site may prevent this from occurring. The bony defect at the fistula site is apparent on coronal CT images. Depending on the fistula size, treatment may be limited to a maxillary antrostomy with the intent that the fistula will close with surgical drainage of the maxillary sinus, or may require soft tissue repair of the fistula defect itself (**Fig. 2.25**) (**see Video 2.5**).

The advent of functional endoscopic sinus surgery (FESS) has made Caldwell–Luc surgery a rare procedure, used primarily as a last resort in patients who have failed prior surgical interventions. Many patients who have undergone this procedure, however, have done well. In fact, a success rate of over 90% has been reported when used in the appropriate patients.[43] It is imperative that otolaryngologists be able to distinguish the healthy post Caldwell–Luc maxillary sinus from the acutely infected sinus, or one with a retained abscess. Approximately half of patients who undergo the Caldwell Luc procedure will reform their maxillary sinus lining after its surgical stripping; the other half will develop scar tissue filling the sinus. Scar tissue, in these latter pa-

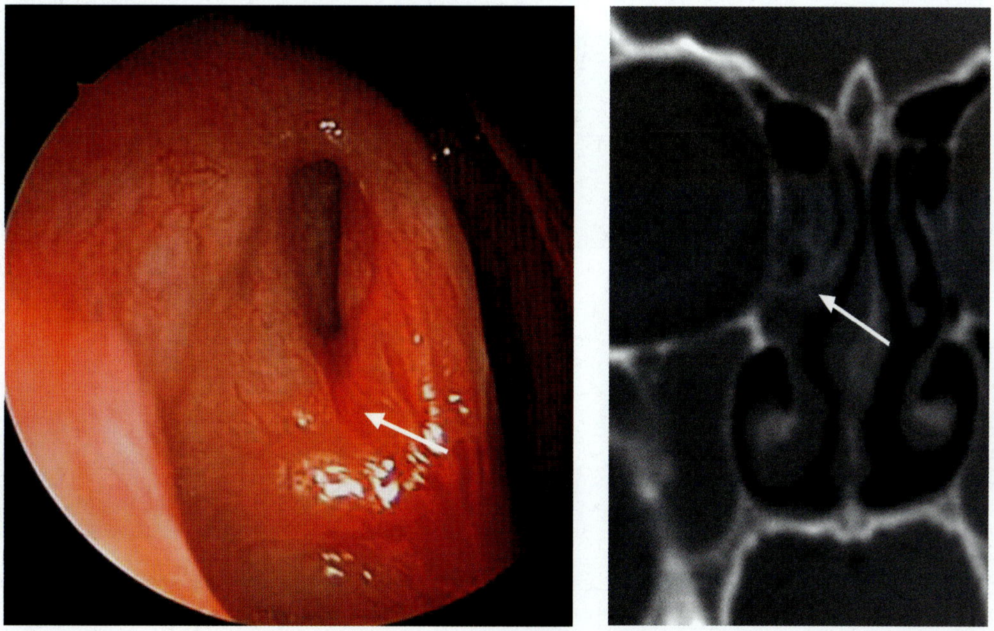
A B

Fig. 2.24 **(A,B)** Middle turbinate lateralization can be recognized on computed tomography (CT) as well as nasal endoscopy. Solid white arrows point to scar tissue on endoscopic view and on coronal CT.

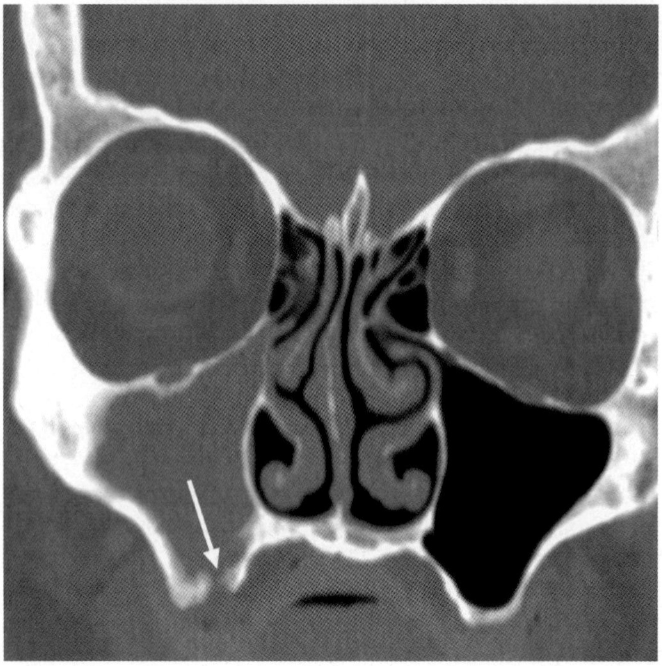

Fig. 2.25 In this coronal computed tomography (CT) image, an oral-antral fistula is demonstrated in the right maxillary sinus (*solid white arrow*).

tients, should not be mistaken for active infection. As with all patient evaluations, patient examination with nasal endoscopy is critical to helping interpret the CT imaging of patients who have undergone the Caldwell–Luc procedure. Images of post-Caldwell–Luc sinuses are shown (**Fig. 2.26**).

One notable complication of Graves disease is exophthalmos in which an autoimmune-mediated inflammatory process of the orbital tissues leads to an increase in the intraorbital volume, specifically increasing orbital fat and the size of the extraocular muscles (**Fig. 2.27**). Treatment may require surgical intervention, notably orbital decompression (see Chapter 20) usually of the medial and/or inferior walls of the orbit. In some cases of decompression, the orbital soft tissues may expand into the maxillary sinus itself, or may block the infundibulum leading to maxillary sinus disease.

The maxillary sinus lift procedure has become an increasingly common adjunctive procedure performed by dentists and oral surgeons to compensate for natural bone loss prior to the placement of dental implants. Autologous and synthetic implants have been used for this procedure, which involves creation of an antral window and submucosal placement of the implant. It behooves the contemporary otolaryngologist to recognize the radiologic appearance of these implants so as to not mistake them for any other type of pathology. On CT, the implants may have a varying appearance based on the material used. Synthetic, silastic materials are radiolucent, whereas autologous bone and hydroxyapatite based implants appear radiopaque and—in most cases—homogeneous. The sinus itself is diminished in volume and should be air-filled. Fluid-filled sinuses should be evaluated for infection and inflammation, as in any other case.

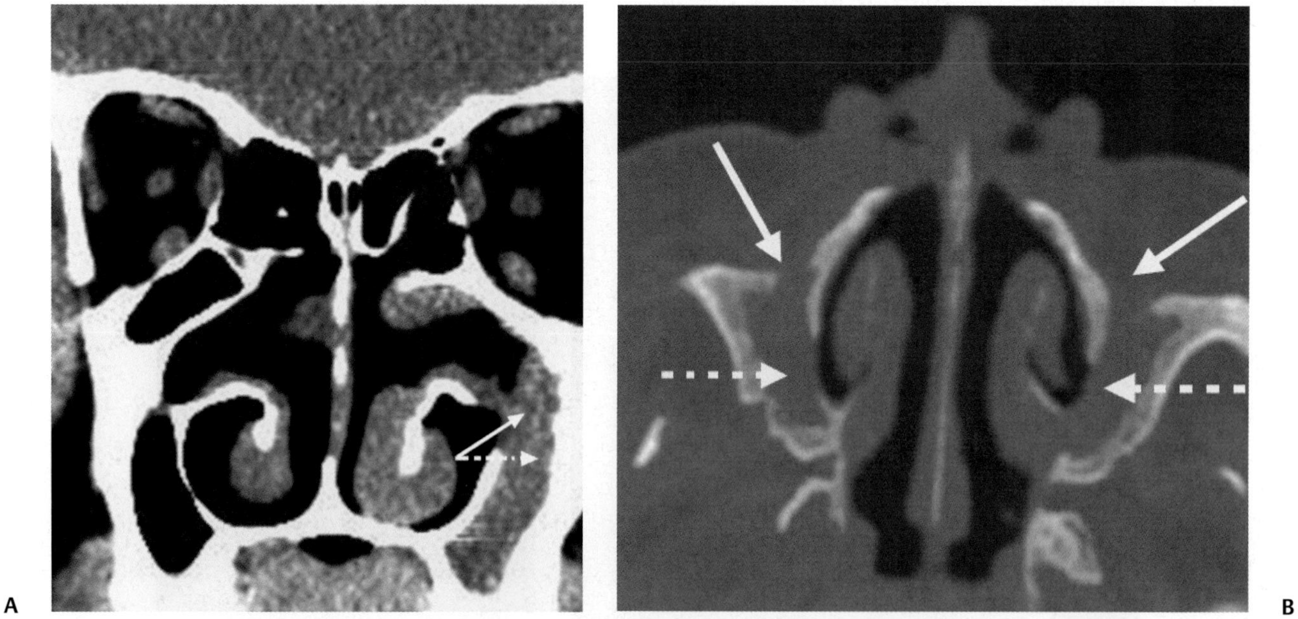

Figs. 2.26 **(A,B)** These sinus computed tomography (CT) scans are of patients who have undergone prior Caldwell–Luc procedures. **(A)** A coronal view, seen in soft tissue windowing, of a patient with a prior Caldwell–Luc procedure. Note the bony defect at the site of the inferior meatal antrostomy (*solid white arrow*), which was made for gravity drainage of the sinus. Note also the scar tissue filling the sinus (*dotted white arrow*). **(B)** An axial view, seen in bony windowing, of a patient with a prior Caldwell–Luc procedure. Note the bony defect at the anterior face of the maxilla (*solid white arrows*) where the sinus was entered via an external approach. Note also the scar tissue filling the sinus (*dotted white arrows*).

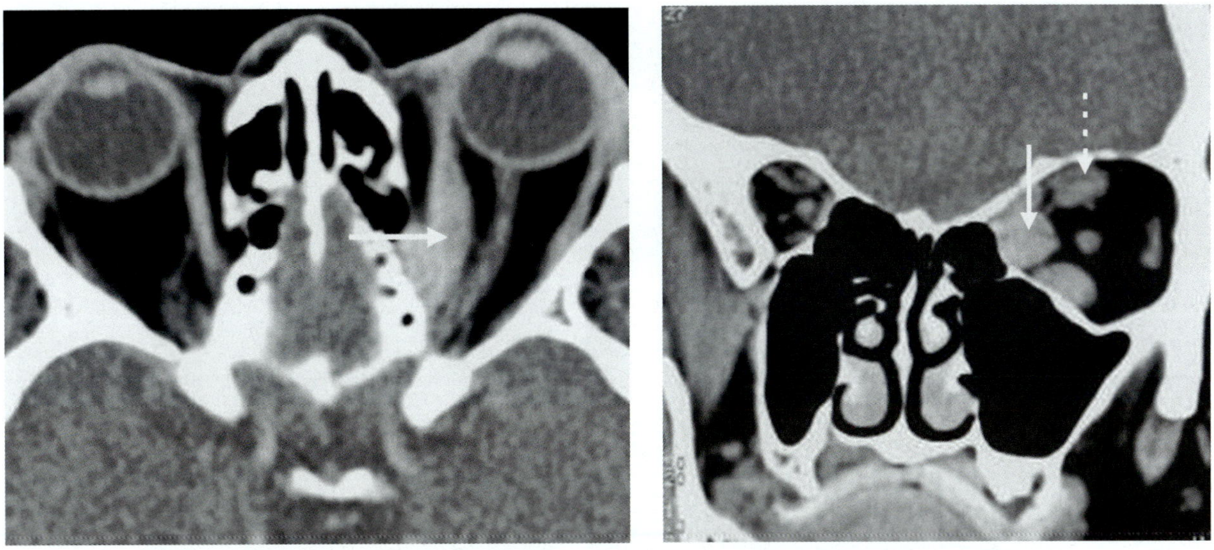

Fig. 2.27 (A,B) Axial and coronal computed tomography (CT) of patient with Graves exophthalmos. Note the enlargement of the eye muscles. In particular, note the enlarged medial rectus (*solid white arrow*) and superior rectus muscles (*dotted white arrow*).

Benign Maxillary Sinus Masses

Many benign masses of the head and neck may occur in the maxillary sinus. Mucous retention cysts are products of obstructed submucosal mucinous glands, and are a common incidental finding in maxillary sinuses. They are felt, in most cases, to be asymptomatic except in cases where they impact on sinus drainage patterns. Their ovoid, nongravity-dependent shape is clearly recognizable on CT, especially on coronal imaging. They occur anywhere on a mucosal surface, including along complete or incomplete bony septations in the maxillary sinus (**Fig. 2.2**). Polyps cannot be differentiated from mucous retention cysts, except that polyps may sometimes be suggested if a stalk is present (**see Video 2.6**).

Mucoceles are cysts lined by flattened, pseudostratified, ciliated columnar epithelium. They are expansile in nature and, unlike retention cysts, are more commonly symptomatic. On CT, mucoceles typically occupy the entire sinus and expand it. A localized mucocele may fill and expand a compartment within a sinus, such as a Haller cell, or may construct its own space in conjunction with a bony septation. Localized mucoceles may appear similar to retention cysts; however, retention cysts do not expand and thin bone, whereas mucoceles do (**Fig. 2.28**).

Antrochoanal polyps (**Fig. 2.29**) are inflammatory lesions that arise within the maxillary sinus and herniate into the nasal cavity via the natural or commonly through the accessory sinus ostia extending to the nasopharynx through the choana (**see Video 2.7**). Histologically, antrochoanal polyps contain numerous inflammatory cells including a few eosinophils and may exhibit surface epithelial squamous metaplasia.[44] Radiologically, there is often complete or near-complete opacification of the maxillary sinus by the antrochoanal polyp alone or in combination with sinus infection or secretions. Enlargement of the maxillary native or accessory ostium, displacement of the inferior and middle turbinates, and medial bulging of the medial maxillary sinus wall are hallmark features.[45] Localized expansion of the maxillary sinus should be distinguished from a mucocele. MRI can sometimes assist in this regard by evaluating the internal sinus contents, displaying the polyp itself as very bright on T2-weighted images.

Simple hematomas may also occur in the maxillary sinus, but are infrequent without a history of trauma or surgery. The radiologic appearance is affected by the duration of time that the hematoma has been present.[46] Over time, hematomas may form an abscess-like collection, and on CT, appear as expansile, heterogeneous masses. Bony erosion may be present in some cases. These characteristics can make a chronic hematoma difficult to differentiate from a benign or malignant tumor, including a mucocele. The ability of MRI to identify hemorrhagic breakdown products can lead to the correct diagnosis.

Allergic fungal sinusitis (AFS) is the most common form of fungal paranasal sinus disease and often involves the maxillary sinus. It is a noninfectious, immune-mediated response to fungi. On gross examination, the fungal mucin is thick, heterogeneous, and of peanut-butter like consistency. Radiologically, the CT scan typically demonstrates rhinitis and multiple sinus involvement. Individual sinuses are usually completely opacified with bony erosion or remodeling due to the expansile nature of the fungal mucin. The mucin itself is heterogeneous with areas of hyperdensity due to the presence of obstructed inspissated mucous as well as calcifications.[47] In fact, often one of the only radiographic clues to distinguish AFS from simple chronic inspissated mucous is the unilateral and expansile nature of the areas with AFS, although this is an inconstant finding. MRI may be useful in the evaluation of AFS, with T2-weighted images typically reveal-

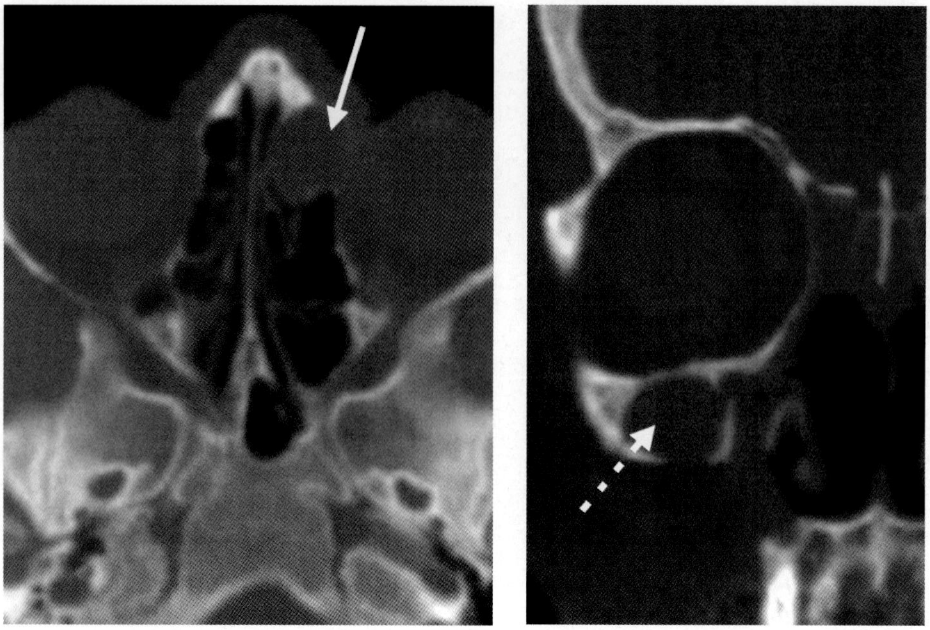

A B

Fig. 2.28 Mucoceles may appear similar to retention cysts; however, retention cysts do not generally erode into adjacent structures, whereas mucoceles often do. **(A)** An axial CT image of an anterior ethmoid mucocoele (*solid white arrow*) which has eroded away the bone which houses the orbit. **(B)** A maxillary sinus mucocoele (*dotted white arrow*) can be seen on coronal CT image of a patient who has undergone prior Caldwell-Luc surgery.

ing a signal void within the sites of allergic fungal sinusitis secondary to elevated protein concentrations in a desiccated environment, plus increased iron, magnesium, and manganese concentrations.[48] The surrounding, inflamed mucosa is bright on T2-weighted images and contrast enhancements. T1-weighted images are more variable, but often display hyperintensity due to the high protein content of the allergic mucin and internal desiccation.

Mycetomas, or fungus balls, are characterized histologically by matted, dense conglomerations of fungal hyphae lacking allergic mucin. The maxillary sinus is the most common sinus to harbor a fungus ball. Radiographically, mycetomas present as a hyperdense mass on CT, sometimes with internal punctuate calcifications. They may cause adjacent bony sclerosis, thinning, erosion, or expansion. On MRI, fungus balls are diminished or increased in signal intensity on T1-weighted images and decreased in signal intensity on T2-weighted images.

Invasive fungal infections, due to organisms such as Mucormycosis and Aspergillosis, may be acute or chronic. The

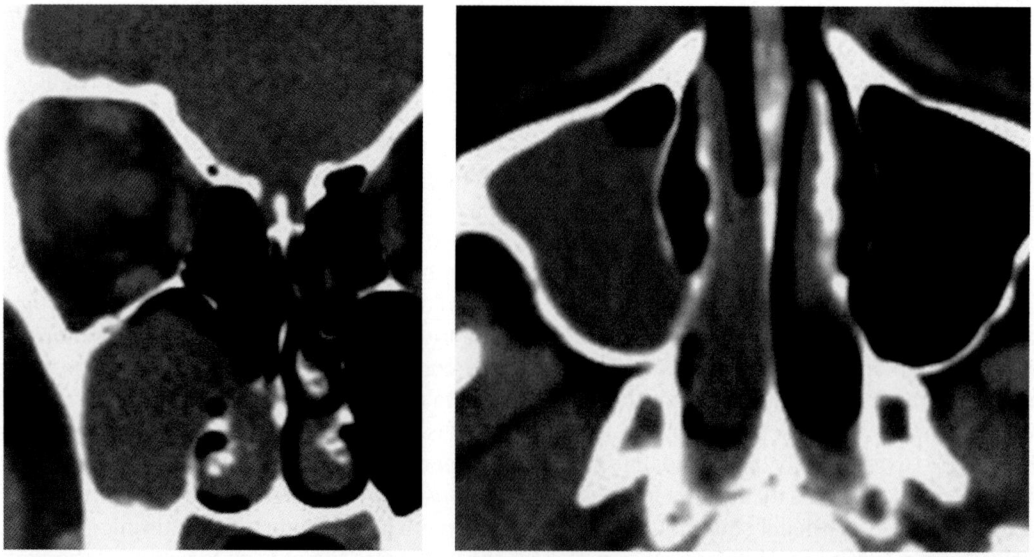

A B

Fig. 2.29 **(A,B)** In these computed tomography (CT) images, an antrochoanal polyp is seen filling the right maxillary sinus and spilling over into the nasal cavity. Note the homogeneity of the polyp. Also, note how it distorts the medial maxillary wall.

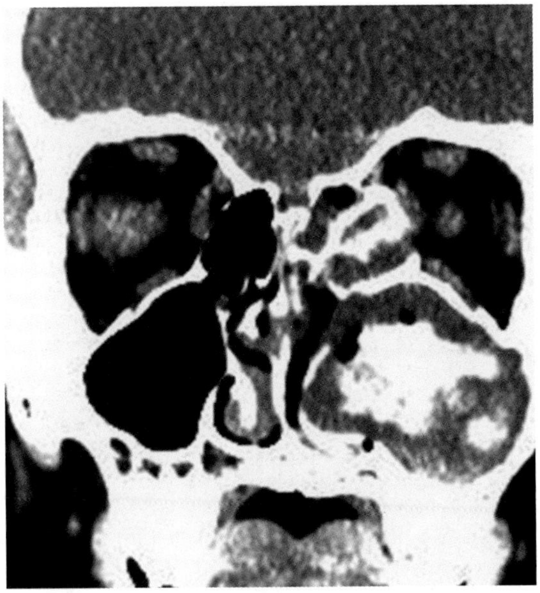

Fig. 2.30 On this coronal computed tomography (CT) image, an opacified left maxillary sinus with central hyperdensity is appreciated. This is a mycetoma, or fungus ball. The lesion is adjacent to, but does not involve the surrounding sinus mucosa.

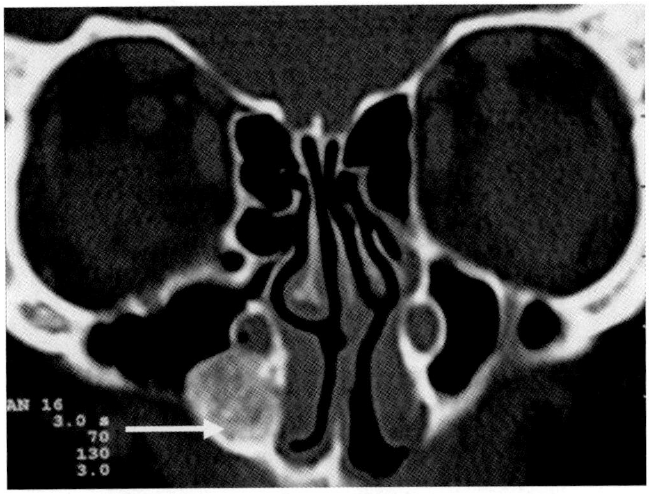

Fig. 2.31 This coronal computed tomography (CT) image demonstrates a case of right maxillary sinus fibrous dysplasia with the characteristic ground glass appearance (*solid white arrow*). The lesion was incidental and stable.

acute variety is most often seen in diabetics and immunocompromised patients. Because the Zygomycetes fungi grow along blood vessels, mortality reaches 50 to 80%.[49] Chronic invasive fungal sinusitis has a more protracted, indolent course. Both acute and chronic forms usually extensively involve nasal mucosa as well as the sinuses and can be classified as rhinosinusitis. Invasive fungal infections may present with heterogeneous imaging findings ranging from soft tissue density to hyperattenuation on CT. MRI findings are typical of fungal infections. Characteristic bone and regional soft tissue invasion are more ominous features, although chronic invasive fungal sinusitis may also produce bony sclerosis (**Fig. 2.30**). The chronic variety may be difficult to differentiate from a malignancy.

Fibroosseous lesions also occur in the maxillary sinus. Osteomas are the most common benign neoplasms of the paranasal sinuses, composed of variable proportions of cancellous and cortical bone. They are most commonly found in the frontal sinus, with maxillary sinus lesions occurring less frequently. Maxillary sinus osteomas may be a component of Gardner syndrome, an inherited autosomal dominant syndrome of intestinal polyposis, soft tissue and cutaneous tumors, and osteomas.[50] Radiologically, osteomas are of solid bone density and are usually circular or ovoid in shape. Fibrous dysplasia is another fibroosseous lesion, which is characterized by replacement of bone with fibrous tissue and immature bone. The maxilla and mandible are the most commonly affected sites in the head and neck. Radiographically, the lesions are most commonly noted to have a "ground-glass" appearance with diffuse, indistinct margins (**Fig. 2.31**). In some cases, it may be difficult to distinguish fibrous dysplasia from an aplastic sinus, which has often been replaced by immature bone. Osteoblastomas are painful, rare lesions of the maxillary sinus that may be difficult to differentiate from fibrous dysplasia and ossifying fibromas. Ossifying fibroma is a slowly expansive lesion containing varying degrees of calcification, bone, and cementum. Radiologically, there is a well-defined bony rim with a heterogeneous central cavity. The bony rim is distinct from the surrounding bone, and in most cases this is evident on CT. In some cases an air–fluid level may be present due to the fluid within the fibroma and internal communication with a normally aerated space. Ossifying fibromas are expansile and may erode the surrounding bone (**Fig. 2.32**).

Inverted papilloma is discussed in great detail in Chapters 9 and 11, and so will be mentioned only briefly here. These benign lesions are most distinctive on endoscopy, with their inverting, mulberry-like formations. This pattern can be appreciated on CT on occasion; however, these lesions may be difficult to distinguish from other benign or malignant masses in this location. CT and MRI do, however, play an important role in defining the extent of disease and the involvement of surrounding structures. CT can best delineate commonly encountered bony erosion or remodeling and intratumoral calcification.[51] It has been suggested that the point of greatest osteitis on CT corresponds to the point of attachment of the papilloma and knowledge of this point of attachment/point of origin can play a useful role in preoperative planning.[52,53] On MRI, the inverted papilloma is isointense on T1-weighted MR images and on T2-weighted MR images is isointense to hypointense. Lesion intensity and contrast enhancement are homogeneous or heterogeneous. The identification of a convoluted cerebriform pattern on T2-weighted or con-

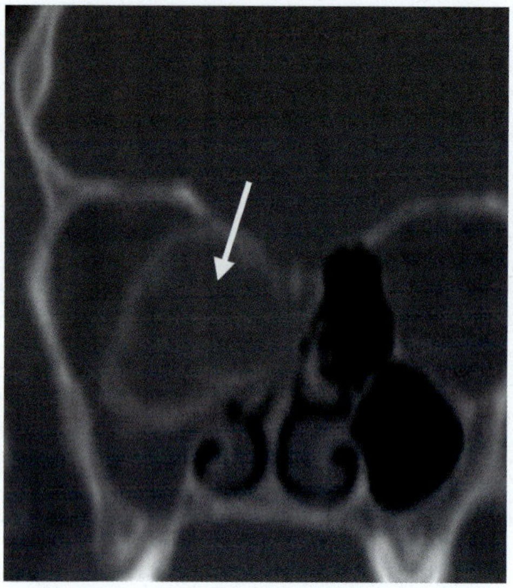

Fig. 2.32 A well-circumscribed ossifying fibroma is seen on coronal computed tomography (CT) (*solid white arrow*). The expansile lesion has compressed and remodeled the surrounding bony structures.

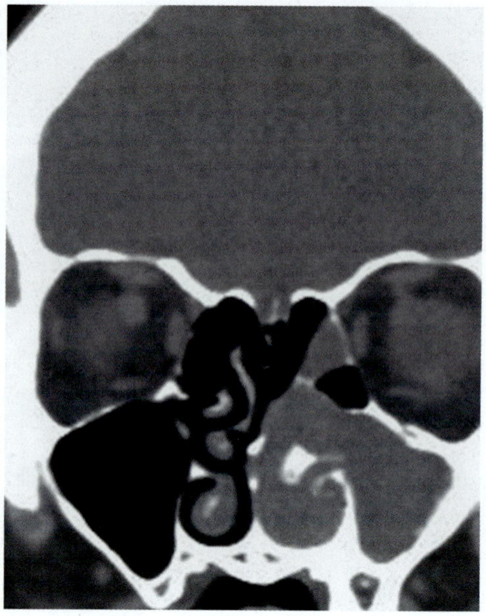

Fig. 2.33 This coronal computed tomography (CT) image shows an expansile lesion filling the left maxillary sinus and extending into the nasal cavity. This is an inverted papilloma that was pedicled to the medial maxillary wall necessitating an endoscopic medial maxillectomy.

trast enhanced T1-weighted MR images can make the diagnosis more certain.[54,55] MRI is useful in distinguishing the solid papilloma itself from postobstructive sinusitis (**Fig. 2.33**) (**see Video 2.8**).

Due to the proximity of the oral cavity to the maxillary sinus, odontogenic processes may impact the maxillary sinus. Odontoma, ameloblastoma, Pindborg tumor, and dentigerous or odontogenic cysts are just a few of the many masses of dental origin that may erode, or otherwise involve, the maxillary sinus. Details of these dental masses fall outside the purview of this chapter; however, the contemporary otolaryngologist should be aware of the close relationship between these neighboring anatomic sites and be prepared to evaluate isolated maxillary sinus pathology arising from an odontogenic source.

Malignant Maxillary Sinus Masses

Practically any malignancy of the head and neck can develop in the sinonasal cavity. Some of the more common varieties are discussed below. Unfortunately, many maxillary sinus malignant neoplasms are not diagnosed until they are in a late stage. Radiology studies are a key tool in the T System staging of malignancy of the paranasal sinuses.[56] Bony destruction, extension to adjacent, often critical structures, and involvement of surrounding nerves and vessels can usually be appreciated with a high degree of accuracy on CT and MRI. CT best demonstrates bony destruction, which is seen in the majority of maxillary sinus malignancies. MRI best demonstrates soft tissue extension and involvement of adjacent structures such as the orbit, skull base, and intracranial contents including the dura. MRI also helps differentiate benign sinus disease from malignancy. MRI best evaluates perineural spread because of pathologic enhancement of the involved nerve, optimally demonstrated when using fat-suppression techniques. Occasionally, this appearance can be mimicked by a postoperative neuroma. CT in perineural spread would demonstrate an enlarged neuroforamen, a relatively late sign.

The most common malignancy of the maxillary sinus is a squamous cell carcinoma originating in the mucosa. 80% of all paranasal sinus squamous cell carcinomas arise in the maxillary sinus.[57] Patients are usually older than 50 and there is a male predominance. Squamous cell carcinomas typically demonstrate diminished signal intensity on T2-weighted images. The hypointensity on T2-weighted MR images is often heterogeneous, usually different than inspissated secretions and fungal infection. Contrast enhancement may be solid or heterogeneous, but usually not peripheral as seen in benign sinus disease, retention cysts, mucoceles, and some polyps. Squamous cell carcinomas may demonstrate internal necrosis, hemorrhage, or calcification and may have mixed adenocarcinoma features.

Minor salivary gland tumors include adenoid cystic carcinoma, mucoepidermoid carcinoma, adenocarcinoma, and undifferentiated carcinoma. Adenoid cystic carcinoma is the most common of these and can present in numerous locations in the sinuses and neck. Not only do minor salivary gland tumors avidly enhance, but they have a predilection for perineural spread. They may be increased or decreased in signal intensity on T2-weighted MR images due to the underlying histologic cell pattern. Adenocarcinomas often demonstrate diminished signal intensity on T2-weighted

MR images as do any neoplasms with increased cellular density or of gastrointestinal origin, including the sinonasal undifferentiated carcinoma (SNUC), another neoplasm rarely seen in the maxillary sinus.

Metastatic disease to the maxillary sinus is uncommon. The most common primary is renal cell carcinoma followed by lung, breast, colon, and prostate carcinomas. Melanoma may be metastatic or primary. Melanoma is typically of increased signal intensity on T1-weighted images and decreased signal intensity on T2-weighted images, although amelanotic melanoma may reverse these imaging findings. Primary maxillary sinus melanomas are usually reported as case studies. B cell or T cell non-Hodgkin lymphoma is not infrequent and its appearance is usually of diminished T2-signal intensity. It demonstrates marked uptake on positron emission tomography (PET) scans. The chloroma of leukemia can mimic a mucous retention cyst or fungus mycetoma.

Rhabdosarcomas rarely originate in the maxillary sinus and more often involve it by contiguous extension. Sarcomas, carcinomas, and meningiomas may be radiation induced.[58] Primary bone tumors are included to be complete and include plasmacytomas and myelomas, plus osteogenic (e.g., osteosarcoma), chondroid (e.g., chondrosarcoma), and fibrous (e.g., malignant fibrous histiocytoma) neoplastic categories.

Pearls

- Radiologic imaging allows the otolaryngologist to appreciate abnormalities of and around the maxillary sinus and surrounding structures.
- Many anatomic abnormalities can be appreciated on preoperative imaging. Awareness of these abnormalities (i.e., silent sinus/atelectatic uncinate process, Haller [infraorbital ethmoid] cells, etc.) can help the surgeon to perform complete, safe, and effective surgery.
- It can be difficult to distinguish acute from chronic sinus disease; however, imaging techniques can be of use in certain circumstances.
- It is useful for the surgeon to learn to appreciate normal from abnormal post-operative images. Maxillary sinus recirculation, lateralized middle turbinates, and mucous retention cysts (for instance) can all be recognized on imaging and may help in the diagnosis of persistent sinus disease. In addition, the appearance of the postoperative sinus after a Caldwell-Luc procedure should be appreciated.
- CT and MRI can help define the extent of tumor disease and the impact on surrounding structures (i.e., bone erosion), as well as distinguish tumor from postobstructive sinus disease.
- Certain masses (i.e., juvenile nasopharyngeal angiofibroma, fibrous dysplasia, osteoma) have characteristic imaging profiles, which are reviewed in this chapter.

References

1. Dammann F, Bode A, Heuschmid M, et al. [Multislice spiral CT of the paranasal sinuses: first experiences using various parameters of radiation dosage]. Rofo 2000;172(8):701–706
2. Zammit-Maempel I, Chadwick CL, Willis SP. Radiation dose to the lens of eye and thyroid gland in paranasal sinus multislice CT. Br J Radiol 2003;76(906):418–420
3. Shellock FG, Kanal E, Moscatel M. Bioeffects and safety considerations. In: Atlas S, ed. Magnetic Resonance Imaging of the Brain and Spine. 2nd ed. Philadelphia, PA:Lippincott-Raven; 1996:109–148
4. Bolger WE, Woodruff WWJr, Morehead J, Parsons DS. Maxillary sinus hypoplasia: classification and description of associated uncinate process hypoplasia. Otolaryngol Head Neck Surg 1990;103(5 (Pt 1)): 759–765
5. Kim HJ, Friedman EM, Sulek M, Duncan NO, McCluggage C. Paranasal sinus development in chronic sinusitis, cystic fibrosis, and normal comparison population: a computerized tomography correlation study. Am J Rhinol 1997;11(4):275–281
6. Haetinger R. Imaging of the nose and paranasal sinuses. In: Stamm A, Draf W, eds. Micro-Endoscopic Surgery of the Paranasal Sinuses and Skull Base. Heidelberg/Berlin/New York: Springer; 2000:53–82
7. Berger G, Balum-Azim M, Ophir D. The normal inferior turbinate: histomorphometric analysis and clinical implications. Laryngoscope 2003;113(7):1192–1198
8. Selcuk A, Ozcan KM, Ozcan I, Dere H. Bifid inferior turbinate: a case report. J Laryngol Otol 2008;122(6):647–649
9. Taggarshe D, Quraishi MS, Dugar JM. Inferior turbinate angiofibroma: an atypical presentation [correction of preservation]. Rhinology 2004;42(1):45–47
10. Yariktaş M, Doğru H, Döner F, Tüz M, Yasan H. Choanal polyp originating from the inferior turbinate presenting as nasal polyposis. Kulak Burun Bogaz Ihtis Derg 2006;16(1):37–40
11. Mesolella M, Galli V, Testa D. Inferior turbinate osteoma: a rare cause of nasal obstruction. Otolaryngol Head Neck Surg 2005;133(6):989–991
12. Ozcan KM, Akdogan O, Gedikli Y, Ozcan I, Dere H, Unal T. Fibrous dysplasia of inferior turbinate, middle turbinate, and frontal sinus. B-ENT 2007;3(1):35–38
13. Mirante JP, Christmas DA, Yanagisawa E. Epistaxis caused by hemangioma of the inferior turbinate. Ear Nose Throat J 2006;85(10):630–632, 632
14. Khnifies R, Fradis M, Brodsky A, Bajar J, Luntz M. Inferior turbinate schwannoma: report of a case. Ear Nose Throat J 2006;85(6):384–385
15. Unlu HH, Celik O, Demir MA, Eskiizmir G. Pleomorphic adenoma originated from the inferior nasal turbinate. Auris Nasus Larynx 2003;30(4):417–420
16. Uzun L, Ugur MB, Savranlar A, Mahmutyazicioglu K, Ozdemir H, Beder LB. Classification of the inferior turbinate bones: a computed tomography study. Eur J Radiol 2004;51(3):241–245
17. Egeli E, Demirci L, Yazýcý B, Harputluoglu U. Evaluation of the inferior turbinate in patients with deviated nasal septum by using computed tomography. Laryngoscope 2004;114(1):113–117

18. Golub JS, Parikh SL, Budnick SD, Bernardino CR, DelGaudio JM. Inverted papilloma of the nasolacrimal system invading the orbit. Ophthal Plast Reconstr Surg 2007;23(2):151–153
19. Wladis EJ, Frempong T, Gausas R. Nasolacrimal metastasis from hepatocellular carcinoma masquerading as dacryocystitis. Ophthal Plast Reconstr Surg 2007;23(4):333–335
20. Xiao MY, Tang LS, Zhu H, Li YJ, Li HL, Wu XR. Adult nasolacrimal sac mucocele. Ophthalmologica 2008;222(1):21–26
21. Maini S, Raghava N, Youngs R, et al. Endoscopic endonasal laser versus endonasal surgical dacryocystorhinostomy for epiphora due to nasolacrimal duct obstruction: prospective, randomised, controlled trial. J Laryngol Otol 2007;121(12):1170–1176
22. Yoon JH, Kim KS, Jung DH, et al. Fontanelle and uncinate process in the lateral wall of the human nasal cavity. Laryngoscope 2000;110(2 Pt 1):281–285
23. Kazkayasi M, Ergin A, Ersoy M, Bengi O, Tekdemir I, Elhan A. Certain anatomical relations and the precise morphometry of the infraorbital foramen—canal and groove: an anatomical and cephalometric study. Laryngoscope 2001;111(4 Pt 1):609–614
24. Chandra RK, Kennedy DW. Surgical implications of an unusual anomaly of the infraorbital nerve. Ear Nose Throat J 2004;83(11):766–767
25. Walsh W, Kern R. Sinonasal anatomy, function, and evaluation. In: Bailey B, Johnson J, eds. Head and Neck Surgery—Otolaryngology. Vol. 1, 4th ed. Philadelphia, PA: Lippincott Williams & Wilkins
26. Milczuk HA, Dalley RW, Wessbacher FW, Richardson MA. Nasal and paranasal sinus anomalies in children with chronic sinusitis. Laryngoscope 1993;103(3):247–252
27. Bolger WE, Butzin CA, Parsons DS. Paranasal sinus bony anatomic variations and mucosal abnormalities: CT analysis for endoscopic sinus surgery. Laryngoscope 1991;101(1 Pt 1):56–64
28. Tonai A, Baba S. Anatomic variations of the bone in sinonasal CT. Acta Otolaryngol Suppl 1996;525:9–13
29. Zinreich SJ, Kennedy DW, Rosenbaum AE, Gayler BW, Kumar AJ, Stammberger H. Paranasal sinuses: CT imaging requirements for endoscopic surgery. Radiology 1987;163(3):769–775
30. Wanamaker HH. Role of Haller's cell in headache and sinus disease: a case report. Otolaryngol Head Neck Surg 1996;114(2):324–327
31. Sebrechts H, Vlaminck S, Casselman J. Orbital edema resulting from Haller's cell pathology: 3 case reports and review of literature. Acta Otorhinolaryngol Belg 2000;54(1):39–43
32. Stackpole SA, Edelstein DR. The anatomic relevance of the Haller cell in sinusitis. Am J Rhinol 1997;11(3):219–223
33. Parsons DS, Stivers FE, Talbot AR. The missed ostium sequence and the surgical approach to revision functional endoscopic sinus surgery. Otolaryngol Clin North Am 1996;29(1):169–183
34. Das S, Kim D, Cannon TY, Ebert CS Jr, Senior BA. High-resolution computed tomography analysis of the greater palatine canal. Am J Rhinol 2006;20(6):603–608
35. Douglas R, Wormald PJ. Pterygopalatine fossa infiltration through the greater palatine foramen: where to bend the needle. Laryngoscope 2006;116(7):1255–1257
36. Methathrathip D, Apinhasmit W, Chompoopong S, Lertsirithong A, Ariyawatkul T, Sangvichien S. Anatomy of greater palatine foramen and canal and pterygopalatine fossa in Thais: considerations for maxillary nerve block. Surg Radiol Anat 2005;27(6):511–516
37. Chan LL, Chong J, Gillenwater AM, Ginsberg LE. The pterygopalatine fossa: postoperative MR imaging appearance. AJNR Am J Neuroradiol 2000;21(7):1315–1319
38. Tomura N, Hirano H, Kato K, et al. Comparison of MR imaging with CT in depiction of tumour extension into the pterygopalatine fossa. Clin Radiol 1999;54(6):361–366
39. Musy PY, Kountakis SE. Anatomic findings in patients undergoing revision endoscopic sinus surgery. Am J Otolaryngol 2004;25(6):418–422
40. Friedman M, Schalch P. Middle turbinate medialization with bovine serum albumin tissue adhesive (BioGlue). Laryngoscope 2008;118(2):335–338
41. Lindemann J, Keck T, Rettinger G. Septal-turbinate-suture in endonasal sinus surgery. Rhinology 2002;40(2):92–94
42. Bolger WE, Kuhn FA, Kennedy DW. Middle turbinate stabilization after functional endoscopic sinus surgery: the controlled synechiae technique. Laryngoscope 1999;109(11):1852–1853
43. Cutler JL, Duncavage JA, Matheny K, Cross JL, Miman MC, Oh CK. Results of Caldwell-Luc after failed endoscopic middle meatus antrostomy in patients with chronic sinusitis. Laryngoscope 2003;113(12):2148–2150
44. Ozcan C, Zeren H, Talas DU, Küçükoğlu M, Görür K. Antrochoanal polyp: a transmission electron and light microscopic study. Eur Arch Otorhinolaryngol 2005;262(1):55–60
45. Chung SK, Chang BC, Dhong HJ. Surgical, radiologic, and histologic findings of the antrochoanal polyp. Am J Rhinol 2002;16(2):71–76
46. Nishiguchi T, Nakamura A, Mochizuki K, Tokuhara Y, Yamane H, Inoue Y. Expansile organized maxillary sinus hematoma: MR and CT findings and review of literature. AJNR Am J Neuroradiol 2007;28(7):1375–1377
47. Mukherji SK, Figueroa RE, Ginsberg LE, et al. Allergic fungal sinusitis: CT findings. Radiology 1998;207(2):417–422
48. Aribandi M, McCoy VA, Bazan C III. Imaging features of invasive and noninvasive fungal sinusitis: a review. Radiographics 2007;27(5):1283–1296
49. Waitzman AA, Birt BD. Fungal sinusitis. J Otolaryngol 1994;23(4):244–249
50. Alexander AA, Patel AA, Odland R. Paranasal sinus osteomas and Gardner's syndrome. Ann Otol Rhinol Laryngol 2007;116(9):658–66217926587
51. Head CS, Sercarz JA, Luu Q, Collins J, Blackwell KE. Radiographic assessment of inverted papilloma. Acta Otolaryngol 2007;127(5):515–520
52. Yousuf K, Wright ED. Site of attachment of inverted papilloma predicted by CT findings of osteitis. Am J Rhinol 2007;21(1):32–36
53. Lee DK, Chung SK, Dhong H-J, Kim HY, Kim H-J, Bok KH. Focal hyperostosis on CT of sinonasal inverted papilloma as a predictor of tumor origin. AJNR Am J Neuroradiol 2007;28(4):618–621
54. Maroldi R, Farina D, Palvarini L, Lombardi D, Tomenzoli D, Nicolai P. Magnetic resonance imaging findings of inverted papilloma: differential diagnosis with malignant sinonasal tumors. Am J Rhinol 2004;18(5):305–310
55. Jeon TY, Kim H-J, Chung S-K, et al. Sinonasal inverted papilloma: value of convoluted cerebriform pattern on MR imaging. AJNR Am J Neuroradiol 2008;29(8):1556–1560
56. Greene FL, Page DL, Fleming ID, et al, eds. AJCC Cancer Staging Manual. 6th ed. New York: Springer-Verlag;2002: 61
57. Grossman RI, Yousem DM. Neuroradiology: The Requisites. 2nd ed. Philadelphia, PA: Elsevier; 2003: 633–638
58. Abrigo JM, King AD, Leung SF, et al. MRI of radiation-induced tumors of the head and neck in post-radiation nasopharyngeal carcinoma. Eur Radiol 2009;19(5):1197–1205

3 Microbiology of Acute and Chronic Maxillary Sinusitis

Eugene A. Chu and Andrew P. Lane

The majority of community-acquired sinusitis is self-limited and caused by upper respiratory viral infections rather than bacteria. With a history of a cold or "influenza-like" illness that has not improved beyond 7 to 10 days, however, there is a significant likelihood of a bacterial etiology, and antimicrobial therapy is indicated. Infectious maxillary sinusitis is categorized as acute or chronic based on the duration of symptoms. Acute maxillary sinusitis is defined as up to 4 weeks of purulent nasal drainage that occurs in the setting of nasal obstruction and/or facial pain, pressure, or fullness; the diagnosis of chronic maxillary sinusitis requires the presence of symptoms or radiographic findings consistent with sinusitis being present for more than 12 weeks.[1]

An appreciation of the bacteriology of acute and chronic maxillary sinusitis is important to guide empiric therapy, confirm successful treatment, and limit the inappropriate use of antibiotics that can promote the development of resistant strains. Furthermore, as a research tool, analysis of sinus bacteriology is essential to documenting the effectiveness of antibiotics and of surgical treatment, as well as developing new treatment modalities.

■ Sources of Maxillary Sinus Cultures

Because the maxillary sinus is relatively easy and safe to access, it has been the primary site of investigation for the microbiology of sinusitis. Traditional approaches used to sample maxillary sinus contents directly have increasingly been supplanted by minimally invasive techniques as endoscopic technology has evolved.

Direct Aspiration

Under normal conditions, the sinuses are believed to be sterile; however, the upper airway is colonized with bacteria and thus may contaminate simple nasal swabs. Before the advent of endoscopes, the gold standard for sinus cultures has been the maxillary sinus puncture (MSP) through either the canine fossa or inferior meatus. Typically, the planned entry site is prepped and then entered with a large bore needle or trocar, and the contents either directly aspirated or lavaged and aspirated. The majority of pharmaceutical trials of antibiotic efficacy rely on these techniques. In fact, the Food and Drug Administration has stated that "... endoscopically guided cultures are not a currently acceptable means of establishing microbiological diagnosis because they may be contaminated by nasal cavity flora."[2]

Besides the obvious discomfort and minimal risk associated with the procedure, MSPs have several limitations. The real or perceived pain associated with the procedure may result in selection bias during studies and, if a lavage technique is used, it may actually be therapeutic and confound the results. Additionally, MSPs fail to sample the key watershed area of the middle meatus.[3]

Endoscopic-guided Middle Meatal Culture

Blind nasal swabs have been notoriously prone to contamination and have found little use in the management of bacterial sinusitis. However, with the introduction of sinonasal endoscopy in the 1980s, endoscopic directed cultures became a feasible option. In endoscopically guided middle meatal (EGMM) cultures, a small flexible wire calcium alginate-tipped swab is used to swab the middle meatus under direct endoscopic visualization (**Fig. 3.1**). Several authors have reviewed the literature comparing endoscopically EGMM

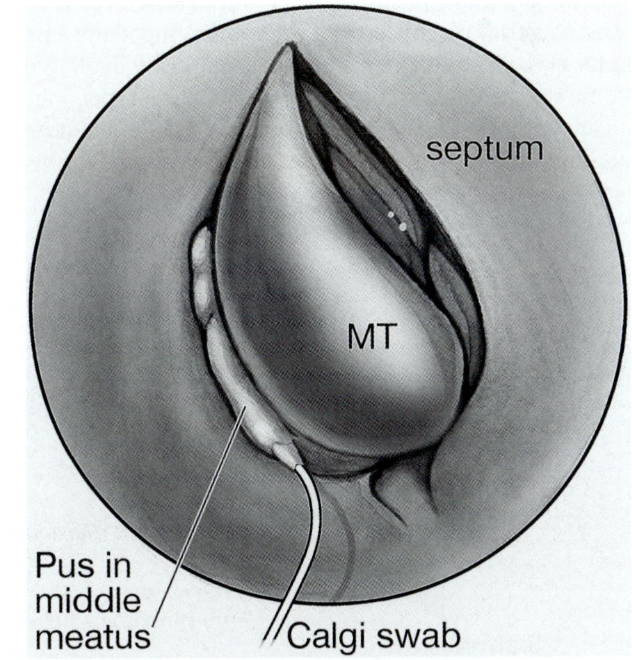

Fig. 3.1 Illustration of endoscopic-directed middle meatal culture utilizing a calcium alginate-tipped swab.

cultures to MSP. One recent meta-analysis found EGMM cultures to have a sensitivity of 80.9% and a specificity of 90.5% compared with MSP, whereas another meta-analysis established an 82% concordance with MSP.[4,5]

With some experience, EGMM cultures can be obtained simply with little morbidity, low risk of contamination, and excellent patient acceptance. At this point, endoscopically directed cultures have found their greatest utility in the clinical setting; however, the majority of research studies continue to rely on the maxillary sinus puncture as the gold standard.

Review of Basic Microbiology

A brief review of basic microbiology will facilitate our discussion of the bacteriology of acute and chronic maxillary sinusitis. Bacteria are broadly categorized based on morphologic characteristics, cell wall composition, and metabolic requirements. Recognized shapes include cocci (round), bacilli (rod), and spirochetes (spiral). Furthermore, their arrangement may also be classified into pairs (diplococci), chains (streptococci), and clusters (staphylococci). Gram-positive and gram-negative bacteria differ in the structure, chemical composition, and thickness of their cell walls (**Fig. 3.2**). Gram-positive organisms have a thick multilayered peptidoglycan cell wall, whereas gram-negative organisms have a thinner but more complex peptidoglycan layer that contains endotoxin and lipopolysaccharides. Between the outer membrane and cytoplasmic membrane of gram-negative organisms, is the periplasmic space, which in some species harbors β-lactamases. Penicillin-binding proteins, enzymes essential for cell-wall synthesis, are found in the cytoplasmic membranes of both gram-positive and gram-negative organisms.

The bacterial response to oxygen is an important criterion for classification and also of practical value in allowing the appropriate culture and isolation of bacterial specimens. Obligate aerobes require oxygen to grow while facultative anaerobes utilize oxygen if present but may use the fermentation pathway to generate energy in the absence of sufficient oxygen. Obligate anaerobes, as the name suggests, cannot grow in the presence of oxygen although some bacteria may survive in an environment with low levels of oxygen.

Bacteriology of Acute Maxillary Sinusitis

Adults

The microbiology of acute maxillary sinusitis is well established, with aerobic and facultative anaerobic bacteria comprising the majority of pathogens. *Haemophilus influenzae* and *Streptococcus pneumoniae* are the two most common isolates, with *Moraxella catarrhalis* a distant third.[6–11] The relative prevalence of the different organisms varies depending on the study population and available culture techniques. **Figure 3.3** combines the results of several studies in demonstrating the bacterial species identified in acute maxillary sinusitis in adults.

Haemophilus Influenzae

H. influenzae is a facultative gram-negative coccobacillus. Strains may be encapsulated or unencapsulated. Six serotypes based on the antigenicity of the capsular polysaccharide are recognized with type b causing the most serious infections—meningitis and sepsis. Unencapsulated (nontypeable) strains cause upper respiratory infections such as sinusitis, otitis media, and bronchitis. Antimicrobial resistance is mediated by the production of β-lactamases, which hydrolyze the amide bond of the β-lactam ring thereby inactivating the antiobiotic.[12,13]

Streptococcus Pneumoniae

Pneumococci are facultative anaerobic gram-positive lancet-shaped cocci typically arranged in pairs of short chains. *S.*

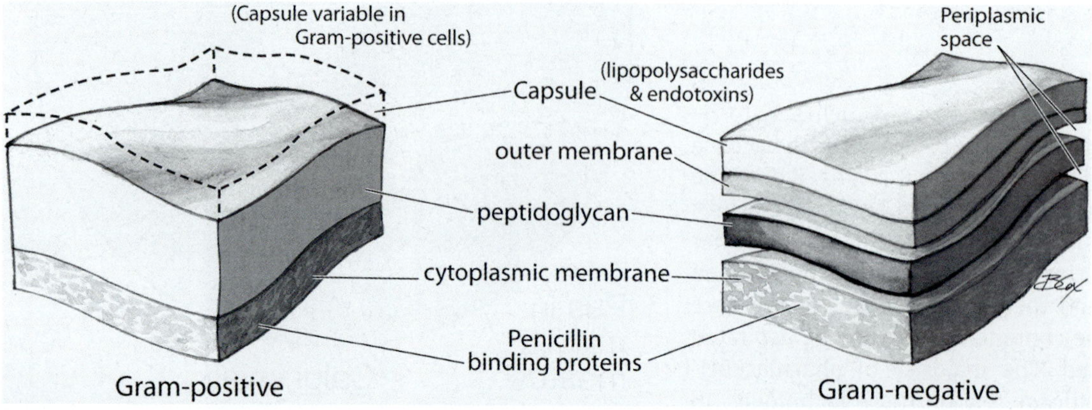

Fig. 3.2 Cell walls of gram-positive and gram-negative bacteria.

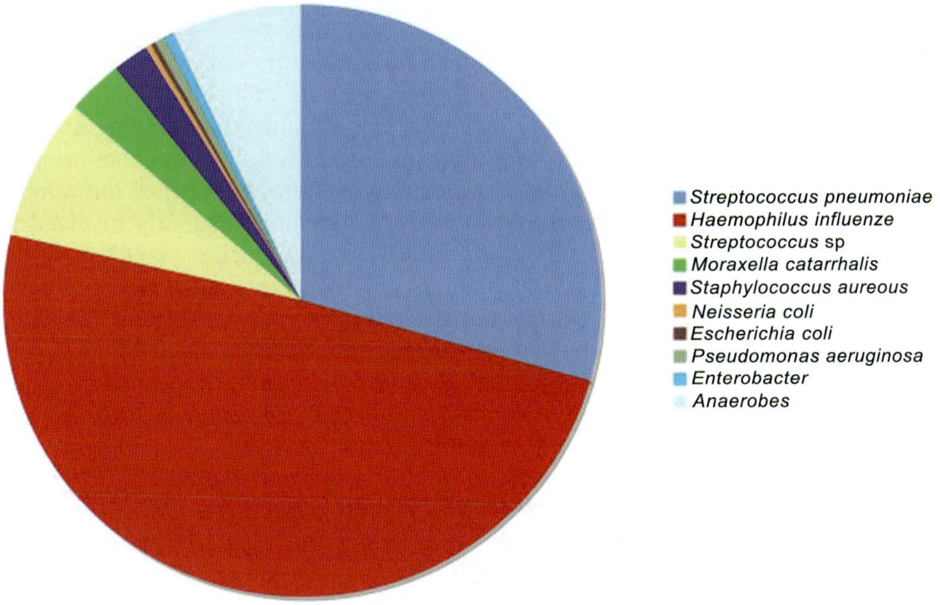

Fig. 3.3 Bacterial causes of acute maxillary sinusitis in adults.

pneumoniae, a member of the α-hemolytic group of streptococci, can be distinguished from *S. viridans* by its bile solubility and growth inhibition by Optochin. Pneumococci possess more than 90 antigenically distinct polysaccharide capsular serotypes that can be used for classification. The incidence of invasive pneumococcal disease varies with serotype and is largely determined by the capsular composition, which is the most important virulence factor. In the United States, seven serotypes account for more than three fourths of all isolates middle ear effusions from children's blood, cerebrospinal fluid, and middle ear and are present in the 7-valent conjugated pneumococcal vaccine utilized in America.[14,15]

S. pneumoniae have developed resistance to multiple forms of antibiotics. Resistance to β-lactams is mediated through the stepwise alteration in penicillin-binding proteins, which alter the binding affinities of β-lactams.[16] Macrolide resistance results from alterations in ribosomal binding sites or expression of an efflux mechanism.[17,18] Fluoroquinolone, trimethoprim, and sulfonamide resistance have developed following mutations to the respective binding sites of these agents (fluoroquinolone → DNA gyrase and topoisomerase IV; trimethoprim→ dihydropteroate synthase; sulfonamides → dihydrofolate reductase).[19]

Moraxella Catarrhalis

M. catarrhalis is an aerobic, gram-negative coccobacilli similar to neisseriae. Most clinical isolates produce β-lactamases, which are distinct from those produced by *H. influenzae*. Thus, antibiotic resistance of one isolate does not necessarily mean that the other will be resistant as well. *M. catarrhalis* has been shown to be intrinsically resistant to trimethoprim.[13,20]

Children

The microbiology of acute maxillary sinusitis in children is very similar to the adult population. *H. influenzae*, *S. pneumoniae*, and *M. catarrhalis* remain the most frequent isolates; however, *M. catarrhalis* infections are more frequent in children than in the adult population.[21,22] *M. catarrhalis* infection is spread by respiratory aerosol; so day-care and school settings may account for the relative increased prevalence compared with adults.

Bacteriology of Chronic Maxillary Sinusitis

Adults

Bacteria are believed to play a major role in the pathogenesis of chronic maxillary sinusitis, although the disease is more heterogeneous than the acute form. In many cases, an underlying inflammatory process may predispose the patient to bacterial colonization, rather than the bacterial infection initiating the inflammation. In either event, all of the same pathogens implicated in acute maxillary sinusitis occur in chronic sinusitis, but are shifted in their relative prevalence. Chronic maxillary sinusitis patients have a repeatedly damaged mucosal lining with resultant inflammation and tissue edema. This can result in decreased oxygen tension within the sinus, as well as a decrease in the mucosal blood flow with resultant decreased antibiotic penetration and a depression in ciliary action.[6,23,24] Decreased pH within the sinus can also reduce the efficacy of some antimicrobial agents such as aminoglycosides and fluoroquinolones and provides anaerobes with an optimal oxidation-reduction potential.[25] Not surprisingly, this milieu favors a different assortment of bacteria than in an acute infection.

Brook et al demonstrated the transition from acute to chronic maxillary sinusitis in five patients who initially presented with acute sinusitis that failed initial antimicrobial therapy.[26] Serial endoscopic cultures were obtained and antibiotics adjusted accordingly. Initial cultures were largely aerobic or facultative organisms (*S. pneumoniae, H. influenzae, and M. catarrhalis*); failure to respond to antibiotic therapy was associated with the emergence of resistant aerobic and anaerobic bacteria such as methicillin-resistant *S. aureus* (MRSA), *Fusobacterium, Prevotella,* and *Peptostreptococcus* in subsequent aspirates.

Anaerobes, gram-negative rods, and *S. aureus* are the predominant microorganisms involved in chronic maxillary sinusitis.[6,10,27–29] **Figure 3.4** combines the results of several studies in demonstrating the bacterial causes of chronic maxillary sinusitis in adults. Compared with acute sinusitis, chronic maxillary sinusitis is more often polymicrobial, and in many cases, the infection may be synergistic.[27]

Anaerobes

Chronic sinus infections caused by anaerobes are of particular concern because they are often responsible for the more severe complications of sinusitis including abscess, mucocele formation, and osteomyelitis. Anaerobes are part of the normal oropharyngeal flora where they outnumber aerobic bacteria 100:1.[30] They are frequently involved in dental-related infections including acute maxillary sinusitis of odontogenic origin. Their emergence as major players in chronic maxillary sinusitis may be related, in part, to the selective pressure of antimicrobial agents, and also to the development of conditions within the sinus associated with chronic inflammation that are conducive to anaerobic growth. Of the gram-negative anaerobes, *Bacteroides* sp and *Fusobacterium* sp are the most frequent isolates.[6,10,27–29] *Peptostreptococcus* sp is the most frequent gram-positive anaerobe isolated.[6,10,27–29] *B. fragilis* and *Fusobacterium* sp isolated in chronic sinusitis have been found to be β–lactamase producers. They are not only able to protect themselves, but can also protect other penicillin-susceptible bacteria in the

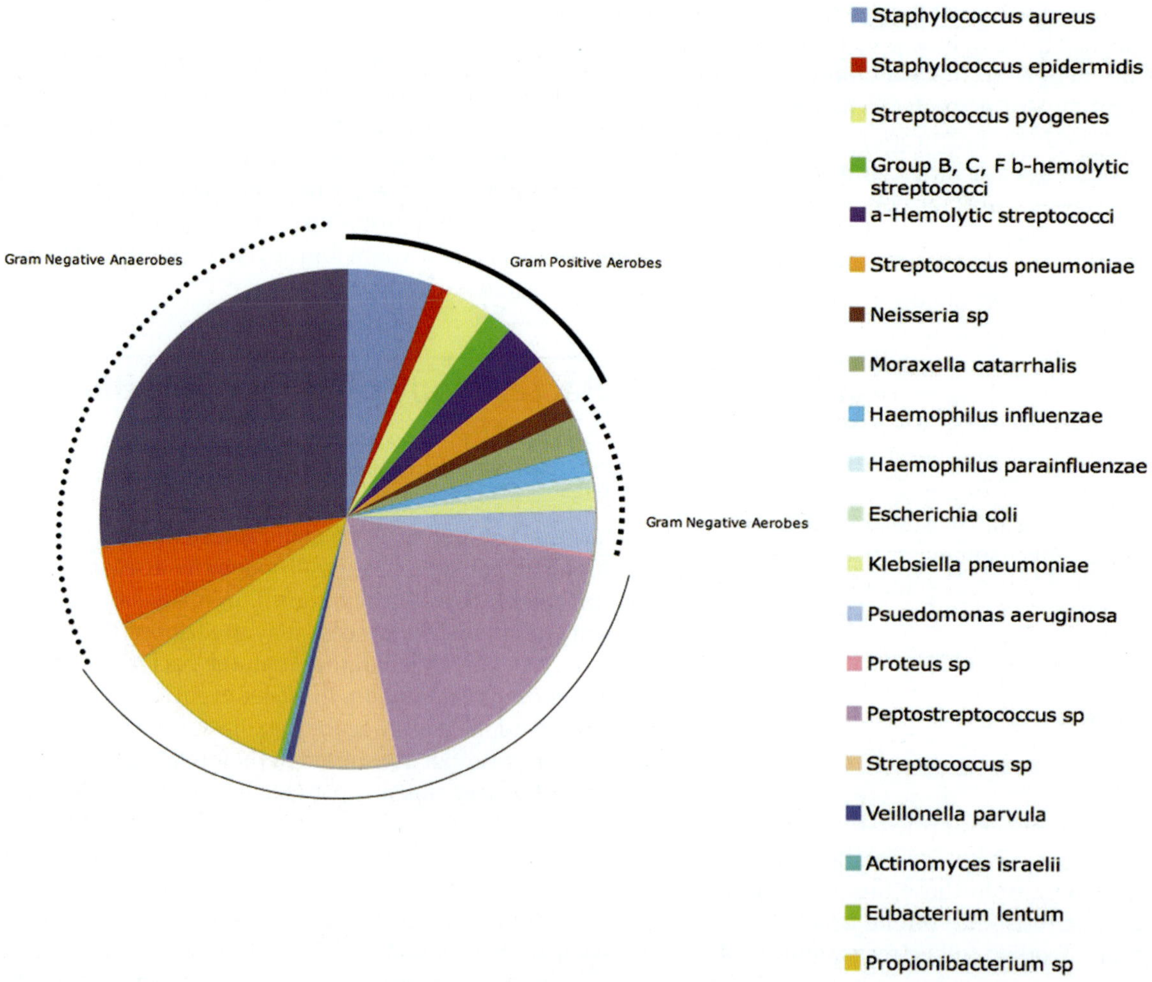

Fig. 3.4 Bacterial causes of chronic maxillary sinusitis in adults.

sinus when the β-lactamase enzyme is present in infected tissue or abscess fluid in sufficient quantity.[31]

Gram-negative Rods

Gram-negative rods are a diverse group of organisms that can be broadly categorized by their primary reservoir: human versus animal, enteric versus respiratory. The majority of gram-negative rods implicated in chronic maxillary sinusitis are of enteric origin and include *Pseudomonas aeruginosa, Klebsiella pneumoniae, Escherichia coli, Proteus mirabilis, and Enterobacter* sp. Because these microorganisms are rarely isolated from middle meatal cultures of normal individuals,[32] their presence in cases of symptomatic chronic sinusitis suggests a pathogenic role.

Antibiotic resistance is common among enteric gram-negative rods due to the production of β-lactamases and other drug-modifying enzymes. These organisms also frequently undergo conjugation and can thus acquire plasmids (R factors) that can mediate multiple-drug resistance.[12]

Staphylococcus Aureus

Staphylococci are gram-positive cocci arranged in irregular grapelike clusters. All staphylococci produce catalase, an important virulence factor, which degrades hydrogen peroxide into oxygen and water. More than 90% of *S. aureus* strains contain plasmids that encode β-lactamase.[15] MRSA strains are resistant to β-lactamase-resistant penicillins by virtue of changes in the penicillin-binding protein in their cell wall. *S. aureus* has several important cell wall components and antigens including protein A (virulence factor), teichoic acids (mediate adherence to cell walls), and peptidoglycan (endotoxin-like properties).

Although *S. aureus* is a frequent isolate in chronic maxillary sinusitis, its exact role in its pathogenesis is unknown. *S. aureus* is frequently found in the nasal passages of normal subjects. Nadel et al,[32] in a study of 25 healthy subjects, isolated *S. aureus* in 24% of middle meatal cultures. It is possible that *S. aureus* is simply a component of normal nasal flora, but its role in sepsis, pneumonia, and surgical wound infections suggests careful consideration of its role as a potential pathogen. Some staphylococcal species produce superantigens that can directly act upon the variable β-region of T-cell receptors to stimulate an inflammatory response. Additionally, organization of staphylococci into biofilms may serve to convert a typically commensal microorganism into one that is pathogenic. In the case of postsurgical patients, changes to the sinus mucosa or underlying bone may also contribute to the pathogenesis of *S. aureus*-related sinus infections.[33,34]

The presence of MRSA in infected sinuses may not only contribute to antibiotic failure, but may also serve as a nidus for the spread of these organisms to other body sites or individuals. Furthermore, as seen with β-lactamase producing anaerobes, the β-lactamase produced by MRSA can also protect penicillin-susceptible pathogens within the same sinus from penicillins.

Several studies have suggested an increase in the recovery of MRSA in both acute and chronic sinusitis.[35,36] A recent study of over 400 patients with acute and chronic maxillary sinusitis between 2001–2003 and 2004–2006 demonstrated a significant increase in the rate of recovery of MRSA in patients with acute and chronic maxillary sinusitis; however, the rates of *S. aureus* recovery were relatively unchanged.[37]

Children

As in acute maxillary sinusitis, the microbiology of chronic maxillary sinusitis in children is very similar to the adult population. Anaerobes, gram-negative enterics, and *S. aureus* remain the most frequent isolates.[21,22,38,39] However, in children *S. pyogenes*-related chronic maxillary sinusitis is more frequent than in the adult population and is about equivalent to that of *S. aureus*.[21,22,38,39] This is not surprising given the prevalence of β-hemolytic group A streptococci, like *S. pyogenes*, in childhood infections. *S. pyogenes* is the most common cause of bacterial pharyngitis,[40] and a frequent cause of childhood skin infections.

Special Considerations

Acute Exacerbation of Chronic Sinusitis

Acute exacerbation of chronic sinusitis (AECS) has been defined as a sudden change in baseline chronic sinusitis with either worsening or new symptoms.[41] Not surprisingly, the microbiology of AECS is largely similar to that of chronic maxillary sinusitis with a predominance of anaerobes and gram-negative enterics. However, AECS may also have some of the typical pathogens associated with acute infections. A study of 32 patients with chronic maxillary sinusitis and 30 patients with acute exacerbations of chronic maxillary sinusitis demonstrated a statistically significantly higher percentage of aerobes typically found in acute sinusitis (*H. influenzae*, *S. pneumoniae*, and *M. catarrhalis*) in patients with acute exacerbations as compared with patients with baseline chronic maxillary sinusitis.[41]

Maxillary Sinusitis of Odontogenic Origin

The proximity of the teeth of the upper jaw to the floor of the maxillary sinus allows for the spread of infection from the oral cavity to the sinus and vice versa. Anaerobes outnumber aerobes in the oral cavity nearly 100 to 1.[42] Not surprisingly, sinusitis of an odontogenic origin is primarily anaerobic in nature. Common causes of odontogenic maxillary sinusitis include periapical abscess, periodontal disease perforating the Schneiderian membrane, sinus perforations during tooth extraction, or irritation and secondary infection caused by intra-antral foreign bodies.[43]

A study of 20 patients with acute maxillary sinusitis and 28 patients with chronic maxillary sinusitis associated with odontogenic infection demonstrated that mixed aerobic–anaerobic polymicrobial infections were most commonly followed by purely anaerobic infection.[44] There was little distinction in the bacteriology of acute and chronic maxillary sinusitis of odontogenic origin. In both cases, the typical aerobic causes of acute sinusitis were seldom seen. The predominant anaerobes seen were gram-negative bacilli, *Peptostreptococcus*, and *Fusobacterium* sp. The predominant aerobes in the mixed infections were α-hemolytic streptococci and *S. aureus*.

The association between odontogenic infections and maxillary sinusitis underscores the importance of a thorough oral cavity examination in patients with sinusitis. Concomitant management of the dental infection is necessary for complete resolution of the maxillary sinusitis.

Immunocompromised Host

The bacteriology of maxillary sinusitis in immunocompromised hosts is difficult to determine because the distribution of pathogens is dependent on the type of immunodeficiency as well as the timing of the infection (i.e., during remission or an active disease state). Empirically, the same bacterial agents and respiratory viruses that cause sinusitis in immunocompetent hosts are also responsible for infections in (1) patients with cancer or leukemia in remission, (2) patients with acquired or congenital immunodeficiencies, and (3) recipients of organ transplants beyond the immediate post-transplant period.[21]

The availability of antiretroviral therapy has significantly improved the survival rates of human immunodeficiency virus- (HIV-) infected patients. As these patients live longer, otolaryngologists are increasingly called upon to treat acute and chronic sinus infections. Many case reports highlight unusual infections associated with HIV; however, most patients' immune status is not an issue until CD4 counts drop below 200 cells per cubic millimeter. Below 50 cells per cubic millimeter, patients become vulnerable to a multitude of opportunistic infections and neoplasms. In general, the bacteriology of maxillary sinusitis in HIV-infected patients is similar to that of the immunocompetent population except for a significantly increased incidence of *staphylococcal* and *pseudomonal* infections in acute and chronic rhinosinusitis.[45,46] Their susceptibility to these organisms likely reflects a compromise of their cellular immunity. With a diagnosis of acquired immunodeficiency syndrome (AIDS) and associated CD4 below 50 cells per cubic millimeter, viruses, bacteria, protozoa, and fungi all enter the mix. Documented causes of sinusitis in AIDS patients include Group G streptococcus, *Rhizopus arrhizus, Legionella pneumophila, Candida albicans, Microsporidian* sp, *Acanthamoeba castellani, Aspergillus fumigatus, Mycobacterium avium-intracellulare, Mycobacterium kansasii, Schizophyllum commune, Cryptococcus neoformans,* and cytomegalovirus.[21]

Maxillary sinus fungal infections are covered in detail in Chapter 5. It should be mentioned here, however, that patients with leukemia and solid malignancies who are febrile and neutropenic, patients on high-dose steroid therapy, patients with severe impairment of cell-mediated immunity, and diabetics are at higher risk for fungal sinusitis. The most common cause of fungal sinusitis in immunocompromised patients is *Aspergillus*; the less frequent *Mucormycosis* has a predilection for diabetic patients.[47,48]

Nosocomial Infections

Nosocomial maxillary sinusitis is associated with patients who require extended periods of hospital care, often in the intensive care unit. These patients typically have prolonged endotracheal or nasogastric intubation. Compared with orotracheal intubation, nasotracheal intubation poses a substantially higher risk for nosocomial sinusitis. Nearly 25% of patients requiring nasotracheal intubation beyond 5 days go on to develop nosocomial sinusitis.[49] The typical organisms are similar to those that cause other nosocomial infections, namely gram- negative enterics (i.e., *P. aeruginosa, K. pneumoniae, Enterobacter* sp, *Proteus mirabilis*) and gram-positive cocci (occasionally streptococci and staphylococci).

It is unclear if all organisms cultured from a hospitalized patient's sinuses are necessarily pathogenic, given that colonization with environmental bacteria is inevitable in the setting of impaired mucociliary clearance, particularly when a foreign body is present. Interestingly, the bacteriology of nosocomial sinusitis is much more similar to chronic sinusitis, where tissue inflammation and edema play a significant role, than acute sinusitis. A study of 24 patients with ventilator-associated sinusitis by computed tomography (CT) found that 39% of the organisms cultured through maxillary sinus punctures were sensitive to antibiotics that the patients were already receiving.[50] However, another study demonstrated that the systematic search for maxillary sinusitis in nasotracheally ventilated patients by CT scan with appropriate antibiotic treatment lowered the incidence of ventilator-associated bronchopneumonia. At this time, clinical judgment and the judicious use of sinus cultures may be the best means of determining the need to treat nosocomial maxillary sinusitis.[51]

Future Directions

In recent years, advances in molecular biology have permitted new insights into the microbiology of human infectious diseases beyond what traditional cell cultures can reveal. *Metagenomics* is a term used to describe the genetic analysis of whole microbial communities, rather than only those grown in culture. DNA may be isolated from noncultured patient samples and sequenced, providing genomic identification of all microbial species present, even when they are very few in numbers (**Fig. 3.5**). This powerful method has not yet been systematically applied to the study of acute and chronic sinusitis, but it is likely that novel microbes will soon be revealed with this technique. Additionally, the importance of biofilms in the pathogenesis of upper airway infections has achieved significant attention in the past 5–10 years.[52,53] It is now recognized that many bacteria in nature exist preferentially within the complex aggregated structure of biofilms, rather than in a free-floating or planktonic state. In one study of chronic sinusitis patients, a poor correlation was observed between bacteria isolated by culture and bacteria identified within mucosal biofilms using in situ hybridization and confocal scanning microscopy.[54] Future research will be needed to determine the relative importance of previously unrecognized sinus microorganisms and to elucidate the impact that biofilms may have in antibiotic resistance or disease persistence. It remains unknown whether biofilms are a cause of sinus inflammation, or if they form only as a consequence of preexisting inflammation. Ongoing research into the innate immunity of the sinonasal tract may ultimately help answer such critical questions about host-microbial interactions in health and disease.[55]

Conclusion

Maxillary sinusitis is associated with a variety of bacterial pathogens, whose patterns may differ with disease chronicity and with certain patient characteristics. Acute sinus infections are primarily caused by aerobic and facultative organisms, whereas chronic sinus infections are primarily caused by anaerobes and gram-negative rods. The bacteriologies of adult and pediatric sinusitis are very similar. Special circumstances such as odontogenic infection, immunocompromise, or nasotracheal intubation often narrow the field of suspected organisms. An appreciation of the bacteriology of acute and chronic maxillary sinusitis will guide empiric therapy and help limit the inappropriate use of antibiotics. Cultures can confirm successful treatment and are critical for research and the development of new drugs. New compounds and devices designed to disrupt bacterial biofilms may eventually find a place in the armamentarium against recalcitrant chronic sinus infections. In addition, modern molecular techniques are beginning to facilitate the discovery of previously unrecognized bacterial species, which may provide future targets for maxillary sinusitis pharmacotherapy.

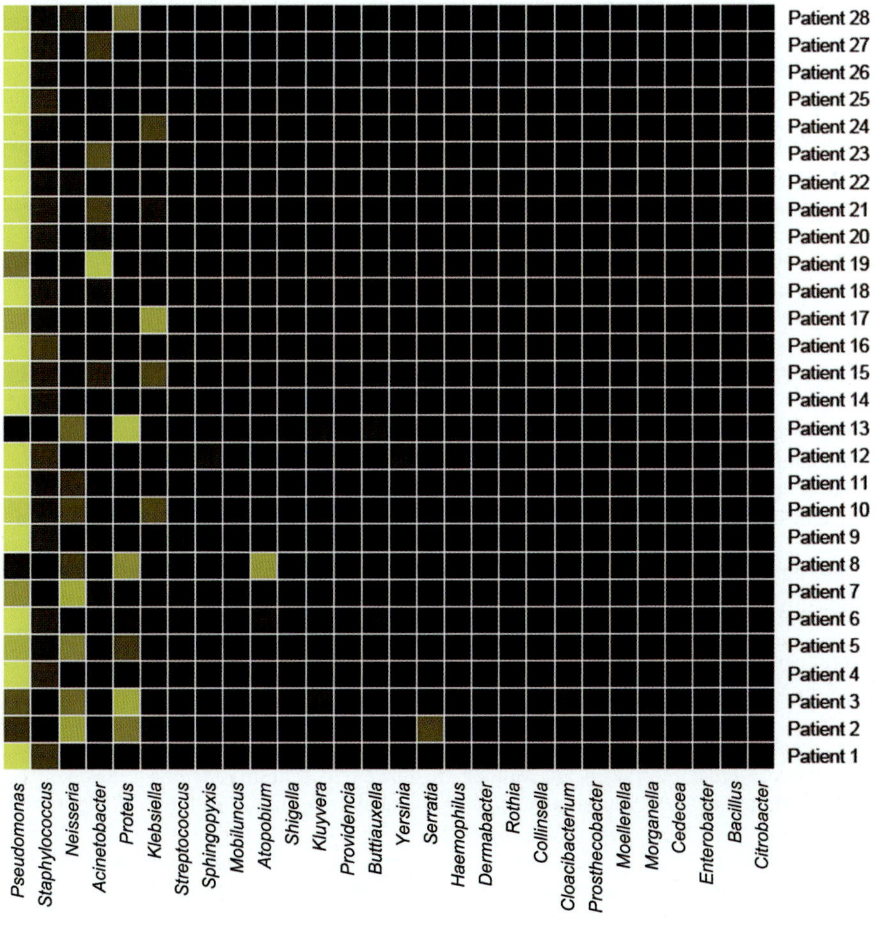

Fig. 3.5 Heat map analysis of multibacterial sinus sample. Increasing color intensity corresponds to a higher prevalence of the particular bacterial genus. The bacterial prevalence data are obtained using real-time polymerase chain reaction (qPCR), microarray, or sequencing analysis.

Pearls

- The bacteriology of adult and pediatric sinusitis is similar.
- Acute maxillary sinus infections are predominantly caused by *Haemophilus influenzae*, *Streptococcus pneumoniae*, and *Moraxella catarrhalis*.
- Anaerobes, gram-negative rods, and *Staphylococcus aureus* are the predominant microorganisms involved in chronic maxillary sinusitis.
- Chronic maxillary sinusitis often has a significant underlying inflammatory component in addition to bacterial infection.
- Endoscopic-guided middle meatal cultures have similar sensitivity and specificity compared with maxillary sinus puncture and may be useful in patients who have failed empiric therapy, are immunocompromised, or are in an inpatient hospital setting.

References

1. Pearlman AN, Conley DB. Review of current guidelines related to the diagnosis and treatment of rhinosinusitis. Curr Opin Otolaryngol Head Neck Surg 2008;16(3):226–230
2. Federal Drug Administration Draft Guidance for Industry: Acute Bacterial Sinusitis: Developing Antimicrobial Drugs for Treatment. Available at: http://www.fda.gov/Drugs/GuidanceComplianceRegulatoryInformation/Guidances/ucm064980.htm. Accessed January 9, 2010
3. Benninger MS, Appelbaum PC, Denneny JC, Osguthorpe DJ, Stankiewicz JA. Maxillary sinus puncture and culture in the diagnosis of acute rhinosinusitis: the case for pursuing alternative culture methods. Otolaryngol Head Neck Surg 2002;127(1):7–12
4. Benninger MS, Payne SC, Ferguson BJ, Hadley JA, Ahmad N. Endoscopically directed middle meatal cultures versus maxillary sinus taps in acute bacterial maxillary rhinosinusitis: a meta-analysis. Otolaryngol Head Neck Surg 2006;134(1):3–9
5. Dubin MG, Ebert CS, Coffey CS, Melroy CT, Sonnenburg RE, Senior BA. Concordance of middle meatal swab and maxillary sinus aspirate in acute and chronic sinusitis: a meta-analysis. Am J Rhinol 2005;19(5):462–470
6. Brook I. The role of anaerobic bacteria in sinusitis. Anaerobe 2006;12(1):5–12
7. Gwaltney JM Jr, Scheld WM, Sande MA, Sydnor A. The microbial etiology and antimicrobial therapy of adults with acute community-acquired sinusitis: a fifteen-year experience at the University of Virginia and review of other selected studies. J Allergy Clin Immunol 1992;90(3 Pt 2):457–461, discussion 462
8. Hamory BH, Sande MA, Sydnor A Jr, Seale DL, Gwaltney JM Jr. Etiology and antimicrobial therapy of acute maxillary sinusitis. J Infect Dis 1979;139(2):197–202
9. Jousimies-Somer HR, Savolainen S, Ylikoski JS. Bacteriological findings of acute maxillary sinusitis in young adults. J Clin Microbiol 1988;26(10):1919–1925
10. Moungthong G, Suwas A, Jaruchida S, Chantaratchada S, Phonphok Y, Rangsin R. Prevalence of etiologic bacteria and beta-lactamase-producing bacteria in acute and chronic maxillary sinusitis at Phramongkutklao Hospital. J Med Assoc Thai 2005;88(4):478–483
11. Ylikoski J, Savolainen S, Jousimies-Somer H. The bacteriology of acute maxillary sinusitis. ORL J Otorhinolaryngol Relat Spec 1989;51(3):175–181
12. Levinson W, Ernest J. Gram-negative rods related to the enteric tract. In: Foltin J, Lebowitz H, & Panton N, eds. Medical Microbiology and Immunology. 7th ed. New York: McGraw-Hill; 2002:115–132
13. Felmingham D, Washington J. Trends in the antimicrobial susceptibility of bacterial respiratory tract pathogens—findings of the Alexander Project 1992-1996. J Chemother 1999;11(Suppl 1):5–21
14. Scott JA, Hall AJ, Dagan R, et al. Serogroup-specific epidemiology of *Streptococcus pneumoniae*: associations with age, sex, and geography in 7,000 episodes of invasive disease. Clin Infect Dis 1996;22(6):973–981
15. Levinson W, Ernest J. Gram-positive cocci. In: Foltin J, Lebowitz H, & Panton N, eds. Medical Microbiology and Immunology. 7th ed. New York: McGraw-Hill; 2002:91–102
16. Appelbaum PC. Epidemiology and in vitro susceptibility of drug-resistant *Streptococcus pneumoniae*. Pediatr Infect Dis J 1996;15(10):932–934
17. Sutcliffe J, Grebe T, Tait-Kamradt A, Wondrack L. Detection of erythromycin-resistant determinants by PCR. Antimicrob Agents Chemother 1996;40(11):2562–2566
18. Fasola EL, Bajaksouzian S, Appelbaum PC, Jacobs MR. Variation in erythromycin and clindamycin susceptibilities of *Streptococcus pneumoniae* by four test methods. Antimicrob Agents Chemother 1997;41(1):129–134
19. Anon JB, Jacobs MR, Poole MD, et al; Sinus And Allergy Health Partnership. Antimicrobial treatment guidelines for acute bacterial rhinosinusitis. Otolaryngol Head Neck Surg 2004; 130(1, Suppl)1–45
20. Jacobs MR, Felmingham D, Appelbaum PC, Grüneberg RN; Alexander Project Group. The Alexander Project 1998-2000: susceptibility of pathogens isolated from community-acquired respiratory tract infection to commonly used antimicrobial agents. J Antimicrob Chemother 2003;52(2):229–246
21. Wald ER. Microbiology of acute and chronic sinusitis in children and adults. Am J Med Sci 1998;316(1):13–20
22. Wald ER, Milmoe GJ, Bowen A, Ledesma-Medina J, Salamon N, Bluestone CD. Acute maxillary sinusitis in children. N Engl J Med 1981;304(13):749–754
23. Aust R, Drettner B. Oxygen tension in the human maxillary sinus under normal and pathological conditions. Acta Otolaryngol 1974;78(3-4):264–269

24. Carenfelt C, Lundberg C. Purulent and non-purulent maxillary sinus secretions with respect to pO2, pCO2 and pH. Acta Otolaryngol 1977;84(1-2):138–144
25. Carenfelt C, Eneroth CM, Lundberg C, Wretlind B. Evaluation of the antibiotic effect of treatment of maxillary sinusitis. Scand J Infect Dis 1975;7(4):259–264
26. Brook I, Frazier EH, Foote PA. Microbiology of the transition from acute to chronic maxillary sinusitis. J Med Microbiol 1996;45(5):372–375
27. Brook I, Thompson DH, Frazier EH. Microbiology and management of chronic maxillary sinusitis. Arch Otolaryngol Head Neck Surg 1994;120(12):1317–1320
28. Erkan M, Aslan T, Ozcan M, Koç N. Bacteriology of antrum in adults with chronic maxillary sinusitis. Laryngoscope 1994;104(3 Pt 1): 321–324
29. Kamau JK, Macharia IM, Odhiambo PA. Bacteriology of chronic maxillary sinusitis at Kenyatta National Hospital, Nairobi. East Afr Med J 2001;78(7):343–345
30. Gibbons RJ, Socransky SS, Dearaujo WC, Vanhoute J. Studies of the predominant cultivable microbiota of dental plaque. Arch Oral Biol 1964;11:365–370
31. Brook I, Yocum P, Frazier EH. Bacteriology and beta-lactamase activity in acute and chronic maxillary sinusitis. Arch Otolaryngol Head Neck Surg 1996;122(4):418–422, discussion 423
32. Nadel DM, Lanza DC, Kennedy DW. Endoscopically guided sinus cultures in normal subjects. Am J Rhinol 1999;13(2):87–90
33. Bhattacharyya N, Gopal HV, Lee KH. Bacterial infection after endoscopic sinus surgery: a controlled prospective study. Laryngoscope 2004;114(4):765–767
34. Khalid AN, Hunt J, Perloff JR, Kennedy DW. The role of bone in chronic rhinosinusitis. Laryngoscope 2002;112(11):1951–1957
35. Huang WH, Hung PK. Methicillin-resistant *Staphylococcus aureus* infections in acute rhinosinusitis. Laryngoscope 2006;116(2):288–291
36. Manarey CR, Anand VK, Huang C. Incidence of methicillin-resistant *Staphylococcus aureus* causing chronic rhinosinusitis. Laryngoscope 2004;114(5):939–941
37. Brook I, Foote PA, Hausfeld JN. Increase in the frequency of recovery of methicillin-resistant *Staphylococcus aureus* in acute and chronic maxillary sinusitis. J Med Microbiol 2008;57(Pt 8):1015–1017
38. Erkan M, Ozcan M, Arslan S, Soysal V, Bozdemir K, Haghighi N. Bacteriology of antrum in children with chronic maxillary sinusitis. Scand J Infect Dis 1996;28(3):283–285
39. Brook I. Bacteriologic features of chronic sinusitis in children. JAMA 1981;246(9):967–969
40. Pichichero ME. Group A streptococcal tonsillopharyngitis: cost-effective diagnosis and treatment. Ann Emerg Med 1995;25(3):390–403
41. Brook I. Bacteriology of chronic sinusitis and acute exacerbation of chronic sinusitis. Arch Otolaryngol Head Neck Surg 2006;132(10):1099–1101
42. Aas JA, Paster BJ, Stokes LN, Olsen I, Dewhirst FE. Defining the normal bacterial flora of the oral cavity. J Clin Microbiol 2005;43(11):5721–5732
43. Mehra P, Murad H. Maxillary sinus disease of odontogenic origin. Otolaryngol Clin North Am 2004;37(2):347–364
44. Brook I. Microbiology of acute and chronic maxillary sinusitis associated with an odontogenic origin. Laryngoscope 2005;115(5):823–825
45. Milgrim LM, Rubin JS, Rosenstreich DL, Small CB. Sinusitis in human immunodeficiency virus infection: typical and atypical organisms. J Otolaryngol 1994;23(6):450–453
46. Tami TA. The management of sinusitis in patients infected with the human immunodeficiency virus (HIV). Ear Nose Throat J 1995;74(5):360–363
47. Anselmo-Lima WT, Lopes RP, Valera FC, Demarco RC. Invasive fungal rhinosinusitis in immunocompromised patients. Rhinology 2004;42(3):141–144
48. Corey JP, Romberger CF, Shaw GY. Fungal diseases of the sinuses. Otolaryngol Head Neck Surg 1990;103(6):1012–1015
49. O'Reilly MJ, Reddick EJ, Black W, et al. Sepsis from sinusitis in nasotracheally intubated patients. A diagnostic dilemma. Am J Surg 1984;147(5):601–604
50. Souweine B, Mom T, Traore O, et al. Ventilator-associated sinusitis: microbiological results of sinus aspirates in patients on antibiotics. Anesthesiology 2000;93(5):1255–1260
51. Holzapfel L, Chastang C, Demingeon G, Bohe J, Piralla B, Coupry A. A randomized study assessing the systematic search for maxillary sinusitis in nasotracheally mechanically ventilated patients. Influence of nosocomial maxillary sinusitis on the occurrence of ventilator-associated pneumonia. Am J Respir Crit Care Med 1999;159(3):695–701
52. Psaltis AJ, Ha KR, Beule AG, Tan LW, Wormald PJ. Confocal scanning laser microscopy evidence of biofilms in patients with chronic rhinosinusitis. Laryngoscope 2007;117(7):1302–1306
53. Post JC, Stoodley P, Hall-Stoodley L, Ehrlich GD. The role of biofilms in otolaryngologic infections. Curr Opin Otolaryngol Head Neck Surg 2004;12(3):185–190
54. Sanderson AR, Leid JG, Hunsaker D. Bacterial biofilms on the sinus mucosa of human subjects with chronic rhinosinusitis. Laryngoscope 2006;116(7):1121–1126
55. Ramanathan M Jr, Lane AP. Innate immunity of the sinonasal cavity and its role in chronic rhinosinusitis. Otolaryngol Head Neck Surg 2007;136(3):348–356

4 Medical Management of Acute and Chronic Maxillary Sinusitis

Bradley A. Otto and Berrylin J. Ferguson

The treatment of maxillary sinusitis generally follows that of rhinosinusitis. The term rhinosinusitis has by convention largely replaced the term sinusitis, due to the frequent concomitant occurrence of nasal and paranasal sinus inflammation. Broadly defined, rhinosinusitis is an inflammatory disorder of the nose and paranasal sinuses. Although this text is dedicated to the maxillary sinus, the status of the mucosa of the maxillary sinus and of the ostiomeatal complex is generally interdependent, especially in the nonoperated sinuses or those where a large antrostomy has not been created. Accordingly, many of the treatments offered in this chapter are aimed not only at the maxillary sinus mucosa, but also the mucosa of the ostiomeatal complex and other affected sinonasal tissues.

This chapter focuses on the medical management of maxillary sinusitis. The diagnosis and classification (acute versus chronic) of maxillary sinusitis have been described elsewhere in this text. Acute maxillary sinusitis (AMS) is generally an infectious condition. However, the etiology of chronic maxillary sinusitis (CMS) is incompletely understood and is likely multifactorial. Accordingly, the management of AMS is aimed at reducing symptoms and clearing infection. The management of CMS is, however, more complex. The approach to the patient with CMS must take into account any concomitant immunodeficiency, atopy, anatomical abnormalities or other factors that contribute to persistent inflammation or impaired mucosal function. Therefore, patients with CMS generally require long-term management and frequent reassessment of the efficacy of each intervention. The medications discussed in this chapter, except antibiotics, are listed in **Table 4.1**.

Table 4.1 Overview of Current Medications for Acute and Chronic Maxillary Sinusitis

Category	Examples
Antiinflammatory	
Steroids	
Intranasal corticosteroids	Mometasone furoate, fluticasone propionate, fluticasone furoate, budesonide, flunisolide, triamcinolone acetonide, ciclesonide
Topical steroid preparations	Budesonide respules
Oral corticosteroids	Prednisone, methylprednisolone
Antihistamines	
Oral first-generation	Diphenhydramine, hydroxyzine, chlorpheniramine, brompheniramine
Oral second-generation	Loratadine, desloratadine, cetirizine, levocetirizine, fexofenadine
Topical intranasal	azelastine, olopatadine
Leukotriene modifiers	
Leukotriene receptor antagonist	Montelukast, zafirlukast
5-lipoxygenase inhibitor	Zileuton
Mast cell stabilization	Cromolyn sodium
Monoclonal antibodies	
Antiimmunoglobulin E	Omalizumab
Antiinterleukin-5	Mepolizumab
Allergen-specific treatment	
Food elimination	Most commonly soy, wheat, eggs, dairy, and corn
Immunotherapy	Specific allergens as determined by skin testing
Decongestants and mucus modulation	
Decongestants	
Oral	Phenylephrine, pseudoephedrine
Topical	Oxymetazoline, phenylephrine
Mucus modulation	
Nasal saline	Mist spray, irrigation, nebulization
Mucolytics	Guaifenesin, acetylcysteine
Anticholinergics	Ipratropium bromide

An Overview of Acute and Chronic Maxillary Sinusitis

Acute Maxillary Sinusitis

Acute rhinosinusitis (ARS) is one of the most common conditions treated in the United States, occurring an estimated 20 million times per year and accounting for ~21% of all antibiotics prescribed annually.[1] The maxillary sinus is the paranasal sinus most frequently involved in rhinosinusitis and its accessibility, via antral or inferior meatal taps, makes it a common target for culture acquisition in studies for antibiotic indications in AMS and in recalcitrant infections.

In addition to facial pain or pressure, common symptoms of AMS include anterior and/or posterior nasal drainage, nasal obstruction, and maxillary tooth pain. These symptoms overlap with ARS, and in the nonoperated patient, identifying maxillary sinus involvement in ARS by endoscopy alone may not be possible. However, AMS is suggested by the presence of pus emanating from the middle meatus. Historical techniques, such as maxillary sinus illumination, may provide additional information, but are not routinely used and show poor intraobserver reliability.[2] Sinus computed tomography (CT) is the imaging modality of choice in the evaluation of the paranasal sinuses. However, CT is not utilized in uncomplicated AMS because over 80% of patients with a common cold show CT abnormalities.[3]

Most episodes of ARS are secondary to viral infection (the common cold). Acute viral rhinosinusitis (AVRS) is generally a self-limited process that resolves within 7 to 10 days. AVRS is complicated by acute bacterial infection in only an estimated 0.5 to 2% of cases. Untreated acute bacterial rhinosinusitis (ABRS) will also resolve spontaneously in 75% of cases, with progression to acute complicated sinusitis a rare occurrence.[1] Nevertheless, antibiotics are frequently prescribed to patients with symptoms suggestive of AVRS or uncomplicated ABRS. This not only sends the wrong message to the patient who, in most cases, would have improved without antibiotics, but also potentially contributes to the emergence and progression of bacterial resistance patterns.

Although the majority of AMS is associated with viral upper-respiratory tract infections, other etiologies, particularly dental disease, should be included in the differential of any patient presenting with symptoms suggestive of AMS, particularly those with persistent, recurrent AMS or unilateral disease (**Fig. 4.1**). The identification of concomitant dental disease not only aids in appropriate antibiotic selection, but also facilitates improved long-term outcomes.[4,5] In a recent study, over 80% of CTs with a fluid level exceeding over two-thirds of a maxillary sinus with mucosal thickening had dental pathology, compared with a baseline level of dental pathology in normal maxillary sinuses of less than 10%.[6]

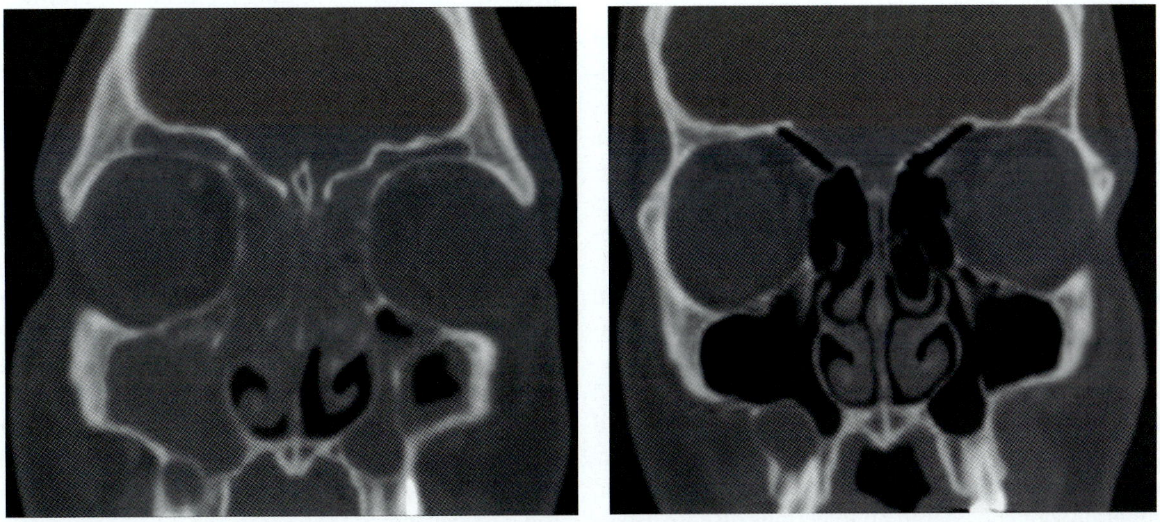

A B

Fig. 4.1 **(A,B)** Computed tomography (CT) scans of a patient who presented with acute rhinosinusitis complicated by preseptal cellulitis. He was treated with antibiotics and referred for follow-up. **(A)** Review of the CT scan taken on admission revealed a cyst arising from the root of the right maxillary second molar. **(B)** After treatment and clinical improvement, the cyst was excised.

Chronic Maxillary Sinusitis

CMS is a syndrome represented by a constellation of symptoms associated with chronic inflammation of the maxillary sinus mucosa. The demographics, clinical presentation, and effects of CMS on quality of life, as well as the tremendous economic burden of CMS, have been described elsewhere in this book. Despite the burden of CRS/CMS, the underlying series of events that lead to chronic mucosal inflammation remains unclear. Several theories (fungal, biofilm, *S. aureus* exotoxin) have been proposed as etiological factors of CRS (with and without nasal polyps). However, no definitive demonstration of a pathogen's ability to permanently modulate the inflammatory profile of sinonasal mucosa has been demonstrated.

Several studies investigating the immunologic aberrancies between chronic rhinosinusitis with nasal polyps (CRSwNP) and chronic sinusitis without nasal polyps (CRSsNP) have been published. Generally, the former is thought to be associated with, a T-helper 2 (Th2) cytokine profile associated with eosinophilic predominance. The latter has been characterized by a T-helper 1 (Th1) cytokine profile and neutrophilic predominance. However, most information regarding underlying pathophysiology remains observational and underlying mechanisms leading to these observed differences are not completely understood. The treatment of CMS is therefore complex and is somewhat hindered by an incomplete understanding of the underlying molecular pathophysiology. Currently, no medication has been approved by the Food and Drug Administration (FDA) for the treatment of CRS/CMS.

Treatment

The mainstay of the management of AMS involves expectant management of symptoms resulting from mucosal inflammation. Accordingly, treatment should be aimed at resolving the underlying inflammation, reducing nasal congestion, and decreasing excess mucus production. Antiinflammatory agents, decongestants, and mucolytics are mainstays of therapy. Pain control is usually achieved with over-the-counter analgesics. Narcotics are rarely necessary. Antimicrobial therapy, when indicated, should be culture-directed if possible. Current guidelines regarding appropriate antibiotic use are described below.

Similar to AMS, medical therapy for CMS should be aimed at reducing chronic inflammation, relieving symptoms, and eradicating microbial pathogens. Although bacterial infection may be an underlying etiology or exacerbating factor, CMS is generally not considered an infectious disease. However, bacterial infection frequently coexists with CRS, either as an inciting event or as a consequence of chronic mucosal inflammation and edema. Additional consideration must also be given to whether a patient has already undergone endoscopic sinus surgery, whether or not an antrostomy was performed, the size of the antrostomy, and the amount of postoperative scarring. Additionally, an understanding of underlying comorbid disorders, especially immunodeficiency and allergic disorders is paramount. Finally, an understanding of what has been previously tried and what has or has not worked will save time and aid in selecting the most appropriate regimen.

Every patient to whom ESS will be recommended in the treatment of CMS should first have tried and failed maximal medical therapy. However, maximal medical therapy varies for each patient, depending on the underlying cause of pathology. Often maximal medical therapy is a rational experiment, in which each antiinflammatory therapeutic intervention is tried one at a time to assess efficacy. Maximal medical therapy should be aimed at reducing sinonasal mucosal inflammation, treating allergy, avoiding irritants, relieving symptoms, and treating clinically evident infection.

Corticosteroids

Corticosteroids are frequently utilized in the management of various otolaryngic disorders, including inflammatory sinonasal disorders. The complex mechanism of action of steroids begins with diffusion into the cell and attachment to the glucocorticoid receptor (GR). Following receptor binding, the steroid-receptor complex translocates to the nucleus where gene expression can be directly or indirectly upregulated or downregulated.[7] Components that are generally downregulated by steroids include inflammatory cytokines, metalloproteinases, inflammatory peptides, and nitric oxide. Components commonly induced by steroids include soluble interleukin receptors, membrane functional proteins, membrane regulatory proteins, and intracellular regulatory proteins.[7] Steroids also reduce the number of inflammatory cells in tissue, an effect that is dependent on the tissue concentration of the steroid.[8]

Intranasal Corticosteroids

Intranasal corticosteroids (INCSs) are approved for management of allergic rhinitis and in some cases, chronic rhinosinusitis with nasal polyps. INCSs have demonstrated good safety profiles, based primarily on low systemic absorption and effective first-pass liver metabolism, whereby 99% of swallowed steroid is cleared.[9] Because ARS is usually a self-limited process, the primary goal of treatment is symptom relief, which can be more effectively achieved by targeting the underlying inflammation. Accordingly, interest in the efficacy of INCSs in the treatment of ARS/AMS has mounted in the past decade.

Recently, several studies have been published investigating the role of INCSs in treating ARS. Fluticasone added to cefuroxime showed improved clinical success and shorter time to clinical resolution of symptoms than cefuroxime alone in patients with recurrent acute sinusitis or acute-onset chronic rhinosinusitis.[10] Other studies have demonstrated improved symptom resolution utilizing mometasone furoate nasal spray in addition to oral antibiotics.[11,12] Although antiinflammatory effects are the likely contributors to these results, in vitro analysis of mometasone demonstrates antimicrobial activity against streptococci.[13] In another study, mometasone furoate nasal spray dosed at 200 mg twice daily was well tolerated and induced significantly greater, sustained relief of most ARS symptoms compared with amoxicillin and placebo.[14] Given low systemic absorption (<0.1%), lack of systemic drug-related effects, and good safety profile, INCSs may be a good alternative to antibiotics as initial therapy of patients presenting with symptoms suggestive of uncomplicated AMS. Alternatively, INCSs may augment the therapeutic effectiveness of antibiotics when prescribed. Based on current evidence in support of INCS therapy, the European Position Paper on Rhinosinusitis and Nasal Polyps 2007 Guidelines and a recent Cochrane meta-analysis recommend using INCSs in the treatment of ARS, both as monotherapy and as an adjunct to antibiotics.[15,16]

Topical steroids are an important component of the medical regimen in the treatment of CMS. INCSs have been shown to reduce symptoms in patients with CRS without nasal polyps.[17,18] The advantage of topical delivery of steroids (low absorption, efficient first-pass metabolism, and low rate of significant side effects) is especially important in patients with CMS, where long-term antiinflammatory regimens are generally necessary.

In a double-blind placebo controlled study on postoperative patients with CRS, topical budesonide instilled into the maxillary sinus via a catheter for 21 days was successful in reducing clinical symptoms. Furthermore, a significant decrease in CD-3 cells, eosinophils, and cells expressing interleukin 4 (IL-4) and IL-5 messenger ribonucleic acid (mRNA) was also demonstrated in the sinuses treated with budesonide, suggesting an improved inflammatory profile in the treated sinuses.[19] Although these results are promising, the ability to effectively administer products to the maxillary sinus mucosa using conventional devices, in both nonoperated and postoperative sinuses, is questionable.[20,21] Therefore, application of INCS using standard metered dose sprays likely limits application to the middle meatus at best. Regardless, INCSs remain an attractive first option in the treatment of CMS due to their relative safety and low cost.

Side effects associated with INCSs are generally limited to nasal dryness and bleeding. Bleeding is generally limited to blood-tinged mucus and may be tolerated by many patients, especially with the addition of agents aimed at preserving mucosal hydration. Rarely, improper use and/or the vasoconstrictive effect of topical steroids can lead to septal perforation. To address this, patients should be instructed to aim the spray along the nasal floor and slightly lateral. Patients may achieve this trajectory more easily by using the contralateral hand to spray each nare.[22]

Alternative methods of topical steroid administration for CMS are generally based on off-label use of nebulized steroids traditionally used in the treatment of asthma. Commercially available products for nasal nebulization for a variety of medications, including antibiotics and steroids, have recently become available.[23,24] However, as noted above, the ability to direct products into the maxillary sinuses using traditional sprays or nebulizers is questionable. An alternative approach involves the use of saline irrigation kits to deliver mixtures of steroid (budesonide respules) and saline at various concentrations. Saline irrigation kits have been shown to deliver significantly more solution to the maxillary sinus than nebulizers and sprays, especially in postoperative cases.[21,25] Alternatively, nondiluted budesonide drops can be placed into the nose directly from the respule container. The most effective method of delivering drops to the maxillary sinus is somewhat controversial. Several studies have been published describing various positions that most optimally deliver drops to various sinonasal regions. The results of cadaver study utilizing latex suggested that the Mygind and Ragan's positions best delivered material to the middle meatus.[26] Several other positions for maximizing delivery of drops to various sinonasal regions have been described.[27] The benefit of using nondiluted budesonide is the potential to deliver a higher concentration of steroid to the maxillary sinus, while maintaining the same total dose per application. However, the optimal dose delivery to the maxillary sinus, based on concentration and total amount actually delivered to the sinus, has not been clearly identified.

Oral Steroids

The use of oral steroids in the management of AMS is limited to cases where patients present with severe pain in the setting of acute bacterial sinusitis. Although systemic steroids appear to more effectively relieve pain in the acute setting, no beneficial long-term effects have been noted.[15,28] Similarly, the use of oral steroids to treat CMS is less common than that of topical steroids. Although an in vitro study using cultured nasal mucosa from patients with CRS demonstrated significantly reduced inflammatory cytokines,[29] there have been no clinical randomized controlled trials evaluating the effectiveness of systemic steroids in the management of CRS / CMS. Therefore, in patients with CMS oral steroids should generally be employed for acute exacerbations of CMS associated with severe pain or in situations where severe maxillary sinus edema is recalcitrant to topical therapy.

Potential side effects associated with short-term use of systemic steroids include hypothalamic–pituitary–adrenal axis suppression, steroid withdrawal syndrome (uncommon when used <2 weeks), gastrointestinal effects (peptic ulcer disease), and psychiatric effects (mood alteration to frank psychosis). Long-term use of steroids may be associated with osteoporosis, cushingoid features, early cataracts, purpura, and avascular necrosis of the hip.[8] Interestingly, coadministration of statins may reduce the risk of avascular necrosis.[30] Although these side effects are generally uncommon with short-term use, the lack of long-term benefit from use of oral steroids should encourage judicious use. Oral steroids should be reserved for those cases where severe pain is a dominant feature.

Decongestants

Mucosal edema associated with sinonasal inflammation is likely a significant factor in both the development and symptoms of AMS. In addition to potential molecular and cellular changes induced by viral infection, mucosal edema may contribute to the development of bacterial maxillary sinusitis through blockage of the maxillary ostium. Reduced mucociliary clearance and stasis of secretions within the maxillary sinus then lead to optimal conditions for bacterial growth. Furthermore, edema within the nasal cavity associated with acute maxillary sinusitis leads to nasal airflow restriction, a symptomatic hallmark of ARS/AMS. The rationale for the use of decongestants from the patient's perspective is generally for symptomatic relief. In addition to symptom resolution, physicians frequently recommend decongestants based on the presumption that reduction in mucosal edema improves maxillary sinus drainage.

Oral Decongestants

Oral decongestants are commonly used, over-the-counter components of many "cold" and "sinus and allergy" preparations. Today, the most commonly used oral decongestants include pseudoephedrine and phenylephrine. A recent amendment to the USA Patriot Act requires that pseudoephedrine be kept "behind-the-counter" because it has been used to illegally manufacture methamphetamine.[31]

Systemic decongestants are frequently used to treat AMS; however, limited data regarding their effectiveness exists. Although a recent meta-analysis of phenylephrine suggested a single dose was effective in decreasing nasal congestion associated with the common cold,[32] another systematic review concluded phenylephrine had no effect as a nasal decongestant.[31] Regardless, there is currently no definitive evidence for the use of systemic decongestants in the treatment of AMS. If patients prefer to use these medications, they should be warned about potential side effects including hypertension, tachyarrhythmia, wakefulness, and urinary retention. These potential side effects make this group of medications even less desirable for use in the elderly. One oral decongestant, phenylpropanolamine, is no longer available due to increased risk of hemorrhagic stroke, especially in the young female population.[9] Oral decongestants are generally not utilized in the long-term management of CMS. Short-term use in acute exacerbation of CMS (AECMS) should be based on the same principles used in the management of AMS.

Topical Decongestants

Topical decongestants, such as oxymetazoline and phenylephrine, also have widespread use in the treatment of nasal congestion. Topical decongestants are commonly recommended as adjuncts in the treatment of ARS/AMS to reduce edema and improve drainage of affected sinuses. Oxymetazoline used in conjunction with antibiotics has been shown to improve mucociliary transport in patients with acute rhinosinusitis; however the effect was not statistically better than concomitant use of fluticasone or nasal saline.[33] Otherwise, there is no significant clinical evidence based on human trials to support the use of topical decongestants in the treatment of ARS/AMS. A study examining the histologic effects of oxymetazoline on rabbit maxillary sinus mucosa after induced sinusitis revealed increased inflammation in sinuses treated with oxymetazoline versus control sinuses. The authors suggested that decreases in mucosal blood flow affected normal local defense mechanisms during bacterial sinusitis.[34] Nevertheless, topical decongestants are commonly recommended by physicians and no significant association with impaired healing secondary to such use has been described. Topical decongestants have a rapid onset of action; however, their use can result in rebound and tachyphylaxis. Therefore, these medications should be used for no longer than 3 to 5 days. As such, topical decongestants have no role in the long-term management of patients with CMS.

Mucus Modulation

Topical Anticholinergics

Ipratropium bromide, a topical anticholinergic nasal spray, provides an effective blockade of parasympathetic input to mucosal mucus glands. It is efficacious in reducing rhinorrhea in both allergic and nonallergic rhinitis and is often used in conjunction with topical nasal steroids. Additionally, it has been approved for use in viral upper respiratory tract infections. However, the role of ipratropium bromide in treating AMS and CMS has not been extensively investigated. Although decreased mucus production in the setting of an acute infection seems desirable, long-term use of anticholinergic medications is generally not recommended due to concern that such use leads to retained, thick secretions. Based on a paucity of data regarding its use to treat AMS and CMS, recommendations for or against ipratropium bromide cannot be clearly argued. However, due to an excellent safety profile, use should not be discouraged in patients who perceive a benefit.

Mucolytics

Mucolytics, such as guaifenesin or acetylcysteine, decrease the viscosity of secretions in the upper airway, theoretically improving mucociliary transport. Guaifenesin has been approved for use by the FDA since 1952 and is another common component of over-the-counter cough and cold formulations. Although little data regarding clinical efficacy exists, guaifenesin has an excellent safety profile and should be utilized in patients with AMS who perceive a benefit. In patients with concomitant cough, guaifenesin may aid in expectoration.

Nasal Saline

Nasal saline irrigation is widely used in the management of patients with inflammatory sinonasal disorders. Saline can be administered in isotonic or hypotonic form by a variety of methods including spray, nebulization, and irrigation. Although isotonic saline has been shown to improve mucociliary clearance in acute sinusitis,[35] there is a relative paucity of clinical data to support its use. A recent study investigating the role of isotonic or hypertonic nasal spray demonstrated no significant effect versus observation in patients with ARS.[36] However, nasal sprays are much less effective than irrigator kits in flushing the nasal cavity. Although there is limited, contradictory data regarding its efficacy in treating AMS, nasal saline irrigation is cheap, safe, and well tolerated and therefore may be recommended for patients who perceive a benefit.

The most commonly studied method of saline administration, relevant to CMS, is irrigation. Nasal saline irrigation has been shown to improve Rhinosinusitis Disability Index scores,[37] and a recent Cochran Database Review concluded that nasal saline is likely to improve symptom control in patients with persistent sinonasal disease.[38] Nasal saline irrigation frequently serves as a vehicle for topical administration of medications such as steroids or antibiotics. Several other substances have been added to saline, however, including shampoo, sodium hypochlorite, xylitol, Dead Sea salts, and Betadine. As noted previously, little product actually enters the nonoperated maxillary sinus. Therefore, in most cases, the treatment effect of saline irrigation is limited to the nasal cavity.

Hypertonic saline is more efficacious than isotonic saline for pulmonary nebulization in patients with cystic fibrosis (CF).[39] Because up to 8% of patients with CRS are heterozygotes for CF, compared with a 1% incidence of CF heterozygosity in the normal population, it may be that these CF carriers do better with hypertonic saline irrigations, whereas other patients do better with isotonic irrigations.

Allergy Management

The management of concomitant allergic rhinitis (AR) is an important component of the overall management of maxillary sinusitis, especially CMS. Allergic rhinitis is a prevalent disorder, affecting ~20% of the adult population of the United States. Similar to rhinosinusitis, AR is an enormous quality of life and economic burden.[40] Like CMS, AR is associated with an altered mucosal immune profile and mucosal edema. Accordingly, many of the symptoms associated with these two conditions, such as rhinorrhea, nasal congestion, and facial pressure, tend to overlap. Recent studies suggest a concordance of AR and rhinosinusitis, with some implicating AR as a predictive factor for decreased quality of life and poorer surgical outcomes in patients with CRS. The structural mucosal changes secondary to AR can lead to obstruction of the maxillary sinus ostium, increased mucus production, and altered mucociliary clearance, all of which can negatively impact CMS. Therefore, it is prudent to search for, and appropriately treat, concomitant AR in patients with CMS. INCSs are generally used as first-line therapy for AR due to a wide range of clinical benefits, including reduction in nasal congestion, rhinorrhea, sneezing, itching, and even some eye symptoms. Therefore, in many patients with CMS, allergy may be appropriately managed with INCS monotherapy. However, in patients whose allergy symptoms are not abated by INCSs, several topical and systemic medical options exist. As in the treatment of CMS, the management of AR is an experiment and not all patients respond similarly. Therefore, we prefer to send most patients home with a treatment algorithm that generally includes a progressive addition or replacement of the various medications described in this section (including ICNSs), to arrive at a treatment regimen that is optimal for the individual patient. The cornerstone of this "rational patient experiment" is that the patient only introduce one medication variable at a time and for long enough to determine whether that medication improves the patient's symptoms.

Immunotherapy is generally reserved for those patients who fail to achieve comprehensive relief with medical therapy or who have symptoms for at least 6 months of the year so that the potential of curing the patient with desensitization is worth the time and small risks of immunotherapy. A detailed discussion of immunotherapy is beyond the scope of this chapter, however, it should be noted that immunotherapy is currently the only allergy treatment option that offers a chance for a cure.

Antihistamines

The release of histamine from mast cells is the hallmark of type 1, immunoglobulin E- (IgE-) mediated sensitivity. Accordingly, the blockade of histamine receptors using antihistamines is a logical and frequently employed method of pharmacotherapy for AR. Of the three types of histamine receptors, H1, H2, and H3, the H1 receptor is responsible for the early-phase symptoms of AR (sneezing, itching, and edema). Histamine type-1 receptor antagonists, commonly known as antihistamines, are one of the oldest forms of pharmacotherapy for AR. First released in 1937, antihistamines were not widely available in the United States until 1946, with the introduction of diphenhydramine and tripelennamine.[41] First-generation antihistamines, such as diphenhydramine, hydroxyzine, chlorpheniramine, and brompheniramine have significant side effects, most notably sedation and performance impairment (10 to 40% of users). It should be noted, that this performance impairment may persist even in those taking first generation antihistamines prior to sleep.[41] First-generation antihistamines also possess anticholinergic effects and therefore are effective in reducing rhinorrhea. However, these anticholinergic side effects also preclude their use in patients with narrow angle glaucoma or prostatic hypertrophy. Additional potential side effects include seizures, insomnia, irritability, and appetite stimulation. Furthermore, the anticholinergic effects of first-generation antihistamines can cause drying of the oral and nasal mucosa, which can be not only uncomfortable but also can potentially hinder mucociliary clearance.

Second-generation antihistamines are currently the preferred antihistamine group and are currently available as prescription and over-the-counter preparations. Second-generation antihistamines do not cross the blood–brain barrier; therefore, they are generally free from sedative effects, although cetirizine and levocetirizine can be mildly sedating. Furthermore, they do not have significant anticholinergic effects. These second-generation antihistamines are generally effective in relieving sneezing, nasal pruritus, rhinorrhea, and eye symptoms. The onset of action is relatively quick, and many patients without persistent daily symptoms take these medications on an as-needed basis. However, their effect on nasal congestion is minimal. Current over-the-counter second-generation antihistamines include loratadine and cetirizine. Prescription second-generation antihistamines include fexofenadine, levocetirizine, and desloratadine.

Topical nasal antihistamines, available by prescription, have similar effects on nasal allergy symptoms in addition to potential decongestant and antiinflammatory properties. Currently, three preparations are available. Azelastine HCL is available in two formulations, Astelin and more recently, azelastine formulated with sorbitol and sucralose (Astepro; Meda Pharmaceuticals, Somerset, NJ). One of the major drawbacks to azelastine is the bitter taste and slight incidence of sedation. These adverse side effects are significantly reduced in Astepro and the third available topical antihistamine, olopatadine (Patanase; Alcon Laboratories, Hünenberg, Switzerland). In CMS patients with concomitant nasal allergy symptoms, topical antihistamines are an appropriate alternative to oral antihistamines. Side effects include nasal dryness and bleeding as well as drowsiness in a small percentage of patients. When prescribing these medications, it is wise to instruct the patient to perform a trial application 2 hours before planned sleep to determine if drowsiness occurs. In the absence of this side effect, these sprays can be used twice daily if needed. These sprays have an onset of action within 30 minutes, much more quickly than a nasal steroid spray. Thus, antihistamine nasal sprays are more attractive agents for rescue therapy than nasal steroid sprays.

Leukotriene Receptor Antagonists

Leukotrienes are produced by inflammatory cells in the late-phase allergic response. Leukotriene synthesis begins with the formation of arachidonic acid from membrane phospholipids by the enzyme phospholipase A2. Once coupled to their receptor, leukotrienes can elicit several responses, including bronchoconstriction, increased vascular permeability, and leukocyte recruitment. The arachidonic acid pathway and site of action of the therapeutic agents targeting this pathway are shown in **Fig. 4.2**. Montelukast, a leukotriene receptor antagonist (LTRA) is approved for the treatment of AR and has been used extensively in the treatment of AR. Montelukast may be as efficacious as loratadine in treating AR, although symptomatic improvement has shown to be improved using both drugs concomitantly.[42] Improved symptom scores were also noted in a study that evaluated the addition of montelukast to standard medical therapy in patients with CRS (all received INCSs).[43] Montelukast is also approved for the treatment of asthma; therefore, it may be an excellent addition to the medical regimen of patients with concomitant AR and/or allergic asthma.

Leukotriene Synthesis Inhibition

Zileuton, a 5-lipoxygenase inhibitor, is currently indicated for prophylaxis and treatment of asthma in adults and children over 12 years of age. As opposed to montelukast and zafirlukast that block leukotriene receptors, zileuton partially prevents the synthesis of leukotrienes by inhibiting the 5-lipoxygenase enzyme. Ying et al[44] recently showed a significant histologic reduction in cysLT receptor expression on inflammatory cells in patients with CRS given zileuton. Although slightly less than half of the 19 patients enrolled in the nonblinded study reported improvement, primarily in olfaction, this did not correlate with histologic changes, perhaps because the study was underpowered.[44] Currently, the role of zileuton in the management of CMS is unknown.

Mast Cell Stabilizers

Mast cells are an integral component of IgE-mediated allergy. Upon antigen exposure, the allergic response is initiated by attachment of the antigen to two adjacent IgE molecules on the mast cell surface in patients who have been previously exposed to that antigen. Following IgE cross-linking, histamine, present in preformed granules, is released from the mast cells and the allergic cascade is initiated. The role of mast cell stabilizers is to prevent the release of histamine from mast cells exposed to antigens. The mechanism of action is thought to be secondary to calcium channel modulation. Because the medications do not affect the downstream effects of histamine, they are only effective if used in prophylaxis. Furthermore, cromolyn sodium has a short half-life and must be taken up to four times daily. For these reasons, cromolyn sodium is generally not convenient for long-term

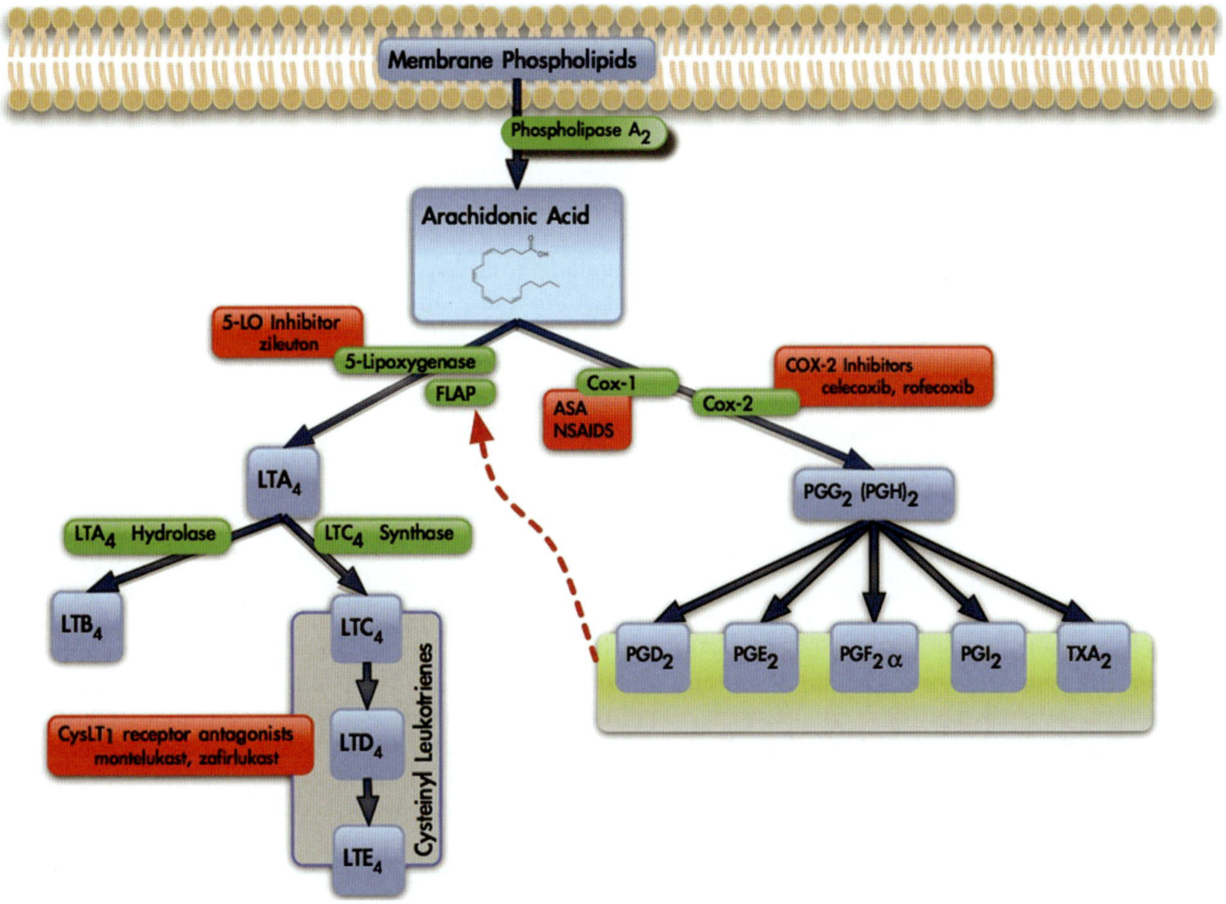

Fig. 4.2 Overview of the arachidonic acid metabolism pathway. Key enzymes (green) that serve as therapeutic targets for currently prescribed medications (red) are shown.

use. However, they do remain an effective measure of prophylaxis in patients predicting brief exposure to antigens.

Monoclonal Antibody Therapy

Omalizumab is a monoclonal antibody that prevents cell binding of IgE. Omalizumab is currently approved for use in adults and adolescents (≥12 years old) with moderate to severe persistent asthma who have a positive skin test or in vitro reactivity to perennial aeroallergens and whose symptoms are inadequately controlled with inhaled corticosteroids. More recently, studies have demonstrated improvement in other inflammatory conditions such as AR[45] and CRSwNP.[46] However, omalizumab is rarely used in otolaryngology today because of high cost, potential severe side effects, and inconvenience. The drug is administered subcutaneously in one to three injections every 2 to 4 weeks. Due to a small risk of anaphylaxis, the company currently requires that it be administered by the patient's healthcare professional.

Mepolizumab is a monoclonal antibody against IL-5 protein. It currently has orphan drug status and its use remains investigational for the treatment of hypereosinophilic syndrome. In a recent randomized, double-blind, placebo-controlled study, mepolizumab decreased blood and sputum eosinophil levels in patients with moderate persistent asthma; however, no significant clinical benefit to these patients was observed.[47] However, another study evaluating the role of mepolizumab in the treatment of hypereosinophilic syndrome demonstrated clinically significant reductions (or discontinuation) of steroid use in the mepolizumab group. The primary endpoint, prednisone use less than 10 mg or less per day, was reached in 17 of 19 patients with respiratory disorders related to hypereosinophilic syndrome.[48] Although these data are encouraging for eosinophil-predominant disorders, such as AR, the role of mepolizumab in the treatment of CMS and AR is unknown and remains investigational.

Food Allergy

Food allergy is defined as an adverse immunologic reaction to ingested foods. In addition to anaphylaxis, reactions to various food may cause mucocutaneous (oral allergy syndrome, urticaria, angioedema, flush, pruritus), respiratory (AR, allergic bronchial asthma), and gastrointestinal (nausea, vomiting, diarrhea) symptoms.[49] Food allergy may be more prevalent in patients with nasal polyps,[50,51] even in asymptomatic patients.[52] The diagnosis of food allergy can be problematic, often due to an inability to clearly define inciting foods. However, it should be kept in the differential diagnosis of all allergy patients, especially those whose symptoms persist despite treatment. Skin prick tests and in vitro testing may be employed, but the gold standard for diagnosis of food allergy is a double-blind, placebo-controlled oral challenge. Although this method provides valuable in vivo evaluation, it is generally not practical. However, patients without life-threatening reactions can perform a similar elimination-challenge procedure at home that, although not blinded or controlled, allows the patient to essentially self-diagnose themselves. The most common "masked" food allergens in adults include wheat, dairy, soy, corn, and eggs. Patients are educated with this information, but are also advised to identify any other food sources that tend to cause symptoms. They are then instructed to completely eliminate that food from their diet for 5 to 7 days. After the elimination period, they are instructed to reintroduce the food into their diet and keep a log of their symptoms. Patients will generally notice symptoms within 15 minutes to 4 hours of the challenge. These symptoms may be nonnasal (abdominal cramping, pruritus, etc.). Regardless of the results of this test, patients are instructed to complete the test for the five food types listed above. Patients who test positive are instructed to eliminate the food from their diet for approximately 3 months, after which time the food can be slowly reintroduced into their diet.

Antimicrobials

Acute Maxillary Sinusitis

AMS is the fifth most common diagnosis for which antibiotics are written.[1] Frequently, they are prescribed empirically based on symptoms. Although recommendations exist regarding the use of antimicrobials in AMS, practical application of these recommendations can be made difficult due to patient expectations, ambiguous diagnostic criteria, and medicolegal concerns regarding potential complications of ongoing infection. The role of antibiotics in the treatment of acute bacterial rhinosinusitis has more recently been questioned. A Cochrane Review analyzed the effectiveness of antibiotics in treating AMS in adults. The review included 6 placebo-controlled studies and 51 studies involving comparisons of different antibiotic classes. The authors concluded that there was a slight treatment effect in patients with uncomplicated acute sinusitis when symptoms last longer than 7 days. However, the placebo group in the analysis had an 80% cure rate compared with a 90% cure rate in the treatment group. There was no statistically significant difference in efficacy among antibiotic classes.[53] Another recent meta-analysis similarly concluded that antibiotics have an approximate 10% added benefit in resolution of ABRS versus placebo. However, this was associated with a similar rise in adverse events, such as gastrointestinal side effects.[54] The recommendations outlined in the European Position Paper on Rhinosinusitis and Nasal Polyps 2007 include the use of antibiotics to treat ABRS in patients whose symptoms worsen after 5 days or in severe cases.[15]

The microbiology of AMS in nonoperated patients has historically followed that of acute otitis media. *Streptococcus pneumoniae* and *Haemophilus influenza* are common pathogens. *Moraxella* is also common in children, but is less of a factor in adults. Although these patterns should be taken into account when using antibiotics empirically, it should be noted that antibacterial resistance patterns are increasing worldwide and vary from region to region. Recently, increases in methicillin-resistant *Staphylococcus aureus* (MRSA) isolates in patients with ARS were demonstrated.[55] MRSA emergence has been associated with previous antibiotic use and may be linked to fluoroquinolone and macrolide use.[56] These data underscore the importance of judicious antibiotic use for AMS in the primary care setting.

When possible, antibiotics should be culture directed. Maxillary sinus taps (MSTs) remain the gold standard for culture acquisition in research. However, endoscopically directed middle meatal (EDMM) cultures are better tolerated and are used more commonly in clinical practice. A recent meta-analysis found that EDMM culture acquisition, when compared with MSTs, had a sensitivity of 80.9%, a specificity of 90.5%, and an overall accuracy rate of 87%.[57] Instruments used in culture acquisition are shown in **Fig. 4.3**. The collection of pus from the right maxillary sinus using our preferred method is shown in **Video 4.1**.

In choosing empiric antibiotics, either for cure or during the window following culture acquisition and results, the local resistance patterns should be considered. Furthermore, the resistance mechanisms of commonly encountered pathogens should be taken into account. For example, *Streptococcus pneumoniae* acquires resistance through alteration of penicillin-binding proteins, changes in efflux cellular mechanisms, and changes in ribosomal configuration. *Haemophilus influenza* is increasingly β-lactamase positive, necessitating the utilization of β-lactamase-resistant antibiotics. Taking this into consideration, most current guidelines recommend amoxicillin as the first choice for uncomplicated bacterial sinusitis in patients who have not recently received antibiotics. Amoxicillin is cheap and is active against *Streptococcus pneumoniae* and *Haemophilus influenzae*. High-dose amoxicillin can be used in cases of *S. pneumoniae* resistance conferred by altered penicillin-binding proteins. The addition of clavulanic acid improves efficacy in treating β-lactamase-producing strains of *H. flu* or other β-lactamase-producing bacteria. Second- or third-generation cephalosporins, trimethoprim-sulfamethoxazole (TMP-SMX), macrolides, and doxycycline are appropriate alternatives as first-line therapy in patients for whom amoxicillin is not appropriate. Emerging resistance patterns should

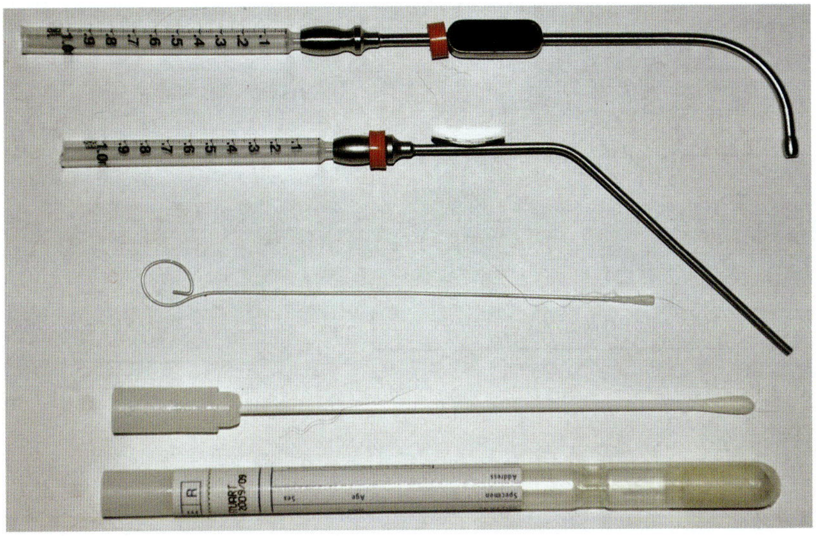

Fig. 4.3 Instruments commonly used for maxillary sinus aspirate culture. **(A)** The curved or **(B)** Frasier-tipped suction is securely attached to a tuberculin syringe, which, in turn, is attached to the suction source. The flanged end of the tuberculin syringe must first be cut so that the suction tubing can fit. Once the sample is collected in the syringe, the end of the syringe that was attached to the suction is cut off with scissors to prevent contamination from the tubing. **(C,D)** The plunger is then placed back into the tuberculin syringe and the sample is expressed onto a cotton swab, which is **(E)** then placed into the culture tube.

be kept in mind when considering alternative antibiotics. For example, *S. pneumoniae* and *H. influenzae* have both become increasingly resistant to TMP-SMX,[58] and indiscriminate use of TMP-SMX has been identified as a factor in the emergence of drug-resistant *S. pneumoniae*.[59] In patients who do not show improvement in 48 to 72 hours, second-line therapy should be initiated. Fluoroquinolones, amoxicillin-clavulanate, or rifampin plus doxycycline (or other agents in combination) are commonly used.[60] Furthermore, TMP-SMX or doxycycline (with or without rifampin) may be used to treat most community-acquired MRSA infections. A flow sheet demonstrating the our use of antibiotics in the management of AMS is shown in **Fig. 4.4**.

Chronic Maxillary Sinusitis

Although CMS is not currently considered an infectious disease, chronic and/or recurrent bacterial infections are frequently encountered in patients with CMS. Although the general treatment principles are similar to AMS, the different microbiologic profile of CMS, coupled with the chronic mucosal inflammation, bear some consideration when prescribing antimicrobials for this condition.

As previously described, most cases of AMS are secondary to viral infection. Only a small percentage of patients develop secondary bacterial infection. The majority of acute infections are dominated by facultative aerobic bacteria. However, in unresolved subacute to chronic infections, anaerobic bacteria of oral flora origin become predominant.[61] The most common isolates in CMS include *Staphylococcus aureus, S. epidermidis,* and anaerobic and gram-negative bacteria. *S. epidermidis* (coagulase-negative staph) is usually considered a contaminant because it colonizes the nasal cavity. Polymicrobial infection is common in CMS, usually necessitating the use of broad-spectrum antibiotics. Gram-negative rods that are commonly found in CMS include *Pseudomonas aeruginosa, Klebsiella pneumoniae, Proteus mirabilis, Enterobacter* species, and *Escherichia coli*.[61]

Antibiotic selection for CMS (or acute exacerbation of CMS) should take into account these general microbial trends as well as local resistance patterns. As in AMS, culture directed therapy is preferred. Recently, one study demonstrated that culture acquisition changed the choice of antibiotic in 50% of patients with CRS for whom antibiotics were prescribed.[62] There are no placebo-controlled studies that validate the use of short-term antibiotics in treating CMS, and short-term use of antimicrobials for CMS is not recommended.[15] For example, uncomplicated acute exacerbation of CMS (AECMS) may respond well to short-term antibiotics; however, no double-blind controlled data for such use exist[15] and patients with AECMS should be followed closely as therapy is finished to confirm clearance of the active infection. Based on the increased presence of anaerobes associated with CMS, the American Academy of Otolaryngology–Head and Neck Surgery (AAO-HNS) recommends amoxicillin-clavulanate for primary treatment of AECMS.[63] Alternatives include metronidazole plus levofloxacin, clindamycin plus rifampin, or TMP-SMX. Alternatively, ciprofloxacin may be added to metronidazole for better potential coverage of *Pseudomonas*. Knowledge of the common pathogens of AECMS may aid in the most appropriate antibiotic selection in patients whose condition necessitates prompt antibiotic coverage, but for whom culture results are pending. A list of Gram stain characteristics of common pathogens in AECMS is presented in **Fig. 4.5**.

Long-term antibiotic therapy is commonplace in the management of CMS. Many otolaryngologists consider long-term antibiotics a necessary component of maximal medical therapy. However, an incomplete understanding of the pathogenesis of CMS, coupled with potential side effects and resistance patterns associated with antibiotic use, has led to difficulties in establishing universal recommendations for maximal medical therapy. Recent interest in the antiinflam-

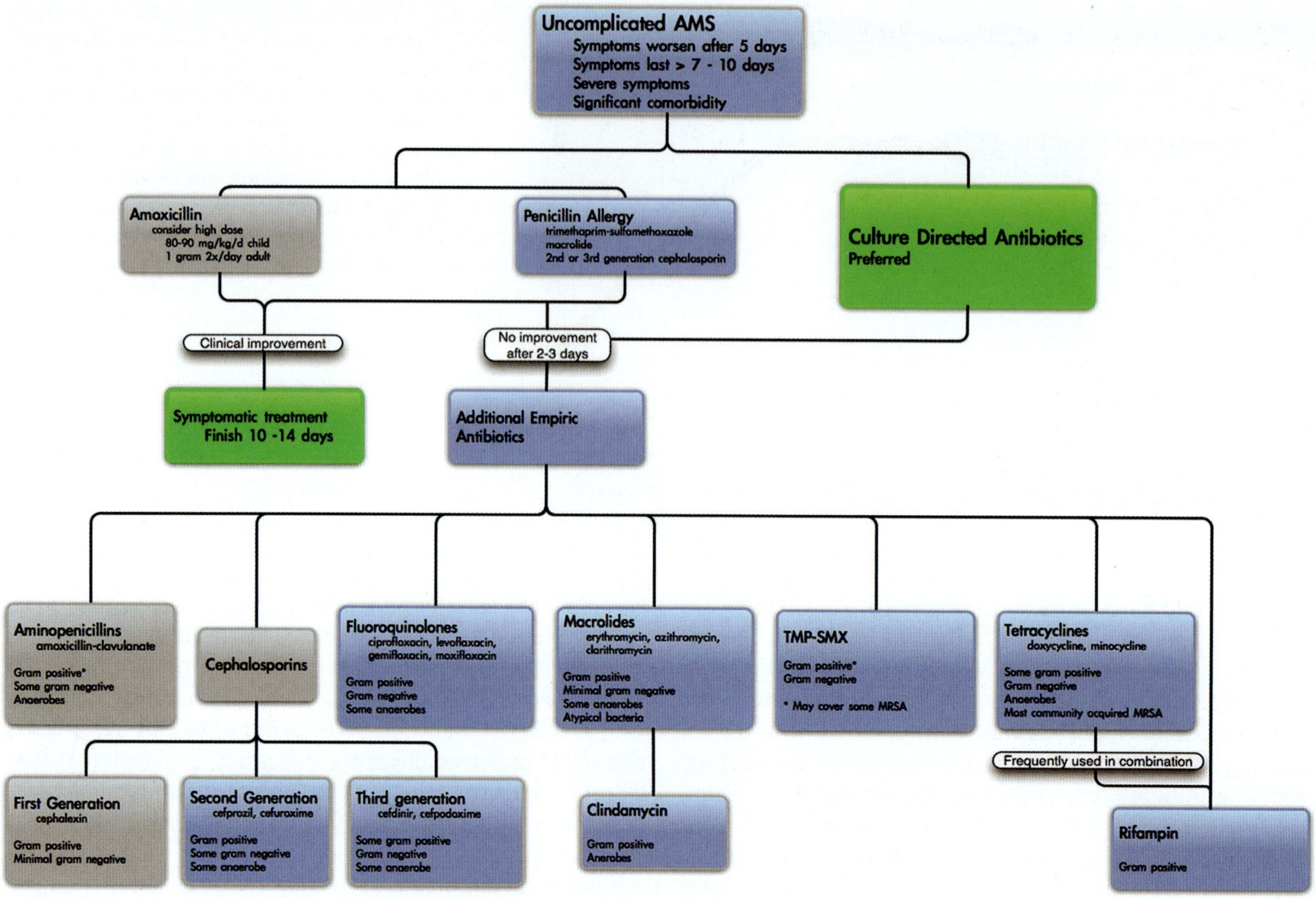

Fig. 4.4 Flowchart demonstrating a rational algorithm for the administration of empiric antibiotics in uncomplicated acute maxillary sinusitis. Whenever possible, culture-directed antibiotics are preferred over empiric therapy. Blue boxes represent antibiotic choices that may be used in penicillin-allergic patients, gray boxes represent commonly used antibiotics in patients without penicillin allergy.

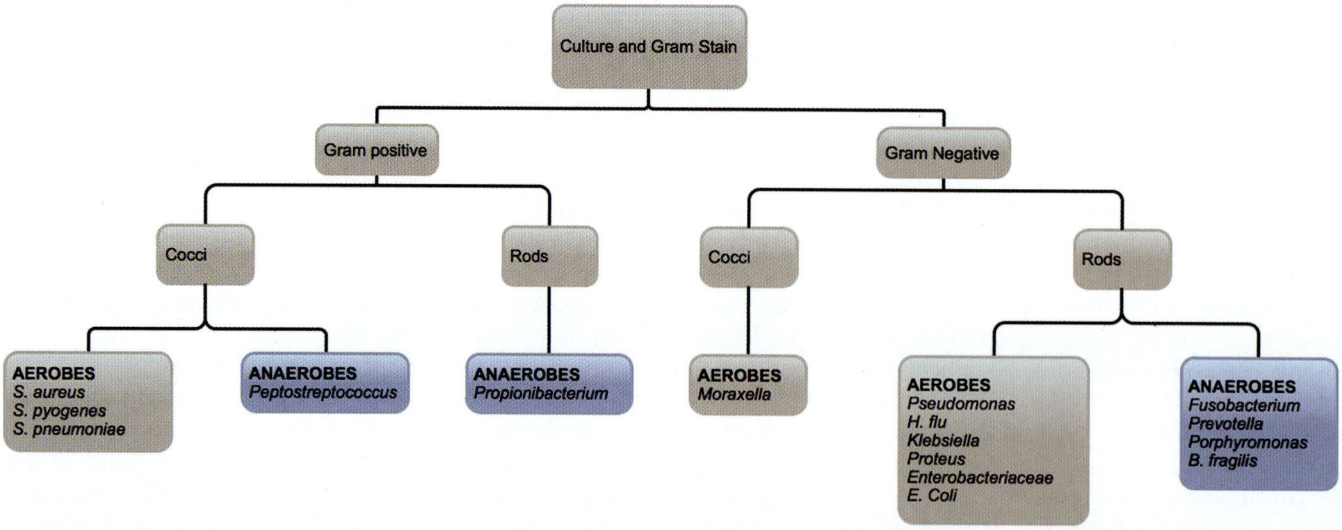

Fig. 4.5 Flowchart demonstrating common pathogens encountered in acute exacerbation of chronic maxillary sinusitis (AECMS). An understanding of the common pathogens associated with AECMS can aid in the administration of empiric antibiotics in the window between Gram stain results and culture identification.

matory effects of macrolides (discussed below) has led to more widespread acceptance of this class of antibiotics as a component of maximal medical therapy. In determining the appropriate antibiotic for each patient, several elements should be considered, such as cost, dosing schedule, potential side effects, and local resistance patterns. Furthermore, any worsening of symptoms during antimicrobial therapy should prompt an expedient evaluation for the presence of an opportunistic infection caused by resistant bacteria. The AAO-HNS currently recommends clindamycin as the first-line therapy for CRS. Alternatives include amoxicillin-clavulanate, TMP-SMX, or doxycycline plus rifampin.[63] Rifampin should not be used alone due to the relatively high potential for resistance after monotherapy.

Macrolide Antibiotics

Macrolides, a group of bacteriostatic antimicrobials isolated from *Streptomyces erythreus*, exert their antimicrobial effects through binding to the 50s ribosomal unit of bacteria. Macrolides are active against gram-positive cocci (including anaerobes) and intracellular pathogens such as *Chlamydia* and *Mycoplasma*. Recently, 14-membered and 15-membered ring macrolides have received clinical interest due to a growing body of evidence supporting antiinflammatory properties. The first clinically relevant publication related to this antiinflammatory property was from Japan. Treatment of patients with panbronchiolitis with long-term low-dose erythromycin results in improved symptoms, oxygenation, chest radiographs, and survival.[64] More recent interest in macrolides related to CRS is based on several beneficial properties not directly related to microbial eradication. In addition to reducing bacterial virulence, macrolides have been shown to decrease inflammatory cytokines, alter the structure of biofilms, reduce leukocyte adhesion, and improve mucociliary clearance.[65] Macrolides are currently recommended in the guidelines set forth in the European Position Paper on Rhinosinusitis and Nasal Polyps.[15] Most clinical studies investigating outcomes after macrolide use in CRS are small. However, improvement is seen in 50 to 88% of patients. Response appears to improve with duration of therapy and some physicians recommend treatment for up to 12 months.[65] It should be noted that resistance to erythromycin appears to be emerging at a higher rate than for other antibiotics.[66] More studies are needed to determine the long-term benefit of macrolide use in treating CMS and the effect on locoregional resistance patterns. Prior to long-term treatment with macrolides, a culture should be obtained and pathogens not susceptible to macrolides should be treated concomitantly.

Topical Antimicrobials

Topical antimicrobial therapy is less likely to be helpful in the unoperated maxillary sinus because drug delivery will necessarily be impaired. Topical antimicrobial therapy is therefore discussed in the chapter on postoperative medical care of the maxillary sinus.

Conclusion

The management of AMS and CMS can be complex and definitive protocols based on hard evidence cannot be defined due to the heterogeneity of causes and the differences in individual's response to various therapeutic interventions. In fact, in most refractory cases our current understanding of the underlying pathophysiology is certainly incomplete. The aforementioned summary of mainstream medical therapy for AMS and CMS will undoubtedly change as these pathogenic mechanisms are learned and targeted.

Pearls

Acute Maxillary Sinusitis

- Most cases of AMS are self-limited viral infections and resolve spontaneously in 7 to 10 days
- Intranasal corticosteroids may be a useful adjunct to antimicrobial therapy in the treatment of AMS
- Culture-directed antibiotics (via antral tap or endoscopically guided aspirate) are preferred for acute bacterial maxillary sinusitis
- Local resistance patterns should be considered when administering empiric antibiotics for AMS

Chronic Maxillary Sinusitis

- The etiology of CMS is incompletely understood and medical therapy is generally an experiment consisting of various agents used individually to assess response.
- Current evidence supports the use of INCS for the initial treatment of CMS
- Topical inhaled corticosteroids, applied via nasal nebulizer or dripping from a respule (off-label use), may improve delivery of steroid to sinonasal cavity and be associated with increased efficacy.
- Isotonic saline irrigation (hypertonic solution for patients with cystic fibrosis) is cheap, well-tolerated, and has been shown to reduce symptoms.
- Topical therapy for CMS may require surgery to optimize delivery of topical medications to the sinonasal cavity.
- The role of allergy in CMS is conflicting, yet optimization of allergy management will often improve symptoms of CMS in patients with concomitant AR.
- Immunotherapy may offer substantial allergy control, and even cure, for those patients who fail to improve on, or cannot tolerate, medical regimens for AR.
- As in AMS, use of antibiotics for AECMS or CMS should be culture directed.
- Based on antiinflammatory properties, long-term use of macrolide antibiotics may augment traditional medical regimens.
- Consider a dental etiology in cases of unilateral maxillary sinusitis, especially when mucosal thickening occupies over two-thirds of the maxillary sinus volume.

References

1. Rosenfeld RM, Andes D, Bhattacharyya N, et al. Clinical practice guideline: adult sinusitis. Otolaryngol Head Neck Surg 2007; 137(3, Suppl)S1–S31 PubMed
2. Williams JWJ Jr, Simel DL, Roberts L, Samsa GP. Clinical evaluation for sinusitis. Making the diagnosis by history and physical examination. Ann Intern Med 1992;117(9):705–710
3. Gwaltney JMJ Jr, Phillips CD, Miller RD, Riker DK. Computed tomographic study of the common cold. N Engl J Med 1994;330(1):25–30
4. Brook I. Microbiology of acute sinusitis of odontogenic origin presenting with periorbital cellulitis in children. Ann Otol Rhinol Laryngol 2007;116(5):386–388
5. Legert KG, Zimmerman M, Stierna P. Sinusitis of odontogenic origin: pathophysiological implications of early treatment. Acta Otolaryngol 2004;124(6):655–663
6. Bomeli SR, Branstetter BFIV, Ferguson BJ. Frequency of a dental source for acute maxillary sinusitis. Laryngoscope 2009;119(3):580–584
7. Schleimer RP. Pharmacology of glucocorticoids in allergic disease. In: Adkinson Jr. NF, Yunginger JW, Busse WW, Bochner BS, Simons FER, Lemanske Jr. RF, eds. Middleton's Allergy Principles and Practice (7th ed). Philadelphia: Mosby; 2009: 1549–1573
8. Cope D, Bova R. Steroids in otolaryngology. Laryngoscope 2008;118(9): 1556–1560
9. Pershall KE, Krouse JH. In: Pharmacotherapy for allergic rhinitis. Mabry RL, Ferguson BJ, Krouse JH, eds. Allergy: The Otolaryngologist's Approach. Washington, DC: The American Academy of Otolaryngic Allergy, 2005: 53–65
10. Dolor RJ, Witsell DL, Hellkamp AS, Williams JW Jr, Califf RM, Simel DL; Ceftin and Flonase for Sinusitis (CAFFS) Investigators. Comparison of cefuroxime with or without intranasal fluticasone for the treatment of rhinosinusitis. The CAFFS Trial: a randomized controlled trial. JAMA 2001;286(24):3097–3105
11. Meltzer EO, Charous BL, Busse WW, Zinreich SJ, Lorber RR, Danzig MR; The Nasonex Sinusitis Group. Added relief in the treatment of acute recurrent sinusitis with adjunctive mometasone furoate nasal spray. J Allergy Clin Immunol 2000;106(4):630–637
12. Nayak AS, Settipane GA, Pedinoff A, et al; Nasonex Sinusitis Group. Effective dose range of mometasone furoate nasal spray in the treatment of acute rhinosinusitis. Ann Allergy Asthma Immunol 2002;89(3):271–278
13. Neher A, Gstöttner M, Scholtz A, Nagl M. Antibacterial activity of mometasone furoate. Arch Otolaryngol Head Neck Surg 2008;134(5):519–521
14. Meltzer EO, Bachert C, Staudinger H. Treating acute rhinosinusitis: comparing efficacy and safety of mometasone furoate nasal spray, amoxicillin, and placebo. J Allergy Clin Immunol 2005;116(6):1289–1295
15. Fokkens W, Lund V, Mullol J; European Position Paper on Rhinosinusitis and Nasal Polyps group. European position paper on rhinosinusitis and nasal polyps 2007. Rhinol Suppl 2007;20(20):1–136
16. Zalmanovici A, Yaphe J. Steroids for acute sinusitis. Cochrane Database Syst Rev 2007; (2):CD005149
17. Lund VJ, Black JH, Szabó LZ, Schrewelius C, Akerlund A. Efficacy and tolerability of budesonide aqueous nasal spray in chronic rhinosinusitis patients. Rhinology 2004;42(2):57–62
18. Sykes DA, Wilson R, Chan KL, Mackay IS, Cole PJ. Relative importance of antibiotic and improved clearance in topical treatment of chronic mucopurulent rhinosinusitis. A controlled study. Lancet 1986;2(8503):359–360
19. Lavigne F, Cameron L, Renzi PM, et al. Intrasinus administration of topical budesonide to allergic patients with chronic rhinosinusitis following surgery. Laryngoscope 2002;112(5):858–864
20. Hwang PH, Woo RJ, Fong KJ. Intranasal deposition of nebulized saline: a radionuclide distribution study. Am J Rhinol 2006;20(3):255–261
21. Wormald PJ, Cain T, Oates L, Hawke L, Wong I. A comparative study of three methods of nasal irrigation. Laryngoscope 2004;114(12):2224–2227
22. Benninger MS, Hadley JA, Osguthorpe JD, et al. Techniques of intranasal steroid use. Otolaryngol Head Neck Surg 2004;130(1):5–24
23. Kanowitz SJ, Batra PS, Citardi MJ. Topical budesonide via mucosal atomization device in refractory postoperative chronic rhinosinusitis. Otolaryngol Head Neck Surg; 2008;139(1):131–136
24. Videler WJ, Drunen CM, Reitsma JB, Fokkens WJ. Nebulized bacitracin/colimycin: a treatment option in recalcitrant chronic rhinosinusitis with Staphylococcus aureus? A double-blind, randomized, placebo-controlled, cross-over pilot study. Rhinology; 2008; 46(2):92–98
25. Harvey RJ, Goddard JC, Wise SK, Schlosser RJ. Effects of endoscopic sinus surgery and delivery device on cadaver sinus irrigation. Otolaryngol Head Neck Surg 2008;139(1):137–142
26. Raghavan U, Logan BM. New method for the effective instillation of nasal drops. J Laryngol Otol 2000;114(6):456–459
27. Cannady SB, Batra PS, Citardi MJ, Lanza DC. Comparison of delivery of topical medications to the paranasal sinuses via "vertex-to-floor" position and atomizer spray after FESS. Otolaryngol Head Neck Surg 2005;133(5):735–740
28. Gehanno P, Beauvillain C, Bobin S, et al. Short therapy with amoxicillin-clavulanate and corticosteroids in acute sinusitis: results of a multicentre study in adults. Scand J Infect Dis 2000;32(6):679–684
29. Wallwork B, Coman W, Feron F, Mackay-Sim A, Cervin A. Clarithromycin and prednisolone inhibit cytokine production in chronic rhinosinusitis. Laryngoscope 2002;112(10):1827–1830
30. Wright ED, Agrawal S. Impact of perioperative systemic steroids on surgical outcomes in patients with chronic rhinosinusitis with polyposis: evaluation with the novel perioperative sinus endoscopy (POSE) scoring system. Laryngoscope 2007; 117(11 Pt 2, Suppl 115)1–28
31. Hatton RC, Winterstein AG, McKelvey RP, Shuster J, Hendeles L. Efficacy and safety of oral phenylephrine: systematic review and meta-analysis. Ann Pharmacother 2007;41(3):381–390
32. Kollar C, Schneider H, Waksman J, Krusinska E. Meta-analysis of the efficacy of a single dose of phenylephrine 10 mg compared with placebo in adults with acute nasal congestion due to the common cold. Clin Ther 2007;29(6):1057–1070
33. Inanli S, Oztürk O, Korkmaz M, Tutkun A, Batman C. The effects of topical agents of fluticasone propionate, oxymetazoline, and 3% and 0.9% sodium chloride solutions on mucociliary clearance in the therapy of acute bacterial rhinosinusitis in vivo. Laryngoscope 2002;112(2):320–325
34. Bende M, Fukami M, Arfors KE, Mark J, Stierna P, Intaglietta M. Effect of oxymetazoline nose drops on acute sinusitis in the rabbit. Ann Otol Rhinol Laryngol 1996;105(3):222–225
35. Ural A, Oktemer TK, Kizil Y, Ileri F, Uslu S. Impact of isotonic and hypertonic saline solutions on mucociliary activity in various nasal pathologies: clinical study. J Laryngol Otol 2009;123(5):517–521
36. Adam P, Stiffman M, Blake RLJ Jr. A clinical trial of hypertonic saline nasal spray in subjects with the common cold or rhinosinusitis. Arch Fam Med 1998;7(1):39–43
37. Rabago D, Pasic T, Zgierska A, Mundt M, Barrett B, Maberry R. The efficacy of hypertonic saline nasal irrigation for chronic sinonasal symptoms. Otolaryngol Head Neck Surg 2005;133(1):3–8

38. Burton MJ, Eisenberg LD, Rosenfeld RM. Extracts from The Cochrane Library: Nasal saline irrigations for the symptoms of chronic rhinosinusitis. Otolaryngol Head Neck Surg 2007;137(4):532–534
39. Elkins MR, Robinson M, Rose BR, et al; National Hypertonic Saline in Cystic Fibrosis (NHSCF) Study Group. A controlled trial of long-term inhaled hypertonic saline in patients with cystic fibrosis. N Engl J Med 2006;354(3):229–240
40. Ahmad N, Zacharek MA. Allergic rhinitis and rhinosinusitis. Otolaryngol Clin North Am 2008;41(2):267–281, v
41. Ferguson BJ. Cost-effective pharmacotherapy for allergic rhinitis. Otolaryngol Clin North Am 1998;31(1):91–110
42. Meltzer EO, Malmstrom K, Lu S, et al. Concomitant montelukast and loratadine as treatment for seasonal allergic rhinitis: a randomized, placebo-controlled clinical trial. J Allergy Clin Immunol 2000;105(5):917–922
43. Wilson AM, White PS, Gardiner Q, Nassif R, Lipworth BJ. Effects of leukotriene receptor antagonist therapy in patients with chronic rhinosinusitis in a real life rhinology clinic setting. Rhinology 2001;39(3):142–146
44. Ying YL, Ferguson BJ, Seethala RR, Rubinstein E. Effects of zileuton on leukotriene receptor expression on nasal mucosal inflammatory cells. Paper presented at: Eastern Section of the Triological Society; January 23–25, 2009; Boston, MA
45. Humbert M, Boulet LP, Niven RM, Panahloo Z, Blogg M, Ayre G. Omalizumab therapy: patients who achieve greatest benefit for their asthma experience greatest benefit for rhinitis. Allergy 2009;64(1):81–84
46. Penn R, Mikula S. The role of anti-IgE immunoglobulin therapy in nasal polyposis: a pilot study. Am J Rhinol 2007;21(4):428–432
47. Flood-Page P, Swenson C, Faiferman I, et al; International Mepolizumab Study Group. A study to evaluate safety and efficacy of mepolizumab in patients with moderate persistent asthma. Am J Respir Crit Care Med 2007;176(11):1062–1071
48. Rothenberg ME, Klion AD, Roufosse FE, et al; Mepolizumab HES Study Group. Treatment of patients with the hypereosinophilic syndrome with mepolizumab. N Engl J Med 2008;358(12):1215–1228
49. Werfel T. Food allergy. J Dtsch Dermatol Ges 2008;6(7):573–583
50. Collins MM, Loughran S, Davidson P, Wilson JA. Nasal polyposis: prevalence of positive food and inhalant skin tests. Otolaryngol Head Neck Surg 2006;135(5):680–683
51. Pang YT, Eskici O, Wilson JA. Nasal polyposis: role of subclinical delayed food hypersensitivity. Otolaryngol Head Neck Surg 2000;122(2):298–301
52. Doğru H, Tüz M, Uygur K, Akkaya A, Yasan H. Asymptomatic IgE mediated food hypersensitivity in patients with nasal polyps. Asian Pac J Allergy Immunol 2003;21(2):79–82
53. Ahovuo-Saloranta A, Borisenko OV, Kovanen N, et al. Antibiotics for acute maxillary sinusitis. Cochrane Database Syst Rev 2008;(2):CD000243
54. Falagas ME, Giannopoulou KP, Vardakas KZ, Dimopoulos G, Karageorgopoulos DE. Comparison of antibiotics with placebo for treatment of acute sinusitis: a meta-analysis of randomised controlled trials. Lancet Infect Dis 2008;8(9):543–552
55. Brook I, Foote PA, Hausfeld JN. Increase in the frequency of recovery of meticillin-resistant *Staphylococcus aureus* in acute and chronic maxillary sinusitis. J Med Microbiol 2008;57(Pt 8):1015–1017
56. Gerencer RZ. Successful outpatient treatment of sinusitis exacerbations caused by community-acquired methicillin-resistant *Staphylococcus aureus*. Otolaryngol Head Neck Surg 2005;132(6):828–833
57. Benninger MS, Payne SC, Ferguson BJ, Hadley JA, Ahmad N. Endoscopically directed middle meatal cultures versus maxillary sinus taps in acute bacterial maxillary rhinosinusitis: a meta-analysis. Otolaryngol Head Neck Surg 2006;134(1):3–9
58. Dagan R. Treatment of acute otitis media - challenges in the era of antibiotic resistance. Vaccine 2000;19(Suppl 1):S9–S16
59. Kärpänoja P, Nyberg ST, Bergman M, et al; Finnish Study Group for Antimicrobial Resistance (FiRe Network). Connection between trimethoprim-sulfamethoxazole use and resistance in *Streptococcus pneumoniae, Haemophilus influenzae, and Moraxella catarrhalis*. Antimicrob Agents Chemother 2008;52(7):2480–2485
60. Marple BF, Brunton S, Ferguson BJ. Acute bacterial rhinosinusitis: a review of U.S. treatment guidelines. Otolaryngol Head Neck Surg 2006;135(3):341–348
61. Brook I. The role of bacteria in chronic rhinosinusitis. Otolaryngol Clin North Am 2005;38(6):1171–1192
62. Cincik H, Ferguson BJ. The impact of endoscopic cultures on care in rhinosinusitis. Laryngoscope 2006;116(9):1562–1568
63. Fairbanks DNF. Antimicrobial Therapy in Otolaryngology–Head and Neck Surgery. 13th ed. Alexandria, VA: American Academy of Otolaryngology–Head and Neck Surgery;2007
64. Kudoh S, Uetake T, Hagiwara K, et al. [Clinical effects of low-dose long-term erythromycin chemotherapy on diffuse panbronchiolitis]. Nihon Kyobu Shikkan Gakkai Zasshi 1987;25(6):632–642
65. Cervin A, Wallwork B. Anti-inflammatory effects of macrolide antibiotics in the treatment of chronic rhinosinusitis. Otolaryngol Clin North Am 2005;38(6):1339–1350
66. Bhattacharyya N, Kepnes LJ. Assessment of trends in antimicrobial resistance in chronic rhinosinusitis. Ann Otol Rhinol Laryngol 2008;117(6):448–452

5 Fungal Disease in the Maxillary Sinus

Jacquelyn M. Brewer and Bradley F. Marple

Our understanding of nasal fungal disease has increased exponentially over the past three decades. An adequate understanding of the variable presentations of fungal disease in the nose is important for diagnosis, management, and prognosis. Recent advances in medical therapies as well as endoscopic surgical therapy have dramatically altered the treatment and prognosis of this disease. Fungal disease in the nose is not specific to the maxillary sinus and in fact, may involve any combination of paranasal sinuses. It is often difficult to separate disease of the maxillary sinus from those occurring elsewhere in the nose and in other sinuses. For this reason, this chapter will focus on fungal disease in general in the paranasal sinuses with identification of those with a predilection for the maxillary sinus.

■ Medical Mycology

Fungi are eukaryotic organisms that are ubiquitous in nature. Scientists estimate that there exist somewhere between 20,000 and 1.5 million different fungal species. Up to one tenth of Earth's entire biomass may be made up of fungi. Yet only a tiny fraction of these fungal organisms are responsible for human disease; in fact, most fungi benefit humankind. Fungi are a major source of carbon, nitrogen, and other nutrients in soil. They play an important role in biodegradation and ecologic recycling. They have even produced byproducts that are responsible for some of medicine's greatest advancements, such as penicillin. Though fungi are widely distributed and a vital component to life on earth, they may infrequently be the cause of human disease. The incidence of mycotic infections is on the rise, and each year some additional species are found to cause human illnesses.

Given the diversity and number of potential fungal pathogens, fungal terminology can be quite confusing. Adding to the confusion that underlies fungal taxonomy, fungi can exist in several forms. A basic understanding of fungal nomenclature is important for an accurate diagnosis, to prevent confusion, and to allow for a clear dialogue among practitioners. The term *yeast* refers to a unicellular fungal organism, which is able to reproduce asexually via budding. *Mold* denotes a multicellular filamentous colony of fungi. Some fungal species are dimorphic, indicating the capability to grow as both yeast and a mold, depending on environmental conditions. A *spore* is a small, usually unicellular body, which is highly resistant to adverse conditions but retains the ability to germinate and produce a new organism once conditions are more favorable. Spores enable fungal dispersion over great distances, survival in seemingly scarce environments, and massive reproduction.[1]

An elementary awareness of fungal taxonomy is important when studying the role of fungal diseases in human inflammatory processes. Currently, in the fungal kingdom there are seven fungal phyla: Chytridiomycota, Blastocladiomycota, Neocallimastigomycota, Zygomycota, Glomeromycota, Basidiomycota, and Ascomycota. The most medically relevant of these groups in regards to fungal disease of the paranasal sinuses include Zygomycota and Ascomycota. Zygomycota include the *Mucor* and *Rhizopus* species, which are often aggressive etiologic organisms in invasive fungal sinusitis. Ascomycota include *Aspergillus, Fusarium,* and *Candida* species. Dematiaceous fungi refer to a heterogeneously diverse population of fungi, which have a dark appearance due to the production of melanin. Colonies may appear gray, brown, or black. Many human inflammatory diseases such as those in the sinuses and lungs are caused by dematiaceous fungi. Soil, wood, and decomposing plants are often satiated with these fungi.[1]

All fungi have a rigid cell wall that determines the shape of the fungus and also mediates attachment to host cells. The majority of fungal antigens are polysaccharides and glycoproteins within the cell wall. The cell wall is resistant to degradation and confers staining properties to fungi allowing for early identification of the presence of fungi. This is useful to begin early treatment if necessary, while awaiting final culture and speciation.[1]

Fungi can be cultured from almost any nose.[2] Silver-based stains, such as Gomori methenamine silver (GMS), stain cell walls black and is the most commonly used method of detecting fungal organisms. Silver ions in GMS bind to polysaccharides in fungal cell walls allowing for the clear identification of fungal elements (**Fig. 5.1**). Alternatively, GMS requires an experienced pathologist to avoid over- or understaining or silver precipitate, which may make identification more difficult. Glycogen stains, such as periodic acid-Schiff (PAS), bestow a red appearance to the polysaccharide filled fungal cell walls. This method is simple and reliable; however, the stain is not limited to polysaccharides in the cell wall. Staining of intracellular components with PAS may be distracting when trying to identify fungal elements. Hematoxylin and eosin (H&E) stain produces variable characteristics in different fungal species and therefore, is not a reliable indicator of

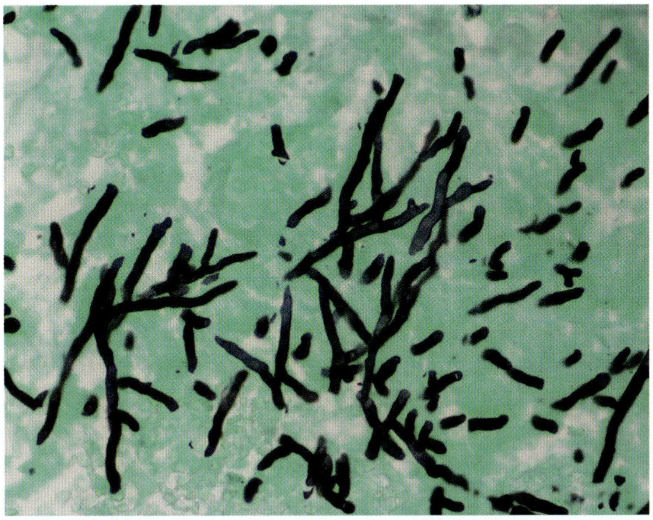

Fig. 5.1 Branching septate hyphae as seen with Gomori methenamine silver (GMS) stain.

fungal presence. Chitin is a unique protein that can be found in the cell walls of most fungi, but not in other organisms. A monoclonal antibody to chitin can be used to very specifically identify fungi. However, this is the most costly and time-consuming method of fungal identification.[3]

Fungal Infection

Paltauf was the first to describe upper airway fungal disease when he presented the case of a patient with mucor infection in 1885. Soon after, parallels of upper respiratory fungal disease and bronchopulmonary aspergillosis appeared in the literature. In 1894, Mackenzie published the first article specifically on fungal sinusitis.[4] However, it wasn't until the 1970s that fungal disease in the sinuses became widely recognized and studied. Given its aggressive nature and shocking virility, the early literature focused mainly on invasive fungal sinus disease. In 1983, however, Katzenstein described a distinct disease entity characterized by fungal hyphae, eosinophilic mucin, and Charcot-Leyden crystals.[5] This article paved the way for a better understanding of the spectrum of fungal sinus disease and the importance of disease identification and stratification. Since then, an abundance of literature has arisen on the different manifestations of fungal disease in the maxillary sinus and other paranasal sinuses.

Despite the prevalence of fungi, human fungal disease is relatively rare. Competent host immune systems usually keep fungal growth at bay. As will be demonstrated, however, fungal growth can sometimes occur despite adequate immunity. Inhalation of spores is likely the instigator of fungal rhinosinusitis in susceptible individuals. It is unlikely that fungal rhinosinusitis occurs as spread from a preexisting infection in the lungs or other site of infection within the body.

Most sinus fungal infections are caused by *Aspergillus* species. *Aspergillus flavus* is the most common cause of sinus fungus ball. Infections by dematiaceous fungi such as *Bipolaris*, *Curvularia*, or *Alternaria*, are commonly seen in patients with allergic fungal sinusitis. Zygomycetes, such as *Mucorales* or *Rhizopus* are well-described aggressive organisms implicated in many cases of invasive fungal sinusitis.[6–8]

The patients' immune response to inhaled spores determines the manifestation of the fungal disease. Fungal rhinosinusitis can be classified as invasive or noninvasive (**Fig. 5.2**). The prognosis of fungal sinus infections is more

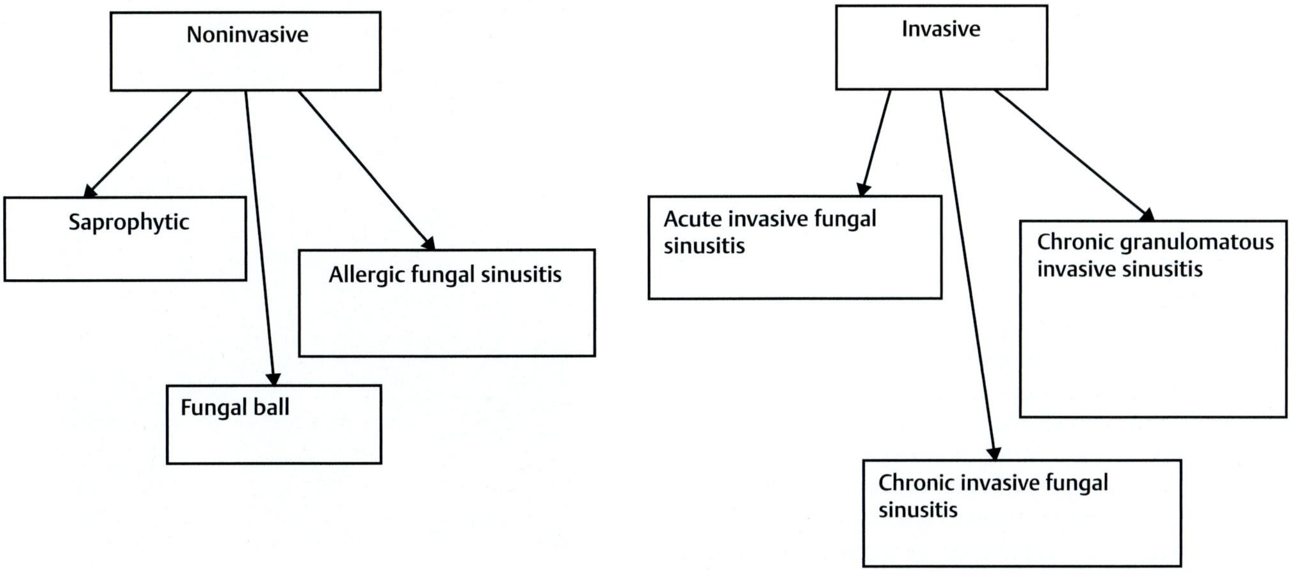

Fig. 5.2 Classifications of fungal sinusitis.

dependent on the manifestation of the disease than on the specific causative species. Noninvasive fungal sinus infections include saprophytic fungal growth, fungus ball, and allergic fungal sinusitis. Invasive sinus disease includes acute and chronic invasive sinusitis and chronic granulomatous invasive sinusitis.

Saprophytic Fungal Growth

Saprophytic fungal growth refers to the proliferation of fungi on a nutritional substrate from which it derives sustenance. In the nose, it may present as a visible growth of fungi on dried mucous or crusts within the sinonasal cavity in an asymptomatic patient. The true incidence of this process is unknown. Fungal growth often occurs postoperatively. Following nasal surgery, disruption in the mucociliary transport pathways may lead to the formation of crusts. These crusts provide the ideal environment to support fungal growth.

Saprophytic growth can be diagnosed on nasal endoscopy as the fungi can often easily be seen flourishing on crusts. Though culture of fungal colonies is likely to generate positive identification, it is of little clinical relevance. Treatment is generally simple and includes office debridement and daily nasal saline irrigations until the process is resolved.[9] Antifungal irrigations have not been adequately studied, but likely provide no additional benefit in this easily treatable process.[10,11] Radiographic imaging provides no additional information.

Fungus Ball

Sinus fungal ball, previously referred to a mycetoma, refers to a fungal mass that is usually unilateral and most often occurs in the maxillary sinus. It presents in immunocompetent persons with equal sex distribution.[12] Most studies agree that this process is mainly seen in the older population, most often occurring in the seventh decade. There may be a geographic predisposition; however, this has not been adequately studied. Fungal ball likely results from fungal exposure in a poorly ventilated sinus. Other theories include accessory ostia and recirculation, which traps spores within the sinus. Those individuals who develop sinus fungal ball are not any more likely than the general population to be atopic. It is not associated with aspirin sensitivity or peripheral eosinophilia. Although some have proposed that allergic rhinitis may be a predisposing factor, the literature does not support a higher incidence of allergic rhinitis in patients who develop sinus fungal ball.

Clinical presentation is often nonspecific. Patients often present with symptoms similar to chronic rhinosinusitis though with a prolonged course, which is refractory to medical management. Patients rarely complain of allergic symptoms. They may complain of facial pain and pressure, congestion, cacosmia (fetid smells), or report blowing a "gravel-like" substance from their nose.[12,13] Associated nasal polyposis is seen in up to 10% due to the chronic inflammatory response. As the fungal ball grows, mass effect resulting in sinus obstruction and worsening symptoms may occur.[14]

Nasal endoscopy is often normal or may reveal mild mucosal edema. Radiographic assessment is often required to make the diagnosis due to nonspecific symptoms and paucity of physical exam findings. Computed tomography (CT) of the sinuses is often ordered to evaluate refractory symptoms. Unilateral, single sinus involvement is seen in 59 to 94% (**Fig. 5.3**). Of the paranasal sinuses, the maxillary sinus is most often involved. Complete or subtotal opacification of the involved sinus is not uncommon. Up to 41% demonstrated heterogeneous opacification with calcifications. Bony erosion or sclerosis from mass effect can be identified in 17 to 36%.[15–17]

Treatment involves endoscopic surgical removal of the disease and restoration of sinus aeration (**see Video 5.1**). Antifungal medications are not indicated because recurrence rates are less than 4 to 7% after adequate endoscopic management.[15,18] Fungal cultures taken from the specimen are often negative because most of the fungal elements within the ball are nonviable. Only 23 to 50% of cultures are positive.[13,15] When identification is successful, however, the pathogen most commonly responsible is *Aspergillus*.

Histopathologically, the sinus fungal ball consists of a dense accumulation of fungal hyphae (**Fig. 5.4**). No sinus

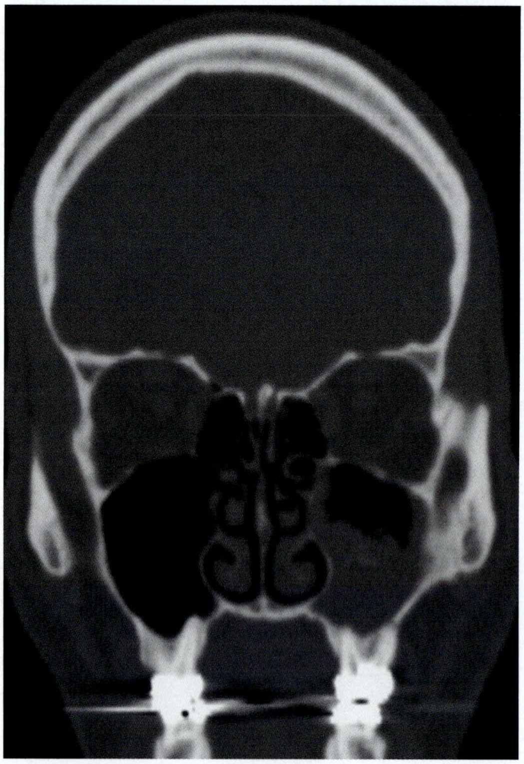

Fig. 5.3 A computed tomography (CT) scan of a left maxillary fungus ball demonstrating areas of heterogeneity within the maxillary sinus.

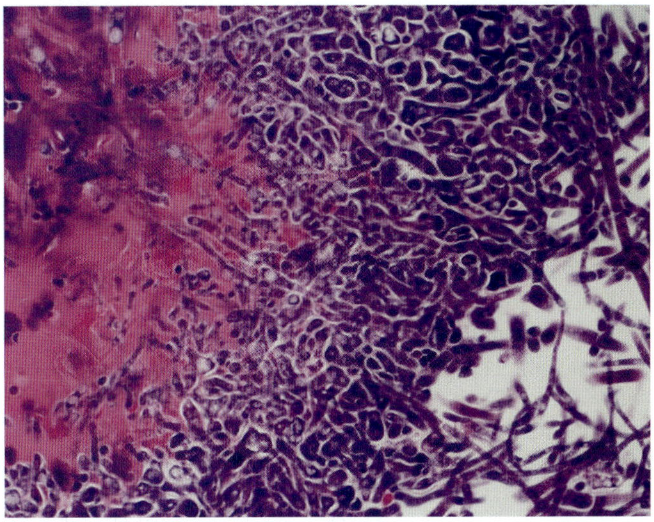

Fig. 5.4 Histologic appearance of fungal ball demonstrating densely packed fungal hyphae.

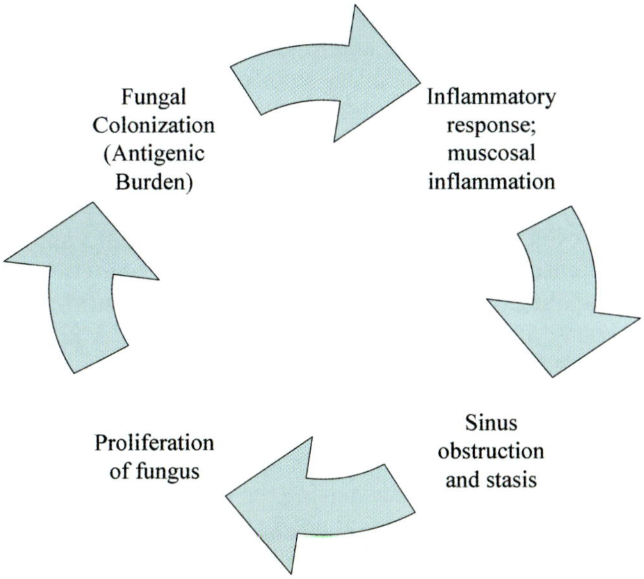

Fig. 5.5 The allergic fungal sinusitis (AFS) cycle.

mucosal invasion or granulomatous reaction can be identified. A chronic inflammatory response is indicated by the mucosal accumulation of plasma cells and lymphocytes. The fungus may be visualized on routine H&E staining; however, special stains may be required in certain cases.[15]

Long-term follow-up is not necessary after the postoperative period given that the incidence of recurrence is so low and no chronic medical management is needed postoperatively.

Allergic Fungal Sinusitis

Allergic fungal sinusitis (AFS) is characterized by fungal sinusitis and allergic mucin in an immunocompetent, but atopic individual. It is now recognized to be an immunologic process as opposed to an infectious one, although its etiology and pathogenesis are incompletely understood. Atopy can be clinically defined as having two of the following conditions: asthma, allergic rhinitis, eczema; or having one of the previous conditions and elevated immunoglobulin E (IgE).[19] AFS is seen in 7% of patients undergoing nasal sinus surgery.[20] It most commonly afflicts pediatric and younger patients; however, any age group can be affected.

Patients with AFS often have asthma, eosinophilia, and increased fungus-specific IgE. Elevated IgE is not limited to fungal antigens, however.[21] The disease is characterized by a self-perpetuating cycle of inflammation (**Fig. 5.5**). An antigenic challenge begins the cycle when colonizing fungi cause allergic mucosal inflammation within the paranasal sinuses. Although this was originally thought to trigger an IgE-mediated response, it now appears that the inflammatory cascade may be much broader than simple IgE-mediated fungal sensitivity.[22] Resulting inflammation leads to anatomic sinus obstruction and stasis ultimately creating an ideal environment for proliferation of fungus. Fungal proliferation then propagates a continuous and mounting antigenic challenge.[23]

Fungal-specific IgE levels have been found to be elevated in the vast majority of patients with AFS, even those in the postoperative period after adequate treatment.[24] Fungal-specific IgE frequently fails to decrease after immunotherapy, which is expected with other diseases mediated by IgE hypersensitivity.[25] Elevated total IgE (>1,000 U/mL) has been shown to be a good predictor of AFS recurrence following initial management.

Patients often present with clinical symptoms similar to those of chronic rhinosinusitis, including facial pressure, headaches, nasal congestion or discharge, and cough. AFS should be suspected in individuals with intractable sinusitis and polyposis. A nonspecific indicator of paranasal sinus inflammation, polyposis is present in nearly 100% of patients with AFS.[26] Bent and Kuhn have developed a set of four diagnostic criteria to accurately define AFS, see **Table 5.1**.[27]

Radiographic exam of the sinuses is often performed due to the chronic nature of the symptoms. Proteinaceous al-

Table 5.1 Diagnostic Criteria in Allergic Fungal Sinusitis

1. Type I hypersensitivity reaction as demonstrated by skin test, history, or serology
2. Nasal polyposis
3. Characteristic radiographic findings
4. The presence of eosinophilic mucin

lergic mucin has a typical radiographic appearance. Characteristic serpiginous, heterogeneous signal intensity is present within the maxillary sinus on CT (**Fig. 5.6**). The accumulations of heavy metals such as iron and manganese and calcium salt precipitation within inspissated allergic fungal mucin are responsible for this heterogenous signal. Longstanding expansile growth of polyps and/or mucin may result in bony remodeling or even erosion. AFS appears isointense to hypointense on T1-weighted magnetic resonance imaging (MRI) and a signal void corresponding to inspissated mucous is seen on T2-weighted MRI. MRI is not indicated in the routine workup of AFS.[28]

Allergic mucin has a very distinctive appearance when encountered endoscopically. It may be variable in color, ranging from green to brown or black. It is thick and tenacious; often described as having the consistency of peanut butter. The thick mucin and polyps form an expansile mass which may widen natural ostia. Although this results in sinus obstruction, it also facilitates complete debridement during surgery. Histologic exam of allergic mucin reveals intact and degenerating eosinophils in sheets, Charcot-Leyden crystals (a product of eosinophil degeneration), cellular debris, and noninvasive fungal elements (**Fig. 5.7**). Sinus mucosal specimens often have a mixed cellular inflammatory infiltrate.[19]

A variety of dematiaceous fungi are responsible for AFS. *Bipolaris* are the most commonly represented; however, *Curvularia* and *Alternaria* are also frequently identified.[29]

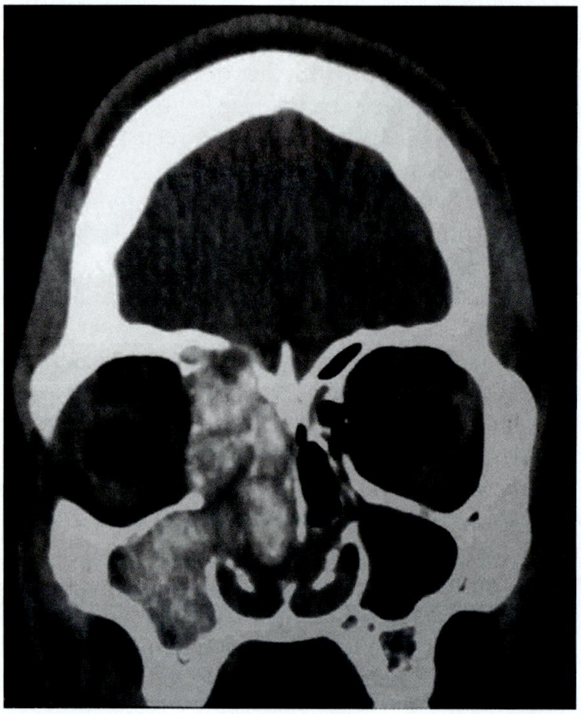

Fig. 5.6 A computed tomography (CT) scan of allergic fungal sinusitis (AFS) involving the right maxillary and ethmoid sinuses and demonstrating characteristic heterogeneity.

Fungal cultures may be difficult to obtain given that allergic mucin usually contains few fungal organisms. When an organism is isolated, its role in AFS cannot be determined absolutely. Depending on the methods used, fungal organisms can be isolated from virtually any nose, even those that are healthy. This makes interpretation of fungal cultures difficult in cases of AFS. Therefore, histologic examination of allergic mucin for fungal elements is required to confirm a positive fungal culture or to reject a negative culture.[29]

The pathophysiology of allergic fungal sinusitis involves antigen exposure in an atopic individual and resulting inflammation. Therefore, AFS is best controlled when these three areas of the disease are addressed: antigen exposure, atopy, and inflammatory response. Surgical debridement of mucin and polyps is indicated to decrease the antigenic burden and to reestablish sinus aeration and wide drainage pathways. Surgery also provides improved access to the paranasal sinuses allowing for postoperative irrigation and clinical surveillance with thorough outpatient endoscopy (**see Video 5.2**). Oral steroids are routinely given 1 week preoperatively and continued 3 weeks postoperatively. Several studies have supported the use of systemic corticosteroids in the perioperative period as they have been shown to extend the time before revision surgery.[30,31] Some advocate low-dose steroid taper over 3 months in intractable cases. In addition, topical nasal steroids and nasal salt water rinses are routinely prescribed for postoperative care. No studies have specifically evaluated the role of nasal steroids in patients with AFS; however, they are generally accepted as a standard part of postoperative therapy.

Following surgical removal of disease, some practitioners will elect to refer patients with AFS for antigen-specific immunotherapy. Immunotherapy for multiple fungal and nonfungal antigens may dramatically reduce the need

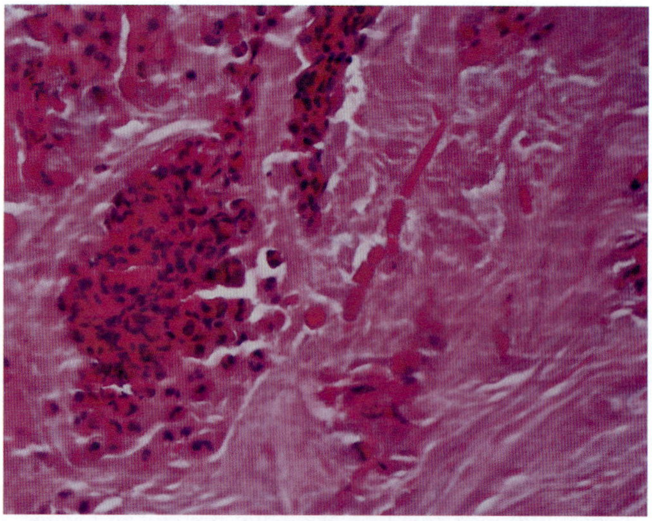

Fig. 5.7 High-powered hematoxylin and eosin (H&E) stain demonstrating allergic mucin and clusters of eosinophils.

for further systemic corticosteroids and revision surgery, especially during the early stages of postoperative management.[24] Most important, patients also require long-term clinic follow-up for maintenance of the sinus cavity. Thorough endoscopic exam with debridement if necessary is important to identify recurrent disease early. A short course of systemic steroids should be given for signs of relapse. Topical nasal steroids are often continued through several immunotherapy treatments.

Some studies have advocated for the use of intranasal antifungal treatments, such as amphotericin B. There are few studies that suggest antifungal irrigations or spray may be beneficial in the treatment of AFS. Studies to date have not verified any benefit from this treatment. However, intranasal antifungal treatment appears intuitively reasonable and may prove appropriate in certain cases.[32] The benefits of systemic antifungals are generally outweighed by the side effects and their use does not appear to significantly alter the course of AFS.

Interestingly, fungal sensitivity also may play a role in chronic rhinosinusitis (CRS). Unlike patients with AFS, patients with CRS do not consistently have IgE-mediated allergy. Ponikau was able to obtain positive fungal identification in nearly all patients with CRS and 100% of healthy controls using very sensitive testing strategies. In those patients with CRS, however, isolated peripheral blood monocytes exposed to *Alternaria* extract in an ex vivo experimental model resulted in statistically significant elevations in interleukin (IL-) 5, IL-8, and interferon- (IFN-) γ when compared with normal controls. This suggests that the underlying cause of CRS may be related to fungal sensitization with or without an IgE mediated response.[22] Although these findings support a fungal role in CRS, the extent to which fungus is involved is yet to be determined. Alternatively, CRS and AFS may exist in a spectrum of sinonasal disease; both occurring because of the bodies variable immunologic response to fungal and nonfungal antigens.

Invasive Fungal Sinusitis

Persons with impaired cellular immunity are even more susceptible to mycotic infections. There is a growing population of immunocompromised people in the United States, and in the world, including those with impaired neutrophil function, hematogenous dyscrasias, diabetes mellitus, AIDS or those taking immunosuppressant medications such as certain chemotherapeutic agents and systemic corticosteroids. One must maintain a high level of suspicion for invasive fungal sinusitis (IFS) in these patients. There are rare reports of IFS occurring in immunocompetent persons.

Invasive fungal sinusitis implies mucosal invasion by fungal elements. It should be suspected in any immunocompromised patient with fever and paranasal sinus symptoms. Like other forms of sinusitis, headache, congestion, orbital swelling, and facial pain may all be present. If suspected, swift action to confirm the diagnosis and begin treatment is necessary.[33] IFS can be classified into three groups depending on the time course of disease progression and histology: acute IFS, chronic IFS, and chronic granulomatous fungal sinusitis (**Table 5.1**).

Acute Invasive Fungal Sinusitis

Acute invasive fungal sinusitis (AIFS) occurs almost exclusively in the immunosuppressed population. Any patient with symptoms referable to the paranasal sinuses and fever deserves a complete head and neck physical examination. Fever is the most consistent sign in patients later diagnosed with AIFS.[34] Intraoral examination may reveal invasion of the disease through the hard palate. Evaluation of facial sensation is important because anesthesia in the distribution of V2 is an early sign of invasive sinus disease. Nasal endoscopy is variable. Findings may range from edematous mucosa to the presence of frankly necrotic material. It is important to follow the nasal mucosa examination over time for changes or the development of suspicious lesions. Nasal exam findings will often change dramatically in a short period in patients with AIFS. The evolution of lesions or the development of frank necrosis should be identified early.

Radiologic evaluation is not diagnostically specific; however, it is necessary for evaluating the extent of the disease and for surgical planning. It also can be used to objectively assess disease progression over time. CT findings of early AIFS are similar to those of bacterial sinusitis. Unfortunately, abnormalities on sinus CT are relatively common in immunocompromised individuals. In a study by Kavanagh, up to 42% of patients with leukemia and no evidence of fungal sinusitis were found to have abnormal findings on sinus CT.[35] The most consistent, albeit nonspecific radiographic finding in IFS is severe unilateral sinus mucosal edema.[36] In advanced cases, bony erosion or extranasal spread may be present. Orbital or intracranial involvement is best evaluated using MRI. When AIFS specifically involves the maxillary sinus, the possibility for orbital extension must be examined.

Urgent endoscopic biopsy should be obtained and sent for frozen section evaluation and culture. If possible, a specimen for culture should be taken prior to initiation of systemic antifungals; however, delay of treatment when AIFS is suspected is not acceptable. Biopsies are best performed in the operating room (OR), as patients are often thrombocytopenic and at high risk for bleeding. It is advisable to correct the thrombocytopenia to a platelet count of at least 60 billion per liter.[37] Specimens from frankly necrotic areas are less likely to be pathologically diagnostic. Biopsies should be exact, and performed at the edge of ischemic mucosa to increase the likelihood of visible fungal elements.[37] When biopsies from suspicious areas fail to provide the diagnosis, directed biopsies of apparently normal mucosa should be sent for frozen examination. IFS involves the middle turbinate in 67% and the nasal septum in 24%.[36,37]

The pathologist should be informed of the suspected diagnosis prior to preparing the frozen sections because special staining techniques are required. Under microscopic examination, fungal elements may be observed in the mucosa, submucosa, blood vessels, or bone (**Fig. 5.8**). If frozen sections are confirmed, appropriate antifungal treatment should be started and extensive surgical resection performed. It is unlikely to obtain fungal speciation on frozen section, however, permanent sections usually allow for specific fungal species to be identified. Culture can often take weeks to grow.

Extensive surgical debridement is advised immediately after diagnosis and on an as-needed basis as the disease progresses and more necrotic tissue appears. Angioinvasion by the fungal elements results in ischemic and devitalized tissue (**Fig. 5.9**). This allows the infection to flourish and further propagate as fungal growth is accelerated in acidotic environments. Mucosa that is pale and does not bleed normally indicates ischemia and likely affected tissue, which should also be resected even though it is not grossly necrotic.[37]

The most important intervention affecting disease outcome in AIFS is reversal of the condition causing the immunodeficiency.[37] If possible, diabetic ketoacidosis should be corrected, immunosuppressant medications discontinued or other methods of reversing immunosuppression employed. Amphotericin B is the initial systemic antifungal therapy of choice. Doses range from 0.8 to 1.5 mg/kg per day. Toxic side effects determine the dosage the patient can tolerate. Nephrotoxicity is often the dose-limiting factor.

Systemic antifungals have high toxicity; therefore, routine prophylaxis of immunocompromised patients is not recommended. However, hospital protocols for early detection of IFS allow for early treatment and can dramatically reduce morbidity and mortality. Prophylactic systemic antifungals are given to patients with a history of IFS who are expected to become immunocompromised again.[33]

AIFS can be caused by any number of fungal species; however, the most common culprits are *Aspergillus* species and members of the family Mucoraceae (*Mucor, Rhizomucor, Absidia*). *Aspergillus* species have narrow hyphae with regular septations that occur at 45-degree branching angles. *Aspergillus fumigatus* is the most common species identified in IFS and often results in the most virulent cases. Mucormycosis is characterized by broad, ribbon-like hyphae, which are irregular with rare septations. Mucoraceae grow rapidly and cultures can often be confirmed within 24 hours. *Mucor* has a propensity for early vascular invasion and obliteration resulting in rapidly progressive ischemia. Mucormycosis is the most acutely fatal fungal infection in humans. Other possible but less common species that may be identified include *Fusarium, Alternaria, Pseudallescheria boydii, Candida*, and *Bipolaris*.[38,39]

Chronic Invasive Fungal Sinusitis

Chronic invasive fungal sinusitis (CIFS) is a slowly progressing form of invasive fungal sinus disease with similar histopathologic findings to AIFS. Symptoms often evolve over 4 to 6 weeks before clear evidence of the sinonasal process is identified. Much like AIFS, patients complain of nonspecific symptoms that resemble CRS. However, symptoms are prolonged and refractory to medical management. In fact,

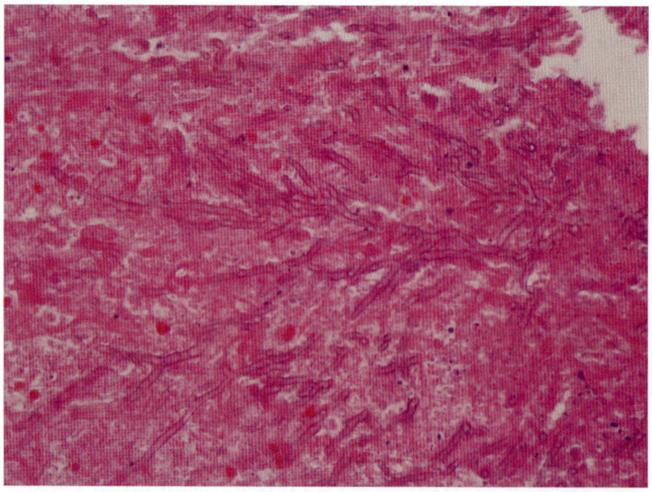

Fig. 5.8 High-powered hematoxylin and eosin (H&E) stain of fungal elements invading into mucosa.

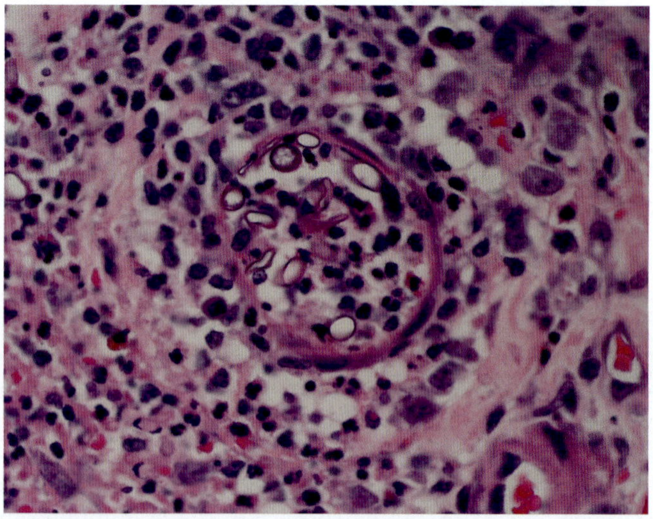

Fig. 5.9 High-powered hematoxylin and eosin (H&E) stain of fungal elements demonstrating intravascular invasion.

diagnosis may be difficult until complications of the disease, such as sensory dysfunction, proptosis, or altered mental status occur.

Diagnosis of CIFS requires the same diligence as when AIFS is suspected. A complete head and neck exam, including nasal endoscopy is warranted. Biopsies should be performed if the physical exam suggests possible fungal disease. Frank necrosis is unlikely in CIFS, and the nasal exam is better characterized by nonspecific findings such as mucous or inflammatory mucosa.

A CT scan should be obtained in the patient with paranasal sinus symptoms and immunocompromise or in patients with suspicious exam findings. Despite the often nonspecific findings, imaging is more useful in patients with CIFS because it can exclude other processes. MRI may be useful when dural or orbital invasion is suspected or denoted on CT. When CIFS is suspected in an immunocompromised patient with refractory nasal symptoms, imaging can be most useful in identifying areas in which the most high-yield biopsies could be obtained.

In contrast to AIFS, CIFS is most often caused by *Aspergillus* species. Again, fungal elements are angioinvasive resulting in mucosal ischemia and eventually necrosis. Although this can be viewed in pathologic specimens, the process is much slower than seen in AIFS. Diagnostic biopsies may be difficult to obtain due to the slowly progressive nature of the disease.

In general, CIFS is treated in a similar manner to AIFS. Once invading fungal elements are identified, debridement of involved sinonasal mucosa is performed and systemic antifungal therapy is begun. Boundaries for surgical debridement may be more difficult to delineate given the disease shows a less dramatic progression. Most would agree that complete debridement of grossly involved mucosa is warranted. This may require several trips to the OR as the disease progresses.

Long-term outcomes following CIFS are scarce in the literature. Absolute mortality has not been adequately examined; however, it is likely improved compared with AIFS. Recurrences of CIFS are common, especially in patients who become recurrently immunocompromised. Repeat nasal endoscopy and imaging following surgical debridement is likely to augment early detection of recurrence. Like AIFS, patients with a history of CIFS who are expected to become immunocompromised again should be treated with prophylactic systemic antifungal medication. Otherwise, the routine prophylactic use of systemic antifungals is not warranted given the side effect profile of these medications.

Prevention of invasive fungal disease, whether acute or chronic, is important in all immunocompromised patients. High-efficiency particulate air filter systems (HEPA) may eliminate fungal exposure. Sources of fungi, such as plants, should be removed from the patient's immediate environment.

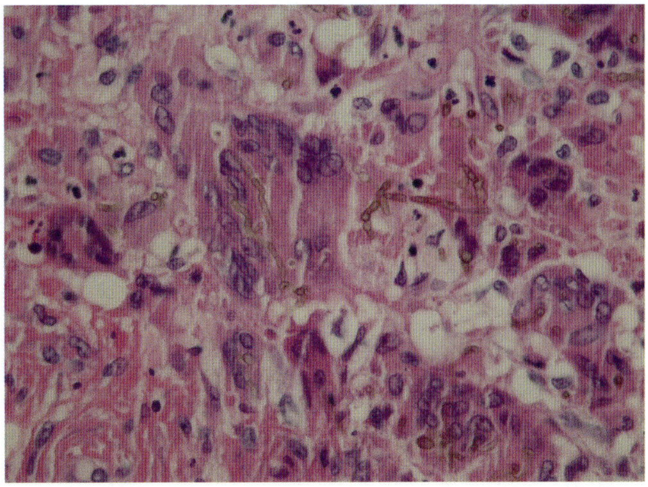

Fig. 5.10 High-powered hematoxylin and eosin (H&E) stain demonstrating chronic granulomatous invasive fungal sinusitis. Multinucleated giant cell granulomas, eosinophilia, and invasive fungal elements can be seen.

Patients may have significant complications related to IFS even after remission is obtained. The most common of these is bacterial rhinosinusitis. Chronic osteomyelitis has been reported. Long-term follow-up with routine nasal endoscopy should be arranged.[40]

Chronic Granulomatous Fungal Sinusitis

Although invasive fungal sinus disease is exceedingly rare in immunocompetent individuals, fungal growth may sometimes occur despite adequate immunity. This is a distinct entity characterized by invasive fungal sinusitis which occurs in an immunocompetent individual. It is almost exclusively encountered in Sudan and Northern India. As opposed to invasive fungal sinusitis, chronic granulomatous fungal sinusitis is less fulminant, and progresses over months to years. Symptoms, clinical presentation, and physical exam are similar to patients with chronic invasive sinusitis; however, disease rarely invades the skull base or dura. The etiologic agent is almost invariably found to be *Aspergillus flavus*. The diagnosis is made intraoperatively by histologic exam of multinucleated giant cell granulomas, which are centered on an eosinophilic core (**Fig. 5.10**). Treatment involves surgical debridement. There is controversy over the role of postoperative systemic antifungal therapy. There is a paucity of outcome studies in the literature supporting routine use of antifungal medications in chronic granulomatous fungal sinusitis. Many would advocate for its use, especially in advanced cases.[41]

Pearls

- There are several manifestations of fungal disease in the maxillary sinuses. Noninvasive fungal diseases include allergic fungal sinusitis, fungal ball, and saprophytic fungal infections. Invasive fungal disease includes acute and chronic invasive fungal sinusitis or chronic granulomatous fungal sinusitis.
- Maxillary sinus fungal ball often presents with unilateral sinus disease and unrelenting symptoms of rhinosinusitis. Treatment involves complete surgical removal of fungal elements.
- Allergic fungal sinusitis is characterized by the presence of allergic mucin in patients with symptoms of chronic rhinosinusitis, polyposis, and an IgE-mediated hypersensitivity reaction to fungal elements resulting in a self-perpetuating inflammatory cascade.
- Both medical therapy and surgical intervention are employed in the treatment of AFS. Surgery is performed to reestablish sinus aeration and to promote improved sinus access for medical therapy. Medical therapy, including immunotherapy, is imperative to lengthen time between, or even prevent, recurrences.
- A high index of suspicion for invasive fungal sinusitis is necessary in patients with immunodeficiency, fever, and symptoms referable to the paranasal sinuses. Immediate endoscopic wide debridement of necrotic debris and fungal elements as well as intervenous antifungals is indicated.
- If possible, reversal of the underlying cause of immunodeficiency is the most important treatment aspect affecting survival.

References

1. Mitchell TG. Overview of basic medical mycology. Otolaryngol Clin North Am 2000;33(2):237–249
2. Manning SC, Schaefer SD, Close LG, Vuitch F. Culture-positive allergic fungal sinusitis. Arch Otolaryngol Head Neck Surg 1991;117(2):174–178
3. Taylor MJ, Ponikau JU, Sherris DA, et al. Detection of fungal organisms in eosinophilic mucin using a fluorescein-labeled chitin-specific binding protein. Otolaryngol Head Neck Surg 2002;127(5):377–383
4. Mackenzie JJ. Preliminary report on *Aspergillus mycosis* of the antrum maxillare. Bull Johns Hopkins Hosp 1893;3:9–10
5. Katzenstein AL, Sale SR, Greenberger PA. Pathologic findings in allergic aspergillus sinusitis. A newly recognized form of sinusitis. Am J Surg Pathol 1983;7(5):439–443
6. Deshazo RD. Syndromes of invasive fungal sinusitis. Med Mycol 2009;47(Suppl 1):S309–S314
7. Michael RC, Michael JS, Ashbee RH, Mathews MS. Mycological profile of fungal sinusitis: An audit of specimens over a 7-year period in a tertiary care hospital in Tamil Nadu. Indian J Pathol Microbiol 2008;51(4):493–496 Abstract
8. Olszewski J, Miłoński J. [The analysis of the bacterial and fungal flora in maxillary sinuses in patients operated due to FESS method]. Otolaryngol Pol 2008;62(4):458–461
9. Ferguson BJ. Definitions of fungal rhinosinusitis. Otolaryngol Clin North Am 2000;33(2):227–235
10. Ponikau JU, Sherris DA, Kephart GM, Adolphson C, Kita H. The role of ubiquitous airborne fungi in chronic rhinosinusitis. Clin Rev Allergy Immunol 2006;30(3):187–194
11. Kuhn FA, Javer AR. Allergic fungal rhinosinusitis: perioperative management, prevention of recurrence, and role of steroids and antifungal agents. Otolaryngol Clin North Am 2000;33(2):419–433
12. Corey JP, Romberger CF, Shaw GY. Fungal diseases of the sinuses. Otolaryngol Head Neck Surg 1990;103(6):1012–1015
13. deShazo RD, O'Brien M, Chapin K, et al. Criteria for the diagnosis of sinus mycetoma. J Allergy Clin Immunol 1997;99(4):475–485
14. Lee KC. Clinical features of the paranasal sinus fungus ball. J Otolaryngol 2007;36(5):270–273
15. Ferguson BJ. Fungus balls of the paranasal sinuses. Otolaryngol Clin North Am 2000;33(2):389–398
16. Ferreiro JA, Carlson BA, Cody DT III. Paranasal sinus fungus balls. Head Neck 1997;19(6):481–486
17. Klossek JM, Serrano E, Péloquin L, Percodani J, Fontanel JP, Pessey JJ. Functional endoscopic sinus surgery and 109 mycetomas of paranasal sinuses. Laryngoscope 1997;107(1):112–117
18. Grosjean P, Weber R. Fungus balls of the paranasal sinuses: a review. Eur Arch Otorhinolaryngol 2007;264(5):461–470
19. Fergusion BJ. Fungal rhinosinusitis: A spectrum of disease. Otolaryngol Clin North Am 2000;33(2):227–235
20. Kuhn FA, Javer AR. Allergic fungal rhinosinusitis: perioperative management, prevention of recurrence, and role of steroids and antifungal agents. Otolaryngol Clin North Am 2000;33(2):419–433
21. Wise SK, Ahn CN, Lathers DM, Mulligan RM, Schlosser RJ. Antigen-specific IgE in sinus mucosa of allergic fungal rhinosinusitis patients. Am J Rhinol 2008;22(5):451–456
22. Ponikau JU, Sherris DA, Kern EB, et al. The diagnosis and incidence of allergic fungal sinusitis. Mayo Clin Proc 1999;74(9):877–884
23. Manning SC, Holman M. Further evidence for allergic pathophysiology in allergic fungal sinusitis. Laryngoscope 1998;108(10):1485–1496
24. Mabry RL, Mabry CS. Allergic fungal sinusitis: the role of immunotherapy. Otolaryngol Clin North Am 2000;33(2):433–440
25. Marple B, Newcomer M, Schwade N, Mabry R. Natural history of allergic fungal rhinosinusitis: a 4- to 10-year follow-up. Otolaryngol Head Neck Surg 2002;127(5):361–366
26. Schubert MS, Goetz DW. Evaluation and treatment of allergic fungal sinusitis. I. Demographics and diagnosis. J Allergy Clin Immunol 1998;102(3):387–394
27. Bent JP III, Kuhn FA. Antifungal activity against allergic fungal sinusitis organisms. Laryngoscope 1996;106(11):1331–1334
28. Houser SM, Corey JP. Allergic fungal rhinosinusitis: pathophysiology, epidemiology, and diagnosis. Otolaryngol Clin North Am 2000;33(2):399–409
29. Manning SC, Schaefer SD, Close LG, Vuitch F. Culture-positive allergic fungal sinusitis. Arch Otolaryngol Head Neck Surg 1991;117(2):174–178
30. Marple BF. Allergic fungal rhinosinusitis: surgical management. Otolaryngol Clin North Am 2000; 33(2):409–419

31. Marple BF, Mabry RL. Comprehensive management of allergic fungal sinusitis. Am J Rhinol 1998; 12(4):263–268
32. Ponikau JU, Sherris DA, Weaver A, Kita H. Treatment of chronic rhinosinusitis with intranasal amphotericin B: a randomized, placebo-controlled, double-blind pilot trial. J Allergy Clin Immunol 2005;115(1):125–131
33. Delguadio JM, Clemson JA. An early detection protocol for invasive fungal sinusitis in neutropenic patients successfully reduces extent of disease at presentation and long term morbidity. Laryngoscope 2009;119(1):180–183
34. Gillespie MB, O'Malley BW Jr, Francis HW. An approach to fulminant invasive fungal rhinosinusitis in the immunocompromised host. Arch Otolaryngol Head Neck Surg 1998;124(5):520–526
35. Kavanagh KT, Hughes WT, Parham DM, Chanin LR. Fungal sinusitis in immunocompromised children with neoplasms. Ann Otol Rhinol Laryngol 1991;100(4 Pt 1):331–336
36. DelGaudio JM, Swain RE Jr, Kingdom TT, Muller S, Hudgins PA. Computed tomographic findings in patients with invasive fungal sinusitis. Arch Otolaryngol Head Neck Surg 2003;129(2):236–240
37. Gillespie MB, O'Malley BW. An algorithmic approach to the diagnosis and management of invasive fungal rhinosinusitis in the immunocompromised patient. Otolaryngol Clin North Am 2000;33(2):323–334
38. Schell WA. Unusual fungal pathogens in fungal rhinosinusitis. Otolaryngol Clin North Am 2000;33(2):367–373
39. Ferguson BJ. Mucormycosis of the nose and paranasal sinuses. Otolaryngol Clin North Am 2000;33(2):349–365
40. Otto KJ, Delgaudio JM. Invasive fungal rhinosinusitis: what is the appropriate follow-up? Am J Rhinol 2006;20(6):582–585
41. Stringer SP, Ryan MW. Chronic invasive fungal rhinosinusitis. Otolaryngol Clin North Am 2000;33(2):375–387

6 Special Considerations for Pediatric Maxillary Sinusitis

Matthew Whitley, Zoukaa Sargi, and Ramzi T. Younis

Pediatric sinusitis is a relatively common problem in the offices of both pediatricians and otolaryngologists. The average child has six to eight upper respiratory tract infections per year and it is estimated that 5 to 10% of these are complicated by rhinosinusitis.[1,2] Despite being relatively common, the sinus disease represents somewhat of an enigma for both parents and primary care physicians, leading to confusion as to the exact scope of the disease. Pediatric sinus disease, including disease specific to the maxillary sinus, can be classified into three categories: acute, subacute, and chronic. Acute rhinosinusitis (ARS) is defined as an upper respiratory infection (URI) that persists without significant improvement for longer than 10 days. This creates some confusion as a viral URI can last longer than 7 to 10 days. A key feature of ARS is that symptoms tend to worsen at 7 to 10 days versus the typical improvement seen with viral illness during this time. Chronic rhinosinusitis (CRS) is a chronic, low-grade infection that persists beyond 3 months. Recurrent acute rhinosinusitis describes recurrent bouts of ARS with interposed symptom-free periods,[2] in contrast with acute exacerbations of chronic rhinosinusitis.

Clinical Presentation

The key diagnostic dilemma is differentiating a viral URI from true rhinosinusitis, the duration and timing being key factors. ARS presents in children with signs and symptoms of nasal discharge and obstruction, persistent cough, and bad breath (halitosis). These symptoms persist beyond 10 days. A small subset present with a more fulminant condition featuring high fevers and purulent rhinorrhea, and a few children will have complications as presenting symptoms for acute maxillary sinusitis. Unlike adult patients, facial pain and headache are less common, especially in younger children (although adolescents may have these complaints as well).[1,2] Although rhinosinusitis pathophysiology is tied closely to allergy, most parents deny signs and symptoms of allergy. Despite this, a family history of allergy and asthma are common in these patients.[3]

One classic symptom of pediatric sinusitis is a chronic cough that worsens at night, although this symptom is also common with chronic adenoiditis. This should be differentiated from chronic cough worse in the daytime, which is more suggestive of asthma (although the two entities are closely related).[3] Fiberoptic exam may be within normal limits, although frank purulence is sometimes seen (**Fig. 6.1**).

The role of imaging studies in the diagnosis of sinusitis is different in children versus adults. Plain radiographs are rarely used due to low sensitivity to detect sinusitis. Although computed tomography (CT) is the gold standard for sinus imaging, it is less useful for diagnostic purposes in the pediatric population. Manning et al showed that 47% of children without chronic sinusitis had abnormalities on CT scans. These patients often had resolving URI or allergic symptoms (i.e., very low specificity).[4] Another study showed that 46% of random CT scans in asymptomatic patients showed mucoperiosteal thickening.[5] Despite this, several specific imaging findings probably do correlate with severity of disease: air fluid levels/bubbles, expansion of the maxillary sinus outflow tract through the infundibulum, and thickened bony septations.[3] Based on the above, CT and plain film imaging serve little purpose in the diagnosis of rhinosinusitis. One exception is the use of lateral neck plain imaging to evaluate the size of the adenoid pad. Many advocate reserving CT imaging until the patient has failed maximal medical therapy. In this context, imaging is used in preoperative planning and serves as a road map for the surgical procedure.

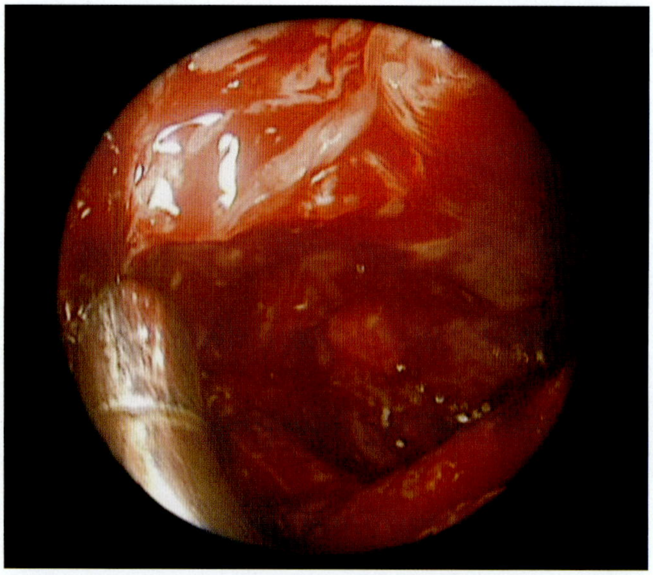

Fig. 6.1 Endoscopic view of diseased mucosa in a left maxillary sinus during episode of acute on chronic maxillary sinusitis in a 10-year-old boy after wide maxillary antrostomy.

Predisposing Factors

The pathophysiology of pediatric maxillary sinusitis is multifactorial and represents the end point of many possible predisposing conditions. In essence, sinusitis is a presumed bacterial infection of a previously damaged underlying mucosa. This damage can be caused by and altered by many factors. In children, rhinosinusitis is generally a problem of mucosal defense more so than one of anatomic obstruction, although these two factors both come into play. A full discussion of the pathophysiology of sinus disease is beyond the scope of this chapter. Some of the factors that lead to maxillary sinus disease are described below.

Allergy

There is a well-established relationship between pediatric sinusitis and allergy and allergic rhinitis. Although the rate of allergy in the general population is only 15 to 20%, more than 80% of children with rhinosinusitis have a positive family history of allergy.[2] The role of allergy in the development of sinusitis is twofold. First, allergic congestion can lead to obstruction of the ostiomeatal complex and block outflow of the maxillary sinus. Second, allergic mediators may have direct effects on the sinus mucosa itself.[2,3]

Environmental Toxins

The development of sinusitis can be exacerbated by the presence of certain airway pollutants. The most common of these is exposure to second-hand tobacco smoke, but other environmental irritants can also have similar effects. These substances have direct irritant effects on the nasal and sinus mucosa leading to impaired ciliary function.[2]

Chronic Adenoiditis

The adenoid pad serves as a bacterial reservoir that may play a part in the pathogenesis of both chronic otitis media and chronic sinusitis. An association has been shown between adenoid bacterial load and sinusitis symptom scores. There did not appear to be a relationship between the size of the adenoid pad and the bacterial load.[6] In addition, there is an 89% correlation between cultures taken from the adenoid pad and the middle meatus, further supporting this as a reservoir for infection.[7]

Gastroesophageal Reflux

Gastroesophageal reflux disease (GERD) has also been implicated as a contributing factor in CRS. Phipps et al studied 30 patients with CRS with dual pH probe monitoring and found that 63% had GERD. Furthermore, 32% of the patients had reflux that reached the nasopharynx; 79% of the patients' sinusitis improved with treatment of their GERD.[8] Another study by Bothwell et al showed when 30 patients that were candidates for sinus surgery were treated with antireflux measures, 89% improved such that surgery was avoided. This was a retrospective review, however.[9] When evaluating patients with CRS, the presence of GERD should be appreciated and included in the medical treatment.

Bacteriology

The microbiology of pediatric maxillary sinusitis does differ greatly from the adult population and consists mainly of *Streptococcus pneumoniae*, *Haemophilus influenzae*, and *Moraxella catarrhalis*, as well as *Staphylococcus aureus* and occasionally anaerobes. Drug-resistant organisms are becoming an increasingly common problem. Risk factors for the development of resistance include age younger than 2 years, day-care exposure, and frequent antibiotic treatment. Knowledge of resistance patterns in the community is a powerful tool.[1] See Chapter 3 for a full discussion of the microbiology of maxillary sinusitis. See below for the bacteriology of sinuses in cystic fibrosis.

Special Populations

Primary Immunodeficiency

All very young children essentially have a physiologic immunodeficiency, which will improve as the child's immune system matures.[3] In addition, a subset of patients have true primary immunodeficiency. The four most common immunodeficiencies in pediatric patients are transient hypogamma-globulinemia of infancy, immunoglobulin G (IgG) subclass deficiency, impaired polysaccharide responsiveness (partial antibody deficiency), and selective IgA deficiency. These patients have defects in the humoral immune system, with maintained function of the cellular, phagocytic, and complement systems. All are heterogeneous and include as a component recurrent bacterial upper respiratory infections, including sinusitis (as well as otitis media).[10] In addition, they normally present with recurrent lower respiratory infections including bronchitis and pneumonia.[2] The genetic factors underlying these conditions are poorly understood and the etiologies are felt to be multifactorial.[10] If one of these conditions is suspected, the physician should order total immunoglobulin, IgG subclasses, and vaccine response testing and should consider referral to a pediatric immunologist.[1]

Primary Ciliary Dyskinesia

Primary ciliary dyskinesia is a disorder of respiratory ciliary function. The patients present with recurrent respiratory tract infections, including pneumonia, bronchitis, otitis media, and sinusitis. The incidence is 1:16,000 live births.[3] The disorder originates from disorganization of the 9+2 microtubule organization of cilia or a defect in the dynein arms.[11] This creates an anatomic distortion in the structure of the cilia and also results in a functional defect noted with decreased ciliary beat frequency.[12] The disease can occur in isolation or as part of Kartagener syndrome (with situs inversus) in ~50% of cases.[2] The diagnosis is made with electron microscopy of nasal turbinate brushing or formal respiratory tract mucosa biopsy.

Cystic Fibrosis

Cystic fibrosis merits special mention in the discussion of pediatric maxillary sinusitis. This disease is the most common lethal hereditary disorder in the white population with a frequency of 1 in 2000 live births. Affected patients demonstrate a generalized exocrinopathy associated with progressive pulmonary disease and gastrointestinal tract malabsorption.[13] Patients with cystic fibrosis have almost universal paranasal sinus disease, which is a significant source of morbidity.

Pathophysiology of Sinus Disease in Cystic Fibrosis

The respiratory tree from the nasal cavity and sinuses down to the level of the distal bronchioles is lined with a ciliated pseudostratified epithelium that acts as an effective barrier against foreign particles, irritants, and microorganisms. The key to the effective function of this "mucociliary elevator" is the coordinated beating of the cilia. For this to occur, the overlying mucus layer must also be optimal. The classical hypothesis holds that the mucus layer is in fact two layers, a deep low-viscosity fluid that bathes the cilia (the sol layer) and a superficial more viscous gel layer. The former is made up of water and ions regulated by active transport by the epithelium, thus generating a transepithelial electrical potential difference. The thicker gel layers serve to catch inhaled foreign particles that are transported along the layer by the ciliary beat.[13,14]

Patients with cystic fibrosis have mutations in the cystic fibrosis transmembrane regulator (CFTR) gene on chromosome 7 that encodes for a chloride ion transporter. Secondary to this, chloride ion gradients are altered and the hydration and viscoelastic properties of mucus are altered. How this directly affects ciliary function is not well understood. Nevertheless, patients with cystic fibrosis have decreased mucociliary clearance that ranges from moderate to severe. Long-standing chronic inflammation is thought to produce changes in the mucosa including goblet cell hyperplasia, squamous cell metaplasia, and loss of ciliated cells. This further compromises mucosal function. In addition, bacterial byproducts may directly alter ciliary function.[14] In addition to the impaired mucosal function, patients with cystic fibrosis have mechanical obstruction of sinus ostia due to the altered mucus viscosity. This leads to infection and inflammation that further compromises sinus drainage.[14]

Nasal Polyposis in Cystic Fibrosis

Nasal polyposis is common in patients with cystic fibrosis with a reported incidence from 6 to 48%. Polyps tend to occur in this population between the ages of 5 to 20 years. Interestingly, the histopathology of cystic fibrosis polyps is different from those found in other patients. Specifically, CF polyps have a thin basement membrane, acidic mucin, and an absence of submucosal hyalinization and eosinophilia. In contrast, atopic polyps have a thick basement membrane, neutral mucin, and abundant eosiniphils.[14]

Anatomy of the Cystic Fibrosis Sinus

The maxillary sinus of patients with cystic fibrosis differs anatomically in that they are smaller in volume. This is thought to be secondary to decreased postnatal growth and pneumatization of the sinuses due to chronic inflammation. This is corroborated by the fact that these patients often have absent sphenoid and frontal sinuses (which in contrast to the maxillary sinus, initiate development postnatally).[14] Cystic fibrosis patients also have demineralization of the uncinate process and medial displacement of the lateral nasal wall. In addition, when these patients also have nasal polyposis, erosion or destruction of the lateral nasal wall is common. This has been hypothesized to be secondary to physical pressure of inspissated mucus and polyps on the thin bone or osteitis of the bone itself. These changes are commonly associated with the formation of a maxillary sinus mucocele, which is extremely rare in children and should raise the suspicion of cystic fibrosis in patients without the diagnosis.[14,15]

Bacteriology of Sinuses in Cystic Fibrosis

The bacteriology of sinus cultures in cystic fibrosis patients varies with age. In younger patients, *Staphylococcus aureus* and *Haemophilus influenzae* are most common. In older children and adults, *Pseudomonas aeruginosa* predominates. Cultures are polymicrobial 25 to 44% of the time and include the more typical respiratory pathogens mentioned above.[16]

Treatment

Medical Management

Acute Rhinosinusitis

The primary treatment of both acute rhinosinusitis and chronic rhinosinusitis is medical therapy. The initial treatment should address the appropriate controlling of the risk factors described above. Any treatment that fails to take these into account risks failure.[3] In addition, treatment must be planned in light of the fact that approximately two-thirds of pediatric ARS will resolve spontaneously. An evidence-based consensus practice guideline from the American Academy of Pediatrics in 2001 recommends amoxicillin in normal dose (45 mg/kg) or high dose (90 mg/kg) as first-line treatment in children that have mild to moderate disease. For more severe disease or those with high risk of resistant *Staphylococcus pneumoniae* should be given high-dose amoxicillin/clavulanate (90 mg/kg). Patients with mild penicillin allergy should receive cefdinir, cefuroxime, or cefpodoxime. Severe penicillin allergy warrants use of a macrolide.[2,16] Duration of therapy has not been well studied, but 7 to 10 days is generally regarded as acceptable. These recommendations have not changed substantially since 2001.

Chronic Rhinosinusitis

Chronic rhinosinusitis treatment begins with appropriate antimicrobial treatment. Initial treatment is with high-dose amoxicillin/clavulanate (90 mg/kg) or the above alternatives in the case of penicillin allergy. Unlike ARS, short courses of antibiotics commonly lead to treatment failure. Although there are no well-designed clinical trials supporting it, most experts advocate a duration of therapy ranging from 3 to 6 weeks.[2,3]

Adjuvant medical therapies complement antimicrobial treatment. Nasal saline rinses are used to remove inspissated mucus and secretions and improve patient comfort. Topical nasal steroids are routinely used, although the literature supporting their efficacy in children is sparse. Mometasone furoate is approved for children 2 years and older and has shown no effect on growth or pituitary function in children.[17,18] Fluticasone propionate is approved for children 4 years and older. Other sprays including budesonide and triamcinolone are approved for children 6 years and older. For a complete discussion of the medical treatment of sinusitis, see Chapter 4.

Surgical Management of Pediatric Sinusitis

In a subset of patients, symptoms or sinusitis persist despite maximal medical therapy. Several options exist for the surgical management of these patients. As mentioned above, computed tomography abnormalities are not a sufficient indication for surgical intervention. The criteria for surgery are the failure of prolonged maximal medical treatment after predisposing risk factors have been appropriately addressed.

Adenoidectomy

The first-line surgical treatment for pediatric is adenoidectomy. Several studies have provided support for efficacy in the treatment of rhinosinusitis. A prospective study of 37 children with chronic rhinosinusitis treated with adenoidectomy demonstrated a significant decrease in episodes of sinusitis and improvement in nasal obstruction.[19] A recent meta-analysis examined the effect of adenoidectomy on sinusitis. The review found improvement in pediatric sinusitis after adenoidectomy in 69.3% of patients.[20] This was based on caregiver-reported symptom scores.

Ramadan et al looked at risk factors for failure of adenoidectomy in the treatment of CRS. In 143 patients treated with adenoidectomy for CRS, 61 children "failed" with persistent symptoms postoperatively and subsequently underwent functional endoscopic sinus surgery. In their analysis, the presence of asthma and age <7 years were statistically significant for adenoidectomy failure. The presence of allergic rhinitis, CT score, and sex were not predictive.[21] In another recent study by the same author, children had improvement in cure rates when adenoidectomy was accompanied at the time of surgery by maxillary sinus washout.[22] Based on the current literature, adenoidectomy is a safe initial treatment for pediatric chronic rhinosinusitis that has failed medical therapy. The procedure is simple, can be done on an outpatient basis, and has little risk.

Functional Endoscopic Sinus Surgery

When medical management and adenoidectomy have failed to control CRS or when the patient has an anatomic or pathologic indication (i.e., mucocele), functional endoscopic sinus surgery (FESS) is a safe and effective therapy. Other indications include suppurative complications, nasal polyposis, neoplasms, and alteration of systemic disease by the presence of sinusitis (see below on cystic fibrosis). One difficulty is that there are currently no studies in the literature using validated outcomes measures to assess outcomes. A meta-analysis of pediatric FESS patients showed positive outcomes in 88.4% of the cases examined. The average combined follow-up time was 3.7 years and the complication rate was 0.6%. Other studies have shown that on longer follow-up, patients have high recurrence rates and lower cure rates.[3] FESS in children has prompted questions about the effect of surgery on subsequent facial growth. Several animal studies suggested this effect[23,24]; human studies have not substantiated this concern.[25,26]

Most authors agree that the concept of "less is more" applies specifically to children undergoing FESS. The two goals of surgery are to (1) restore patent physiologic communication between diseased sinuses and the nasal cavity, and (2) preserve normal anatomy.

Preoperative Evaluation

The most critical aspect of preoperative preparation is setting appropriate expectations for the caregivers. Surgery is generally a mechanism for reducing the severity of symptoms or increasing the time between episodes versus a true cure. Patients with cystic fibrosis and patients on prolonged antibiotics courses may have malabsorption and vitamin K deficiency that can predispose to bleeding.[2]

Maxillary Antrostomy / Uncinectomy

As with adults, the key to success with sinus surgery is successful removal of the uncinate process and the restoration of appropriate clearance through the ostiomeatal complex (OMC). Young children tend to have more narrow ethmoid cavities and a concave middle meatus. The uncinate itself is often immediately apposed to the lamina papyracea, which may project medially (thus predisposing to inadvertent orbital injury). The uncinate is retracted off of the lamina medially and a window created using a back biting forceps. This allows identification of the infundibulum and the natural ostium. The complete uncinate is removed (**see Video 6.1**). If necessary, the maxillary antrostomy in communication with the natural ostium is created in the posterior fontanelle. Care is taken not to disturb the anterior fontanelle of the natural ostium to prevent damage to the nasolacrimal system. Some authors advocate a "mini-FESS" procedure that includes an uncinectomy ± maxillary antrostomy and opening of the ethmoid bullae.[27] Others believe that the minimal surgery indicated is a formal maxillary antrostomy and anterior ethmoidectomy (**Fig. 6.2**).[2]

Postoperative Care

Postoperatively, patients are given nasal saline sprays twice daily and treated with topical nasal steroids. In the past, FESS was a two-stage procedure and the patient was brought back to the operating room 2 to 4 weeks after the initial surgery for debridement under anesthesia. Currently, this second stage is reserved for patients with specific needs for the procedure, including very ill patients and all patients with systemic abnormalities including cystic fibrosis, primary ciliary dyskinesia (PCD), and immunodeficiency.[28]

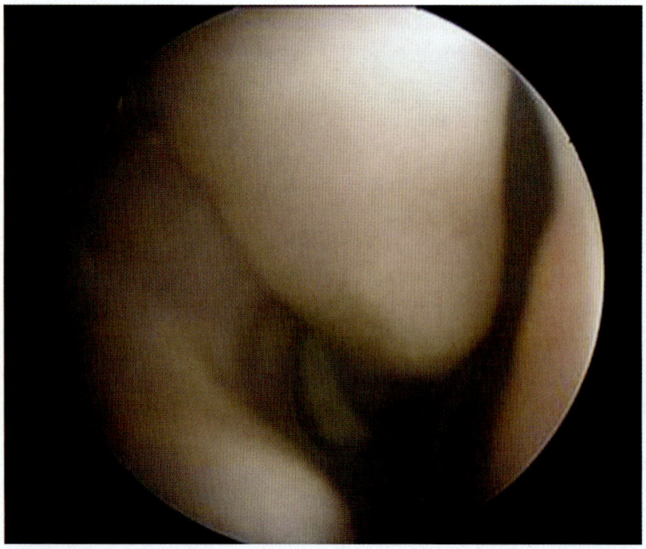

Fig. 6.2 Endoscopic view of frank purulence in the right posterior middle meatus in a 7-year-old child with acute maxillary sinusitis.

Treatment of Chronic Rhinosinusitis in Cystic Fibrosis Patients

Like the disease process itself, the treatment of rhinosinusitis has several unique aspects. Similar to typical patients, medical therapy consists of long-term antibiotics and adjunct treatment with nasal saline irrigation. Only one clinical trial looking at inhaled steroids in the CF population exists in the literature. This study showed significant symptom improvement and a decrease in polyp size in patients treated with 100 µg of betamethasone twice daily for 6 weeks, although the study was in adults with CF and follow-up was limited.[29] Nasally inhaled dornase alfa (Pulmozyme; Hoffmann-La Roche, Basel, Switzerland) is a highly purified solution of recombinant human deoxyribonuclease I that has been used as a mucolytic in CF patients. A trial compared 24 CF patients that underwent FESS and were then randomized to one year treatment with dornase alfa or placebo. The treatment group showed improvement in symptoms, CT appearance, and endoscopic exam score.[30]

The use of topical tobramycin treatment for CRS in CF patients is well described in the literature, specifically in the perioperative period surrounding lung transplant. The sinuses are thought to serve as a reservoir for *Pseudomonas aeruginosa* in these patients, a microorganism that is the cause of several serious postoperative complications in these patients. In one study, patients underwent FESS with the placement of a maxillary sinus irrigation catheter at the end of the case. Tobramycin was given for 10 days postoperatively. Weekly administration was performed under local anesthesia for up to 3 weeks. The study's clinical outcome measures were vague, but they did demonstrate negative sinus *P. aeruginosa* cultures at the completion of treatment.[31] Another study used the same protocol and found dramatically decreased rates of need for revision surgery and recurrence of disease, but no difference in *P. aeruginosa* sinus colonization.[32]

Studies have demonstrated FESS to be a safe procedure for those with cystic fibrosis with low rates of complications such as bleeding.[32] The surgical approach is similar to non-CF patients, although studies have shown better symptom scores and lower rate of recurrence with more extensive surgery. Future research is centered on the use of intranasal gentamicin and low-dose systemic macrolide therapy as novel treatments for CRS in CF patients.[33]

Conclusion

Pediatric maxillary sinusitis is a common problem whose primary medical treatment leads to resolution for the majority of patients. Adenoidectomy and FESS provide safe alternatives for those that fail maximum medical therapy. Physicians treating these patients should be attuned to the specific needs of the pediatric population and those of patients with other systemic diseases.

Pearls

- Unlike adults, chronic sinusitis in children is associated with less headache and facial pain; instead, it commonly presents with cough that is worse at night.
- Computed tomography scans are of limited diagnostic value for chronic rhinosinusitis in children.
- Pediatric sinus disease has a strong correlation with allergy.
- The adenoids are thought to serve as a bacterial reservoir in the pathophysiology of pediatric sinusitis.
- Patients with cystic fibrosis have universal chronic sinusitis, a source of significant morbidity for these patients.
- The maxillary sinus of patients with cystic fibrosis differs anatomically in that they are smaller in volume.
- Cystic fibrosis patients have demineralization of the uncinate process and medial displacement of the lateral nasal wall.
- Maxillary sinus mucocele in children should prompt the physician to rule out CF as a possible diagnosis.
- The first-line treatment for CRS in children is adenoidectomy.
- FESS is reserved for cases of failed medical treatment.

References

1. Lieser JD, Derkay CS. Pediatric sinusitis: when do we operate? Curr Opin Otolaryngol Head Neck Surg 2005;13(1):60–66
2. Goldsmith AJ, Rosenfeld RM. Treatment of pediatric sinusitis. Pediatr Clin North Am 2003;50(2):413–426
3. Manning S. Endoscopic sinus surgery in the pediatric age group. In: Rice D. Endoscopic Paranasal Sinus Surgery. Philadelphia, PA: Lippincott; 2003: 125–144
4. Manning SC, Biavati MJ, Phillips DL. Correlation of clinical sinusitis signs and symptoms to imaging findings in pediatric patients. Int J Pediatr Otorhinolaryngol 1996;37(1):65–74
5. Cotter CS, Stringer S, Rust KR, Mancuso A. The role of computed tomography scans in evaluating sinus disease in pediatric patients. Int J Pediatr Otorhinolaryngol 1999;50(1):63–68
6. Lee D, Rosenfeld RM. Adenoid bacteriology and sinonasal symptoms in children. Otolaryngol Head Neck Surg 1997;116(3):301–307
7. Bernstein JM, Dryja D, Murphy TF. Molecular typing of paired bacterial isolates from the adenoid and lateral wall of the nose in children undergoing adenoidectomy: implications in acute rhinosinusitis. Otolaryngol Head Neck Surg 2001;125(6):593–597
8. Phipps CD, Wood WE, Gibson WS, Cochran WJ. Gastroesophageal reflux contributing to chronic sinus disease in children: a prospective analysis. Arch Otolaryngol Head Neck Surg 2000;126(7):831–836
9. Bothwell MR, Parsons DS, Talbot A, Barbero GJ, Wilder B. Outcome of reflux therapy on pediatric chronic sinusitis. Otolaryngol Head Neck Surg 1999;121(3):255–262
10. Stiehm ER. The four most common pediatric immunodeficiencies. J Immunotoxicol 2008;5(2):227–234
11. Teknos TN, Metson R, Chasse T, Balercia G, Dickersin GR. New developments in the diagnosis of Kartagener's syndrome. Otolaryngol Head Neck Surg 1997;116(1):68–74
12. Chapelin C, Coste A, Reinert P, et al. Incidence of primary ciliary dyskinesia in children with recurrent respiratory diseases. Ann Otol Rhinol Laryngol 1997;106(10 Pt 1):854–858
13. Schulte DL, Kasperbauer JL. Safety of paranasal sinus surgery in patients with cystic fibrosis. Laryngoscope 1998;108(12):1813–1815
14. Gysin C, Alothman GA, Papsin BC. Sinonasal disease in cystic fibrosis: clinical characteristics, diagnosis, and management. Pediatr Pulmonol 2000;30(6):481–489
15. Brihaye P, Clement PA, Dab I, Desprechin B. Pathological changes of the lateral nasal wall in patients with cystic fibrosis (mucoviscidosis). Int J Pediatr Otorhinolaryngol 1994;28(2-3):141–147
16. Wald E, et al; American Academy of Pediatrics. Subcommittee on Management of Sinusitis and Committee on Quality Improvement. Clinical practice guideline: management of sinusitis. Pediatrics 2001;108(3):798–808
17. Schenkel EJ, Skoner DP, Bronsky EA, et al. Absence of growth retardation in children with perennial allergic rhinitis after one year of treatment with mometasone furoate aqueous nasal spray. Pediatrics 2000;105(2):E2210654982
18. Brannan MD, Herron JM, Affrime MB. Safety and tolerability of once-daily mometasone furoate aqueous nasal spray in children. Clin Ther 1997;19(6):1330–1339
19. Ungkanont K, Damrongsak S. Effect of adenoidectomy in children with complex problems of rhinosinusitis and associated diseases. Int J Pediatr Otorhinolaryngol 2004;68(4):447–451
20. Brietzke SE, Brigger MT. Adenoidectomy outcomes in pediatric rhinosinusitis: a meta-analysis. Int J Pediatr Otorhinolaryngol 2008;72(10):1541–1545
21. Ramadan HH, Tiu J. Failures of adenoidectomy for chronic rhinosinusitis in children: for whom and when do they fail? Laryngoscope 2007;117(6):1080–1083
22. Ramadan HH, Cost JL. Outcome of adenoidectomy versus adenoidectomy with maxillary sinus wash for chronic rhinosinusitis in children. Laryngoscope 2008;118(5):871–873
23. Hebert RL II, Bent JP III. Meta-analysis of outcomes of pediatric functional endoscopic sinus surgery. Laryngoscope 1998;108(6):796–799

24. Carpenter KM, Graham SM, Smith RJ. Facial skeletal growth after endoscopic sinus surgery in the piglet model. Am J Rhinol 1997;11(3):211–217
25. Mair EA, Bolger WE, Breisch EA. Sinus and facial growth after pediatric endoscopic sinus surgery. Arch Otolaryngol Head Neck Surg 1995;121(5):547–552
26. Bothwell MR, Piccirillo JF, Lusk RP, Ridenour BD. Long-term outcome of facial growth after functional endoscopic sinus surgery. Otolaryngol Head Neck Surg 2002;126(6):628–634
27. Parsons D, Nishioka G. Pediatric sinus surgery. In: Kennedy D, ed. Diseases of the Sinus. New York: Bolger;2001: 271–280
28. Younis RT. The pros and cons of second-look sinonasal endoscopy after endoscopic sinus surgery in children. Arch Otolaryngol Head Neck Surg 2005;131(3):267–269
29. Hadfield PJ, Rowe-Jones JM, Mackay IS. A prospective treatment trial of nasal polyps in adults with cystic fibrosis. Rhinology 2000;38(2):63–65
30. Cimmino M, Nardone M, Cavaliere M, et al. Dornase alfa as postoperative therapy in cystic fibrosis sinonasal disease. Arch Otolaryngol Head Neck Surg 2005;131(12):1097–1101
31. Lewiston N, King V, Umetsu D, et al. Cystic fibrosis patients who have undergone heart-lung transplantation benefit from maxillary sinus antrostomy and repeated sinus lavage. Transplant Proc 1991;23(1 Pt 2):1207–1208
32. Moss RB, King VV. Management of sinusitis in cystic fibrosis by endoscopic surgery and serial antimicrobial lavage. Reduction in recurrence requiring surgery. Arch Otolaryngol Head Neck Surg 1995;121(5):566–572
33. Robertson JM, Friedman EM, Rubin BK. Nasal and sinus disease in cystic fibrosis. Paediatr Respir Rev 2008;9(3):213–219

7 Medical Management of Maxillary Sinusitis in the Postsurgical Sinus

Nick I. Debnath and Rodney J. Schlosser

Sinus surgery plays an important role in the management of chronic rhinosinusitis (CRS) that is refractory to maximal medical therapy with good success. However, multiple medical therapies continue to be an important part of the postsurgical management of maxillary sinusitis as well. Postoperative patients may remain symptomatic with persistent or recurrent disease, and attention must focus on returning to the original diagnosis and whether surgery has properly addressed the underlying problem. After the proper diagnosis has been made, management of postsurgical CRS is multifaceted, individualized to the patient, and designed to treat the underlying pathology (e.g., mucus recirculation, bacterial biofilms, recurrent nasal polyposis, cystic fibrosis, dental pathology). To this end, the rhinologist's armamentarium is replete with a multitude of systemic and topical medications.

Diagnosis and History

The diagnostic criteria for CRS in the postsurgical patient are the same as for all patients with CRS as defined by the report of the rhinosinusitis task force.[1] There is likely no single pathophysiologic mechanism of CRS in all patients. Biofilms, fungi, superantigens, eosinophil-driven immune processes, and mucociliary dysfunction all represent a diverse group of processes that may lead to the manifestations of CRS. As with any disease process, a careful history must be elicited with special attention to the type and extent of prior surgery and whether that surgery addressed the underlying problem. Patients with persistent or recurrent disease can present a challenge to the rhinologist, and the astute clinician should reassess the original diagnosis and possibly examine preoperative imaging and operative notes. This is especially true for patients who originally present with some of the more nonspecific symptoms of CRS such as sinonasal pain or headache. It is also important to reassess the patient for factors that may modify their management such as asthma, allergic rhinitis, cystic fibrosis, host immunosuppression, and anatomic variations.[2]

Endoscopic sinus surgery has become one successful facet in the overall management of CRS refractory to medical therapy with success rates estimated between 80 to 95%.[3,4] Surgery allows improvement in mucociliary clearance and sinus ventilation by unobstructing and enlarging the natural maxillary ostium. Surgical failure and recurrent disease continue to be a problem, however, with an estimated 2 to 18% of patients undergoing additional revision surgical procedures.[5] Surgical failure may be the result of suboptimal prior surgery or iatrogenic disturbance of mucociliary flow. Several retrospective studies have identified the most common causes of surgical failure to be adhesions, residual air cells, and stenosis or obstruction of the natural maxillary ostium.[5,6] A patient's symptom history may not always be specific for CRS isolated to the maxillary sinus, but the type of prior surgery may provide clues to whether there is residual focal disease in the postsurgical maxillary sinus. For instance, a post-Caldwell-Luc sinus in which all mucosa was stripped is at increased risk for long-term complications from dysfunctional mucociliary clearance and loculated pockets due to scarring within the maxillary sinus itself.[7] A thorough history should help guide the clinician to the underlying pathology and the correct treatment course.

Endoscopic Evaluation

Diagnostic nasal endoscopy in the clinic is always an important part of the complete physical exam of the postoperative patient. It is especially vital in the immediate postoperative period when endoscopy allows the debridement of nasal crusting and the lysis of adhesions to help prevent late inflammatory complications that might contribute to obstructing the maxillary ostium. Diagnostic endoscopy is usually performed in the decongested state with both straight and angled (45 degree or 70 degree) rigid telescopes and/or flexible endoscopes to assess the maxillary sinus in its entirety. Endoscopy affords the opportunity to assess the patency of the maxillary sinus and search for inflammatory signs associated with the patient's symptoms. For instance, the middle meatus is examined for purulence, granulation tissue, synechiae, retained uncinate process, or nasal polyps. It is important to document any stenosis of the maxillary antrostomy and the presence of any accessory ostia. The sinonasal mucosa is also evaluated for edema or polypoid changes. The middle turbinate, if not previously amputated, is evaluated to make certain there is no lateralization with obstruction of the middle meatus. The inferior and lateral limits of the maxillary sinus should also be examined to evaluate for dental pathology or loculated pockets that could be contributing to persistent infections. Given the increase in antibiotic-resistant organisms contributing to sinusitis, mucopurulent secretions apparent on endoscopy should be cultured to direct antibiotic therapy. A recent meta-analysis concluded that culture via the middle meatus had a high concordance rate (82%) with the traditional gold standard of maxillary antral puncture cultures.[8]

Radiographic Evaluation

Noncontrast computed tomography (CT) often proves useful as an additional source of information to supplement a thorough history and physical examination. High-resolution CT scans in coronal as well as sagittal and axial planes excel at evaluating bone detail and anatomy of the paranasal sinuses that may only be partially evident on endoscopic exam.[9] Particular attention should be given to the area of the natural maxillary ostium to assess its patency and to evaluate for anatomic clues that may be contributing to persistent disease (e.g., a residual uncinate process obstructing the infundibulum, accessory ostia that may contribute to mucus recirculation).

At times a subtle finding on CT imaging, recirculation phenomenon in the maxillary sinus involves abnormal flow of mucus between neighboring openings into the maxillary antrum and is a common iatrogenic cause of persistent postsurgical CRS (**see Videos 7.1 and 7.2**). When present, this can often be observed on CT imaging as an opacification in and around the natural or accessory ostium (**Fig. 7.1**).[10] Magnetic resonance imaging (MRI) is usually not necessary to evaluate the maxillary sinus, but MRI is sometimes useful as an adjunct to CT images when distinguishing between tumor, trapped secretions, and allergic fungal mucin.

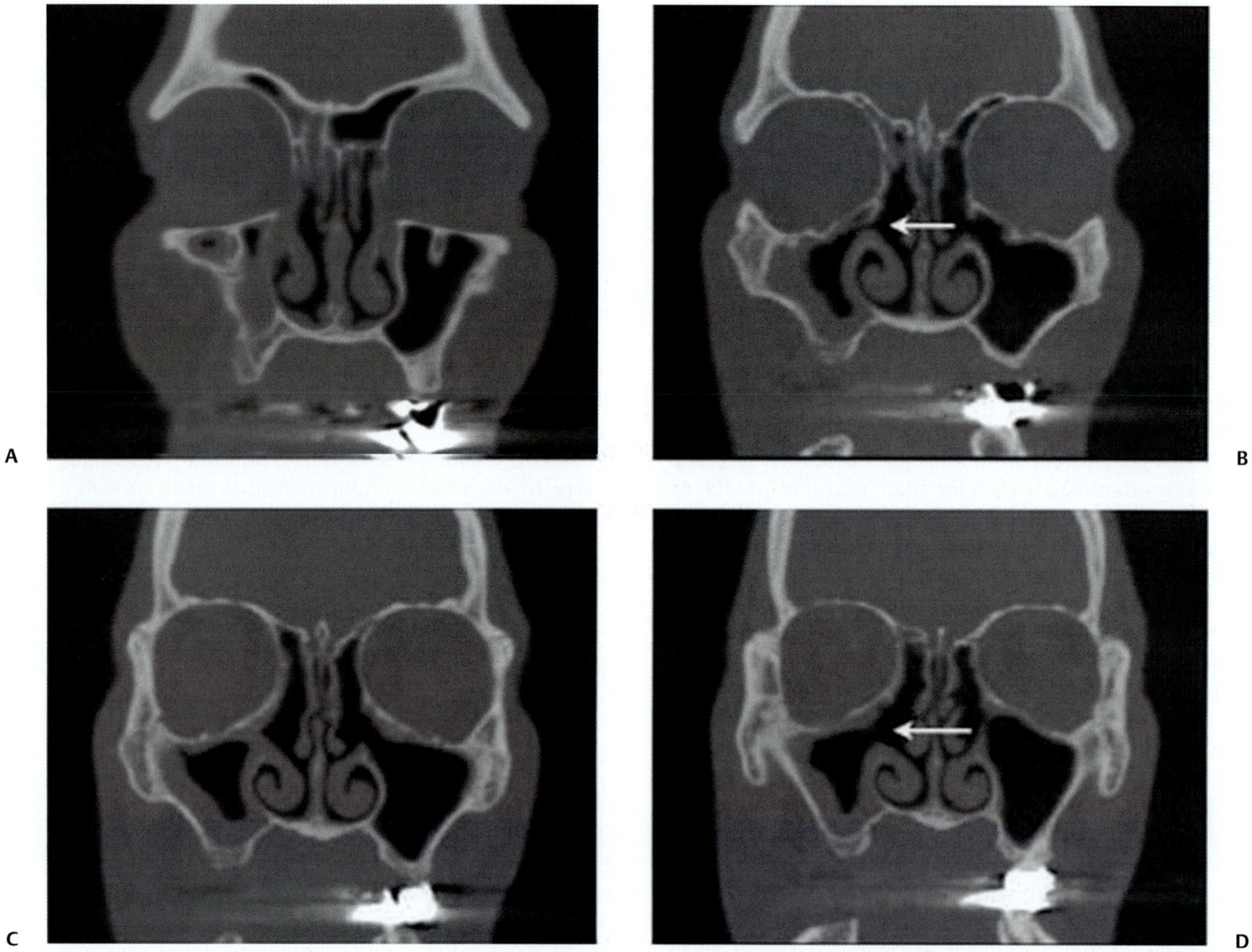

Fig. 7.1 (A–D) Coronal computed tomographic (CT) images of a patient with right maxillary mucus recirculation. **(B)** *Arrow* points to mucus at the natural ostium just inferior to a Haller cell. **(C)** Mucosal bridge is present posterior to the natural ostium with mucosal thickening. **(D)** *Arrow* points to the accessory ostium.

Management of Suboptimal Prior Surgery

If initial evaluation of the patient reveals refractory disease secondary to suboptimal prior surgery or an iatrogenic process, then revision surgery may become necessary to address the problem. Prevention of these problems is fundamental and begins in the operating room to deter the formation of postoperative adhesions, which represent a common source of surgical failure with an incidence from 1 to 36%.[11] Many studies have evaluated the use of a variety of middle meatal packing both for hemostasis and adhesion prevention, and a recent review concluded that resorbable packs [FloSeal (Baxter, Deerfield, IL), Gelfilm (Pfizer Pharmaceuticals, New York, NY), Gelfoam (Pfizer)] have no added benefit over nonresorbable packing (Merocel; Medtronic, Mystic, CT) or no packing. In fact, some resorbable packing (Floseal, Gelfilm) had an increased risk of granulation tissue and adhesions, although it was not clear whether the resulting synechiae were clinically significant.[11] Noting that mitomycin C has been used in other fields to inhibit scar formation, several groups examined topical administration of this agent at the middle meatus to determine whether it would decrease the incidence of stenosis and synechiae. All three studies concluded that mitomycin C offered no significant reduction in stenosis or adhesions.[12–14]

Aggressive postoperative cleaning and debridement also play an important role in preventing postsurgical maxillary CRS. Careful endoscopic inspection in the office should identify any middle meatal debris, crusting, or bone fragments which should be suctioned and removed to prevent an inflammatory reaction and adhesion formation. Localized adhesions between the middle turbinate and the natural ostia may be cut in the clinic with topical and local anesthesia if the patient is tolerant.

In addition to a residual uncinate process, a common cause of a persistent obstructed maxillary ostium was found to be a missed maxillary sinus ostia, which was not connected to the surgically created maxillary antrostomy.[5] This iatrogenic posterior fontanelle antrostomy may result in the mucus recirculation phenomenon (**Fig. 7.2**). This can also occur when an inferior meatal antrostomy was created in addition to a middle meatal antrostomy to cause recirculation between the two openings. The treatment is surgical and leads to resolution of the abnormal mucus flow. The openings involved must be joined into one larger antrostomy by removing the bridge of bone or mucosa between the two. This can often be performed in the clinic with cutting instruments with topical and local anesthesia.[15] In those patients with recirculation between middle and inferior meatal antrostomies, Coleman and Duncavage have described an extended middle meatal antrostomy that connects the two openings by creating a much larger antrostomy.[16]

One procedure that has a high rate of postsurgical failure is the Caldwell–Luc procedure, which usually entails removal of maxillary sinus mucosa. Long-term complications in post-Caldwell–Luc sinuses include abnormal mucociliary function, chronic neuralgia, infraorbital nerve injury, tooth root injury, and delayed mucocele.[7] In their retrospective study of post-Caldwell–Luc patients with persistent disease, Han et al determined that surgical salvage with an endoscopic "mega-antrostomy" was an alternative to repeating the Caldwell–Luc procedure. The mega-antrostomy is created by endoscopically extending the maxillary antrostomy inferiorly to the nasal floor to facilitate sinus ventilation and postoperative irrigation given the disorganized mucociliary clearance in these sinuses.[7] Woodworth et al also showed that 14 patients who had failed a Caldwell–Luc procedure were successfully treated with a modified endoscopic medial maxillectomy.[17]

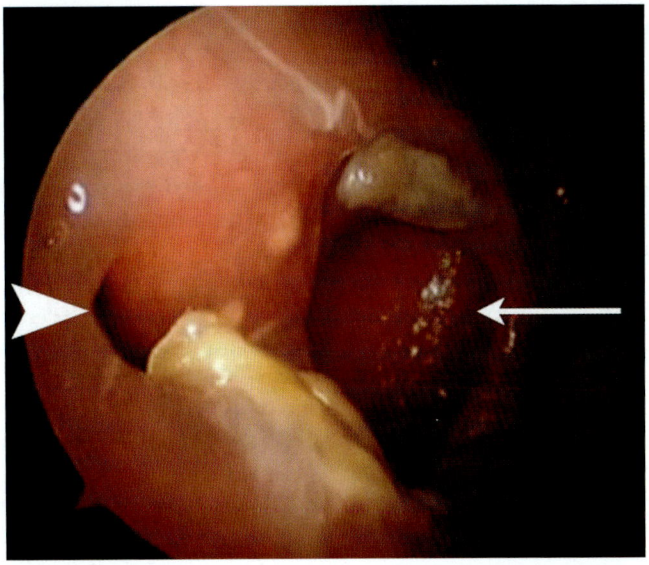

Fig. 7.2 Endoscopic view of mucus recirculation in the same patient shown in Fig. 7.1. Thickened mucus is transported from the natural ostium (*arrowhead*) to the iatrogenic maxillary antrum (*arrow*).

Medical Management

Medical therapies for CRS in postsurgical patients are the same as for the treatment of all CRS patients and can be categorized into topical and systemic therapies ranging from topical saline and antiinflammatory agents to systemic antibiotics and steroids. The choice of medical therapy should be catered to the individual patient on the basis of the underlying pathology. Usually, the treatment is an integrated, multifaceted approach designed to reduce chronic sinus mucosal inflammation and infection. Adjuvant therapy in postsurgical CRS may include nasal saline, antibiotics, antifungals, topical and systemic steroids, antihistamines, decongestants, and topical biofilms inhibitors.

Nasal Saline

The practice of nasal irrigation with saline has a long history stemming from purification rites in ancient India in preparation for yoga. Topical delivery of saline via irrigations, sprays, and nebulizers has been intensively studied recently as an adjunct in the treatment of sinonasal inflammatory disease, and a recent Cochrane review concluded that saline irrigation is beneficial resulting in the improvement of symptoms of CRS.[18] Several investigators have examined the effects of delivery device on penetrating the paranasal sinuses with varying results. Multiple studies have shown that large volume, positive pressure irrigations with syringes or squeeze bottles to be superior to atomizer, nebulizer, and spray in postsurgical sinus delivery,[19–21] and that these large volume irrigations are superior to sprays in reduction of symptom severity and frequency.[22]

There is also growing evidence to support the intuitive claim that saline delivery is greater in the postoperative maxillary sinus compared with the preoperative state. In fact, Grobler et al calculated that a minimum ostial dimension of 3.95 mm is required to attain a 95% probability of topical irrigant penetration.[23] Harvey et al performed an irrigation study using radiocontrast dye in cadavers before surgery, after endoscopic sinus surgery, and after endoscopic medial maxillectomy. The delivery was with a pressurized spray, a squeeze bottle, or a neti pot, and they found that sinus distribution as measured by CT imaging was greater after sinus surgery with additional distribution gained after a medial maxillectomy. Furthermore, irrigation delivery was significantly greater via the neti pot and squeeze bottle techniques compared with the spray, and the neti pot offered the greatest distribution after surgery (**see Video 7.3**).[24]

Based on these reviews and studies, saline irrigation via squeeze bottle or neti pot is recommended to who have postsurgical maxillary CRS. It is especially useful in the immediate postoperative period to help remove crusting and debris, which may contribute to inflammation.[20] This is easily tolerated by most patients and appears to improve overall symptoms. It is important to note, however, that patients should be instructed in the proper sterile care of their irrigation fluid and device to prevent bacterial colonization and possible subsequent infection.

Antibiotics

Although there is considerable variability in the usage of antibiotics and their duration, the microbiology of acute and chronic rhinosinusitis is well established, and the most common organisms cultured in CRS are both aerobes (*Streptococcus pneumoniae, Staphylococcus aureus*, coagulase-negative *Staph*) as well as anaerobes (*Peptostreptococcus* species).[25] However, evidence suggests that the microbiological environment of the maxillary sinus may be different in the postsurgical state. Brook and Frazier found that *Pseudomonas aeruginosa* and gram-negative aerobic bacilli were more often isolated in patients who had previous sinus surgery, and they showed that postsurgical patients had fewer anaerobic isolates.[26] Coagulase-negative *Staph* and *S. aureus* were also found to be common isolates in the postsurgical sinus.[27] Current evidence shows that bacteria contributing to CRS are exhibiting growing resistance to antimicrobial agents. There are more prevalent strains of *S. pneumoniae* resistant to penicillin, trimethoprim-sulfamethoxazole, and macrolides, and there is a documented increase in β-lactamase-producing aerobes.[25] A recent study also found that the rate of recovery of methicillin-resistant *S. aureus* (MRSA) from patients with acute and chronic sinusitis has increased from 2001 to 2003 and from 2004 to 2006.[28]

Because of this variability in microbiology and the rise of antibiotic-resistant organisms, culture-directed therapy individualized to each patient is most likely to provide therapeutic benefit. We prefer culture-directed oral antibiotics administered for at least 3 weeks in addition to adjuvant therapies to reduce infection and inflammation (e.g., topical saline irrigations, antibiotics or steroids).

Antibiotics may also be administered topically in irrigated or nebulized form to deliver the agent directly to the infected mucosa of the postsurgical maxillary sinus. As with topical steroids, this greatly reduces systemic side effects of oral or parenteral antibiotics. Although there are no established clinical criteria for their use, they may serve as a therapeutic adjunct in patients who are recalcitrant to medical and surgical therapy. These patients with postsurgical CRS may suffer from persistent bacterial colonization in the maxillary sinuses secondary to poor mucociliary function, biofilm formation, or other innate host factors, and topical antibiotics may reduce the bacterial load.

One recent study evaluated evidence-based recommendations for topical antibiotic use to find that several agents have reasonable clinical evidence to justify their use: topical mupirocin, levofloxacin, clindamycin, tobramycin, and ceftazidime.[27] In one study of 16 postsurgical patients with persistent *S. aureus* infection, twice daily nasal lavages with 0.05% mupirocin (Bactroban; GlaxoSmithKline, Research Triangle Park, NC) improved endoscopic findings and yielded negative swab results for *S. aureus* after 3 weeks of treatment.[29] Mupirocin has been well studied for its topical activity against MRSA in the nose, and it is ideal as a topical agent because it exceeds the minimum inhibitory concentration (MIC) and retains its anti-*Staphylococcus* activity in nasal secretions for up to 8 hours.[27]

Topical tobramycin is used often in patients with persistent *P. aeruginosa* sinusitis, which is common in cystic fibrosis. Aerosolized tobramycin has been well established in the treatment of pseudomonal pneumonia in cystic fibrosis patients, and several groups have adapted this to treat *Pseudomonas*-positive sinonasal cultures. One study found that topical tobramycin delivered to postsurgical sinuses via nasal lavage in cystic fibrosis patients resulted in a significant decrease in revision surgeries,[30] although others have not found significant improvement with topical tobramycin.[31]

Topical antibiotics may serve to disrupt sinus biofilms as well. A biofilm is a structured community of organized bacterial cells that adhere to both inert and biologic surfaces.[32,33] Studies have begun to establish that biofilms may play a role in chronic sinusitis, although their exact mechanism in the pathophysiology of sinusitis remains elusive.[32] Recent investigations have begun to associate biofilms with clinically significant sinus disease. Bendouah et al showed a correlation between the presence of *P. aeruginosa* and *S. aureus* biofilms and postoperative persistence of sinus disease.[34] In a retrospective study, Psaltis et al found that patients with biofilms had significantly worse postoperative symptoms and mucosal disease. Interestingly, the presence of fungus at the time of surgery also correlated with an unfavorable outcome in this study.[35] With increasing data supporting a role for biofilms in the pathophysiology of recalcitrant CRS, more studies are investigating agents that may disrupt biofilms including topical mupirocin, tobramycin, and moxifloxacin.[36–38]

Topical agents to disrupt biofilms other than antibiotics are also being investigated. For instance, Chiu et al have found that the chemical surfactant baby shampoo delivered as a 1% solution in nasal irrigations for 4 weeks resulted in an improvement in subjective symptoms and in olfaction testing in postsurgical patients.[39]

Antifungals

Like antibiotics, antifungal agents may be delivered systemically or topically. Intravenous antifungal therapies such as amphotericin-B and posaconazole have considerable systemic side effects (nephrotoxicity, hepatotoxicity), and these are usually reserved for the treatment of invasive fungal sinusitis. Oral itraconazole has been used as an adjunct in the treatment of allergic fungal sinusitis,[40] but given its poor therapeutic indices, costs, risks of hepatotoxicity and other systemic side effects, its relative therapeutic benefits should be carefully weighed.[41]

Topical antifungal therapy in the form of amphotericin B has been proposed in the treatment of allergic fungal sinusitis (AFS) as well as CRS. Fungus has been well established in the pathogenesis of AFS as outlined in the diagnostic criteria by Bent and Kuhn.[42] AFS patients are atopic and often have nasal polyps and the allergic fungal mucin that is a rather specific finding for the disease; hence, these patients are usually treated with a combination of systemic or topical steroids as well as immunotherapy directed against fungal antigens. Endoscopic sinus surgery is often necessary for those patients with a large burden of polyp disease or allergic fungal mucin, especially if topical corticosteroids are to reach inflamed mucosa unobstructed.[41]

However, Ponikau et al have proposed that fungal infection is actually a pathologic mechanism in all forms of CRS by either direct infection or secondary inflammatory responses.[43] They demonstrated that fungal cultures were positive in 96% of CRS patients, and they subsequently found that treatment of 51 patients with CRS with topical irrigations of amphotericin-B for 3 months resulted in an improvement in CT and endoscopic findings, but there was no clinical improvement.[44] However, Weschta et al were not able to duplicate this finding in a double-blind randomized controlled trial of 60 patients with CRS (and excluding AFS patients).[45] The position that fungus is the sole mechanism of disease in CRS remains unproven. Most acknowledge the importance of fungus in sinus disease, but the pathogenesis is likely due to multiple etiologic mechanisms leading to the final common result of CRS. The therapeutic benefit of topical antifungals in AFS and CRS will remain controversial until further clinical trials are done.

Steroids

Intranasal and systemic glucocorticoid steroids have been widely used in the treatment of CRS, both before and after sinus surgery. Although many mechanisms may lead to CRS, the multiple actions of glucocorticoid steroids (e.g., reducing eosinophil mucosal infiltration, decreasing mucosal vascular permeability) make them ideal for treating everything from allergic rhinitis to nasal polyposis to postoperative mucosal edema.[46] The use of oral steroids has been found to reduce recurrence of disease, especially in AFS patients. In one retrospective study, oral steroid treatment in AFS patients showed clinical improvement after sinus surgery and reduced the time in between revision surgeries.[47] There were no reported adverse effects from long-term systemic steroid therapy in this study. However, side effects of oral steroids may potentially be severe and undesirable including immunosuppression, psychotropic effects, osteoporosis, diabetes mellitus, Cushing syndrome via suppression of the hypothalamic–pituitary axis, and aseptic joint necrosis. Oral steroids are therefore administered with caution and their use is tailored to the individual patient. Often a short tapering "burst" of oral steroids is necessary as an adjunct to irrigations or culture-directed antibiotics to alleviate postsurgical mucosal edema or to treat an acute exacerbation of CRS secondary to nasal polyps. Sometimes low-dose long-term oral steroid therapy may be necessary to prevent recurrent disease, but with careful consideration of their adverse effect profile.

Topical glucocorticoid steroids have a safer side-effect profile given their more limited systemic bioavailability, and the efficacy of steroid sprays has been well described in the long-term treatment of allergic rhinitis. Topical steroid sprays also have demonstrated improvement in symptom scores and nasal obstruction in the treatment of CRS with nasal polyposis.[46] This class of medication remains a mainstay of treatment in postsurgical patients with AFS, CRS with polyposis, and those patients with persistent reactive hyperplastic mucosal edema.

Investigators have also studied other topical formulations of glucocorticoid steroids. Nebulized budesonide (Pulmicort Respules) has proven benefit in reducing pulmonary inflammation in the treatment of asthmatic patients. Lund et al found that budesonide delivered via an aqueous nasal spray also exhibited efficacy in allergic CRS patients.[48] Kanowitz et al demonstrated that topical budesonide delivered via an atomization device in postsurgical patients exhibited symptomatic relief and a reduction in the need for systemic steroids.[49] We recommend budesonide in nasal irrigations in many of our postoperative patients with AFS and polyposis who are refractory to other treatments.

Topical steroids may also be administered in the form of drops. DelGaudio and Wise reported their experience with topical steroid drops (dexamethasone ophthalmic, prednisolone ophthalmic, and ciprofloxacin-dexamethasone otic) in a cohort of CRS patients who had recent sinus surgery. The drops were anatomically directed with the head hanging off the bed (Mygind's position) to the frontal sinuses in a majority of cases, although they did include one patient in whom they specifically addressed the maxillary sinus. They reported good success with 64% of their cases exhibiting persistent sinus patency, although there was one case of adrenal suppression from drop use.[50]

Sinonasal polyps may also be treated with steroid injections in addition to systemic or topical steroids. Injection of nasal polyps with a steroid (e.g., triamcinolone acetonide) has been shown to be an effective adjunct treatment, although its use is typically guarded due to the rare, but reported complication of permanent visual loss. In a recent report, Becker et al demonstrated in a series of 358 patients that intrapolyp steroid injection compared with surgical excision was associated with a lower rate of complications.[51] In the appropriate patient with nasal polyposis, intermittent steroid injections may play a role in controlling polyp disease.

Other Medical Therapies

Evidence supports the use of maximal medical therapy in the postsurgical patient before proceeding to a revision surgery. The treatment of CRS is as multifaceted as its pathogenesis, so a host of other therapies in addition to antibiotics and steroids is also necessary in some patients. Oral and topical decongestants may temporarily alleviate maxillary sinus obstruction, but their use is limited due to systemic side effects (e.g., hypertension). Long-term use of topical decongestants such as oxymetazoline and phenylephrine also carries the risk of abuse by the patient and rhinitis medicamentosa.

Other medications such as mucolytics and antihistamines may have a limited role in some postsurgical patients. Treatment with a mucolytic such as guaifenesin may alleviate the symptoms of thick nasal secretions. Antihistamines and leukotriene inhibitors have known therapeutic benefit in allergic rhinitis, and these may be recommended in CRS patients with concomitant atopic disease.[52] Laryngopharyngeal reflux disease may play a role in CRS, although evidence in the literature is frequently conflicting. The treatment of reflux with proton-pump inhibitor therapy may certainly be required in a subset of recalcitrant CRS patients.[53]

Allergy testing and possible immunotherapy should be considered in those CRS patients who may be refractory to medical and surgical therapy. In fact, immunotherapy to fungal antigens has become widely accepted as one part of the multifaceted treatment management for AFS patients.[41]

Another subset of challenging patients for the practicing rhinologist is the patient with cystic fibrosis. The incidence of CRS in these patients approaches 100%, and 10 to 20% eventually undergo sinus surgery.[54] Postoperative medical therapies are directed at clearing viscous mucous, maintaining sinus ostial patency, and reducing persistent bacterial colonization. Often these patients require multiple therapies including saline or steroid irrigations, topical and oral antibiotics, and oral steroids. Recent studies have shown encouraging results for some postoperative cystic fibrosis patients who received nasally inhaled dornase alfa, although further study is needed to evaluate its benefit.[55]

Revision Sinus Surgery

When medical management of postsurgical maxillary sinusitis fails, revision surgery may become necessary. Between 2 to 18% of surgical patients require at least a second procedure for recidivistic disease.[5] Patients with CRS with polyposis have a higher rate of refractory disease with one study demonstrating that 27% of these patients required revision sinus surgery to reduce their polyp burden.[56] It should be noted that these challenging patients should be thoroughly evaluated to rule out other mechanisms of disease. For instance, refractory maxillary disease may sometimes have odontogenic origin, most commonly from dental abscesses, but sometimes from unrecognized dentigerous cysts (**Fig. 7.3**), which may require surgical treatment.[57,58] Also refractory disease may be due to mucoceles of the maxillary sinus, which should be evident on careful endoscopic or radiographic evaluation. The treatment of these mucoceles is surgical excision resulting in very low rates of recurrence.[59]

A full discussion of revision sinus surgery is outside the scope of this chapter, but many approaches have been described to address surgical failures of the maxillary sinus including the modified endoscopic medial maxillectomy,[17] the canine fossa puncture,[60] and even the Caldwell–Luc procedure.[61]

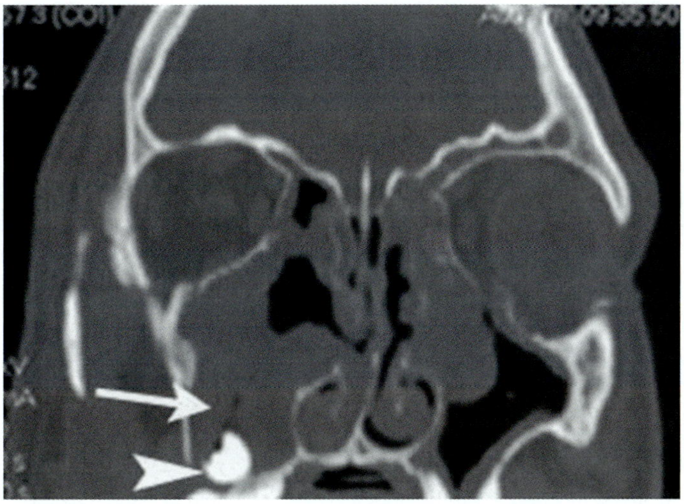

A

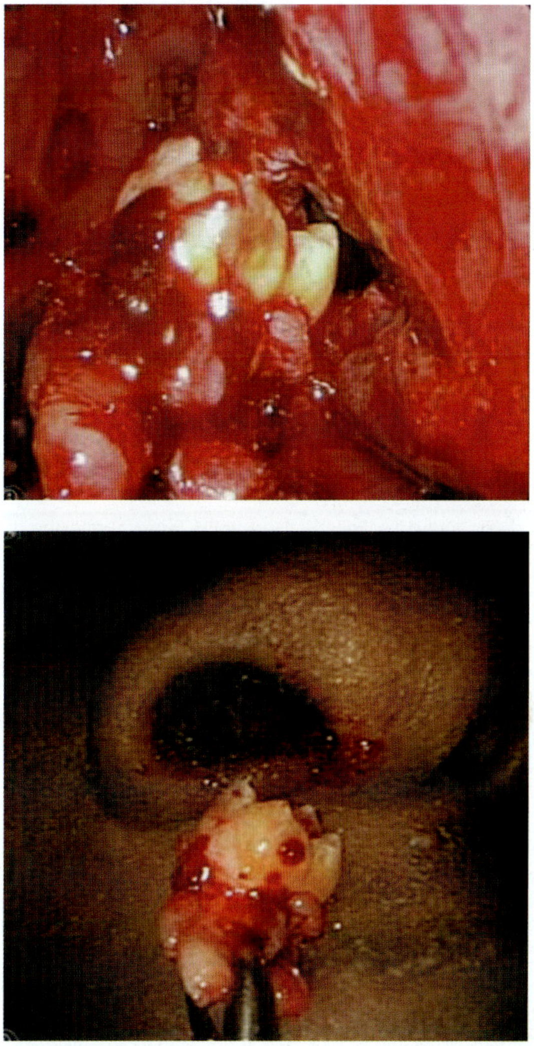

B

C

Fig. 7.3 **(A)** Coronal CT reveals a dentigerous cyst (*arrow*) in the right maxillary sinus arising from the crown of an unerupted tooth (*arrowhead*). **(B)** Endoscopic view of the tooth in the sinus. **(C)** Removal of the cystic unerupted tooth.

■ Conclusion

Treatment of CRS of the maxillary sinus refractory to medical and surgical intervention may be challenging to manage and is best individualized for each patient given the multifactorial etiologies that may result in disease. The clinician should focus on determining the underlying cause to administer the correct therapies, whether medical or surgical. Pathologies such as mucus recirculation or a lateralized middle turbinate may require a revision surgery to correct structural abnormalities. Underlying immunologic abnormalities, such as AFS may rely primarily on a combination of topical steroids and immunotherapy, whereas cystic fibrosis sinusitis may need office debridements, saline and tobramycin irrigations to disrupt biofilms. Achieving the best results in any one patient will require a multifaceted approach. The clinician should return to the basic algorithm of establishing the diagnosis, exhausting medical therapy, followed by surgical treatment only when indicated and when the patient is willing.

Pearls

- Focus on determining the underlying diagnosis in postoperative patients with persistent or recurrent maxillary disease.
- Management of suboptimal prior surgery or an iatrogenic process may require revision surgery.
- The choice of medical therapy should be catered to the individual patient. Usually the treatment is an integrated, multifaceted approach designed to reduce inflammation and infection.

References

1. Benninger MS, Ferguson BJ, Hadley JA, et al. Adult chronic rhinosinusitis: definitions, diagnosis, epidemiology, and pathophysiology. Otolaryngol Head Neck Surg 2003; 129(3, Suppl)S1–S32
2. Rosenfeld RM, Andes D, Bhattacharyya N, et al. Clinical practice guideline: adult sinusitis. Otolaryngol Head Neck Surg 2007; 137(3, Suppl)S1–S31
3. Senior BA, Kennedy DW, Tanabodee J, Kroger H, Hassab M, Lanza D. Long-term results of functional endoscopic sinus surgery. Laryngoscope 1998;108(2):151–157
4. Poetker DM, Smith TL. Adult chronic rhinosinusitis: surgical outcomes and the role of endoscopic sinus surgery. Curr Opin Otolaryngol Head Neck Surg 2007;15(1):6–9
5. Richtsmeier WJ. Top 10 reasons for endoscopic maxillary sinus surgery failure. Laryngoscope 2001;111(11 Pt 1):1952–1956
6. Ramadan HH. Surgical causes of failure in endoscopic sinus surgery. Laryngoscope 1999;109(1):27–29
7. Han JK, Smith TL, Loehrl TA, Fong KJ, Hwang PH. Surgical revision of the post-Caldwell-Luc maxillary sinus. Am J Rhinol 2005;19(5):478–482
8. Dubin MG, Ebert CS, Coffey CS, Melroy CT, Sonnenburg RE, Senior BA. Concordance of middle meatal swab and maxillary sinus aspirate in acute and chronic sinusitis: a meta-analysis. Am J Rhinol 2005;19(5):462–470
9. Branstetter BF IV, Weissman JL. Role of MR and CT in the paranasal sinuses. Otolaryngol Clin North Am 2005;38(6):1279–1299, x.
10. Chung SK, Cho DY, Dhong HJ. Computed tomogram findings of mucous recirculation between the natural and accessory ostia of the maxillary sinus. Am J Rhinol 2002;16(5):265–268
11. Weitzel EK, Wormald PJ. A scientific review of middle meatal packing/stents. Am J Rhinol 2008;22(3):302–307
12. Anand VK, Tabaee A, Kacker A, Newman JG, Huang C. The role of mitomycin C in preventing synechia and stenosis after endoscopic sinus surgery. Am J Rhinol 2004;18(5):311–314
13. Chan KO, Gervais M, Tsaparas Y, Genoway KA, Manarey C, Javer AR. Effectiveness of intraoperative mitomycin C in maintaining the patency of a frontal sinusotomy: a preliminary report of a double-blind randomized placebo-controlled trial. Am J Rhinol 2006;20(3):295–299
14. Chung JH, Cosenza MJ, Rahbar R, Metson RB. Mitomycin C for the prevention of adhesion formation after endoscopic sinus surgery: a randomized, controlled study. Otolaryngol Head Neck Surg 2002;126(5):468–474
15. Kane KJ. Recirculation of mucus as a cause of persistent sinusitis. Am J Rhinol 1997;11(5):361–369
16. Coleman JR Jr, Duncavage JA. Extended middle meatal antrostomy: the treatment of circular flow. Laryngoscope 1996;106(10):1214–1217
17. Woodworth BA, Parker RO, Schlosser RJ. Modified endoscopic medial maxillectomy for chronic maxillary sinusitis. Am J Rhinol 2006;20(3):317–319
18. Harvey R, Hannan SA, Badia L, Scadding G. Nasal saline irrigations for the symptoms of chronic rhinosinusitis. Cochrane Database Syst Rev 2007; (3):CD006394
19. Miller TR, Muntz HR, Gilbert ME, Orlandi RR. Comparison of topical medication delivery systems after sinus surgery. Laryngoscope 2004;114(2):201–204
20. Wormald PJ, Cain T, Oates L, Hawke L, Wong I. A comparative study of three methods of nasal irrigation. Laryngoscope 2004;114(12):2224–2227
21. Valentine R, Athanasiadis T, Thwin M, Singhal D, Weitzel EK, Wormald PJ. A prospective controlled trial of pulsed nasal nebulizer in maximally dissected cadavers. Am J Rhinol 2008;22(4):390–394
22. Pynnonen MA, Mukerji SS, Kim HM, Adams ME, Terrell JE. Nasal saline for chronic sinonasal symptoms: a randomized controlled trial. Arch Otolaryngol Head Neck Surg 2007;133(11):1115–1120
23. Grobler A, Weitzel EK, Buele A, et al. Pre- and postoperative sinus penetration of nasal irrigation. Laryngoscope 2008;118(11):2078–2081
24. Harvey RJ, Goddard JC, Wise SK, Schlosser RJ. Effects of endoscopic sinus surgery and delivery device on cadaver sinus irrigation. Otolaryngol Head Neck Surg 2008;139(1):137–142
25. Brook I. Bacteriology of chronic sinusitis and acute exacerbation of chronic sinusitis. Arch Otolaryngol Head Neck Surg 2006;132(10):1099–1101
26. Brook I, Frazier EH. Correlation between microbiology and previous sinus surgery in patients with chronic maxillary sinusitis. Ann Otol Rhinol Laryngol 2001;110(2):148–151
27. Elliott KA, Stringer SP. Evidence-based recommendations for antimicrobial nasal washes in chronic rhinosinusitis. Am J Rhinol 2006;20(1):1–6
28. Brook I, Foote PA, Hausfeld JN. Increase in the frequency of recovery of meticillin-resistant *Staphylococcus aureus* in acute and chronic maxillary sinusitis. J Med Microbiol 2008;57(Pt 8):1015–1017
29. Uren B, Psaltis A, Wormald PJ. Nasal lavage with mupirocin for the treatment of surgically recalcitrant chronic rhinosinusitis. Laryngoscope 2008;118(9):1677–1680
30. Moss RB, King VV. Management of sinusitis in cystic fibrosis by endoscopic surgery and serial antimicrobial lavage. Reduction in recurrence requiring surgery. Arch Otolaryngol Head Neck Surg 1995;121(5):566–572
31. Desrosiers MY, Salas-Prato M. Treatment of chronic rhinosinusitis refractory to other treatments with topical antibiotic therapy delivered by means of a large-particle nebulizer: results of a controlled trial. Otolaryngol Head Neck Surg 2001;125(3):265–269
32. Palmer J. Bacterial biofilms in chronic rhinosinusitis. Ann Otol Rhinol Laryngol Suppl 2006;196:35–39
33. Harvey RJ, Lund VJ. Biofilms and chronic rhinosinusitis: systematic review of evidence, current concepts and directions for research. Rhinology 2007;45(1):3–13
34. Bendouah Z, Barbeau J, Hamad WA, Desrosiers M. Biofilm formation by *Staphylococcus aureus* and *Pseudomonas aeruginosa* is associated with an unfavorable evolution after surgery for chronic sinusitis and nasal polyposis. Otolaryngol Head Neck Surg 2006;134(6):991–996
35. Psaltis AJ, Weitzel EK, Ha KR, Wormald PJ. The effect of bacterial biofilms on post-sinus surgical outcomes. Am J Rhinol 2008;22(1):1–6
36. Ha KR, Psaltis AJ, Butcher AR, Wormald PJ, Tan LW. In vitro activity of mupirocin on clinical isolates of *Staphylococcus aureus* and its potential implications in chronic rhinosinusitis. Laryngoscope 2008;118(3):535–540
37. Chiu AG, Antunes MB, Palmer JN, Cohen NA. Evaluation of the in vivo efficacy of topical tobramycin against *Pseudomonas* sinonasal biofilms. J Antimicrob Chemother 2007;59(6):1130–1134
38. Desrosiers M, Bendouah Z, Barbeau J. Effectiveness of topical antibiotics on *Staphylococcus aureus* biofilm in vitro. Am J Rhinol 2007;21(2):149–153
39. Chiu AG, Palmer JN, Woodworth BA, et al. Baby shampoo nasal irrigations for the symptomatic post-functional endoscopic sinus surgery patient. Am J Rhinol 2008;22(1):34–37

40. Rains BM III, Mineck CW. Treatment of allergic fungal sinusitis with high-dose itraconazole. Am J Rhinol 2003;17(1):1–8
41. Ryan MW, Marple BF. Allergic fungal rhinosinusitis: diagnosis and management. Curr Opin Otolaryngol Head Neck Surg 2007;15(1):18–22
42. Bent JP III, Kuhn FA. Diagnosis of allergic fungal sinusitis. Otolaryngol Head Neck Surg 1994;111(5):580–588
43. Ponikau JU, Sherris DA, Kern EB, et al. The diagnosis and incidence of allergic fungal sinusitis. Mayo Clin Proc 1999;74(9):877–884
44. Ponikau JU, Sherris DA, Kita H, Kern EB. Intranasal antifungal treatment in 51 patients with chronic rhinosinusitis. J Allergy Clin Immunol 2002;110(6):862–866
45. Weschta M, Rimek D, Formanek M, Polzehl D, Podbielski A, Riechelmann H. Topical antifungal treatment of chronic rhinosinusitis with nasal polyps: a randomized, double-blind clinical trial. J Allergy Clin Immunol 2004;113(6):1122–1128
46. Lund VJ. Maximal medical therapy for chronic rhinosinusitis. Otolaryngol Clin North Am 2005;38(6):1301–1310, x
47. Schubert MS, Goetz DW. Evaluation and treatment of allergic fungal sinusitis. II. Treatment and follow-up. J Allergy Clin Immunol 1998;102(3):395–402
48. Lund VJ, Black JH, Szabó LZ, Schrewelius C, Akerlund A. Efficacy and tolerability of budesonide aqueous nasal spray in chronic rhinosinusitis patients. Rhinology 2004;42(2):57–62
49. Kanowitz SJ, Batra PS, Citardi MJ. Topical budesonide via mucosal atomization device in refractory postoperative chronic rhinosinusitis. Otolaryngol Head Neck Surg 2008;139(1):131–136
50. DelGaudio JM, Wise SK. Topical steroid drops for the treatment of sinus ostia stenosis in the postoperative period. Am J Rhinol 2006;20(6):563–567
51. Becker SS, Rasamny JK, Han JK, Patrie J, Gross CW. Steroid injection for sinonasal polyps: the University of Virginia experience. Am J Rhinol 2007;21(1):64–69
52. Grayson MH, Korenblat PE. The role of antileukotriene drugs in management of rhinitis and rhinosinusitis. Curr Allergy Asthma Rep 2007;7(3):209–215
53. Passàli D, Caruso G, Passàli FM. ENT manifestations of gastroesophageal reflux. Curr Allergy Asthma Rep 2008;8(3):240–244
54. Becker SS, de Alarcon A, Bomeli SR, Han JK, Gross CW. Risk factors for recurrent sinus surgery in cystic fibrosis: review of a decade of experience. Am J Rhinol 2007;21(4):478–482
55. Cimmino M, Nardone M, Cavaliere M, et al. Dornase alfa as postoperative therapy in cystic fibrosis sinonasal disease. Arch Otolaryngol Head Neck Surg 2005;131(12):1097–1101
56. Wynn R, Har-El G. Recurrence rates after endoscopic sinus surgery for massive sinus polyposis. Laryngoscope 2004;114(5):811–813
57. Brook I. Sinusitis of odontogenic origin. Otolaryngol Head Neck Surg 2006;135(3):349–355
58. Haber R. Not everything in the maxillary sinus is sinusitis: a case of a dentigerous cyst. Pediatrics 2008;121(1):e203–e207
59. Busaba NY, Salman SD. Maxillary sinus mucoceles: clinical presentation and long-term results of endoscopic surgical treatment. Laryngoscope 1999;109(9):1446–1449
60. Singhal D, Douglas R, Robinson S, Wormald PJ. The incidence of complications using new landmarks and a modified technique of canine fossa puncture. Am J Rhinol 2007;21(3):316–319
61. Cutler JL, Duncavage JA, Matheny K, Cross JL, Miman MC, Oh CK. Results of Caldwell-Luc after failed endoscopic middle meatus antrostomy in patients with chronic sinusitis. Laryngoscope 2003;113(12):2148–2150

8 Orbital Complications of Maxillary Sinusitis

D. S. Sethi and B. Forer

In this chapter, we will describe the relevant anatomy, physiology, and pathogenesis of orbital complications of maxillary sinusitis. The classification of orbital complications and the diagnostic and therapeutic strategies when dealing with these complications will also be discussed.

Bacterial infection of the paranasal sinuses is one of the most common diseases affecting almost 32 million Americans every year.[1] It almost always is a consequence of a preceding viral infection affecting the upper respiratory tract. The maxillary and ethmoid sinuses are the most common sinuses affected followed by the frontal and sphenoid sinuses. Sinusitis responds to medical treatment in the majority of cases, yet occasionally orbital complications may occur due to spread of infection. The infection may involve the eyelid and the surrounding skin or extend deeper into the orbit and its adnexa. Periorbital cellulitis (POC) refers to an infection involving the eyelid and the surrounding skin, whereas infection affecting the orbit and its contents is called orbital cellulitis (OC). Often POC, a commonly occurring infectious process, may be difficult to distinguish from OC, which is traditionally associated with a high morbidity and potential mortality.

Sinusitis is a frequent cause of periorbital and orbital cellulitis accounting for up to 80% of cases. The ethmoid sinus is the most common source of orbital infection.[2–4] Direct extension of infection from the maxillary sinus to the orbit, though rare, may occur in the presence of a preexisting defect in the orbital floor due to previous trauma or via the various venous channels connecting this structures.[5,6]

More commonly, orbital complications from maxillary sinusitis result when there is extension to or there is concomitant ethmoid involvement. Odontogenic infections are an infrequent but important cause of orbital infections.[7–9] The apices of the maxillary molars and premolars that lie in close proximity to the floor of the maxillary sinus may be the source of ascending infection that progresses from the antrum into the ethmoid labyrinth, then through the lamina into the orbit. Infection from the maxillary sinus may also extend into the orbit through the inferior and the superior orbital fissure resulting in orbital abscesses that are laterally or posteriorly located.

It must be appreciated the POC and OC are two distinct disorders with different etiologies. POC is a more common infectious process limited to the eyelids in the preseptal region. In contrast, OC represents a more severe, but less common, infection of the orbit posterior to the septum. If not diagnosed and treated promptly, OC can have devastating consequences. Permanent visual impairment has been reported resulting from orbital complications due to sinusitis.[10–12] In a recent report of 218 cases of orbital infection, permanent orbital complications were reported in 19 patients including blindness (nine patients), strabismus (six patients), and ptosis (four patients).[4] In another report describing 159 cases of orbital complications due to sinusitis, four patients suffered from permanent blindness.[13] Increased intraorbital pressure due to infection in conjunction with the septic process might lead to blindness from thrombosis of the retinal artery, direct pressure effect on the optic nerve or vasculitis of its vasa vasorum. Visual loss may be gradual or sudden and may occur without any funduscopic abnormality.

Life-threatening intracranial complications may arise from direct extension of the infection from the orbit via retrograde thrombophlebitis of the ophthalmic veins into the cavernous sinus.[14] Infection may also extend intracranially through other anatomic routes, such as the optic foramen, superior orbital fissure, and ethmoid canals, where the periorbita continues as the dura.

Although orbital complication may occur in both adults and children, the latter group is affected more frequently.[4,10,15] Schramm and colleagues collected 303 cases of orbital cellulitis over a 10-year period.[3] Age range was 2 weeks to 66 years. Another study by Shahin showed that 75% of the patients were below age 16 and 33% below 4 years.[16] The severity of the disease may be lesser in children as compared with adults.[17]

Proptosis is a significant finding in orbital cellulitis. In general, the degree of proptosis correlates well with the severity of orbital cellulitis or abscess. The orbit may also be affected in chronic maxillary sinus disease. Chronic osteomyelitis may cause orbital cellulitis. Displacement of the globe and diplopia may also result from an expanding maxillary mucocele. Rarely, enophthalmos may be a sequel of chronic maxillary sinusitis causing its walls to collapse, a condition also described as silent sinus syndrome.[18,19]

Relevant Anatomy

The orbit is a quadrangular pyramidal cavity composed of seven separate bones. Sixty to 80% of the orbit has its contributions from the sinuses, i.e., the roof of the maxillary sinus, the lateral wall of the ethmoids, and the floor of the frontal sinus. The paranasal sinuses are in intimate contact with the orbit, which is separated only by a thin plate of bone from the frontal sinus superiorly, the ethmoid labyrinth medially, and the maxillary sinus inferiorly. The roof of the maxillary sinus forms the inferior orbital wall and is relatively thick. In contrast, the medial wall of the orbit, which is formed by the lateral wall of the ethmoid, is extremely thin, and therefore is called the lamina papyracea. The lamina papyracea may show bony dehiscence that offers little resistance to inflammation and displacing forces. The lamina papyracea also has preformed vascular channels communicating the ethmoid cavity with the orbit. Consequently, acute and chronic inflammatory disease within the sinuses has ready access to the orbit and its adnexa. The orbit is predominantly an osseous socket and any extension of inflammation or the compression of the orbital contents will lead to exophthalmos or proptosis.

The surrounding paranasal sinuses are divided into two groups. The anterior group of paranasal sinuses, the maxillary sinus, the frontal sinus, and the anterior ethmoid cells, are a common source of orbital complications. Direct orbital spread of maxillary sinus disease is uncommon, and usually results when there is concomitant ethmoid involvement or there is extension of the inflammation to the ethmoid labyrinth.

The posterior group of paranasal sinuses includes the posterior ethmoid cells and the sphenoid sinus. These are closely related to the orbital apex, optic nerve, and the cavernous sinus. Inflammatory disease in this region may cause serious complications including impairment of vision, blindness, cranial nerve palsies, and thrombophlebitis of the cavernous sinus.

Venous drainage is the key to the spread of infection from the sinuses to the orbit. The venous drainage forms a vascular network that interconnects with the nasal cavity, orbit, and paranasal sinuses. These veins are valveless allowing retrograde extension of the infection. The superior and inferior ophthalmic veins course throughout the orbit, draining portions of the paranasal sinuses, and eventually empty into the cavernous sinus. The superior ophthalmic vein is continuous with the nasofrontal vein and the inferior ophthalmic vein receives tributaries from the eyelids, lacrimal sac, and orbital muscles. These interconnecting systems of veins permit ready access to the orbit and eyelids from infections in the nose and paranasal sinuses. The cavernous sinus contains several cranial nerves (CNs) including the oculomotor (CN III), trochlear (CN IV), first branch of the trigeminal, and the abducent (CN VI), as well as the internal carotid artery. The communication between the cavernous sinuses on either side, present a pathway for the spread of infection to the opposite side.

Pathophysiology of the Spread of Infection

Orbital extension of infection from the maxillary sinus may occur through a variety of avenues:

- **Direct invasion through compromised bony barriers:** the most common spread of infection is by extension to the ethmoid labyrinth. Within the ethmoids, the lamina papyracea offers little resistance to infection. Often, the lamina papyracea may show various degrees of bone dehiscence that may be congenital or occur secondary to trauma or surgery. The lamina papyracea has two main natural openings along the fronto-ethmoid suture line through which the anterior and posterior ethmoid neurovascular bundles pass. Direct spread of infection can take place through dehiscent areas or through the vascular channels mentioned above. Infection from the maxillary sinus may also reach the orbit via the inferior orbital fissure. A rare route is via the pterygopalatine or the infratemporal fossa and the superior orbital fissure.
- **Retrograde septic thrombophlebitis**: access to the orbit is gained by the ophthalmic vein via the pterygoid venous plexus. The pathogens can also reach the orbit via the facial vein and the angular vein. These veins communicate in the region of the medial canthus via its venous anastomosis with the supratrochlear veins and the supraorbital veins. A report of postmortem dissections have shown septic thrombi to occur in venous channels communicating the paranasal sinuses the orbit and cranial cavity.[20]
- **Erosive osteomyelitis:** osteomyelitic bone erosion of the maxillary sinus may extend to the orbit.

Classification of Orbital Complications of Sinusitis

Chandler's classification, based on the anatomic location of inflammation, is the most widely accepted classification for orbital infections.[21] According to the classification, orbital inflammation is divided into five groups (**Fig. 8.1**): Group I is preseptal cellulitis (PSC), Group II is orbital cellulitis (OC), Group III is subperiosteal abscess (SPA), Group IV is orbital abscess (OA), and Group V is cavernous sinus thrombosis (CST). The anatomic distinction among the various types of orbital infections is important as it significantly influences the selection of therapy and clinical outcome.

Preseptal Cellulitis

In this group, the infection is limited to the skin and the subcutaneous tissue of the eyelid, which is anterior to the orbital septum (**Fig. 8.2**). The orbital septum is the reflection of the periorbita from the orbital margin to the globe and serves as an important barrier to the spread of infection. The orbital adnexa, including the muscles and optic nerve, lies behind the orbital septum and is unaffected by the infectious process. PSC accounts for ~70% of orbital infections.[2,3] Reviewing 119 patients with inflammatory disease about the eye, Goodwin et al found that in 97 cases (81.5%), the

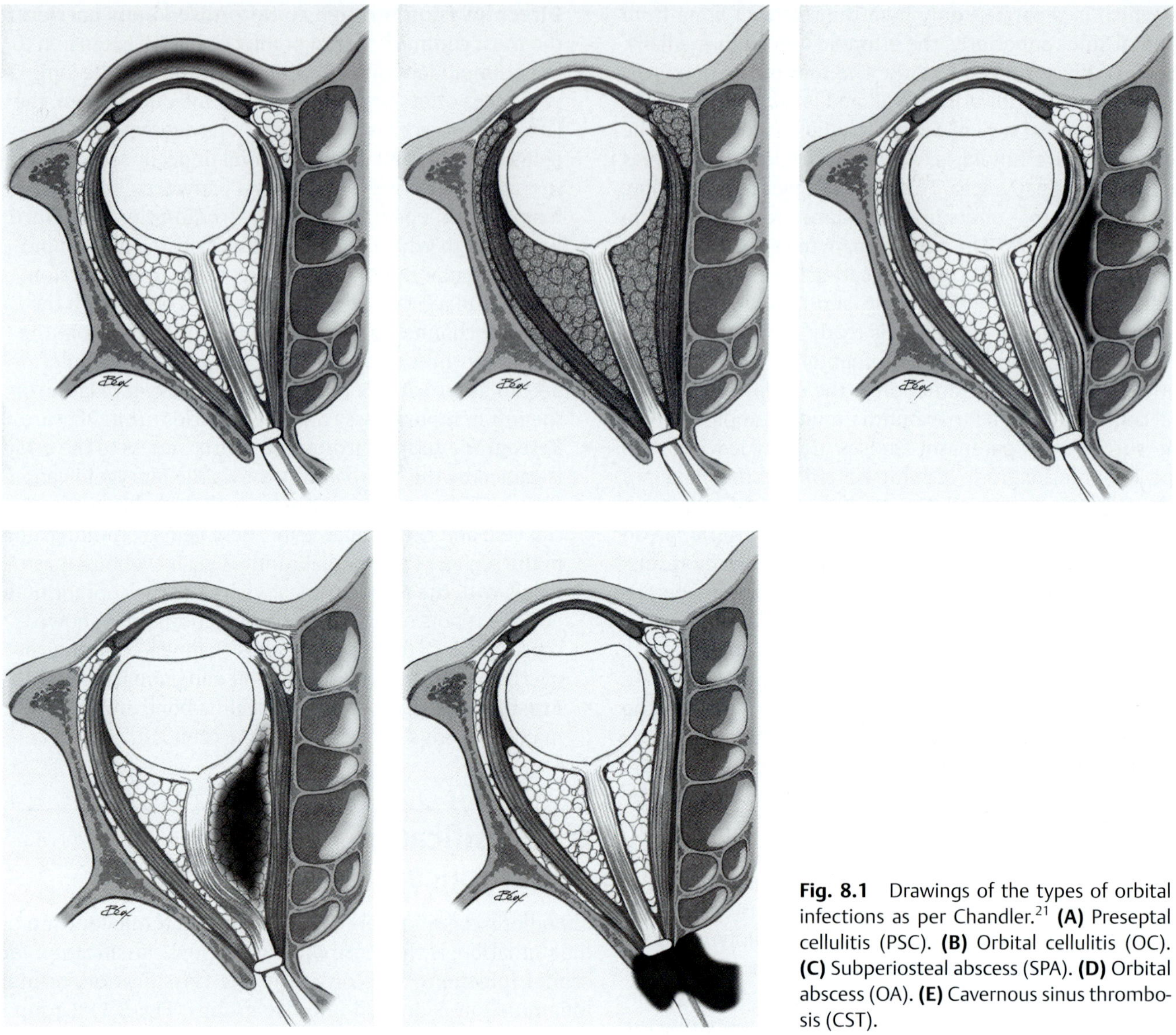

A–C

D,E

Fig. 8.1 Drawings of the types of orbital infections as per Chandler.[21] **(A)** Preseptal cellulitis (PSC). **(B)** Orbital cellulitis (OC). **(C)** Subperiosteal abscess (SPA). **(D)** Orbital abscess (OA). **(E)** Cavernous sinus thrombosis (CST).

infection was preseptal.[22] Clinical findings in PSC include edema and erythema of the eyelid, with or without, conjunctival injection. As the infection is anterior to the orbital septum, there is no limitation of extraocular movement and no impairment of visual acuity. Often the segment of the eyelid involved may suggest the sinus of origin. Ethmoid sinusitis may cause edema of the eyelids medially early in the course of infection and later proceed to involve the entire eyelid. Maxillary sinusitis may produce swelling of the lower eyelid. Frontal or supraorbital ethmoid disease may involve only the upper eyelid. The inflammatory edema may totally close the eye and therefore it is extremely important to force the eyelids apart to evaluate the eye. A computed tomography (CT) scan obtained in this group will demonstrate edema of the eyelid anterior to the orbital septum. The characteristic finding is that the tissues posterior to the orbital septum are radiographically normal. PSC generally resolves with appropriate antibiotic therapy. Persistent swelling may represent the formation of an eyelid abscess, which will require independent drainage.

Subperiosteal Abscess

Subperiosteal abscess (SPA) is defined as a collection of pus between the bony orbital wall and the periorbita. The periorbita, which is loosely attached to the underlying bone, readily separates from it. The circumscribed swelling, resulting from the SPA tends to displace the globe and may cause impairment of ocular motility. SPA is commonly located in the superomedial or inferomedial aspect of the orbit (**Fig. 8.3**), but may occur in the superior, inferior, and even lateral aspects (**Fig. 8.4**).[4] In the early stage, the patient presents with minimal conjunctival congestion and normal visual acuity.

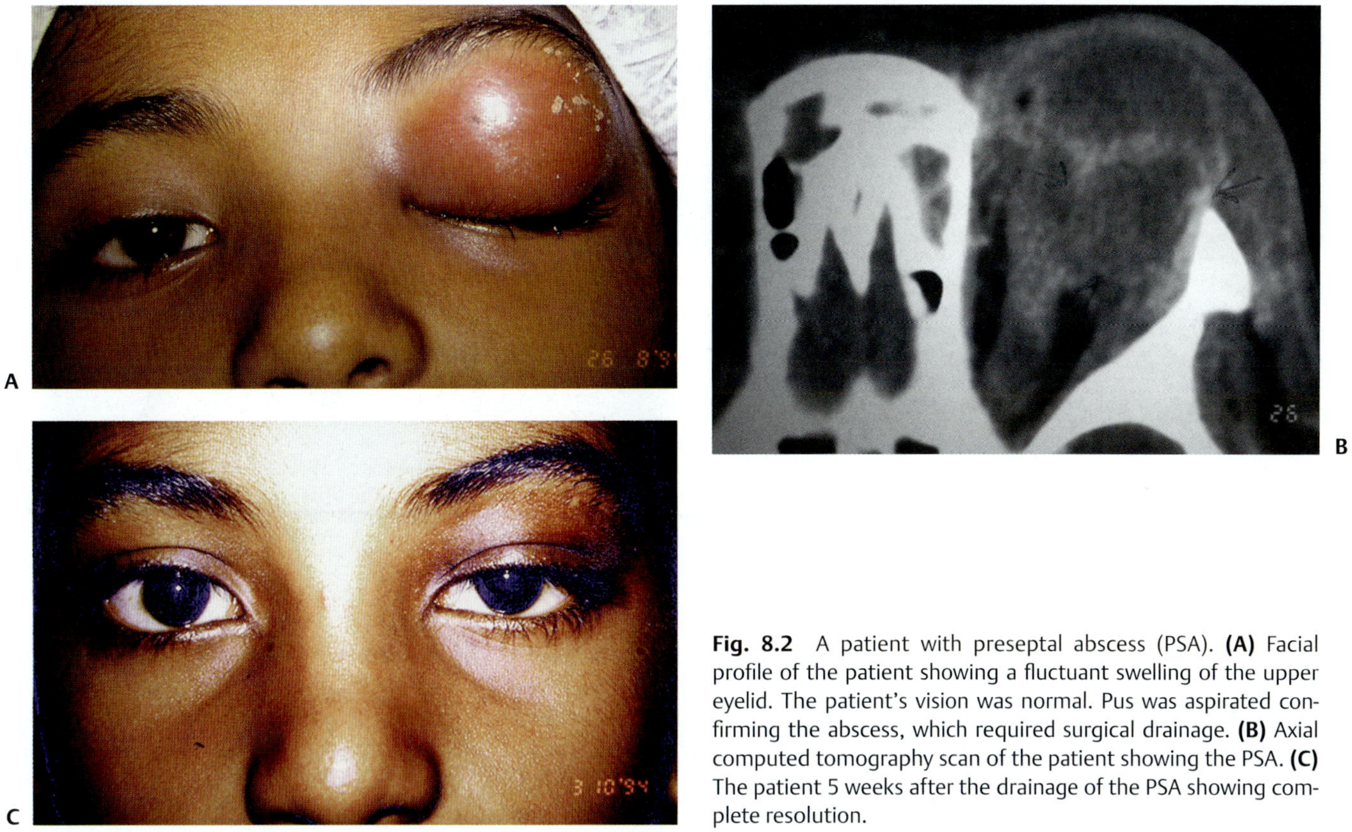

Fig. 8.2 A patient with preseptal abscess (PSA). **(A)** Facial profile of the patient showing a fluctuant swelling of the upper eyelid. The patient's vision was normal. Pus was aspirated confirming the abscess, which required surgical drainage. **(B)** Axial computed tomography scan of the patient showing the PSA. **(C)** The patient 5 weeks after the drainage of the PSA showing complete resolution.

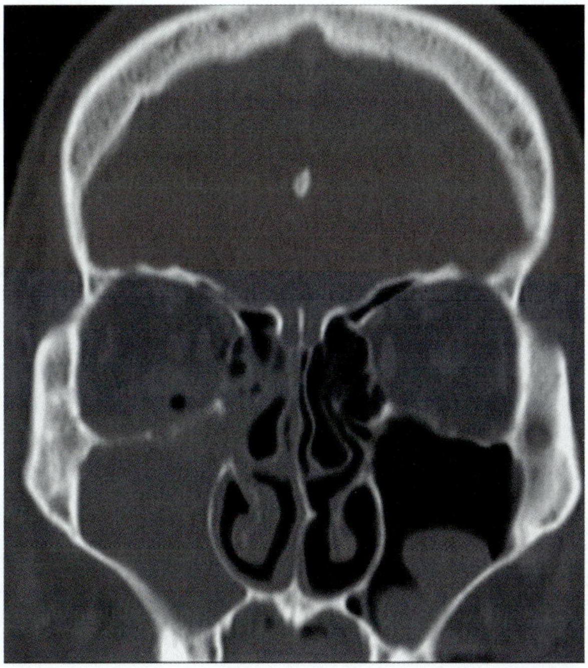

Fig. 8.3 A patient with inferior subperiosteal abscess resulting from maxillary sinusitis. This patient was referred by an ophthalmologist after the computed tomography scan showed a subperiosteal abscess secondary to maxillary sinusitis. Note the air bubble in the abscess and the concha bullosa. This patient had very minimal disease in the ethmoids. The abscess was drained endoscopically. Surgery involved trimming of the lateral lamella of the concha bullosa, uncinectomy, a wide middle meatal antrostomy, ethmoidectomy, exposure of the lamina papyracea, and removal on the lamina papyracea anteriorly to drain the abscess into the nasal cavity.

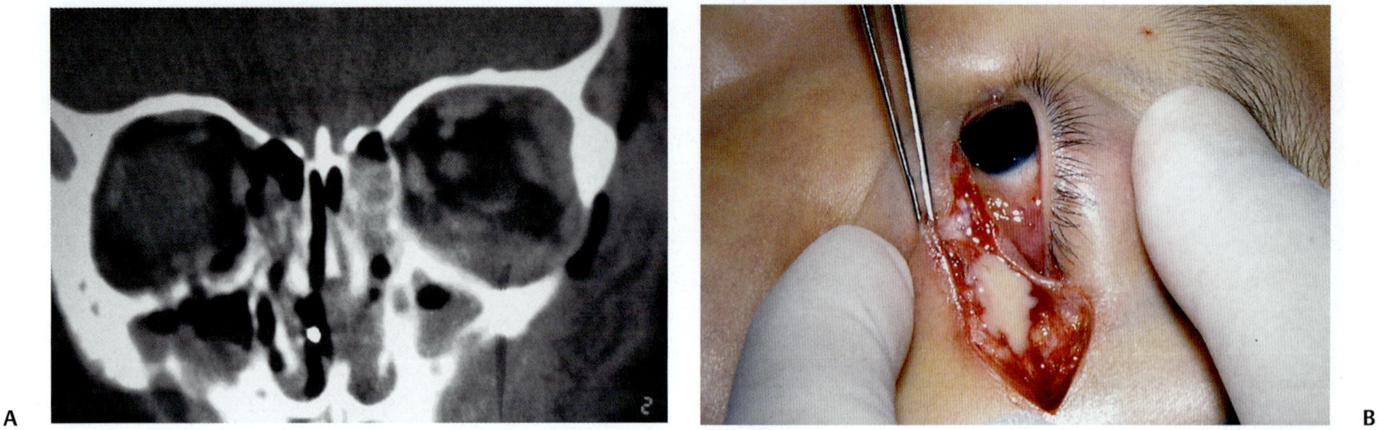

Fig. 8.4 A 16-year-old boy with inferior and lateral abscess secondary to maxillary sinusitis. **(A)** Coronal computed tomography scan of the patient, who presented with proptosis and impairment of vision and eye movements. Note the inferior SPA and lateral extension of the abscess. **(B)** Open drainage of the abscess done by the ophthalmologist.

With progression of the disease, chemosis, proptosis, and limited mobility of extraocular muscles along with some visual loss develops. The abscess may remain localized or may penetrate the periorbita to produce an orbital cellulitis or abscess. On CT scan or magnetic resonance imaging (MRI), SPA is seen as a contrast-enhancing mass in the extraconal space with a ring-enhanced lesion or an air fluid level being pathognomic of an abscess. This is considered by most to be a surgical emergency requiring prompt drainage.

Orbital Cellulitis

Orbital cellulitis (OC) is postseptal cellulitis in which the infectious process spreads to the soft tissue posterior to the orbital septum and penetrates the orbital periosteum to involve the orbital contents (**Fig. 8.5**). There is diffuse edema of the orbital contents with infiltration of the adipose tissue with inflammatory cells and bacteria. In most cases, the patient presents clinically with severe eyelid edema, which may close the eyes. Proptosis and chemosis that result from obstruction of the ophthalmic veins may be so intense that prolapse of the bulbar conjunctiva develops. In most cases, there is impaired ocular mobility that may range from partial to total ophthalmoplegia. Continuous elevation of intraocular pressure leads to progressive visual loss and eventually permanent blindness. Ophthalmologic evaluation in orbital cellulitis might show a decrease in visual acuity and/or limitation of global movements, proptosis, significant chemosis, and eyelid edema. Constitutional symptoms may be prominent, with fever, malaise, and leukocytosis present. Treatment is with intravenous antibiotics and close monitoring of the patient for

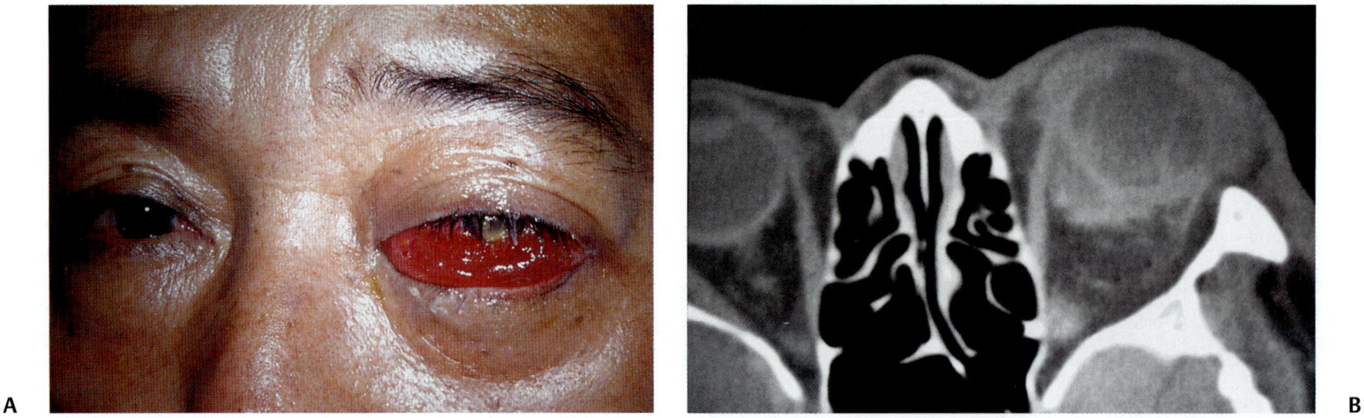

Fig. 8.5 A 52-year-old Chinese man with orbital cellulitis. **(A)** He presented with mild proptosis and gross chemosis of the left eye. The vision was slightly impaired and eye movements restricted. **(B)** Axial computed tomography scan of the patient. Note the inflammatory edema of the orbital fat in the affected eye emits different signals as compared with the normal eye. No obvious orbital abscess was noted. As his vision deteriorated despite antimicrobial therapy, an open surgical drainage was performed by the ophthalmologist. Minimal pus was drained, but the patient's vision improved following the drainage.

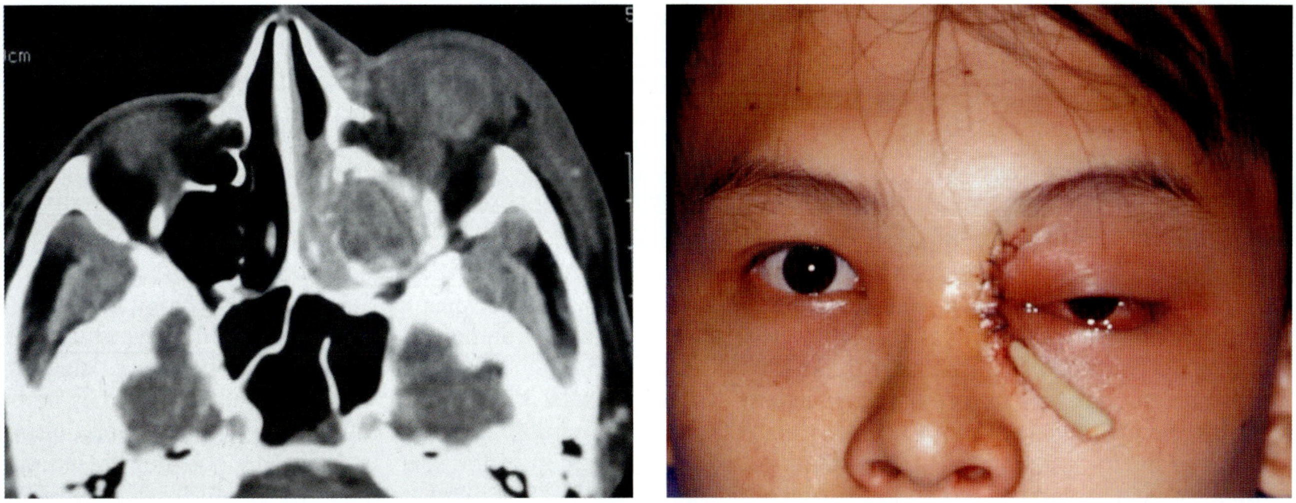

A B

Fig. 8.6 **(A)** A 26-year-old man referred by the ophthalmologist with an orbital abscess documented on computed tomography scan. This patient presented with proptosis, ophthalmoplegia, restricted eye movements, and progressive deterioration of vision. **(B)** The patient underwent combined endoscopic and open surgical drainage of the orbital abscess. Following a complete ethmoidectomy and middle meatal antrostomy, the lamina papyracea was removed as far back as the orbital apex. Three incisions were made in the periorbita extending from posterior to anterior. The abscess was drained externally through an external ethmoidectomy incision.

any progression of the disease. Absence of clinical improvement in the ocular findings, after adequate medical therapy, is an indication for surgical exploration or drainage.

Orbital Abscess

Orbital abscess (OA) is a collection of pus within the orbital tissues (**Fig. 8.6A**). This may arise from an acute sinus infection penetrating the periosteum or from an orbital cellulitis progressing to suppuration. Clinically, the patient presents with marked proptosis, chemosis, and ophthalmoplegia, and intense congestion of the eyelids and conjunctiva. Pus collection in close proximity to the optic nerve results in severe visual loss and even blindness due to compression. Septic or vascular visual loss may result from continued presence of pus within the orbit. Orbital abscess may sometimes be difficult to distinguish from orbital cellulitis. There is diffuse infiltration of the orbital fat with massive proptosis, extraocular enlargement, and occasionally gas formation seen within the orbital tissue on CT or MRI. If an obvious abscess is documented on the CT scan, emergent surgical drainage of the abscess is indicated (**Fig. 8.6B**).

Cavernous Sinus Thrombosis

Cavernous sinus thrombosis (CST) may be caused by retrograde spread of infection through the superior and/or inferior ophthalmic veins into the cavernous sinus causing life-threatening septic thrombophlebitis (**Fig. 8.7**). Because the left and right cavernous sinuses are interconnected, the signs and symptoms of orbital infection may be bilateral in many cases. When the contralateral eye is beginning to be affected by orbital infection, it is most likely that the infection has extended to the cavernous sinus and should prompt the diagnosis of cavernous sinus thrombosis. Patients with CST are extremely ill on presentation, with signs of meningitis and multiple cranial nerve palsies bilaterally. Neglected or inadequately treated orbital infections may progress to cavernous sinus thrombosis. Occasionally, the disease may

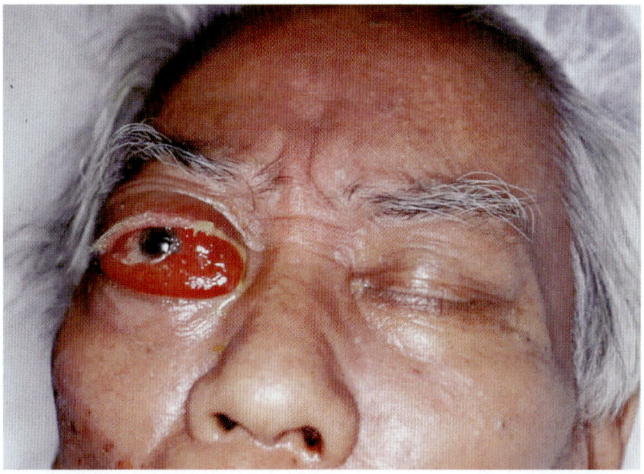

Fig. 8.7 A patient with cavernous sinus thrombosis. This immunocompromised diabetic 76-year-old man with fungal sinusitis presented with marked proptosis, chemosis, ophthalmoplegia, and complete visual loss. Despite aggressive medical therapy and surgical intervention, this patient died of the infection and cavernous sinus thrombosis.

run a fulminant course, especially in the compromised host. This generally involves tissue invasion by opportunistic mycotic organisms.

Microbiology

The organisms that cause these infections are similar to the bacteria that cause acute sinusitis, with the most common being *Streptococcus pneumoniae*, *Haemophilus influenza*, and *Branhamella catarrhalis*. In adults, *Staphylococcus aureus* and mixed cultures including anaerobic organisms such as *Bacteroides* species (sp) gram-negative anaerobic bacilli (*Prevotella*, *Porphyromonas*, and *Fusobacterium*), *Peptostreptococcus* and microaerophilic sp may be implicated.[23,24] Anaerobes could be associated with cellulitis and orbital abscess that develops following chronic sinusitis or following sinusitis associated with odontogenic infection. The orbital infections associated with maxillary sinusitis of odontogenic origin is often polymicrobial and organisms most often isolated are anaerobic gram-negative bacilli, *Peptostreptococcus* sp, *Fusobacterium* sp, and *Streptococcus* sp.[23,25] The organisms isolated in cavernous sinus thrombosis are *S. aureus* (50 to 70% instances), *Streptococcus* sp (20%), and gram-negative anaerobic bacilli. Similar organisms can be recovered from subperiosteal and orbital abscesses and their corresponding maxillary sinusitis.

Diagnosis

History and physical examination is the cornerstone of the diagnosis with emphasis on ophthalmologic examination to document any decrease in visual acuity, limitation of extraocular movement and cranial nerve deficits. A neurologic examination should also be performed to exclude concomitant intracranial complications.

Laboratory Tests

Elevated white blood count and CRP are nonspecific markers of inflammation and support the assumption of infectious process. Blood cultures have low yield yet can be taken when bacteremia is suspected due to chills and temperature elevation.[10] Lumbar puncture is unreliable and should be used judiciously when central nervous system (CNS) involvement is suspected.[24] Cultures from the nasal cavity and eye secretions have limited correlation to the sinus content and thus are not reliable.

Imaging

Plain radiographs are nonspecific yet can show the presence or absence of air fluid level, opacification or bony destruction of the sinuses. This imaging modality is seldom used today. CT is readily available and is the imaging modality of choice. It clearly demonstrates the orbital contents and the anatomy of the adjoining structures. For a more complete evaluation, CT scans are acquired in axial views; triplanar reconstruction permits evaluation in coronal, axial, and sagittal planes and provides detailed information of bone and soft tissue. Based on clinical symptoms, it is impossible to differentiate PSC or OC from an OA. CT scanning with contrast enhancement is capable of localizing an abscess and defining its walls. A CT scan may demonstrate SPA as either homogeneous or ring enhancement, with displacement of the rectus muscle and increased radiodensity of extraconal fat. Gas may be present within an abscess owing to gas-forming organisms or communication with an adjacent sinus. Bone window can outline bone defects that may predispose or result from the inflammatory process. Based on the CT scanning, Zimmerman and Bilaniuk have anatomically divided infections within the orbit proper into (1) intraconal—centrally within the muscle cone; (2) extraconal—peripherally between the periosteum and recti; and (3) subperiosteal—between the orbital wall and its periosteum.[26]

A CT scan has up to 90% accuracy in identifying SPA.[27–29] Skedros et al found CT scans to be accurate predictors of SPA in 80% of their 20 cases, whereas Younis et al reported a diagnostic accuracy of 91% in a series of 43 patients with orbital complications.[28,29] Though CT scans have a high degree of accuracy in identifying SPA, the importance of clinical examination and vigilance in periorbital involvement cannot be overemphasized.[15,30] There have been reports where orbital abscess was not identified on the CT, but found on surgical exploration. Delay in surgery in such cases resulted in visual loss for some patients. Patt and Manning report of four patients, in their series of 159 patients, who developed permanent blindness.[13] The presence of an orbital abscess, which was ultimately found at surgical exploration, was not diagnosed by CT in any of these four patients.

MRI provides superior soft tissue resolution and tissue characterization when compared with CT and is indicated when orbital or intracranial extension of infection is suspected. OC is demonstrated as an increased signal signifying edema and inflammatory infiltrates in the orbital fat on T2-weighted images and with diffuse enhancement postcontrast (gadolinium) administration. On T1-weighted images, the signal of the fat is low due to the high water content within inflammatory process. Both SPA and OA are seen on T2 as ring enhancement with low signal intensity centrally and high signal, peripherally. An air fluid level within the collection is diagnostic of abscess. The role of MRI is useful for soft tissue details, delineating SPA, and early detection of intracranial involvement.

Orbital ultrasound has been used in the diagnosis and in following the progression of intraorbital infection. This is an inexpensive study, does not expose the patient to ionizing radiation, and in most cases can be performed at the bedside if needed.[31] Although its theoretical ability to differentiate severe tissue edema from abscess formation surpasses CT, the limitations of ultrasound are its inability to identify deep orbital as well as intracranial disease extent. Therefore, it is not recommended as a routine diagnostic test.[15,22]

Management

Medical Treatment

Medical treatment should be aggressive from the early stages to prevent progression of the infection. In our institution, the majority of these patients present to the ophthalmologist and are referred to the Otolaryngology service. POC is best managed by a multidisciplinary team including an ophthalmologist, microbiologist, otolaryngologist, radiologist, and a pediatrician, as most patients are in the pediatric age group. The role of the otolaryngologist is extremely important as sinus disease accounts for more than 80% of POC. The management should be as an inpatient and is initiated with blood tests, cultures, and imaging studies of the sinus and orbit. Therapeutic measures should be instituted immediately. Evaluation of the patient should include a comprehensive clinical examination and imaging studies with an attempt to make a distinction between PSC and postseptal infection. Clinical examination should test for changes in visual acuity, papillary reactivity, and evaluation of extraocular mobility. Imaging studies such as the CT scans of the sinuses and orbit facilitate the diagnosis and aid in the distinction of PSC from a postseptal inflammation. Though CT scans are a fairly accurate predictor of SPA, these can sometimes be misleading and should not be the absolute criteria for surgical intervention.[13,30] An MRI scan may be indicated in assessing complex presentations of POC or when intracranial complications are suspected.

Patients with mild inflammatory eyelid edema and PSC can be treated with oral antibiotics such as amoxicillin-clavulanate or a second-generation cephalosporin. Close monitoring of the patient is mandatory, however. Parenteral antimicrobial therapy should be initiated when postseptal involvement is suspected or develops. Drugs that have good blood–brain barrier are preferred. The parenteral agents include ceftriaxone or cefotaxime, and metronidazole or clindamycin should be added for anaerobe cover. Anaerobic bacteria should be suspected when orbital cellulitis is associated with odontogenic infection and chronic sinusitis. Vancomycin should be administered in cases where methicillin-resistant *S. aureus* is present or suspected. When CST is suspected, high doses of parenteral wide-spectrum antimicrobial agents should be used. The role of anticoagulants and corticosteroids is controversial.

Medical therapy of orbital complications of sinusitis must also include supportive therapy with topical and systemic decongestants, humidification, analgesics, and hydration with intravenous fluids. The patient's visual acuity and extraocular muscle mobility should be closely monitored. Sequential CT scans may be needed for follow-up. If there is no improvement with 24 to 36 hours of medical therapy, or there is progression of symptoms within 24 hours, surgical intervention is indicated.

Surgical Management

The majority of preseptal infections generally resolve with medical treatment except for an occasional case that forms an eyelid abscess and may require an incision and drainage. Intraorbital infections, however, are more serious and the majority of them require surgical drainage. A conservative approach for intraorbital abscesses such as SPA and OA is generally not recommended, though few reports in the literature support this.[22,32,33] Goodwin and colleagues reported three patients of a series of 13 with orbital abscess who responded to antibiotic therapy alone.[22] However, the selection criteria for conservative management should include normal visual acuity and some globe motion. Patients on conservative therapy must be vigilantly monitored and repeatedly reexamined during therapy and surgical intervention initiated if the vision is compromised. Souliere et al reported 5 of the 10 patients documented as SPA on CT scan were managed with intravenous antibiotics and nasal decongestion alone.[32] All had complete clinical and radiographic resolution without complications. Handler et al caution that because it may not be possible to differentiate pus-containing abscesses from inflammatory masses seen on CT, a more conservative approach with aggressive medical therapy in such cases is justified.[33] Others also warn of what appears as an orbital abscess on CT scan may not be confirmed at surgery. They advocate careful clinical evaluation and response to antibiotic therapy as important determinants in the decision for surgical intervention.[34] Some authors have also reported a better outcome with conservative treatment in young children, particularly infants, as compared with adults who tend to have a worse prognosis.[17]

The general opinion, however, is that in view of the severe and potentially devastating complications, including visual loss, cavernous sinus thrombosis, and the potential for intracranial progression, surgical drainage should be performed sooner in the disease course. There have been several reports where CT scan had failed to detect intraorbital abscess. These reports express caution in interpreting the CT scan and advocate aggressive surgical therapy in appropriate clinical situations.[13,30,35] Krohel et al report four cases with visual loss to less than 20/200, despite treatment with intravenous antibiotics and surgical drainage. A CT scan had failed to detect orbital abscess in two cases.[35] It must be emphasized that inappropriate or inadequate treatment may result in significant morbidity. Furthermore, partially treated cases may not manifest the expected clinical findings of orbital infection and may present in an insidious fashion with symptoms evolving over weeks to months.

In most cases, surgical intervention is indicated by the presence of an abscess on CT, deterioration of visual acuity, signs of deterioration and progression in the orbital involvement despite adequate medical therapy, relapse of symptoms, or their progression to the contralateral eye. Indicators for deterioration may be radiologic, clinical, or both. Proptosis may be used as an indicator for surgery.

Surgery involves drainage of the abscess and the involved sinuses. Surgical management includes open external drainage, transnasal endoscopic drainage, or combined endoscopic and external drainage. In the past, open external drainage was the modality of choice for a majority of the patients.[2] The diagnostic and treatment trends in orbital infections have changed since the rise in popularity of endoscopic sinus surgery in the mid-1980s.[36] There have been several reports since early 1990 on the use of endoscopic sinus surgery for orbital infections.[25,37–39] Medially located SPA are particularly suitable for endoscopic drainage.[40,41] The main advantage of endoscopic surgery is the simultaneous treatment of causative sinus infection and orbital disease and the ability to explore the orbit with improved illumination and visualization using angled endoscopes when necessary. The added advantage is that of cosmesis given that it avoids the external scar of an open drainage. Though medial SPA is ideal for endoscopic treatment, there have been reports of draining superior and inferiorly located SPA using the endoscopes.[42] Drainage of orbital abscess, particularly intraconal abscess, is best achieved through a combined approach and should not be attempted without the active participation of ophthalmology colleagues.

Surgical Technique

The surgery (see **Video 8.1**) is performed with the patient under general anesthesia and with orotracheal intubation. Nasal decongestion is achieved with neuropatties soaked in 4% cocaine if available, or oxymetazoline. With patient supine on the operating table, the head is elevated by ~20 degrees. During draping of the patient the eyes are left uncovered. The nasal mucosa is allowed to decongest for at least 10 to 15 minutes, after which the neuropatties are removed and the operating field is infiltrated with 1:80000 epinephrine. To avoid bleeding due to mucosal trauma, a 27-gauge needle is used and multiple sites for infiltration are avoided. The two main sites of infiltration are the uncinate process and the basal lamella. Often, the nasal mucosa is severely inflamed and may not respond to decongestion resulting in excessive bleeding during the surgery. Continuous suction provided by the microdebrider assists in clearing the bloody field and maintains optimal visualization intraoperatively.

The majority of the surgery is performed using the zero-degree endoscope; and 30-, 45-, and 70-degree endoscopes are used as and when necessary particularly when working in the maxillary and the frontal sinus. The angled endoscopes are used to visualize laterally and around the corners into the orbit especially in the case of an intraorbital abscess. Maxillary sinusitis by itself is rarely the cause of OA, often it involves other paranasal sinuses. Most patients with orbital complication from maxillary sinusitis have involvement of the ethmoid labyrinth and require an anterior or complete ethmoidectomy with middle meatal antrostomy for drainage of the maxillary sinus. Manipulation of the frontal recess is usually not necessary, and is performed only when the epicenter of the infection is in the frontal recess. In most cases, a complete ethmoidectomy is performed by removing the uncinate process, the ethmoid bulla, only the middle part of the basal lamella to ensure the stability of the middle turbinate, and the posterior ethmoid cells. Depending upon the involvement, a sphenoidotomy is performed. A middle meatal antrostomy is performed to drain the pus within the maxillary sinus. The lamina papyracea is skeletonized from the orbital apex posteriorly to the nasolacrimal system anteriorly. The superior limit of exposure is the skull base and inferiorly is the roof of the maxillary sinus.

The lamina papyracea is gently palpated with a Freer elevator and fractured at its thinnest location. A plane of dissection is established between the lamina papyracea and the periorbita, and the lamina papyracea is dissected off the periorbita using the Freer elevator. The extent of removal of the lamina papyracea and exposure of the periorbita depends on the extent and location of the abscess.

In the situation when there is a circumscribed SPA, lamina papyracea overlying the SPA is removed to drain the abscess. Incision of the periorbita in draining a SPA may not be necessary. However, if there is an OA present, the periorbita is incised to drain the abscess. In case the orbital pressure is persistently elevated, it is prudent to decompress the entire medial orbital wall. This is done by one or several incisions of the periorbita. A sharp sickle knife or a #11 blade on a Bard Parker handle is used to make these incisions. The tip of the knife should remain superficial and the incision made from posterior to anterior. Most extraconal orbital abscesses can be drained by this maneuver. Drainage of an intraconal abscess, however, may require orbital exploration and must be done with an ophthalmologist. A combined approach is necessary in most cases.

It is important to obtain pus for cultures. This should be done in the beginning of the procedure when purulent material is obtained from the middle meatus and the maxillary sinus. Subsequently, purulent material from the SPA or OA should also be obtained and sent for cultures.

Postoperative Care

The patient's general condition, vital signs, vision, and eye movements are monitored postoperatively. Postoperative care is performed as in routine sinus surgery. Patients are instructed to perform nasal irrigations twice a day. Endoscopic debridement is performed on a weekly basis until mucosal healing takes place. In pediatric patients, office debridement may not be tolerated by the patient and a second-look procedure may be necessary. This is individualized depending on the extent of surgery and the mucosal trauma during the operation. Systemic culture directed antimicrobial therapy is continued postoperatively. Once there is improvement and signs of infection have abated, the patient is sent home.

Conclusion

Although infrequent, complications of sinusitis are clinical emergencies and can result in devastating permanent vision and neurologic deficits if not diagnosed and treated promptly. Orbital involvement in sinusitis occurs most commonly by spread of infection from the ethmoid sinuses; yet maxillary sinusitis can spread to the orbit directly through the superior wall of the maxilla or indirectly through extension to the ethmoids and then to the orbit. The main pathophysiologic mechanisms for infection spread to the orbit are direct extension through compromised bony barriers, septic thrombophlebitis, and erosive osteomyelitis. *S. pneumoniae*, *H. influenza*, and *B. catarrhalis* are the most common pathogens in acute sinusitis, yet *S. aureus* and anaerobes in a dental infection can also be the cause.

Chandler et al have described five stages of orbital involvement: less severe infection might cause cellulitis of orbital tissue yet in more serious cases orbital abscess or cavernous sinus thrombosis might form, which carry a high incidence of permanent visual deficiency. When orbital complication of sinusitis is suspected, a CT scan is recommended to define the orbital involvement and detect abscess formation.

In case of cellulitis without pus collection, broad-spectrum intravenous antibiotics can be started under close otolaryngologic and ophthalmologic follow-up. In contrast, abscess formation merits immediate surgical intervention and drainage of the involved sinuses as well as the intraorbital pus collection. In case of cavernous sinus thrombosis, anticoagulant therapy is added to surgical drainage and antibiotic therapy. A multidisciplinary team composed of an ophthalmologist, otolaryngologist, microbiologist, neurosurgeon, and a pediatrician, if the patient is a child, should manage patients together. Though open drainage of orbital abscess is widely practiced by ophthalmologists, endoscopic drainage of SPA and OA has been increasingly reported in the past 15 years. A combined endoscopic and open drainage may be necessary for some intraconal and/or laterally located OA.

Pearls

- Patients with periorbital cellulitis should be carefully evaluated and a distinction made between periorbital and orbital cellulitis.
- A CT scan, generally the recommended imaging modality to differentiate between cellulitis and abscess formation, may not always be reliable. Clinical correlation is essential.
- An MRI should be considered if intracranial complication is suspected.
- Close ophthalmologic follow-up is essential to detect visual impairment, which dictates immediate surgical drainage.
- Blood cultures and lumbar puncture have low yield and therefore are of limited value.
- Dental infection is an important cause of sinusitis and if suspected, anaerobic coverage is recommended.
- Open surgical drainage is widely practiced by the ophthalmologist when surgical drainage is indicated.
- As the majority of orbital infections are caused by paranasal sinus infections, endoscopic surgical drainage of the sinuses should be performed. Endoscopic sinus surgery has the advantage of improved illumination and visualization. Angled endoscopes can be useful to look around the corners while draining the OA.
- Depending upon the extent of the disease a middle meatal antrostomy and anterior ethmoidectomy is performed and if needed, posterior ethmoidectomy and sphenoidotomy can also be done.
- In draining a medial SPA, the lamina papyracea is resected to drain the abscess.
- Incision of the periorbita following removal of the lamina may be done if the abscess is extraconal or the intraorbital pressure is high. It may be combined with an open drainage.
- Intraconal abscess is best drained by open drainage.

References

1. Collins JG. Prevalence of selected chronic conditions. United States, 1983–85 (No 155). Hyattsville, MD: National Center for Health Statistics; 1988
2. Jackson K, Baker SR. Clinical implications of orbital cellulitis. Laryngoscope 1986;96(5):568–574
3. Schramm VL Jr, Curtin HD, Kennerdell JS. Evaluation of orbital cellulitis and results of treatment. Laryngoscope 1982;92(7 Pt 1):732–738
4. Chaudhry IA, Shamsi FA, Elzaridi E, et al. Outcome of treated orbital cellulitis in a tertiary eye care center in the Middle East. Ophthalmology 2007;114(2):345–354
5. Wilkins RB, Kulwin DR. Spontaneous enophthalmos associated with chronic maxillary sinusitis. Ophthalmology 1981;88(9):981–985
6. Ben Simon GJ, Bush S, Selva D, McNab AA. Orbital cellulitis: a rare complication after orbital blowout fracture. Ophthalmology 2005;112(11):2030–2034

7. Allan BP, Egbert MA, Myall RW. Orbital abscess of odontogenic origin. Case report and review of the literature. Int J Oral Maxillofac Surg 1991;20(5):268–270
8. Poon TL, Lee WY, Ho WS, Pang KY, Wong CK. Odontogenic subperiosteal abscess of orbit: a case report. J Clin Neurosci 2001;8(5):469–471
9. Stübinger S, Leiggener C, Sader R, Kunz C. Intraorbital abscess: a rare complication after maxillary molar extraction. J Am Dent Assoc 2005;136(7):921–925
10. Ferguson MP, McNab AA. Current treatment and outcome in orbital cellulitis. Aust N Z J Ophthalmol 1999;27(6):375–379
11. Connell B, Kamal Z, McNab AA. Fulminant orbital cellulitis with complete loss of vision. Clin Experiment Ophthalmol 2001;29(4):260–261
12. Jarrett WH II, Gutman FA. Ocular complications of infection in the paranasal sinuses. Arch Ophthalmol 1969;81(5):683–688
13. Patt BS, Manning SC. Blindness resulting from orbital complications of sinusitis. Otolaryngol Head Neck Surg 1991;104(6):789–795
14. Hartstein ME, Steinvurzel MD, Cohen CP. Intracranial abscess as a complication of subperiosteal abscess of the orbit. Ophthal Plast Reconstr Surg 2001;17(6):398–403
15. Goldberg AN, Oroszlan G, Anderson TD. Complications of frontal sinusitis and their management. Otolaryngol Clin North Am 2001;34(1):211–225
16. Shahin J, Gullane PJ, Dayal VS. Orbital complications of acute sinusitis. J Otolaryngol 1987;16(1):23–27
17. Harris GJ. Subperiosteal abscess of the orbit: older children and adults require aggressive treatment. Ophthal Plast Reconstr Surg 2001;17(6):395–397
18. Hayes EJ, Weber AL. Chronic sinus disease: a rare cause of enophthalmos. Ann Otol Rhinol Laryngol 1987;96(3 Pt 1):351–353
19. Eto RT, House JM. Enophthalmos, a sequela of maxillary sinusitis. AJNR Am J Neuroradiol 1995;16(4, Suppl) 939–941
20. Adams R, Petersdorf R. Pyogenic infections of the central nervous system. In: Adams R, Petersdorf R, Braunwald E, eds. Harrison's Principles of Internal Medicine. New York: McGraw-Hill; 1983:2084–2085
21. Chandler JR, Langenbrunner DJ, Stevens ER. The pathogenesis of orbital complications in acute sinusitis. Laryngoscope 1970;80(9):1414–1428
22. Goodwin WJ Jr, Weinshall M, Chandler JR. The role of high resolution computerized tomography and standardized ultrasound in the evaluation of orbital cellulitis. Laryngoscope 1982;92(7 Pt 1):729–731
23. Brook I, Frazier EH. Microbiology of subperiosteal orbital abscess and associated maxillary sinusitis. Laryngoscope 1996;106(8):1010–1013
24. Antoine GA, Grundfast KM. Periorbital cellulitis. Int J Pediatr Otorhinolaryngol 1987;13(3):273–278
25. Arjmand EM, Lusk RP, Muntz HR. Pediatric sinusitis and subperiosteal orbital abscess formation: diagnosis and treatment. Otolaryngol Head Neck Surg 1993;109(5):886–894
26. Zimmerman RA, Bilaniuk LT. CT of orbital infection and its cerebral complications. AJR Am J Roentgenol 1980;134(1):45–50
27. Towbin R, Han BK, Kaufman RA, Burke M. Postseptal cellulitis: CT in diagnosis and management. Radiology 1986;158(3):735–737
28. Skedros DG, Haddad J Jr, Bluestone CD, Curtin HD. Subperiosteal orbital abscess in children: diagnosis, microbiology, and management. Laryngoscope 1993;103(1 Pt 1):28–32
29. Younis RT, Anand VK, Davidson B. The role of computed tomography and magnetic resonance imaging in patients with sinusitis with complications. Laryngoscope 2002;112(2):224–229
30. McIntosh D, Mahadevan M. Failure of contrast enhanced computed tomography scans to identify an orbital abscess. The benefit of magnetic resonance imaging. J Laryngol Otol 2008;122(6):639–640
31. Kaplan DM, Briscoe D, Gatot A, Niv A, Leiberman A, Fliss DM. The use of standardized orbital ultrasound in the diagnosis of sinus induced infections of the orbit in children: a preliminary report. Int J Pediatr Otorhinolaryngol 1999;48(2):155–162
32. Souliere CR Jr, Antoine GA, Martin MP, Blumberg AI, Isaacson G. Selective non-surgical management of subperiosteal abscess of the orbit: computerized tomography and clinical course as indication for surgical drainage. Int J Pediatr Otorhinolaryngol 1990;19(2):109–119
33. Handler LC, Davey IC, Hill JC, Lauryssen C. The acute orbit: differentiation of orbital cellulitis from subperiosteal abscess by computerized tomography. Neuroradiology 1991;33(1):15–18
34. Gold SC, Arrigg PG, Hedges TR III. Computerized tomography in the management of acute orbital cellulitis. Ophthalmic Surg 1987;18(10):753–756
35. Krohel GB, Krauss HR, Winnick J. Orbital abscess. Presentation, diagnosis, therapy, and sequelae. Ophthalmology 1982;89(5):492–498
36. Younis RT, Lazar RH, Bustillo A, Anand VK. Orbital infection as a complication of sinusitis: are diagnostic and treatment trends changing? Ear Nose Throat J 2002;81(11):771–775
37. Deutsch E, Eilon A, Hevron I, Hurvitz H, Blinder G. Functional endoscopic sinus surgery of orbital subperiosteal abscess in children. Int J Pediatr Otorhinolaryngol 1996;34(1-2):181–190
38. Page EL, Wiatrak BJ. Endoscopic vs external drainage of orbital subperiosteal abscess. Arch Otolaryngol Head Neck Surg 1996;122(7):737–740
39. Wolf SR, Göde U, Hosemann W. Endonasal endoscopic surgery for rhinogen intraorbital abscess: a report of six cases. Laryngoscope 1996;106(1 Pt 1):105–110
40. Pereira KD, Mitchell RB, Younis RT, Lazar RH. Management of medial subperiosteal abscess of the orbit in children—a 5 year experience. Int J Pediatr Otorhinolaryngol 1997;38(3):247–254
41. Fakhri S, Pereira K. Endoscopic management of orbital abscesses. Otolaryngol Clin North Am 2006;39(5):1037–1047, viii
42. Roithmann R, Uren B, Pater J, Wormald PJ. Endoscopic drainage of a superiorly based subperiosteal orbital abscess. Laryngoscope 2008;118(1):162–164

9 Benign Maxillary Sinus Masses

Hesham Saleh and Valerie J. Lund

The maxillary sinus may harbor any of a large number of benign lesions with a different array of etiologies. Being a relatively large cavity within the craniofacial skeleton, long periods may pass before any symptoms manifest themselves. Frequently, patients only present when their lesions have filled the cavity, causing pressure symptoms or spread into surrounding areas such as the nasal cavity. Many pathologies in this area share common presenting symptoms, but some have unique features. The goal of this chapter is to present a detailed overview of these lesions' characteristics, their diagnosis, and treatment.

Differential Diagnosis

Benign lesions of the maxillary sinus can be conveniently divided into nonneoplastic and neoplastic (**Table 9.1**). Nonneoplastic lesions represent a range of inflammatory conditions with varied etiology, some not well understood. Neoplasms can originate from any of the tissues that form the architecture of the maxillary sinus. These include the mucosa, salivary glands, mesenchyme, vessels, muscle, dentition, and bone. They are uncommon tumors: Some are very rarely encountered. Many of these pose significant diagnostic problems requiring a low threshold of suspicion and histopathologic expertise. Lesions of the maxillary sinus affect a wide age range from children to the elderly and some have either sex predilection. Lesions such as fibrous dysplasia have a tendency to stabilize, but others are slowly progressive.

Diagnosis

Clinical Features

Many of the maxillary sinus lesions are initially asymptomatic and only cause symptoms when they reach larger dimensions. They share a common presentation similar to rhinosinusitis such as unilateral nasal obstruction, rhinorrhea, and local discomfort. Some symptoms are more common with certain lesions such as epistaxis in hematomas and hemangiomas. Lesions such as mucoceles and most tumors can lead to expansion of the sinus with the resultant facial swelling. When symptoms due to pressure occur, they can lead to epiphora, diplopia, proptosis, and loose dentition, but paresthesias are rarely encountered. Palatal and gingival swellings are sometimes encountered with salivary gland and odontogenic tumors, respectively.

Imaging

Computed tomography (CT) is the most commonly used modality. Although most lesions share common features of radiopacity in the sinus, some show specific features that are sometimes diagnostic. This is often true for mucoceles,

Table 9.1 Classification of Benign Lesions of the Maxillary Sinus

Nonneoplastic	Neoplastic
Mucosal cyst	Papillomas
Antrochoanal polyp	Salivary gland tumors (pleomorphic adenoma, oncocytoma)
Fungal disease (covered in chap 5)	Mesenchymal tumors (fibroma, lipoma, myxoma)
Mucocele	Vasiform tumors (hemangioma, aneurysmal bone cyst, hemangiopericytoma)
Cholesterol granuloma	Tumors of muscle origin (leiomyoma, rhabdomyoma)
Hematoma	Odontogenic tumors (see also Table 9.3)
Eosinophilic angiocentric fibrosis	Fibroosseous lesions (osteoma, ossifying fibroma, fibrous dysplasia, osteoblastoma)
Granulomatous deposits in sarcoidosis and Wegener granulomatosis	Neuroectodermal tumors (schwannoma, neurofibroma)
Antrolithiasis	

antrochoanal polyps, Wegener granulomatosis, antrolithiasis, and odontogenic and fibroosseous tumors (see below). Magnetic resonance imaging (MRI) can often be helpful in differentiating fluid from soft tissue and contrast enhancement is useful in delineating tumors. Panoramic maxillary x-rays (orthopantomogram [OPG]) can give supplementary information particularly with odontogenic tumors.

Additional Tests

When suspected, blood serology for granulomatous disease (angiotensin converting enzyme [ACE] and cytoplasmic-staining antineutrophil cytoplasmic antibodies [cANCA]) and clotting factors in case of hematomas are done. Some tumors occasionally represent part of a syndrome, which should be suspected and investigated. These include osteoma in Gardner syndrome, fibrous dysplasia in McCune–Albright syndrome, and neurofibromas in type 1 neurofibromatosis (NF1; see below).

Surgery

Surgery is the main treatment of the majority of maxillary sinus lesions except when they are asymptomatic and nonprogressive such as small osteomas and fibrous dysplasia, respectively (see below). Most lesions can be excised through an endoscopic approach with other approaches available for extensive, awkwardly positioned, or recurrent lesions. The surgeon should always be prepared to change the approach to get the optimum result and this must be part of the informed consent.

Endoscopic Resection

Standard endoscopic sinus surgery techniques are often sufficient to excise maxillary sinus lesions.[1] A large middle meatal antrostomy should be fashioned to obtain sufficient access. Angled instruments, specifically designed for the maxillary sinus are invaluable. We also use combinations of 30- and 45-degree rigid endoscopes for removal and 70-degree for final inspection. Occasionally, the antrostomy can be extended inferiorly through to the middle portion of the inferior turbinate if more access is needed. This can also be combined with an inferior antrostomy to access the floor such as in some cases of antrolithiasis. An endoscopic medial maxillectomy is sometimes necessary such as in cases of extensive inverted papilloma of the medial maxillary wall.[2,3] This involves removal of the inferior turbinate and medial wall down to the nasal floor with varying degrees of resection for the bone of pyriform aperture (**see Video 9.1**). The endoscopic resection can also be combined with an anterior antrostomy (Caldwell–Luc approach) when access to the floor and lateral wall is required.

Anterior Antrostomy

Although the use of a Caldwell–Luc approach has considerably declined in the management of chronic rhinosinusitis, it still has a definite role in the management of benign maxillary lesions.[4] We often use it in combination with the endoscopic approach to improve access. A standard gingivobuccal incision is made at the canine fossa after infiltrating the area with 1:80,000 epinephrine and 2% lignocaine. The incision starts at the level of the canine tooth and ends at the first molar, and is carried down to the bone. After retracting the periosteum, a cutting bur is used to drill a window in the bone and then the mucosa of the sinus cavity is opened. The window should be 1 to 2 cm inferior to infraorbital rim and 1 to 2 cm superior to the gingivobuccal sulcus to avoid injuring the infraorbital nerve and dental roots. The gingivobuccal flaps are kept retracted and instruments and/or endoscopes can be introduced through antrostomy. Closure of the soft tissue at the end of the procedure is achieved with a continuous absorbable suture.

Midfacial Degloving

This approach is ideally suited for extensive lesions because it allows direct access to the maxillary sinus, nasal cavity, and infratemporal fossa while avoiding external incisions.[5,6] Complications are infrequent and can generally be avoided by applying meticulous techniques. The procedure is in essence an extension of bilateral gingivobuccal incisions with the inclusion of the nasal dorsum through intercartilaginous and transfixion incisions. First 1:80,000 epinephrine and 2% lignocaine are infiltrated into the gingivobuccal sulcus, intercartilaginous area, and columella. A bilateral gingivobuccal incision is made down to bone running from maxillary tuberosity to tuberosity. The periosteum and soft tissue of the cheek are raised, as for Caldwell–Luc approach, exposing the infraorbital nerves and orbital margin. Intercartilaginous incisions are made as in rhinoplasty and connected to transfixion incision at the caudal end and anterior septum separating it for the medial crura. The incision is continued across the floor of the nose to join the intercartilaginous incisions laterally. Elevation of the nasal soft tissue envelope all the way laterally to the maxillary bones now allows complete degloving of the middle third of the face. At the end of the procedure, closure is achieved with absorbable suture and a nasal plaster is used.

Lateral Rhinotomy and Medial Maxillectomy

Lateral rhinotomy allows direct access to the lateral nasal wall and maxillary sinus.[7] With meticulous techniques an innocuous scar and minimal morbidity is achievable. It has the advantage of being extendable superiorly to gain access to the orbit and frontal sinus if needed. The incision site is infiltrated with epinephrine and lignocaine as above. The curvilinear skin incision begins just below the medial aspect of the brow and extends inferiorly midway between the medial canthus and nasion. It is then carried over just anterior to the nasomaxillary sulcus and alar groove to end in the nasal vestibule. The incision is deepened to the bone then the periosteum is retracted after achieving hemostasis. The medial canthal ligament and lacrimal sac are detached laterally. An osteotomy along the frontal process of the maxilla can then be made using a saw or osteotome. Incising the nasal mucosa and retraction of the bone laterally then allows access into the nasal cavity and lateral nasal wall. A medial maxillectomy can satisfactorily be done through this approach by removing bone at the pyriform aperture from anterior to posterior. Closure of the periosteum is achieved with absorbable sutures after reattaching the medial canthal ligament. Skin closure is done with fine Prolene (Ethicon, Somerville, NJ) sutures.

Other Treatments

In general, surgery is not indicated in active granulomatous disease and the treatment is medical. Bisphosphonates have been used for the treatment of fibrous dysplasia in some centers (see below).

Outcomes

A complete cure can be achieved with a large number of benign lesions of the maxillary sinus. Some lesions are more aggressive and some have higher recurrence rates than others. These will be outlined in the rest of the chapter.

Specific Lesions

Nonneoplastic

Mucosal Cyst

Mucosal cysts of the maxillary sinus are common with an incidence between 12.4 and 35.6% detected on radiography.[8–10] They are broadly classified into secretory and nonsecretory cysts.[11] Obstruction of mucosal glands leads to the formation of secretory cysts, which are less common. The more common nonsecretory cysts are presumably caused by an accumulation of exudates in the sinus mucosa lifting the epithelial lining. The etiologic factors behind cyst formation remain unknown. One study showed high levels of immunoglobulins, complement, and antiproteases in cyst aspirates consistent with an inflammatory process.[12] Levels of immunoglobulin E (IgE) and eosinophils were not raised, suggesting that allergy was not a significant factor. Oral flora was cultured from cyst fluid suggesting a possible dental cause. In another study, dental disease has been found in up to 50% of patients' mucosal cysts.[9] The majority of mucosal cysts originate in the floor of the maxillary sinus.[9] They are mostly unilateral, but can be bilateral in 10 to 20% of cases.[13,14] They are usually seen as homogeneous, dome-shaped opacities on CT scanning and are usually a chance diagnosis on sinus radiography (**Fig. 9.1**).[10] Controversy still exists on the clinical importance of mucosal cysts. Some authors suggest they represent an inflammatory sinus disease; others disagree.[9,10] The variation could be attributed to different patient populations chosen for studies and the methods of interpretation of results. A recent study of a large number of patients undergoing CT scanning for ophthalmologic conditions showed no statistically significant relationship to subjective rhinologic symptoms and objective measurements in the form of Lund–Mackay Scores.[10] The mere presence of the cysts, in the opinion of the authors, is not in itself an indication for surgical intervention. When operating on patients with rhinosinusitis, mucosal cysts are often encountered and can be opened (**Fig. 9.2**). They express yellowish to green transparent fluid and can be removed via a middle meatal antrostomy.

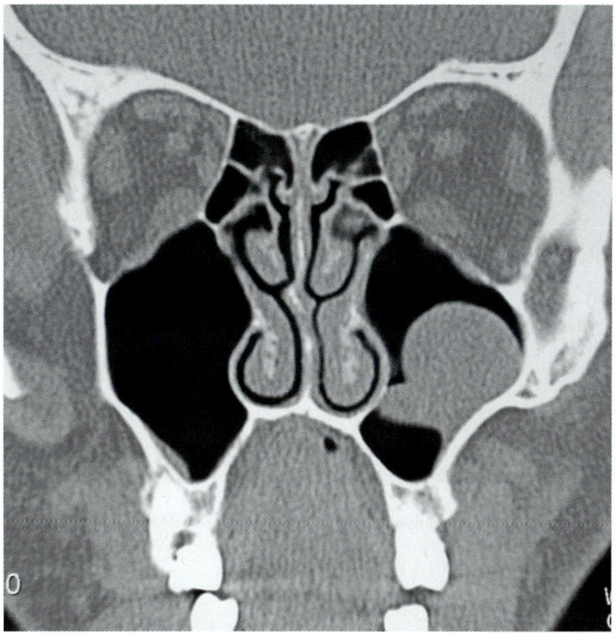

Fig. 9.1 A coronal computed tomography scan showing a mucosal cyst in the left maxillary sinus. Note the typical domed surface and the origin at the floor of the sinus.

Antrochoanal Polyp

An antrochoanal polyp (ACP) is a benign lesion that originates from the mucosa of the maxillary sinus and grows into the nasal cavity to reach the choana. Although the first report of ACP was attributed to Palfyn in 1753, it was Killian who

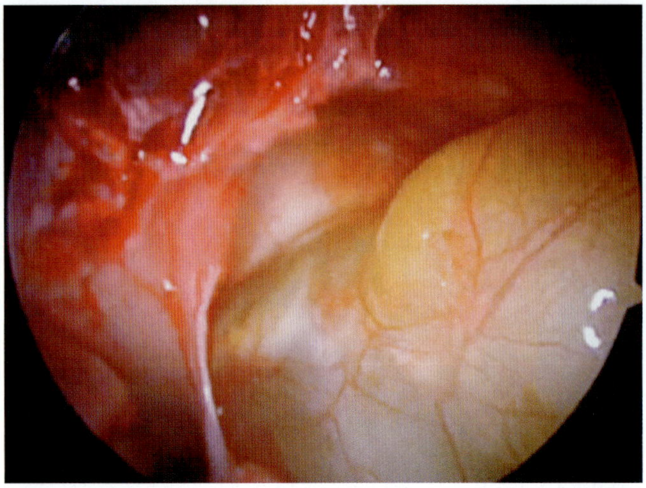

Fig. 9.2 An endoscopic view of a mucosal cyst in the left maxillary sinus seen through an antrostomy.

described the condition in detail in 1906.[15] ACPs account for 4 to 6% of all nasal polyps with increased incidence of 33% in children.[16,17] ACPs are usually unilateral with only a small number of reported cases with bilateral polyps.[16] It has been suggested that most ACPs originate from the posterior antral wall. In a series of 37 cases, 38% originated in the posteromedial wall, 19% in the posterior wall, 8% in the anterior wall, 8% in the anteromedial wall, 8% in the floor, 5% in the lateral wall, 5% in the roof, 3% in the anterolateral wall, 3% in the posterosuperior wall, and 3% in the inferolateral wall.[18] Mean age of presentation is 27 years and it is reported to be twice as common in males than females.[18] However, some have reported no difference in incidence between males and females in a pediatric population.[19,20] An ACP differs from nasal polyps in the fact that it is a solitary lesion that extends into the choana. Stammberger and Hawke[21] found that 70% of ACPs emerge through an accessory ostium. Aydin et al studied 37 patients with ACP and found that 51% originated from an accessory ostium, 43% from the natural ostium, and 6% from both.[18] Macroscopically, it has a cystic part filling the maxillary sinus and a solid part in the nasal cavity.[22] Berg found similarity between both tissues and fluid content in ACP and maxillary mucosal cysts with the resultant hypothesis that ACP is the intranasal form of mucosal cysts. Microscopically, it has a central cavity surrounded by a homogeneous edematous stroma bearing few cells, while the polyp surface is covered with respiratory epithelium.

In contrast to nasal polyps, an ACP has less inflammatory infiltrate and significantly lower eosinophils while edema is essentially the same.[23] An ACP also exhibits significantly higher fibroinflammatory changes with proliferation of fibroblasts and collagen, and a lymphocyte inflammatory infiltrate. It has been postulated that the latter is related to the long evolution of an ACP that leads to a scarring stage.[16] The surface epithelium of an ACP is mostly intact in contrast to some disruption in nasal polyps.[24]

The molecular biology of an ACP has been studied by some authors. Urokinase type plasminogen activator (u-PA), which is related to proliferative changes of the mucous membrane in inflammatory tissue, has been identified in ACP tissue extracts.[25] Others reported that the expression of basic fibroblast growth factor (bFGF) and transforming growth factor (TGF) β was significantly higher in ACPs than in chronic rhinosinusitis and healthy mucosa.[17] Some also showed increased expression of matrix metalloproteinase-9 (MMP-9), which is involved in mucous membrane inflammation, in ACPs, and nasal polyps compared with normal nasal mucosa.[26] Clinical manifestations usually start with unilateral nasal obstruction, but other symptoms have been reported such as epistaxis, purulent rhinorrhea, postnasal drip, snoring, obstructive sleep apnea, dysphonia, and dysphagia.[16,18]

Nasal endoscopy reveals a smooth swelling originating in the middle meatus and extending posteriorly into the choana. Very large ACPs can be seen in the nasopharynx or even in the oral cavity. CT scanning shows a mass filling the maxillary sinus with opacification of the middle meatus and extension into the choana (**Fig. 9.3**). MRI shows a hypointense signal on T1 modality and enhanced signal on T2 modality.

The accepted management of ACPs is surgical removal. Simple avulsion is associated with high rates of recurrence because the maxillary portion is not removed.[16] Endoscopic sinus surgery is used where a large middle meatal antrostomy is created to access the maxillary portion. A nasal snare can be tightened around the nasal portion close to the antrostomy and gradual "to and fro" movement can lead to the

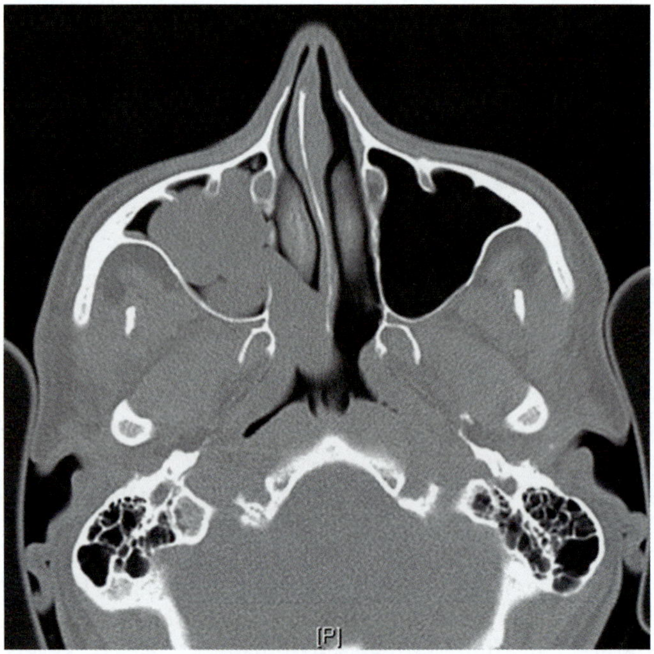

Fig. 9.3 An axial computed tomography scan of a patient with a right antrochoanal polyp showing both maxillary and nasal components with a narrower part passing through an accessory ostium.

complete removal of the whole ACP. The cavity of the maxillary sinus is then inspected with angled endoscopes and any mucosal remnant is removed. For this, angled instruments or a curved microdebrider can be used (**see Video 9.2**). Some advocate the combined use of a Caldwell–Luc approach with an endoscopic procedure.[16,18] We prefer to reserve the combined approach for recurrent cases.

Mucocele

A mucocele is an epithelial-lined mucus-containing sac completely filling a sinus cavity. Its main feature is the capability of expansion by the process of bone resorption and new bone formation.[27] As it expands, it becomes locally destructive and leads to the displacement of adjacent tissues. Maxillary sinus mucoceles are rare in comparison to frontal or frontoethmoidal mucoceles. They account for fewer than 10% of all mucoceles of the paranasal sinuses in the United States and Europe.[28–31] However, they are more commonly reported in Japan, usually as a long-term sequel of Caldwell–Luc surgery.[32] It has traditionally been thought that mucoceles develop as a result of obstruction of sinus outflow resulting in accumulation of mucus and buildup of pressure that gradually causes expansion and destruction.[33] It has been shown that the obstruction in combination with superimposed infection cause the release of cytokines from lymphocytes and monocytes. The cytokine release stimulates fibroblasts to secrete prostaglandins and collagenases, which, in turn, stimulate bone resorption.[34,35] The etiologic factors that lead to the formation of mucoceles have been attributed to previous surgery, trauma, inflammation, and tumors.[28,31] The development of a mucocele is a slow process that can take many years. In one large series, the median interval for the development of maxillary mucoceles after Caldwell–Luc was 15 years.[28] This was the longest when compared with mucoceles in other sinuses. Interestingly, 17 to 36% of patients with mucoceles do not have a history of any of the above.[28,36]

Symptoms and signs are caused by the expansion of the mucocele into the nose and surrounding structures. Patients can present with nasal obstruction, cheek swelling, upward displacement of the globe and proptosis.[28,30,31] Endoscopic examination may reveal pus or occasionally prolapse of the medial sinus wall in the middle meatus. Busaba stated that a triad of a bulging medial wall, prolapsed middle meatal mucosa obliterating the middle meatus, and a streak of mucopurulent drainage in the middle meatal region is suggestive of a maxillary mucocele.[30] CT scanning is the optimum diagnostic modality to show bone expansion and typically the bony outline becomes more rounded as the bone remodels in response to pressure within the sinus cavity (**Fig. 9.4A**).[31] MRI is not always necessary, but will establish the fluid content of the mucocele.[31]

Traditional teaching emphasized the need for complete removal of the mucocele to prevent recurrence.[28,29] It is now well established, however, that the majority of mucoceles can be managed endoscopically. Bockmühl suggested some contraindications to the endoscopic approach, which include far lateral (compartmentalized) or zygomatic bone maxillary mucoceles, the presence of a cutaneous fistula and in cases of associated malignancy.[28] The authors perform a large middle meatal antrostomy of up to 2 cm in diameter to avoid restenosis and recurrence of the mucocele. If needed, a partial medial maxillectomy that involves excising the middle third

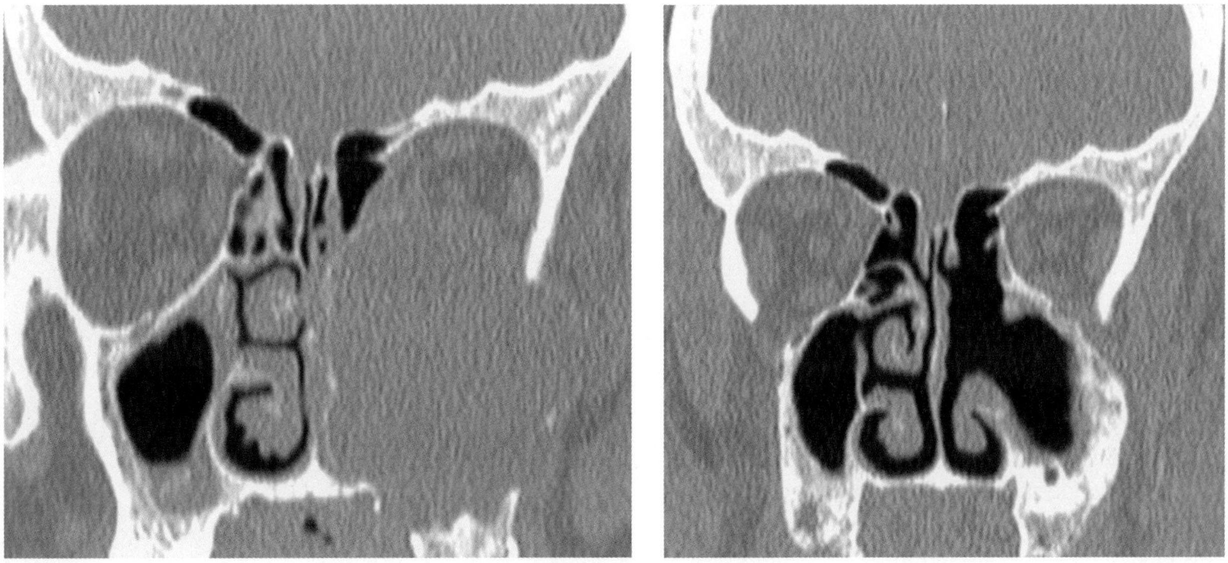

A B

Fig. 9.4 **(A)** A coronal computed tomography scan of a large left maxillary mucocele showing extensive expansion, bone thinning, and pressure on the orbit. The patient presented with cheek swelling and nasal obstruction, but no diplopia due to the slow developing-disease process. **(B)** Same patient in Fig. 9.3A 6 months after drainage of the mucocele through a large middle meatal antrostomy. Note the return of the sinus cavity to its normal contours.

of the inferior turbinate can be done. This would not cause damage to the nasolacrimal duct. It is not necessary to remove the mucosa of the mucocele cavity because it is known that the mucocele epithelium retains its respiratory nature and returns to normal appearance after surgery.[34] Over a period of 3 to 6 months, bone remodeling with shrinkage of the expanded sinus walls occurs (**Fig. 9.4B**).

Cholesterol Granuloma

Cholesterol granuloma (CG) is a histologic term used to describe the coexistence of granulation tissue with cholesterol crystals and foreign body giant cells.[37] The condition is well described in the temporal bone, but is rarely encountered in the paranasal sinuses.[38] Within the small number of published cases, the maxillary sinus is most commonly involved.[38,39] Only one case of bilateral maxillary sinus involvement has been reported.[39] CG has been observed more in men, with 3:1 male to female ratio and an average age of 41 years. The disease duration varied from 6 weeks to 10 years.[39] Only a small number of patients had a history of previous trauma or surgery.[38,39]

It has been suggested that a combination of factors leads to the formation of CG. These include disturbed ventilation in a bony cavity, impaired drainage, and hemorrhage.[38–41] Impaired drainage would increase pressure in the sinus cavity, which, in turn, obstructs venous and lymphatic circulation and predisposes to mucosal hemorrhage. The insufficient lymphatic drainage would fail to eliminate lipid components in red blood cells and contribute to accumulation of cholesterol crystals. These act as foreign material that stimulates the granulomatous reaction in the sinus cavity.[38,39,42]

Patients with CG present with symptoms and signs resembling chronic rhinosinusitis.[38,39] Most of the reported cases presented with nasal obstruction, postnasal drip, rhinorrhea, facial pain, or headaches. Rarely patients present with clear golden yellow rhinorrhea, which is considered suspicious of CG.[39] CT shows a cyst-like opacity, which does not enhance with contrast. Bony erosion or expansion has been reported in a small number of cases.[39,42] The lesion gives a very high signal on all MRI sequences. Therefore, the diagnosis is confirmed on histologic analysis of the removed tissue. This is characterized by a large number of clefts due to the dissolution of cholesterol crystal by alcohol used in staining the tissue.[42] These are surrounded by foreign-body giant cells, and macrophages filled with hemosiderin embedded in fibrous granulation tissue.

Treatment is by surgical excision. Most cases are accessible endoscopically and can be completely removed through this route.[43] The most frequent findings were cystic or partially cystic masses with bluish, yellowish, or brownish colors.[39] It is important to remove the granulation tissue completely to prevent recurrence. A large middle meatal antrostomy and the use of angled instruments will facilitate the procedure. The sinus cavity is inspected with a 70-degree endoscope at the end of the operation to confirm complete removal.

Hematoma

Hematoma of the maxillary sinus is also known as organized hematoma or hemorrhagic pseudotumor.[44–46] It is an uncommon cause of a maxillary sinus mass with only a small number of reported cases. A good number of reports come from Korea and Japan.[45] Although some of the hematomas have been reported in patients with bleeding diathesis such as Von Willebrand disease, there are several patients who present with what appears to be a spontaneous etiology.[45–47] Patients presenting with this condition belong to a wide age range, which probably reflects a varied pathology. It has been suggested that the condition develops in several stages. First a blood clot accumulates in the maxillary sinus secondary to facial trauma, operative bleeding, recurrent epistaxis, or bleeding diathesis. Second, the hematoma develops and because of poor ventilation and obstruction of drainage it transforms into an organized hematoma by means of neovascularization and fibrosis.[45,46] Encapsulation of the blood clot by fibrous tissue prevents reabsorption of the hematoma. Further bleeding causes increasing pressure and progressive expansion, which leads to erosion of adjacent structures.[46,47]

The most common symptom at presentation is epistaxis followed by unilateral nasal obstruction and facial swelling.[44,45] Symptoms due to pressure on adjacent structures such as proptosis and infraorbital hypoesthesia have been reported.[48,49] Clinical examination shows aspects that are generally similar to those of other expansible nasal masses such as medialization of the lateral nasal wall with or without a mass in the middle meatus.[44,45] CT scanning shows the hematoma as a nonenhancing soft tissue mass, which can be heterogeneous or homogeneous. It also demonstrates bony erosion if this has occurred (**Fig. 9.5**).[44,45] The mass is

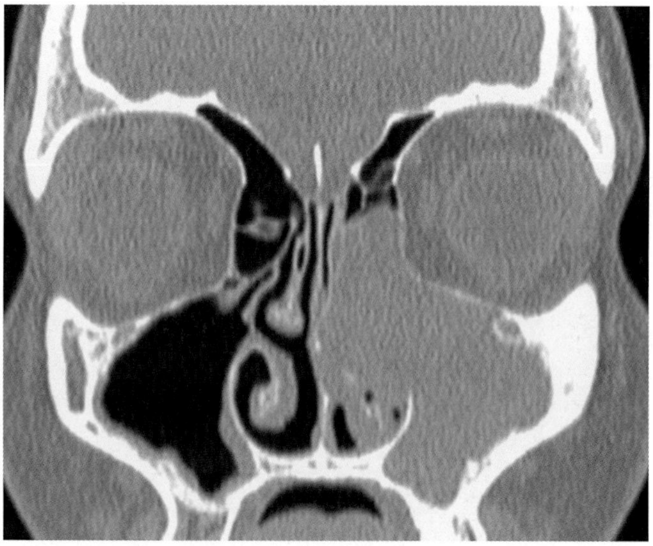

Fig. 9.5 A coronal computed tomography scan of a patient with an organized hematoma in the left maxillary sinus showing expansion with bone remodeling.

nonenhancing on both T1-weighted and T2-weighted MRI sequences.[46,49] Heterogeneous signal intensity on MRI represents different phases of blood products caused by rebleeding into the hematoma.[47] Histologically, the hematoma has a peripheral wall that consists of dense fibrous tissue with spindle-shaped myofibroblast cells. The center of the hematoma consists of loose fibrous tissue, which is relatively acellular and contains some intact erythrocytes.[44,45,49]

Treatment is surgical and is accessible endoscopically. The authors have treated all cases of this condition via this route with no recurrence. A large middle meatal antrostomy is often all that is necessary combined with partial medial maxillectomy if needed (**see Video 9.3**). The hematoma appears as a well-circumscribed nodular mass with no apparent point of origin in the sinus wall (**Fig. 9.6**). After removal, inspection of the sinus cavity with angled scopes should be done to ensure complete removal.

Eosinophilic Angiocentric Fibrosis

Eosinophilic angiocentric fibrosis (EAF) is an uncommon inflammatory fibrotic lesion that affects the submucosa of the nose, larynx, and orbit.[50,51] The pathologic process is manifested by predominantly eosinophilic perivascular inflammation and gradual replacement with progressive fibrosis.[50–53] The condition was first described by Roberts and McCann in 1985; since then a small number of cases have been reported.[53] EAF is found with a slightly higher incidence in young to middle-aged women than men.[50] The etiology of EAF is unknown, but it has been closely linked to granuloma faciale due to similarities in histologic features.[50–54] Some association with allergy and trauma has also been suggested, but has not been substantiated.[50,51] The majority of the lesions involve the nasal septum and lateral nasal wall, with only a small number of reported cases involving the maxillary sinus. Similarly, the disease has very rarely been reported in the larynx and orbit.[50]

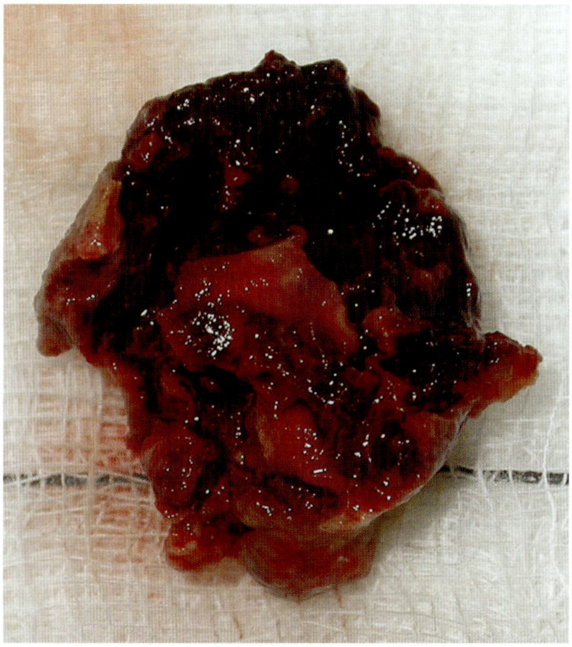

Fig. 9.6 A photograph of the maxillary hematoma just after removal from the sinus of the patient shown in Fig. 9.5.

EAF is slow growing and can take many years to manifest.[50,51] Symptoms are nonspecific and can initially include nasal obstruction, rhinorrhea, epistaxis, and facial pain.[50,53,54] Due to mass expansion the patients will later present with facial swelling.[50,51] Involvement of the orbit can lead to periorbital edema and proptosis.[50] Examination usually reveals thickening of the nasal septum with an intranasal mass.[50,51]

Imaging findings are usually nonspecific and include septal thickening, sinus opacification, and focal bone destruction.[50,52] Histology is diagnostic due to the very specific features: perivascular fibrosis with collagen and reticulin fibers in an "onion-skin like" pattern.[50–52] Single histology specimens may exhibit a spectrum of lesions from early inflammatory to late fibrotic lesions.[50] Early lesions consist of an eosinophilic vasculitis without fibrinoid necrosis involving small blood vessels (capillaries and/or venules). Eosinophils predominate, but they are invariably accompanied by plasma cells and lymphocytes.[50] There are no granulomas, foreign body-type giant cells or necrosis.[50,52] Late lesions show dense fibrous thickening of the subepithelial stroma with obliterative perivascular onion-skin of collagen and reticulin fibers.[50]

Surgical resection appears to be the treatment of choice, but recurrences are common.[50–52] The surgical approach is tailored to the extent of the lesion and lateral rhinotomy is often required.[51] Medical treatment with various agents such as local and systemic steroids, dapsone, hydroxychloroquine, and azathioprine have been unsuccessful.[50,51]

Granulomatous Deposits in Sarcoidosis and Wegener Granulomatosis

Sarcoidosis is a chronic noncaseating granulomatous disease of unknown origin, principally affecting the respiratory tract.[54] The multisystem nature of sarcoidosis was described by Boeck in 1899.[55] The incidence of the condition is estimated between 1.2 and 19 per 100,000 in Caucasians; it is much higher in African Americans with a ratio of 12:1.[56] There is a slight female preponderance with the age of presentation between the third and fifth decades.[56–58] West Indians and Scandinavians appear to be more commonly affected than other racial groups.

There is predilection for lungs and hilar lymph nodes, which are affected in 90% of patients with clinical disease. The disease involves the nose and sinuses in only 1 to 4% of patients.[56–59] A minority present with nasal symptoms without other systemic manifestations of the disease.[56,58,60] Patients complain of nasal stuffiness, blood-stained discharge, crusting, and an offensive postnasal drip. Clinical manifestations include nasal crusting with friable submucosal yellowish granulomas involving the inferior turbinates and septum (**Fig. 9.7**). The inflammation may progress to cause septal ulceration and perforation, which occurs particularly in those who have had previous surgery. Saddling of the nose or skin manifestations (lupus pernio) are occasionally seen (**Fig. 9.8**). Although the sinuses are often involved in patients with nasal disease, it is extremely rare for patients to present with isolated maxillary sinus involvement without nasal symptoms. Only a small number of cases have been reported and certainly this reflects our experience.[56,57] Nevertheless, the condition should be included in the differential diagnosis of maxillary sinus masses. Findings on CT scanning of the sinuses are nonspecific with uniform opacity and occasional bony erosion. Erythrocyte sedimentation rate (ESR), ACE levels, and chest radiography are worth considering in suspected cases. Biopsy only yields positive results when taken from areas with mucosal inflammation.[61] Treatment is medical in a multidisciplinary approach and is tailored to the severity of the condition. This usually includes combinations of oral corticosteroids, macrolide antibiotics, methotrexate, and hydroxychloroquine and more recently infliximab according to the severity of the condition.[62] Local nasal symptoms can be controlled by topical antibiotic ointments, nasal douching, and topical steroids, although the latter often worsens the bleeding episodes. Surgery is contraindicated in the presence of active disease because it will lead to further necrosis followed by excessive scarring and possible atrophic rhinitis. Endoscopic sinus surgery is generally only undertaken for the treatment of selected patients with secondary bacterial infections.[63]

Wegener granulomatosis is a multisystem disease of unknown etiology characterized by necrotizing granulomas of the upper and lower respiratory tracts, systemic vasculitis, and focal necrotizing glomerulonephritis. Wegener granulomatosis was first described by Klinger in 1932, and subsequently by Wegener in 1936 who established the classical triad of the condition.[64,65] The incidence of this disease is difficult to quantify, but it is known to equally affect men and women between the ages 15 and 73 years. It has also been reported in children. The nose and sinuses are involved in 85% of patients, and nasal complaints are the most common presenting symptoms of all age groups.[66] Patients present with nasal crusting, nasal obstruction, and epistaxis.[66] Destruction of the intranasal structures including the nasal septum may follow, leading to nasal collapse. The destructive process is located initially in the midline, affecting the septum and turbinates, then spreads symmetrically to involve the maxillary and the rest of the sinuses.[67] It is extremely rare for patients to present with an isolated lesion in the maxilla.[68] Untreated, the disease may follow a relentless course, leading eventually to renal failure and significant mortality.[62] A limited form of Wegener granuloma has also been described in the upper respiratory tract presenting with purely granulomatous form of the localized disease.[67] It is unknown what proportion of these patients ultimately progress to classical, multisystem disease.[66] A diagnosis of Wegener granulomatosis should be considered in patients who report levels of malaise, which are disproportionate to their upper respiratory tract symptoms and clinical findings.[66] Serology for cANCA is positive in 95% of patients with generalized active disease and 60% of those with localized disease.[66] In a patient without a history of previous sinonasal surgery, a combination of bone destruction and new bone formation on CT is virtually diagnostic of Wegener granulomatosis, especially when accompanied on MRI by a fat signal from the sclerotic sinus wall.[67]

Like sarcoidosis, treatment is medical in a multidisciplinary approach with combination of high-dose systemic corticosteroids and a cytotoxic agent such as azathioprine, cyclophosphamide, or mycophenolate mofetil. Because of its greater side effects, cyclophosphamide is used mainly in patients with severe disease and in those with renal in-

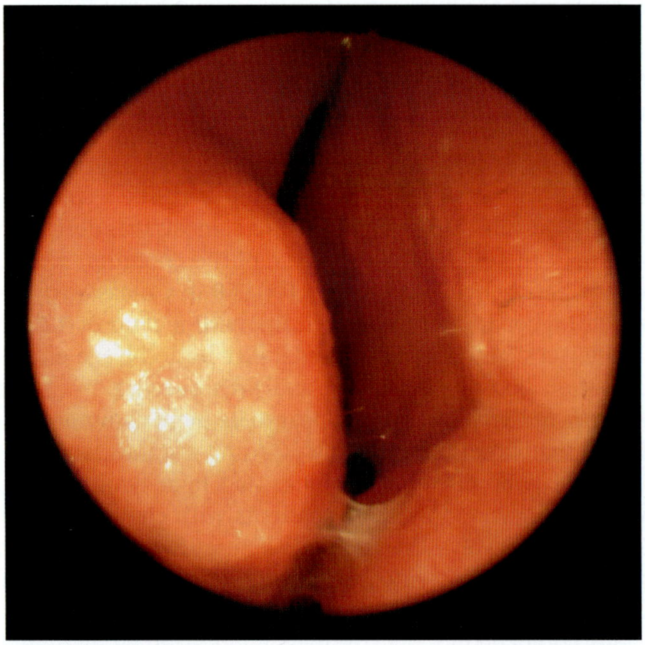

Fig. 9.7 An endoscopic photograph of the right nasal cavity in a patient with nasal sarcoidosis showing crusting, mucosal inflammation, and granulomas.

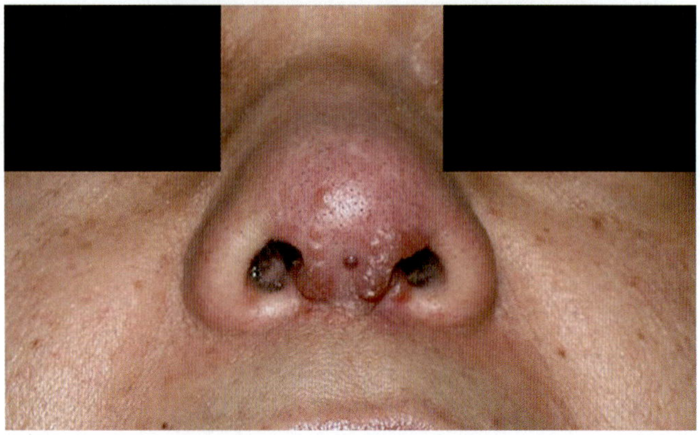

Fig. 9.8 Classical "lupus pernio" with purple skin discoloration and nodules.

volvement. Immunoglobulin infusion and monoclonal antibodies, such as rituximab, are also being used. When the condition is controlled the medication can be reduced, but most patients require a maintenance low-dose corticosteroid. The nasal symptoms are managed as in patients with sarcoidosis. Reconstructive surgery is contraindicated when the disease is still in its active stage, but maxillary sinus exploration is sometimes undertaken in the presence of pain and opacification of imaging.

Antrolithiasis

Antroliths are calcified bodies that are formed from a mineral salt deposition around a nucleus within the maxillary sinus cavity.[69] They are synonymous with rhinoliths, which are reported within the nasal cavity. However, reports of antroliths are very infrequent compared with rhinoliths. It has been postulated that antroliths result from either endogenous or exogenous factors. Endogenous factors may include blood, mucus, or pus; exogenous factors include teeth and their roots or other foreign body material. It is assumed that these would initiate a foreign body reaction that would form the antrolith over a long period. The main components of antroliths are calcium phosphate, calcium carbonate, organic matter, and water.[69] The lesions may also be covered by granulation tissue. The majority of cases reported in the literature had tooth extraction prior to the presentation. The patients can be asymptomatic and may present with symptoms of unilateral chronic maxillary sinusitis. On CT scanning, antroliths are radiopaque masses of varying sizes and shapes and irregular borders. They are usually surrounded by mucosal thickening and occasionally associated polyps or fluid level. Treatment is by surgical removal, which can generally be achieved through the endoscopic approach (**Fig. 9.9**) (**see Video 9.4**).

Neoplastic

Papillomas

Papillomas are the most common benign epithelial tumor found in the sinonasal region, accounting for up to 10% of all neoplasms in this area.[70] Histologically, they are divided into inverted, cylindric, and everted.[71] Everted and cylindric cell papillomas are true papillomas, lined by stratified squa-

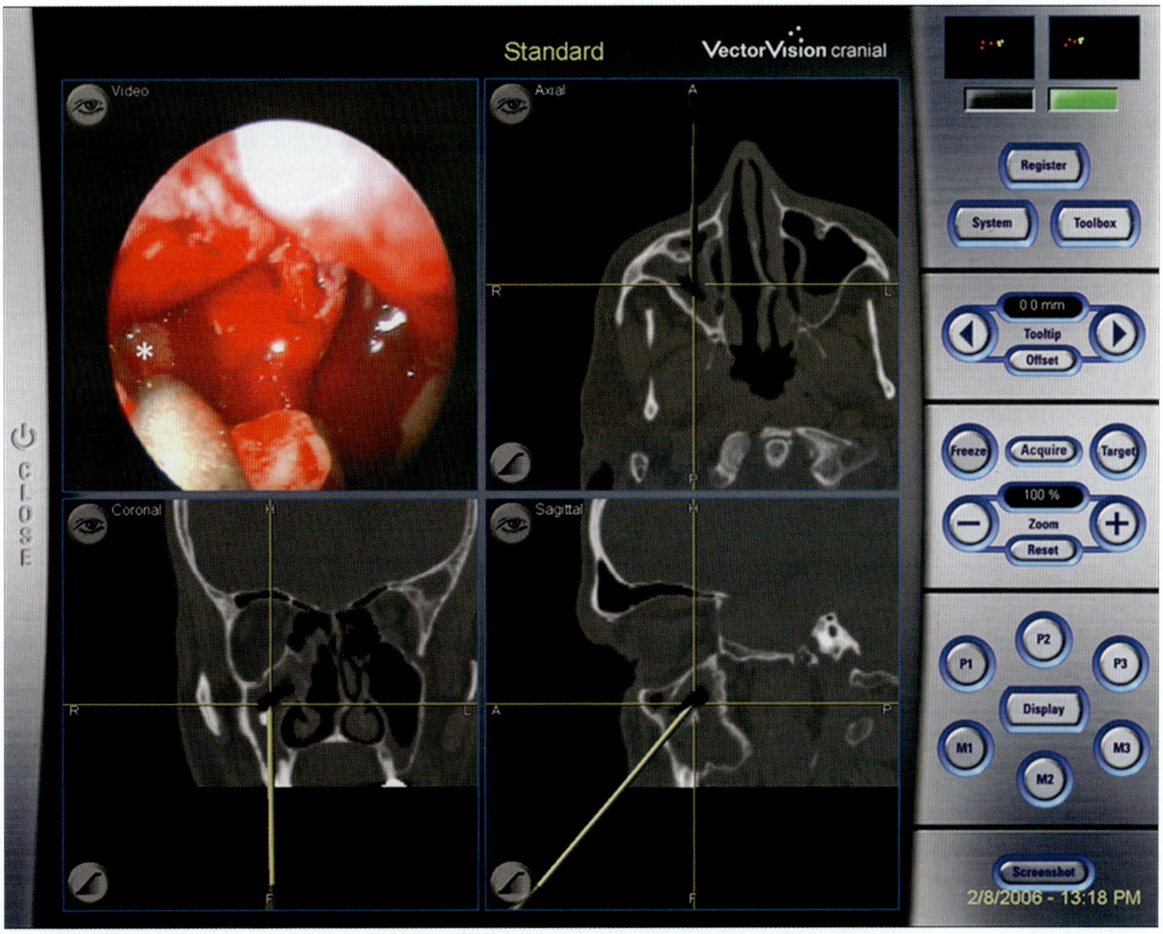

Fig. 9.9 An intraoperative screen shot from an image guidance system during removal of a right maxillary antrolith (asterisk) through a middle meatal antrostomy.

mous and microcyst-laden, columnar, and oncocytic epithelium, respectively.[71] Inverted papillomas are polyps with marked, patchy squamous metaplasia in ductal and surface epithelium with extensive "inversion" of the epithelium into the underlying stroma.

Everted papilloma more often arises on the nasal septum, whereas both inverted and cylindric papillomas mostly arise on the lateral nasal wall within the middle meatus. They most commonly extend into the maxillary sinus through an expanded natural ostium then to the ethmoids or frontal sinuses.[70–73] It is not certain if some papillomas originate within the cavity of the maxillary sinus itself then spread into the middle meatus. The age presentation is from 35 to 60 years with male preponderance of 3.5:1.[70,72] It appears to be more common in Caucasians compared with other racial groups. A viral etiology has been suggested with a link to papilloma viral subtypes 6, 11, 16, and18.[72] Patients generally present with obstructive nasal symptoms, rhinorrhea, and chronic rhinosinusitis.[70,72] Inverted papilloma appears as a firm vascular polyp, which is sometimes mixed with normal nasal polyps. Cylindric papilloma appears as smooth fleshy polypoid mass and is much less common. The diagnosis is suggested on CT scans when there is a mass continuous from the middle meatus into the adjacent maxillary sinus, through an expanded maxillary ostium.[73] The mass may contain areas of apparent calcification and there may be sclerosis of the walls of the sinus (**Fig. 9.10**).[73] The main advantage of MRI is defining the extent of the tumor and differentiating it from adjacent inflammatory tissue.

Both a high recurrence rate and malignant transformation have been quoted repeatedly in the literature. A recurrence rate of up to 75% usually reflects inadequate excision whereas malignant transformation at rates from 0 to 53% suggests that the majority of these cases had squamous carcinoma ab initio. A recent review of the literature of over 200 cases calculated 7.1% synchronous carcinoma and 3.6% metachronous carcinoma.[74]

There is currently a growing body of evidence supporting endoscopic resection of these tumors.[3,72,75] We believe that the approach that allows the most reliable total excision of the lesion is the most appropriate. In general, endoscopic excision (**see Video 9.1**), with or without medial maxillectomy, is suitable for most tumors except for those that invaded the lateral maxillary wall, frontal sinus, orbit, or skull base. Caldwell–Luc, lateral rhinotomy, or midfacial degloving are tailored to the individual lesion. It is most important that the resection is subperiosteal and that all sclerotic bone is removed—whatever the approach—to minimize recurrence. This is of the order of 10 to 15% irrespective of the approach in the larger series. **Table 9.2** shows the overall recurrence rates based on our review of 31 series that included 1574 patients.

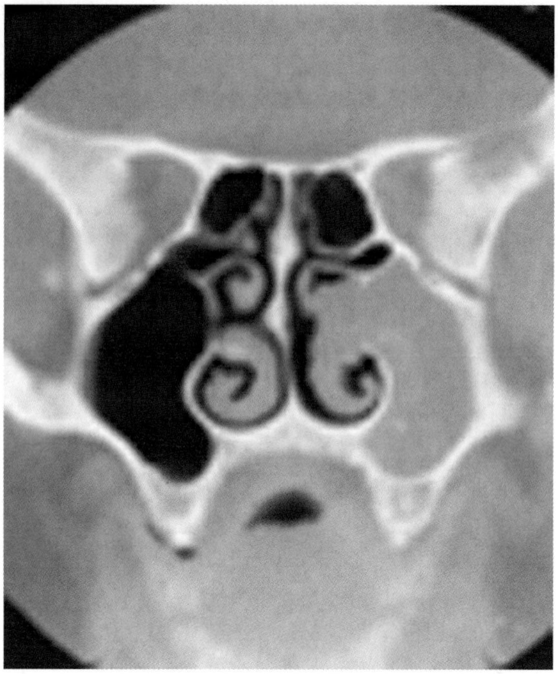

Fig. 9.10 A coronal computed tomography scan showing a inverted papilloma extending from the middle meatus into the maxillary sinus. Small areas of high density are seen within the maxillary component.

Salivary Gland Tumors: Pleomorphic Adenoma and Oncocytoma

Pleomorphic adenoma of the upper respiratory tract occurs almost exclusively in the nasal cavity with a very rare occurrence in the paranasal sinuses.[76–78] There are only a very small number of reports of isolated tumors arising in the cavity of the maxillary sinus.[76,77] Age presentation is usually between the third and sixth decade when occurring in the nasal cavity.[78] Patients with maxillary pleomorphic adenoma present with facial swelling, nasal obstruction, and occasional palatal swelling.[76,77] Bony expansion and erosion have been reported on CT scanning. Histology shows the typical feature of duct-like structures and myoepithelial cells within myxoid stroma.[77] Surgical treatment is tailored

Table 9.2 Overall Recurrence Rates of Inverted Papilloma

Conservative (Polypectomy, Ethmoidectomy, Caldwell–Luc)	External (Lateral Rhinotomy, Midfacial Degloving)	Endoscopic	Endoscopic and External (Combined)
58%	14%	19%	20%

to the extent of the tumor: both endoscopic and open approaches have been used. One series reported a high recurrence rate, highlighting the importance of complete excision via the most suitable route.[76]

Oncocytoma is exceedingly rare in the maxillary sinus.[79] It is reported more frequently in the nasal cavity, but there is only a small number of cases in the literature.[80] Oncocytoma is a term that describes a tumor composed of epithelial cells or myoepithelial cells with abundant granular eosinophilic cytoplasm. The peculiar appearance of these oncocytes is due to the large number of mitochondria in their cytoplasm as demonstrated on electron microscopy.[80] The presentation is similar to pleomorphic adenoma, although oncocytomas can be more aggressive. Malignant transformation has also been reported. Surgical approach should be tailored to the extent of the tumor.

Mesenchymal Tumors: Fibroma, Lipoma, and Myxoma

These rare tumors may be encountered in the nose and sinuses and generally present prior to adulthood. Isolated tumors within the maxillary sinus are very rare. Fibromas result from progressive inflammation or fibroblastic proliferation of the nasal mucosa.[81] They present as slow-growing, gray-white, smooth-surfaced masses producing obstructive nasal symptoms.

Lipoma is the most common soft tissue tumor in adulthood. It can be seen wherever there is adipose tissue. In contrast, intraosseous lipoma is a rare condition. The etiology of intraosseous lipoma is unknown, but infarction, ischemia, trauma, and irradiation may be contributing factors.[82] Cases have been reported within the nasal cavity and very rarely in the maxillary sinus. The presentation is of a facial swelling and possible nasal obstructive symptoms.

Myxoma of the maxillary sinus is very rare, but has been reported more frequently than fibromas and lipomas.[83] The age at presentation is between 2 and 15 years. They may be related to dental malformations or missing teeth, but may also occur without such abnormalities. Histologically, there is a myxomatous background surrounding a hypocellular proliferation of small stellate or spindle-shaped cells with regular nuclei and a variable amount of cytoplasm. They are locally aggressive with a high recurrence rate when locally excised.

Vasiform Tumors: Hemangioma, Aneurysmal Bone Cyst, and Hemangiopericytoma

These benign lesions originate from vascular tissue within the mucosa or bone of the nose and sinuses. Hemangiomas are said to represent 20% of benign nonepithelial tumors of the nasal cavity and paranasal sinuses.[84] Mean age at diagnosis is 40 years and the most frequent presenting symptoms are nasal obstruction and epistaxis. Those that originate in the maxillary sinus have been reported less frequently.[84] Both cavernous and capillary hemangiomas have been reported with no apparent difference in the pattern of presentation.[84,85] CT scanning is nonspecific and show features of expansion similar to other benign conditions. The lesion can bleed profusely during surgical excision and preembolization has been suggested by some.[85]

Aneurysmal bone cysts (ABCs) are expansile lesions of unknown etiology that usually affect long bones and vertebrae of patients younger than 20 years. About 2% of ABCs are encountered in the head and neck region with the jaw being the most frequently involved site. An ABC of the maxillary sinus may be associated with other bone pathology such as fibrous dysplasia; isolated lesions have rarely been reported.[86] They present with facial swelling and obstructive nasal symptoms in the age group between 5 and 23 years. Histologically, ABCs consist of multiple cavities filled with blood and serous fluid, which are separated by septa and surrounded by a rim of bone.[86] The septa are composed of fibroblasts, myofibroblasts, giant cells, osteoid and woven bone and are not lined by endothelium. It is postulated that preexisting bone lesions may cause venous occlusion or an arteriovenous malformation; the consequent change in hemodynamics leads to the ABC formation.[87] CT shows a multiloculated, heterogeneous contrast-enhancing mass surrounded by a thin rim of bone, which expands the maxillary sinus. Fluid-fluid levels may be seen on CT or MRI. ABCs have a "honeycomb" appearance on gadolinium-enhanced MRI studies.[86] The cysts can be treated endoscopically, although the long-term prognosis of these lesions is unknown due to their rarity.

Hemangiopericytoma (HPC) is a rare vascular tumor derived from extracapillary cells (pericytes), which surround normal vascular channels. Less than one-third of HPC occur in the head and neck and 5% are located in the nasal cavity and paranasal sinuses.[88,89] Sphenoid and ethmoid sinuses are involved more frequently than the maxillary sinus. It affects males and females equally and can occur at any age, but it most often develops after the second decade. The patients usually present with epistaxis and nasal obstruction with reddish submucosal nasal mass. CT and MRI show nonspecific features of a nasal mass. Histologically, they are characterized by sheets or randomly scattered ovoid or spindle-shaped cells with indistinct cytoplasm and large nuclei, distributed around normal vascular channels. HPC of the nose is considered benign, but some forms of the tumor affecting other sites are malignant. Late recurrence rates of 25 to 50% have been reported with systemic metastases in up to 10% of patients. Mortality has been reported as high as 50% after 5 to 20 years. Wide local excision is therefore recommended with long-term follow-up.

Tumors of Muscle Origin: Leiomyoma and Rhabdomyoma

Leiomyoma is a smooth muscle tumor that originates in areas of abundance of such muscle like the uterus. It is extremely rare for these tumors to present in the sinonasal tract because of the paucity of smooth muscle. Only a handful of cases of leiomyoma have been reported in the maxillary sinus.[90] When present, it has been suggested that they originate from undifferentiated mesenchyme muscle elements in the wall of blood vessels or both. The presentation is of obstructive nasal symptoms and the tumors seem to be slow-growing and nonaggressive. The few reported cases did not seem to show any evidence of recurrences after excision.

Rhabdomyoma is a skeletal muscle tumor; hence, it is exceedingly rare in the nose and sinuses. Only a handful of historic case reports exist; they describe the rhabdomyoma's benign behavior and low recurrence rate.[91,92]

Odontogenic Tumors

Odontogenic tumors are derived from the epithelial, ectomesenchymal, or mesenchymal components that are part of tooth development.[93] They originate either within the maxillofacial skeleton (intraosseous) or within the gingival or alveolar mucosa overlying the tooth-bearing areas (extraosseous). Odontogenic tumors of the maxillary sinus are usually slow growing and have been associated with the noneruption of teeth. Patients usually present with swelling of the alveolar process along with nasal obstruction and epistaxis. Superior displacement of the globe has been reported with large odontogenic tumors. The location and behaviors of the tumors vary according to their subtype. **Table 9.3** is adapted from the revised World Health Organization's (WHO) classification of odontogenic tumors.[94]

Ameloblastoma is the most common odontogenic tumor. It originates from epithelial components of the embryonic tooth arrested developmentally prior to enamel formation. It is slow growing, locally invasive and has a high rate of recurrence if not treated effectively. Patients between the ages of 16 and 60 years are generally affected, with the region of the canine tooth and maxilla being the most common sites. They are often asymptomatic, but can present with a painless swelling of the cheek, gingiva, and palate that may reach a large size. Radiologically, ameloblastoma presents as a unilocular or multilocular radiolucency that may be associated with an impacted tooth. Treatment includes excision with a margin of uninvolved tissue. This is preferable to enucleation or curettage, which are associated with a high recurrence rate.[93]

Fibroosseous Lesions: Osteoma, Ossifying Fibroma, Fibrous Dysplasia, and Osteoblastoma

Fibroosseous lesions represent a class of bony abnormalities: osteoma, ossifying fibroma, fibrous dysplasia, and osteoblastoma. They are distinct but lie along a continuum from the most to the least bony content. They do have some similarities in appearance, but their clinical implications differ.

Osteomas are a frequent incidental finding in up to 3% of CT scans of the paranasal sinuses.[95] Eighty percent occur in the frontal sinuses followed by the ethmoids; they are least found in the maxillary sinuses. Their etiology is still debated, with suggestions that they are either embryologic, or secondary to traumatic or an infective process. There is an association with Gardner syndrome, which is an autosomal dominant condition characterized by intestinal polyposis and pigmented skin lesions in addition to the osteomas.[96] Maxillary sinus osteomas are slow growing and usually asymptomatic, but they may become symptomatic depending on the location and onset.[97] Treatment is only required if they produce cosmetic problems or symptoms related to mass effect. Depending on their extent and location, this can be done via an endoscopic approach or an open procedure.

Ossifying fibroma (OF) is an expansible well-circumscribed lesion that continues to grow after sexual maturity and can attain dramatic proportions.[95,98] Variants of ossifying fibroma include cementoossifying fibroma, which occurs in relation to dentition; psammomatoid ossifying fibroma and juvenile ossifying fibroma, which can be locally destructive.[95] The vast majority is located in the posterior region of the mandible; those involving the maxillary sinus are uncommon.[99] Patients usually present between the third and fourth decades and the lesion is more common in women.[99] The most common presentation is of a painless cheek swelling, but involvement of the orbit or nasal cavity may be signified by proptosis, loss of visual acuity,

Table 9.3 Classification of Odontogenic Tumors

Epithelial Odontogenic Tumors	Mixed Epithelial and Mesenchymal Odontogenic Tumors	Mesenchymal Odontogenic Tumors
Ameloblastoma	Ameloblastic fibromas	Odontogenic fibromas
Calcifying epithelial odontogenic tumor (Pindborg tumor)	Odontoma Calcifying cystic odontogenic tumor (Gorlin cyst)	Odontogenic myxoma
Adenomatoid odontogenic tumor		
Keratocystic odontogenic tumor		

Source: Data from Barnes L, Eveson JW, Reichart PA, Sidransky D, eds. World Health Organization classification of tumors: pathology and genetics of tumors of the head and neck. Lyon: IARC; 2005.

epiphora, nasal obstruction, and epistaxis.[95,99] Radiologically, the lesion is sharply circumscribed with an eggshell rim and central radiolucency (**Fig. 9.11**). This differentiates it from fibrous dysplasia, which has indistinguishable borders. The histologic features can be difficult to discriminate from those of fibrous dysplasia.[98] Because of the progressive and locally destructive nature of OF complete surgical excision is recommended.

Fibrous dysplasia (FD) is a slow, progressive disorder where normal bone is replaced by fibrous tissue and immature woven bone.[95,98] There are two main forms of FD: monostotic (70–85%) that involves only one bone, and polyostotic (15–30%) where multiple bones are involved. A variant of the polyostotic form is the McCune–Albright syndrome (precocious puberty, FD, and cafe-au-lait spots).[95] The maxilla and mandible are the most commonly involved bones generally in the monostotic form. FD is a disease of young age where patients present in their first or second decade and is assumed to "burn out" as the patients reach skeletal maturity. The usual symptom is of painless facial deformity although other complaints such as loosening of teeth, nasal obstruction, or epistaxis have been encountered.[100] CT scans show lesions with indistinct borders and an homogeneous "ground glass" appearance representing disorganized spicules of bone (**Fig. 9.12**).[95] Histologically normal bone is replaced by fibrous tissue with varying degrees of osseous metaplasia. Diagnosis is undertaken on the combination of the clinical picture, radiology, and histology as the latter can be indistinguishable from ossifying fibroma. Treatment is conservative due to the expected natural cessation of the lesion, usually in the third or fourth decades. Where there are significant symptoms or severe deformity, recontouring of the affected bone can be undertaken. The lesions are usually very vascular and surgical intervention can be difficult. Some authors have showed regression of lesions on using the bisphosphonate pamidronate, but caution is needed as there are case reports of avascular necrosis.[101,102]

Osteoblastoma is an uncommon neoplasm characterized by proliferation of osteoblasts forming bone trabeculae set in a vascularized fibrous connective tissue stroma.[103] The tumor occurs predominantly in vertebrae and long bones and can affect craniofacial bones, with the mandible being the most commonly involved. It is reported less in the maxillary bone and rarely in the maxillary sinus.[104] The majority of patients are under the age of 30 years and present with a facial swelling that is often painful.[103] CT features range from radiolucent to radiopaque lesions and are often mistaken for other fibroosseous lesions (**Fig. 9.13**).[103] Diagnosis is therefore mainly histologic and treatment is by surgical excision.

Neuroectodermal Tumors: Schwannoma and Neurofibroma

Schwannomas are benign peripheral nerve sheath tumors of which 50% occur in the head and neck region. They are very uncommon in the paranasal sinuses with only 4% estimated in this area; a very small number involve the maxillary sinus.[105] The lesion slowly expands in the sinus cavity result-

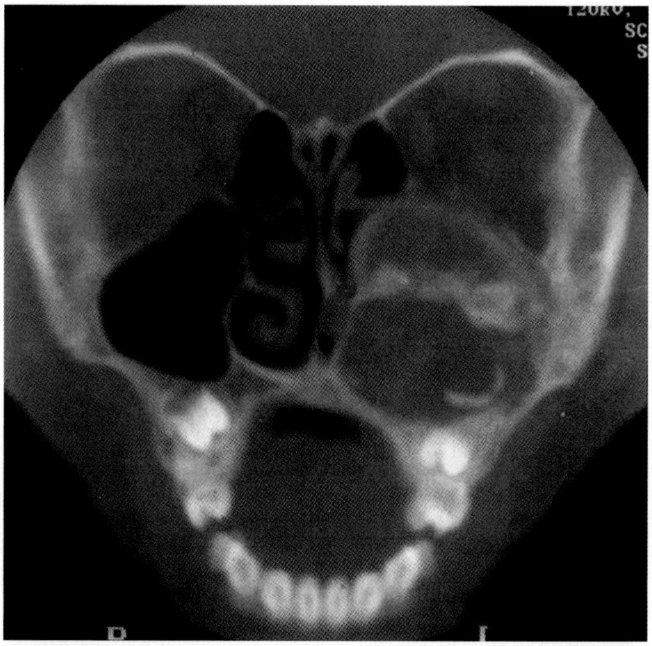

Fig. 9.11 A coronal computed tomography scan of a patient with ossifying fibroma in the left maxillary sinus.

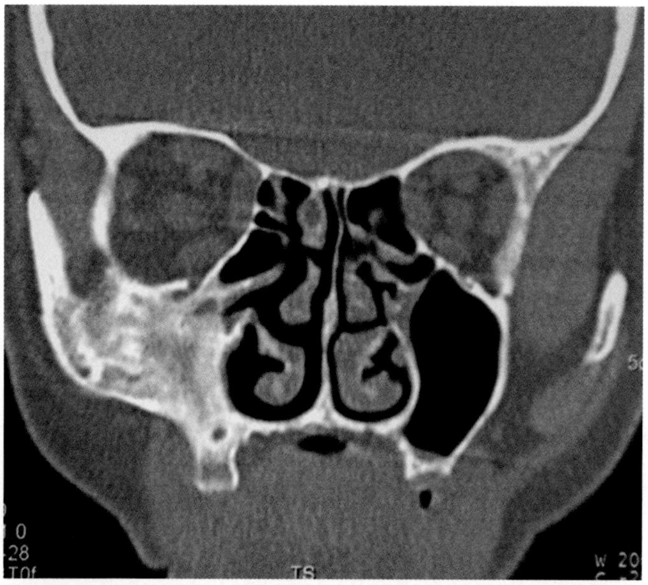

Fig. 9.12 A coronal computed tomography scan showing a typical fibrous dysplasia affecting the right maxillary sinus. Note the "ground glass" appearance and the indistinct borders.

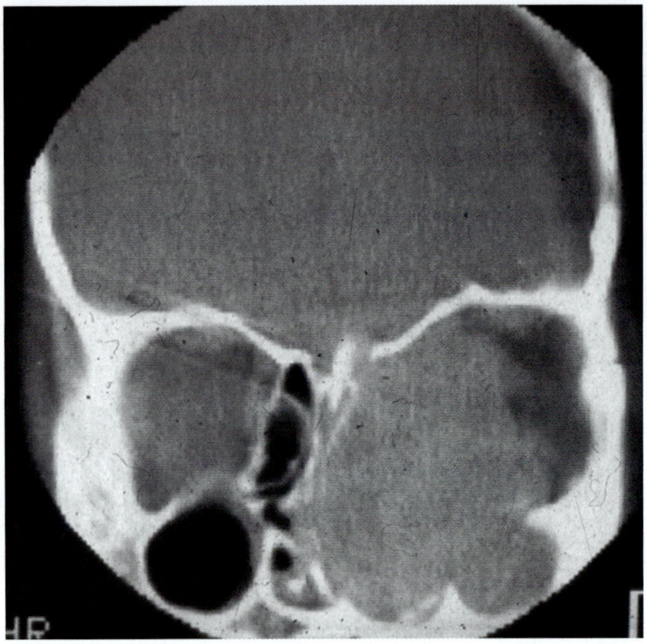

Fig. 9.13 A coronal computed tomography scan of a patient with a very large osteoblastoma in the left maxillary sinus.

ing in swelling, pressure symptoms, and bony necrosis. Cystic lesions that are associated with sudden bursts of worsening symptoms have also been reported.[105] The patients mostly present with nasal obstruction, but other symptoms such as proptosis, epiphora, headaches, facial anesthesia, and epistaxis have been reported.[106] CT scanning shows a homogeneous radiopaque mass with evidence of bone destruction. On MRI they appear as hyperintense well-demarcated masses. Histologically, they exhibit characteristic features of schwannomas and are typically positive to S100 protein. Treatment is by local excision via the most suitable approach.

Neurofibromas are heterogeneous peripheral nerve sheath tumors that arise from the connective tissue of the nerves, especially the endoneurium.[107] They may occur as sporadic lesions but are much more common in association with neurofibromatosis type 1 (NF1). Neurofibromas of the maxillary sinus are exceedingly rare with only a small number of reported cases. As for schwannomas, they slowly grow and expand within the cavity of the sinus causing swelling, pressure symptoms, and bone necrosis. Presentation is similar to other expanding masses in the maxillary sinus. CT scanning shows a well-circumscribed mass with some bony erosion. On MRI, neurofibromas are usually isointense or of lower intensity than gray matter on T1-weighted images and are isointense or of higher signal on T2-weighted images.[107] Histologically, they are differentiated from schwannomas by the lack of the palisade pattern of the nuclei and the lower tumor cell density. Treatment is by local excision.

Conclusion

The maxillary sinus is a unique structure which can be involved in a large number of benign pathologies. Some are more aggressive than others and some have higher recurrence rates. A systematic approach to diagnosis with a high index of suspicion and an awareness of uncommon lesions is therefore essential. An armamentarium of surgical approaches is at our disposal; each is applicable to certain situations. The surgeon should be adept with these techniques and prepared to interchange between them to suit particular lesions. Finally, long-term follow-up is essential in many cases and should not be overlooked.

Pearls

- The maxillary sinus may be affected by a variety of benign pathologies.
- Symptoms are mostly nonspecific and can be similar to maxillary sinusitis.
- Some lesions can lead to facial swelling.
- Imaging is helpful and can be characteristic in some cases, but diagnosis is often based on histopathology.
- Surgery is the mainstay of treatment in the majority of cases.
- Long-term follow-up is often necessary because of the high incidence of recurrence of some pathologies.

References

1. Stammberger H, Posawetz W. Functional endoscopic sinus surgery. Concept, indications and results of the Messerklinger technique. Eur Arch Otorhinolaryngol 1990;247(2):63–76
2. Lund V, Howard DJ, Wei WI. Endoscopic resection of malignant tumors of the nose and sinuses. Am J Rhinol 2007;21(1):89–941
3. Lawson W, Patel ZM. The evolution of management for inverted papilloma: an analysis of 200 cases. Otolaryngol Head Neck Surg 2009;140(3):330–335
4. Matheny KE, Duncavage JA. Contemporary indications for the Caldwell-Luc procedure. Curr Opin Otolaryngol Head Neck Surg 2003;11(1):23–26
5. Howard DJ, Lund VJ. The midfacial degloving approach to sinonasal disease. J Laryngol Otol 1992;106(12):1059–1062
6. Howard DJ, Lund VJ. The role of midfacial degloving in modern rhinological practice. J Laryngol Otol 1999;113(10):885–887
7. Weisman R. Lateral rhinotomy and medial maxillectomy. Otolaryngol Clin North Am 1995;28(6):1145–1156

8. Bhattacharyya N. Do maxillary sinus retention cysts reflect obstructive sinus phenomena? Arch Otolaryngol Head Neck Surg 2000;126(11):1369–1371
9. Harar RPS, Chadha NK, Rogers G. Are maxillary mucosal cysts a manifestation of inflammatory sinus disease? J Laryngol Otol 2007;121(8):751–754
10. Kanagalingam J, Bhatia K, Georgalas C, Fokkens W, Miszkiel K, Lund VJ. Maxillary mucosal cyst is not a manifestation of rhinosinusitis: results of a prospective three-dimensional CT study of ophthalmic patients. Laryngoscope 2009;119(1):8–12
11. Gardner DG. Pseudocysts and retention cysts of the maxillary sinus. Oral Surg Oral Med Oral Pathol 1984;58(5):561–567
12. Berg O, Carenfelt C, Sobin A. On the diagnosis and pathogenesis of intramural maxillary cysts. Acta Otolaryngol 1989;108(5-6):464–468
13. Casamassimo PS, Lilly GE. Mucosal cysts of the maxillary sinus: a clinical and radiographic study. Oral Surg Oral Med Oral Pathol 1980;50(3):282–286
14. Fisher EW, Whittet HB, Croft CB. Symptomatic mucosal cysts of the maxillary sinus: antroscopic treatment. J Laryngol Otol 1989;103(12):1184–1186
15. Killian G. The origin of choanal polipi. Lancet 1906;2:81–82
16. Maldonado M, Martínez A, Alobid I, Mullol J. The antrochoanal polyp. Rhinology 2004;42(4):178–182
17. Mahfouz ME, Elsheikh MN, Ghoname NF. Molecular profile of the antrochoanal polyp: up-regulation of basic fibroblast growth factor and transforming growth factor beta in maxillary sinus mucosa. Am J Rhinol 2006;20(4):466–470
18. Aydin O, Keskin G, Ustündağ E, Işeri M, Ozkarakaş H. Choanal polyps: an evaluation of 53 cases. Am J Rhinol 2007;21(2):164–168
19. Chen JM, Schloss MD, Azouz ME. Antro-choanal polyp: a 10-year retrospective study in the pediatric population with a review of the literature. J Otolaryngol 1989;18(4):168–172
20. Orvidas LJ, Beatty CW, Weaver AL. Antrochoanal polyps in children. Am J Rhinol 2001;15(5):321–325
21. Stammberger H, Hawke M. Essentials of Functional Endoscopic Sinus Surgery. St. Louis, MO: Mosby; 1993: 103–105
22. Berg O, Carenfelt C, Silfverswärd C, Sobin A. Origin of the choanal polyp. Arch Otolaryngol Head Neck Surg 1988;114(11):1270–1271
23. Min YG, Chung JW, Shin JS, Chi JG. Histologic structure of antrochoanal polyps. Acta Otolaryngol 1995;115(4):543–547
24. Ozcan C, Zeren H, Talas DU, Küçükoğlu M, Görür K. Antrochoanal polyp: a transmission electron and light microscopic study. Eur Arch Otorhinolaryngol 2005;262(1):55–60
25. Yamashiro Y, Nakamura M, Huang GW, Kosugi T. Presence of urokinase-type plasminogen activator (u-PA) in tissue extracts of antrochoanal polyp. Laryngoscope 1992;102(9):1049–1052
26. Topal O, Erbek SS, Kiyici H, Cakmak O. Expression of metalloproteinases MMP-2 and MMP-9 in antrochoanal polyps. Am J Rhinol 2008;22(4):339–342
27. Lund VJ. Endoscopic management of paranasal sinus mucocoeles. J Laryngol Otol 1998;112(1):36–40
28. Bockmühl U, Kratzsch B, Benda K, Draf W. Surgery for paranasal sinus mucocoeles: efficacy of endonasal micro-endoscopic management and long-term results of 185 patients. Rhinology 2006;44(1):62–67
29. Har-El G. Endoscopic management of 108 sinus mucoceles. Laryngoscope 2001;111(12):2131–2134
30. Busaba NY, Salman SD. Maxillary sinus mucoceles: clinical presentation and long-term results of endoscopic surgical treatment. Laryngoscope 1999;109(9):1446–1449
31. Lloyd G, Lund VJ, Savy L, Howard D. Optimum imaging for mucoceles. J Laryngol Otol 2000;114(3):233–236
32. Hasegawa M, Saito Y, Watanabe I, Kern EB. Postoperative mucoceles of the maxillary sinus. Rhinology 1979;17(4):253–256
33. Natvig K, Larsen TE. Mucocele of the paranasal sinuses. A retrospective clinical and histological study. J Laryngol Otol 1978;92(12):1075–1082
34. Lund VJ, Milroy CM. Fronto-ethmoidal mucocoeles: a histopathological analysis. J Laryngol Otol 1991;105(11):921–923
35. Lund VJ, Henderson B, Song Y. Involvement of cytokines and vascular adhesion receptors in the pathology of fronto-ethmoidal mucocoeles. Acta Otolaryngol 1993;113(4):540–546
36. Lund VJ. Anatomical considerations in the aetiology of fronto-ethmoidal mucoceles. Rhinology 1987;25(2):83–88
37. Friedmann I, Osborn DA. Pathology of granulomas and neoplasms of the nose and paranasal sinuses. In: WStC Symmers, ed. Systemic Pathology. Edinburgh/London/New York: Churchill Livingstone; 1982: 192–235
38. Astarci HM, Sungu N, Samim EE, Ustun H. Presence of cholesterol granuloma in the maxillary and ethmoid sinuses. Oral Maxillofac Surg 2008;12(2):101–103
39. Chao TK. Cholesterol granuloma of the maxillary sinus. Eur Arch Otorhinolaryngol 2006;263(6):592–597
40. Graham J, Michaels L. Cholesterol granuloma of the maxillary antrum. Clin Otolaryngol Allied Sci 1978;3(2):155–160
41. Niho M. Cholesterol crystals in the temporal bone and the paranasal sinuses. Int J Pediatr Otorhinolaryngol 1986;11(1):79–95
42. Kunt T, Ozturkcan S, Egilmez R. Cholesterol granuloma of the maxillary sinus: six cases from the same region. J Laryngol Otol 1998;112(1):65–68
43. Marks SC, Smith DM. Endoscopic treatment of maxillary sinus cholesterol granuloma. Laryngoscope 1995;105(5 Pt 1):551–552
44. Lim M, Lew-Gor S, Beale T, Ramsay A, Lund VJ. Maxillary sinus haematoma. J Laryngol Otol 2008;122(2):210–212
45. Song HM, Jang YJ, Chung YS, Lee BJ. Organizing hematoma of the maxillary sinus. Otolaryngol Head Neck Surg 2007;136(4):616–620
46. Lee PK, Wu JK, Ludemann JP. Hemorrhagic pseudotumour of the maxillary sinus. J Otolaryngol 2004;33(3):206–208
47. Ozhan S, Araç M, Isik S, Oznur II, Atilla S, Kemaloglu Y. Pseudotumor of the maxillary sinus in a patient with von Willebrand's disease. AJR Am J Roentgenol 1996;166(4):950–951
48. Lee BJ, Park HJ, Heo SC. Organized hematoma of the maxillary sinus. Acta Otolaryngol 2003;123(7):869–872
49. Tabaee A, Kacker A. Hematoma of the maxillary sinus presenting as a mass—a case report and review of literature. Int J Pediatr Otorhinolaryngol 2002;65(2):153–157
50. Kosarac O, Luna MA, Ro JY, Ayala AG. Eosinophilic angiocentric fibrosis of the sinonasal tract. Ann Diagn Pathol 2008;12(4):267–270
51. Paun S, Lund VJ, Gallimore A. Nasal fibrosis: long-term follow up of four cases of eosinophilic angiocentric fibrosis. J Laryngol Otol 2005;119(2):119–124
52. Thompson LD, Heffner DK. Sinonasal tract eosinophilic angiocentric fibrosis. A report of three cases. Am J Clin Pathol 2001;115(2):243–248
53. Roberts PF, McCann BG. Eosinophilic angiocentric fibrosis of the upper respiratory tract: a mucosal variant of granuloma faciale? A report of three cases. Histopathology 1985;9(11):1217–1225
54. Yung A, Wachsmuth R, Ramnath R, Merchant W, Myatt AE, Sheehan-Dare R. Eosinophilic angiocentric fibrosis—a rare mucosal variant of granuloma faciale which may present to the dermatologist. Br J Dermatol 2005;152(3):574–576

55. Boeck C. Multiple benign sarkoid of the skin. J of Cutan and Dis 1899;17:543–553
56. Zeitlin JF, Tami TA, Baughman R, Winget D. Nasal and sinus manifestations of sarcoidosis. Am J Rhinol 2000;14(3):157–161
57. Braun JJ, Gentine A, Pauli G. Sinonasal sarcoidosis: review and report of fifteen cases. Laryngoscope 2004;114(11):1960–1963
58. Fergie N, Jones NS, Havlat MF. The nasal manifestations of sarcoidosis: a review and report of eight cases. J Laryngol Otol 1999;113(10):893–898
59. McCaffrey TV, McDonald TJ. Sarcoidosis of the nose and paranasal sinuses. Laryngoscope 1983;93(10):1281–1284
60. Krespi YP, Kuriloff DB, Aner M. Sarcoidosis of the sinonasal tract: a new staging system. Otolaryngol Head Neck Surg 1995;112(2):221–227
61. Wilson R, Lund V, Sweatman M, Mackay IS, Mitchell DN. Upper respiratory tract involvement in sarcoidosis and its management. Eur Respir J 1988;1(3):269–272
62. Fuchs HA, Tanner SB. Granulomatous disorders of the nose and paranasal sinuses. Curr Opin Otolaryngol Head Neck Surg 2009;17(1):23–27
63. Kay DJ, Har-El G. The role of endoscopic sinus surgery in chronic sinonasal sarcoidosis. Am J Rhinol 2001;15(4):249–254
64. Klinger H. Grenzformen der periarteritis nodosa. Frankf Z Pathol 1932;41:455–480
65. Wegener F. Uber generalisierte septische gefasserkrankungen. Verh Dtsch Ges Pathol 1936;29:202–212
66. Srouji IA, Andrews P, Edwards C, Lund VJ. Patterns of presentation and diagnosis of patients with Wegener's granulomatosis: ENT aspects. J Laryngol Otol 2007;121(7):653–658
67. Lloyd G, Lund VJ, Beale T, Howard D. Rhinologic changes in Wegener's granulomatosis. J Laryngol Otol 2002;116(7):565–569
68. Yanamoto S, Kawasaki G, Yoshida H, et al. Rapidly growing mass of the anterior maxillary gingiva. Oral Surg Oral Med Oral Pathol Oral Radiol Endod 2007;104(2):153–159
69. Güneri P, Kaya A, Calişkan MK. Antroliths: survey of the literature and report of a case. Oral Surg Oral Med Oral Pathol Oral Radiol Endod 2005;99(4):517–521
70. Lund VJ. Optimum management of inverted papilloma. J Laryngol Otol 2000;114(3):194–197
71. Michaels L. Benign mucosal tumors of the nose and paranasal sinuses. Semin Diagn Pathol 1996;13(2):113–117
72. Minovi A, Kollert M, Draf W, Bockmühl U. Inverted papilloma: feasibility of endonasal surgery and long-term results of 87 cases. Rhinology 2006;44(3):205–210
73. Savy L, Lloyd G, Lund VJ, Howard D. Optimum imaging for inverted papilloma. J Laryngol Otol 2000;114(11):891–893
74. Mirza S, Bradley PJ, Acharya A, Stacey M, Jones NS. Sinonasal inverted papillomas: recurrence, and synchronous and metachronous malignancy. J Laryngol Otol 2007;121(9):857–864
75. Cannady SB, Batra PS, Sautter NB, Roh HJ, Citardi MJ. New staging system for sinonasal inverted papilloma in the endoscopic era. Laryngoscope 2007;117(7):1283–1287
76. Lu L, Zhou L, Li X, et al. [Pleomorphic adenoma of nose and accessory nasal sinuses: a report of 15 cases]. Lin Chuang Er Bi Yan Hou Ke Za Zhi 2004;18(9):549–551
77. Berenholz L, Kessler A, Segal S. Massive pleomorphic adenoma of the maxillary sinus. A case report. Int J Oral Maxillofac Surg 1998;27(5):372–373
78. Prager DA, Weiss MH, Buchalter WL, Jacobs M. Pleomorphic adenoma of the nasal cavity. Ann Otol Rhinol Laryngol 1991;100(7):600
79. Handler SD, Ward PH. Oncocytoma of the maxillary sinus. Laryngoscope 1979;89(3):372–376
80. Hamdan AL, Kahwagi G, Farhat F, Tawii A. Oncocytoma of the nasal septum: a rare cause of epistaxis. Otolaryngol Head Neck Surg 2002;126(4):440–441
81. Lin HL, Huang CC, Lee TJ. Endoscopic sinus surgery treatment for a huge sinonasal fibroma. Chang Gung Med J 2004;27(3):233–237
82. Uysal A, Kayiran O, Cuzdan SS, Bektas CI, Aslan G, Caydere M. Maxillary sinus lipoma: an unanticipated diagnosis. J Craniofac Surg 2007;18(5):1153–1155
83. Gregor RT, Loftus-Coll B. Myxoma of the paranasal sinuses. J Laryngol Otol 1994;108(8):679–681
84. Raboso E, Rosell A, Plaza G, Martinez-Vidal A. Haemangioma of the maxillary sinus. J Laryngol Otol 1997;111(7):638–640
85. Mussak E, Lin J, Prasad M. Cavernous hemangioma of the maxillary sinus with bone erosion. Ear Nose Throat J 2007;86(9):565–566
86. Fyrmpas G, Constantinidis J, Televantou D, Konstantinidis I, Daniilidis J. Primary aneurysmal bone cyst of the maxillary sinus in a child: case report and review of the literature. Eur Arch Otorhinolaryngol 2006;263(7):695–698
87. Matt BH. Aneurysmal bone cyst of the maxilla: case report and review of the literature. Int J Pediatr Otorhinolaryngol 1993;25(1–3):217–226
88. Hervé S, Abd Alsamad I, Beautru R, et al. Management of sinonasal hemangiopericytomas. Rhinology 1999;37(4):153–158
89. Stomeo F, Fois V, Cossu A, Meloni F, Pastore A, Bozzo C. Sinonasal haemangiopericytoma: a case report. Eur Arch Otorhinolaryngol 2004;261(10):555–557
90. LaBruna A, Reagan B, Papageorge A. Leiomyoma of the maxillary sinus: a diagnostic dilemma. Otolaryngol Head Neck Surg 1995;112(4):595–598
91. Fu YS, Perzin KH. Nonepithelial tumors of the nasal cavity paranasal sinuses, and nasopharynx: a clinicopathologic study. V. Skeletal muscle tumors (rhabdomyoma and rhabdomyosarcoma). Cancer 1976;37(1):364–376
92. Reitter GS. Rhabdomyoma of nose: Report of case. JAMA 1921;76:22–23
93. Press SG. Odontogenic tumors of the maxillary sinus. Curr Opin Otolaryngol Head Neck Surg 2008;16(1):47–54
94. Barnes L, Eveson JW, Reichart PA, Sidransky D, eds. World Health Organization classification of tumours: pathology and genetics of tumours of the head and neck. Lyon: IARC; 2005
95. Eller R, Sillers M. Common fibro-osseous lesions of the paranasal sinuses. Otolaryngol Clin North Am 2006;39(3):585–600
96. Alexander AA, Patel AA, Odland R. Paranasal sinus osteomas and Gardner's syndrome. Ann Otol Rhinol Laryngol 2007;116(9):658–662
97. Park W, Kim HS. Osteoma of maxillary sinus: a case report. Oral Surg Oral Med Oral Pathol Oral Radiol Endod 2006;102(6):e26–e27
98. Harrison DF. Osseous and fibro-osseous conditions affecting the craniofacial bones. Ann Otol Rhinol Laryngol 1984;93(3 Pt 1):199–203
99. Chong VF, Tan LH. Maxillary sinus ossifying fibroma. Am J Otolaryngol 1997;18(6):419–424
100. Muraoka H, Ishihara A, Kumagai J. Fibrous dysplasia with cystic appearance in maxillary sinus. Auris Nasus Larynx 2001;28(1):103–105
101. Chapurlat RD, Hugueny P, Delmas PD, Meunier PJ. Treatment of fibrous dysplasia of bone with intravenous pamidronate: long-term

effectiveness and evaluation of predictors of response to treatment. Bone 2004;35(1):235–242
102. Marx RE. Pamidronate (Aredia) and zoledronate (Zometa) induced avascular necrosis of the jaws: a growing epidemic. J Oral Maxillofac Surg 2003;61(9):1115–1117
103. Jones AC, Prihoda TJ, Kacher JE, Odingo NA, Freedman PD. Osteoblastoma of the maxilla and mandible: a report of 24 cases, review of the literature, and discussion of its relationship to osteoid osteoma of the jaws. Oral Surg Oral Med Oral Pathol Oral Radiol Endod 2006;102(5):639–650
104. Osguthorpe JD, Hungerford GD. Benign osteoblastoma of the maxillary sinus. Head Neck Surg 1983;6(1):605–609
105. Sarioğlu S, Ozkal S, Güneri A, et al. Cystic schwannoma of the maxillary sinus. Auris Nasus Larynx 2002;29(3):297–300
106. Sheikh HY, Chakravarthy RP, Slevin NJ, Sykes AJ, Banerjee SS. Benign schwannoma in paranasal sinuses: a clinico-pathological study of five cases, emphasising diagnostic difficulties. J Laryngol Otol 2008;122(6):598–602
107. Boedeker CC, Ridder GJ, Kayser G, Schipper J, Maier W. Solitary neurofibroma of the maxillary sinus and pterygopalatine fossa. Otolaryngol Head Neck Surg 2005;133(3):458–459

10 Silent Sinus Syndrome

Jayakar V. Nayak, John Lee, and Alexander G. Chiu

Silent sinus syndrome (SSS), is a rare disorder involving the maxillary antrum, characterized by an indolent course of subclinical maxillary sinusitis that leads to progressive contraction of the maxillary sinus. This process can eventually lead to prolapse of the orbital contents, enophthalmos (recession of the globe into the orbital vault) and ensuing ocular symptomatology. Patients with SSS therefore typically present with complaints of asymmetric facial features and visual changes, rather than symptoms typically associated with chronic maxillary sinusitis. The pathophysiology, presentation, imaging, clinical implications, and treatment of this unusual disorder are discussed in this chapter.

Historical Perspective

The first report of SSS was an article by Montgomery in 1964.[1] In this paper, the author describes his experience with two patients who experienced diplopia and enophthalmos associated with collapse of the maxillary sinus. Of note, the two patients in this report possessed mucoceles of the maxillary sinus. Subsequently in 1981, Wilkins and Kulwin reported a series of five patients, each of whom presented with spontaneous enophthalmos and ptosis unassociated with antecedent orbital trauma.[2] The authors observed that the patients each had unexpected defects in the orbital floor, which was attributed to their chronic, ipsilateral maxillary sinusitis. Thereafter, Wesley et al published another early report of SSS, documenting a single patient who presented with spontaneous enophthalmos without demineralization of the orbital floor.[3]

The term *silent sinus syndrome* was first introduced by Soparkar et al in the ophthalmology literature.[4] In this report, the authors analyzed an impressive series of 14 patients presenting to Baylor College of Medicine with spontaneous, unilateral enophthalmos and hypoglobus (downward displacement of the globe) associated with "asymptomatic, bone thinning, maxillary sinus disease" through extensive correlation of physical exam attributes along with computed tomography (CT) characteristics. This group coined the term *silent sinus syndrome* to describe this constellation of ocular and sinonasal findings. None of their 14 patients had signs or symptoms suggestive of intrinsic inflammatory rhinosinusitis. The authors hypothesized that this phenomenon may have been caused by bone remodeling in the maxillary sinus secondary to ostial obstruction in the setting of "hormonal and local influences" in an attempt to explain the findings of a contracted maxillary sinus without symptoms in younger adults. This publication began to give both credence to, and a more concrete definition for, the clinical entity of SSS.

Terminology

There is some controversy in the literature over whether silent sinus syndrome is a distinct condition or a late manifestation of a process termed *chronic maxillary atelectasis*. The latter condition involves a similar presentation to that seen in SSS, with the exception of associated facial pain, pressure, and nasal congestion in patients diagnosed with chronic maxillary atelectasis. A staging system has been proposed that attempts to annotate the so-called membranous, bony, and clinical progression of deformities in chronic maxillary atelectasis.[5] Brandt and Wright recently performed an exhaustive analysis of the available reports in the otolaryngology and ophthalmology literature on chronic maxillary atelectasis and SSS.[6] They concluded that these two disorders should be considered clinically indistinguishable, and might better be characterized under a single diagnosis. Although these authors proposed that chronic maxillary atelectasis is a more encompassing, umbrella name for the constellation of findings of SSS, this is not a generally accepted term in the rhinology or otolaryngology community at this point. We will therefore use the term silent sinus syndrome and maxillary atelectasis interchangeably in this chapter.

Pathophysiology

Silent sinus syndrome results from atelectasis of the maxillary sinus, and is generally believed to arise as an unusual consequence of obstruction of the maxillary sinus ostium. Initial hypotheses to address the mechanism for this process suggested silent sinus syndrome may arise in the setting of congenital maxillary sinus hypoplasia. However, this theory has been largely discredited by reports of several patients with normal anatomic relationships of the ostiomeatal complex (OMC) and orbit on CT imaging, who later went on to develop SSS.[7–9] These data support the principle that SSS is an acquired condition.

The current paradigm is that obstruction of the OMC of the paranasal sinuses leads to hypoventilation of the maxillary sinus. This enclosed cavity in certain settings is thought to develop air resorption, thus creating a suction effect of negative pressure within the maxillary antrum.[10–12] The development of a negative pressure vacuum within the sinus, in turn, results in the accumulation of mucous into the antrum, subclinical inflammation, and eventual collapse of the maxillary sinus through attenuation of the bony side walls of this structure.

There are experimental reports that provide evidence in support of this theory of the pathophysiology underlying SSS. One study measured inspiratory and expiratory pressures within the maxillary sinus in anesthetized rabbits. The investigators demonstrated that patent, unperturbed ostia had isobaric pressure readings in these animals, but that transient blockade of the maxillary sinus os first produces a spike in elevated antral pressures, followed by a protracted period of measurable negative pressure (>–20 cm H20) within the sinus.[13] The development of negative pressure was attributed to the absorption of respiratory gases into the rich capillary network of the sinonasal mucosa within the occluded sinus at this site. A corollary to this work is a report by Kass et al who introduced pressure-sensitive transducers through the membranous posterior fontanelle of patients with maxillary atelectasis. They compared their measurements to the pressures found in the contralateral, unaffected maxillary antrum in the same patient versus a separate cohort of patients with inflammatory rhinosinusitis. This group documented negative pressures (–8.4 cm H20) in the maxillary sinuses of five patients with SSS, compared with isobaric pressure measurements in maxillary sinuses unaffected by SSS.[14] This result was later supported by an isolated report of manometric recordings from a patient undergoing endoscopic sinus surgery for silent sinus syndrome. The pressure in the maxillary sinus was found to be –23 mm Hg.[11]

Clinical Evaluation and Assessment

An overlying principle in the clinical presentation of silent sinus syndrome is that patients with this disorder essentially *do not* have complaints with regard to their maxillary, or other, paranasal sinuses. Hallmark symptoms of maxillary sinusitis such as infraorbital facial pressure, pain, nasal congestion, and purulent rhinorrhea are notably absent in this patient population. Instead, pathognomonic of SSS is spontaneous enophthalmos and hypoglobus resulting from ipsilateral attenuation of the walls of the maxillary antrum in the distinct absence of clinically evident maxillary sinusitis (**Table 10.1**). With regard to the orbit, patients with SSS will have normal ocular motility and visual acuity, but the majority of patients will complain of some degree of diplopia.

Table 10.1 Clinical and Imaging Findings in Patients with Silent Sinus Syndrome

Clinical findings of silent sinus syndrome:
Spontaneous, gradual enophthalmos (eye recession into globe)
Spontaneous, gradual hypoglobus (inferior descent of eye)
Ocular asymmetry
Absence of sinus-related symptoms
Radiographic findings of silent sinus syndrome:
Ipsilateral contraction of affected maxillary sinus with volume loss
Inferior displacement of ipsilateral orbital floor
Partial to complete opacification of affected maxillary sinus
Increased orbital volume on affected side

In addition to the clinical features described above, radiographic evaluation for characteristic changes to the orbit and the paranasal sinuses via CT imaging is required to confirm the diagnosis of SSS.[8,15] CT is the gold standard imaging modality for the diagnosis of SSS, although magnetic resonance imaging (MRI) is sometimes utilized.[16] The classic CT finding in SSS is the inward retraction of the medial and superior walls of the maxillary sinus associated with a decrease in the maxillary antral volume (**Fig. 10.1**). Additional imaging findings in SSS typically include a well developed, but opacified, maxillary sinus, occlusion of the maxillary infundibulum due to retraction of the uncinate process, and an expanded middle meatus with increased orbital volume (**Fig. 10.2A**).

On external physical examination, patients with SSS will have orbital asymmetry due to unilateral enophthalmos and hypoglobus (**Fig. 10.2B**). This gradual alteration in facial appearance is very commonly the presenting concern for these patients.[17] In tabulating past articles of SSS, one group determined that the average reported orbital recession is 2.96 mm (±0.16 mm) and 53% of those patients presented with hypoglobus with an average orbital decline of 2.78 mm (±0.25 mm).[6] This concurs with the previously discussed landmark publication by Soparkar et al, showing an average enophthalmos of 3 mm, and average hypoglobus of 3.4 mm.[4] Other physical examination findings may include eyelid retraction, narrowing of the palpebral fissure, and lagophthalmos.[6,18] On nasal endoscopic examination, patients may have a normal appearance to the nasal cavity on the affected side, or may have subtle alterations such as a widened middle meatal cavity with inward retraction of the uncinate process. Alternatively, the middle meatus may be obscured on endoscopy due to lateral displacement of the middle turbinate toward the uncinate process.[15]

SSS most commonly presents in the third to fourth decades of life, and appears to affect both genders equally with the exception of one small case series that demonstrated

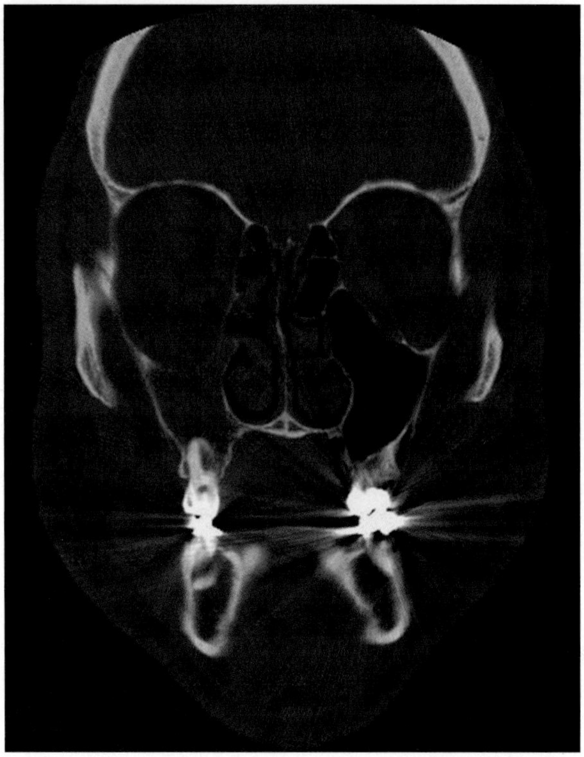

Fig. 10.1 Coronal computed tomography scan of a patient with silent sinus syndrome. Classic imaging findings seen here include atelectasis of right maxillary sinus walls compared with the left side, reduced right maxillary antral volume and opacification, and increased right orbital volume with clear descent of orbital floor.

an increased incidence in males.[6,10,15] SSS also has a similar incidence in the left and right maxillary sinuses. The average duration of the progressive, characteristic orbitopathies until presentation is 3 months (range 10 days–2 years).[4] Although the vast majority of patients with SSS present as adults, it should be noted that there have been a limited number of case reports of this disorder in children. There are isolated case reports of SSS with classic findings of facial asymmetry and enophthalmos in teenagers presenting with findings suggestive of SSS.[19–21] The above reports indicate that, although quite rare, SSS may occur in pediatric patients and should be considered when treating a young patient with facial asymmetry or enophthalmos.

The fact that SSS is an uncommon entity should prompt clinicians and surgeons alike to consider a wide range of disease processes in the evaluation of a patient presenting with enophthalmos and hypoglobus. The differential diagnosis for SSS includes relatively common clinical causes of enophthalmos such as trauma to the orbit (especially blowout fracture of the orbital floor), chronic sinusitis, osteomyelitis, Wegener granulomatosis, orbital metastasis, human immunodeficiency virus (HIV) lipodystrophy, and prior orbital radiation therapy. Several exceedingly rare disorders in the differential include orbital fat atrophy, Recklinghausen disease (absence of the sphenoid wing), linear scleroderma, Parry–Romberg syndrome (progressive hemifacial atrophy), and pseudoenophthalmos.[10,18]

As we have noted previously, there will be a subset of patients who have classic orbital findings of SSS, but in fact also suffer from symptoms of nasal congestion, rhinorrhea, facial pain, and facial pressure. These patients have, by convention, been considered to have chronic maxillary atelectasis. Except for nomenclature, these patients possess the cardinal signs and symptoms of SSS, and would be treated in the same fashion as SSS. Again, the distinction between SSS and chronic maxillary atelectasis has been largely refuted by recent reports. The finding of sinus symptomatology in the presence of the ocular and radiologic findings discussed should not alter the assessment or interventions employed for patient care.[6,22]

A

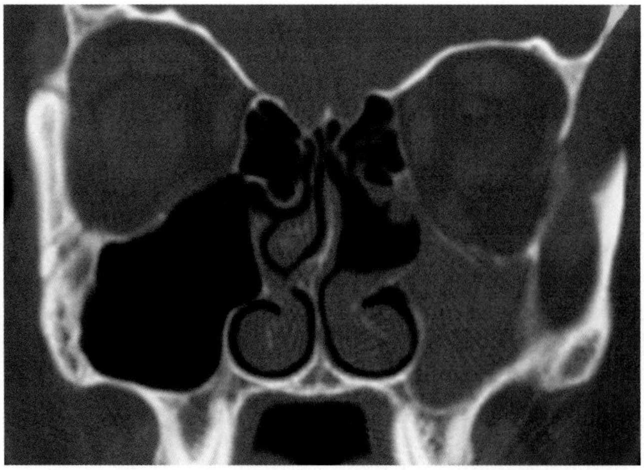

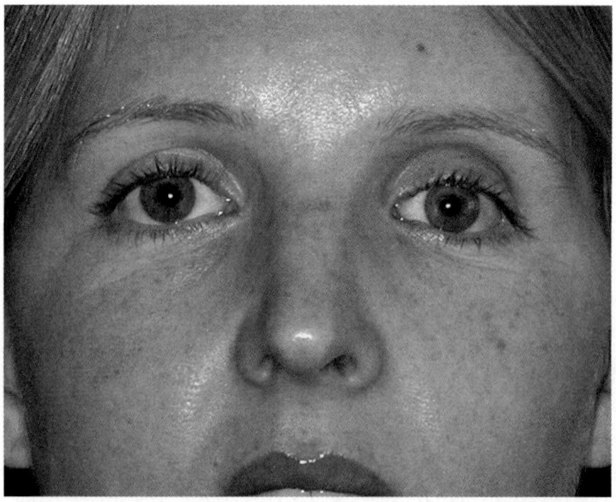

B

Fig. 10.2 **(A)** Atelectatic uncinate process. In addition to other classic imaging findings of silent sinus syndrome (SSS), this computed tomography scan demonstrates a retracted left uncinate process that is often found on imaging of the maxillary sinus. **(B)** Clinical presentation of the same patient presented in Fig. 10.2A with left SSS. Especially notable is this young adult's facial asymmetry and hypoglobus of the left orbit compared with the right.

Treatment

Treatment of SSS is focused on correcting the causative problem that has produced SSS (i.e., maxillary sinus negative pressure leading to structural collapse). Historically, SSS was treated using a Caldwell–Luc approach to enter the anterior face of the affected maxillary sinus. However, as the techniques and technology employed in endoscopic sinus surgery have been refined, this has clearly become the primary treatment modality for SSS.[6,10] Key principles of endoscopic surgery in the treatment of SSS are summarized in **Table 10.2**.

When treating SSS via endoscopic techniques (**see Video 10.1**), it is critical to first obtain detailed preoperative CT scans to best assess the anatomic relationships present to reduce the possibility of unintended orbital entry during surgery. The surgeon should plan to perform a complete uncinectomy with a wide maxillary antrostomy to expose the entire maxillary sinus to prevent recurrence. The surgeon must be mindful during any endoscopic instrumentation of the uncinate and maxillary sinus in patients with SSS, due to the inferior displacement of the orbital contents in this disorder. With an atelectatic uncinate process lateralized to the medial orbital wall, there is an elevated risk of inadvertent entry into the orbit. Traditional uncinectomy techniques such as the use of a sickle knife to incise the uncinate at its anterior attachment to the lacrimal bone is discouraged in SSS because this practice may result in penetration through the lamina papyracea. A safer technique is to insert endoscopically a ball-tip probe posterior to the free margin of the uncinate and anterior to the lamina papyracea. By dissecting in a location anterior to the lamina papyracea, the uncinate process can be reflected forward and away from the orbit, thereby allowing for safe resection with the use of cutting instruments or a microdebrider. In isolated maxillary sinus involvement, an anterior ethmoidectomy procedure is usually warranted to further expose the landmark of the medial orbital wall, and to liberate the hiatus semilunaris region of the middle meatus from obstruction.

Table 10.2 Key Points in the Endoscopic Treatment of Silent Sinus Syndrome

Preoperative review of computed tomography (CT) scan imaging to determine relationship of uncinate and maxillary os to affected orbit
Preoperative CT scan obtained using image-guidance protocol
Complete uncinectomy with wide maxillary antrostomy
Anterior ethmoidectomy for added exposure of hiatus semilunaris and medial orbital wall
Inferior meatal antrostomy with possible endoscopic medial maxillectomy in select cases

A notable concern arises during endoscopic sinus surgery if the inferior displacement of the orbit is significant, or more likely, if the acquired atelectasis in the maxillary sinus has precluded safe uncinectomy due to scarring and edema between the uncinate and medial orbital wall/lamina papyracea. In this predicament, the surgeon may need to consider safely exposing the maxillary antrum through an inferior meatal antrostomy, and converting to an endoscopic medial maxillectomy procedure to halt progression of the SSS disease process, ensure a safe sinus, and allow for optimal postoperative examination and debridement in the office setting.

Studies have confirmed the superiority of an endoscopic approach in the treatment of other forms of sinus disease, and the majority of case reports on silent sinus syndrome have indicated good outcomes using endoscopic techniques.[6] Complications are essentially the same as would be expected for routine endoscopic sinus surgeries and include infection, bleeding, unintended entry into the orbit with injury to the orbital musculature and/or optic nerve.

In addition to relieving the obstruction of the maxillary sinus ostium, a second surgical procedure to restore the height of the orbital floor may need to be entertained. The indication for this surgery would be persistent orbitopathy after endoscopic maxillary antrostomy and uncinectomy, to restore orbital volume and symmetry. There is some debate regarding whether a one-stage or two-stage surgical approach should be utilized in the treatment of SSS. Vander Meer et al describe successful orbital correction of a series of four patients who received simultaneous endoscopic sinus surgery and orbital floor repair using Medpor malleable mesh (Porex Technologies, Fairburn, GA).[9] Preoperative enophthalmos by Hertle exophthalmometry ranged between 1 to 4 mm for these patients. Rose et al followed 14 patients with SSS (termed imploding antrum syndrome in this work), and found that several patients progressed in severity of enophthalmos over time without surgery.[16] Six patients eventually underwent silicone block placement to restore orbital floor height. Unfortunately, this group did not document the degree of enophthalmos using standardized measurement criteria, and it is unclear how many of these patients received endoscopic sinus surgery prior to open orbital surgery.

In contrast, Thomas et al followed four patients with SSS, each with a preoperative enophthalmos of 3 mm by Hertle exophthalmometry.[23] Two of these patients developed spontaneous resolution of their enophthalmos after endoscopic sinus surgery, to a final displacement of 1 mm over a 6-month period. The latter patients were reportedly content with the resolution in their facial asymmetry, and did not require corrective surgery for the affected orbital floor. In contrast, the remaining two patients in this report each had a residual, persistent enophthalmos of 2 mm after a similar 6-month postoperative interval, and orbital floor reconstruction through placement of an implant was undertaken in a second procedure. For one of these same two patients, volumetric calculations using CT scans were performed with spontaneous resolution of enophthalmos, showing a rebound recovery from 16.9 to 19.6 cubic millimeters of maxillary sinus volume 6 months after endoscopic surgery alone. These data provide objective evidence that after an endoscopic approach for SSS, some patients have natural, progressive improvement in orbital ptosis and maxillary sinus characteristics, thus obviating the need for corrective orbital floor surgery. The benefit of avoiding orbital correction for this disease process has been shown in several other case series as well.[24,25]

We advocate a two-stage approach; that is, to delay any intervention for augmentation of the orbital floor for at least 6 to 12 months after endoscopic sinus surgery for SSS. This allows for full resolution of any possible infectious agents found in the operated antrum prior to placement of a foreign material implant, and also allows for the possibility of natural resolution of orbital findings and subjective complaints.

The approaches and materials optimal for repair of the orbital floor are beyond the scope of this chapter, but are well described by others.[18] Complications resulting from the orbital floor repair include persistence or worsening of diplopia, under- or overcorrection of enophthalmos and a foreign body reaction to materials used in the reconstruction of the orbital floor.

Conclusion

Silent sinus syndrome is a rare condition in which patients present with enophthalmos and hypoglobus due to subclinical disease of the maxillary sinus. Patients with SSS usually present with facial asymmetry and visual disturbances and, by definition, lack subjective complaints associated with acute or chronic sinus disease. The physical examination of a patient with SSS will demonstrate enophthalmos and hypoglobus, and may have subtle findings of asymmetry on nasal endoscopy. The diagnosis of SSS can be stamped after appropriate CT imaging studies confirm atelectasis of the ipsilateral maxillary sinus. Silent sinus syndrome is effectively treated using endoscopic sinus surgical techniques and image guidance without simultaneous repair of the affected orbital floor. It is important for ophthalmologists, radiologists, oromaxillofacial surgeons, and otolaryngologists to be aware of this condition and its characteristics to make an appropriate diagnosis and offer patients salient options for intervention.

Pearls

- SSS is a clinical entity characterized by progressive, spontaneous changes to the ipsilateral maxillary sinus and orbit in the absence of typical symptoms of maxillary sinusitis.
- Presenting complaints in SSS typically involve the affected orbit, and include diplopia, enophthalmos, and hypoglobus.
- Several reports lend support to the hypothesis that negative pressure within an obstructed maxillary sinus eventually produces antral atelectasis and orbital floor descent in SSS.
- To confirm the diagnosis of SSS and assist with possible surgical planning, CT is required.
- Endoscopic sinus surgery is a safe and effective strategy to treat the pathophysiologic disease process in SSS appropriately.
- Orbital floor reconstruction can be considered at a separate future surgery if the affected sinus and orbital floor in SSS remain collapsed, and/or if the patient's orbital complaints persist after confirmed endoscopic surgical correction of the underlying disease.

References

1. Montgomery WW. Mucocele of the maxillary sinus causing enophthalmos. Eye Ear Nose Throat Mon 1964;43:41–44
2. Wilkins RB, Kulwin DR. Spontaneous enophthalmos associated with chronic maxillary sinusitis. Ophthalmology 1981;88(9):981–985
3. Wesley RE, Johnson JJ II, Cate RC. Spontaneous enophthalmos from chronic maxillary sinusitis. Laryngoscope 1986;96(4):353–355
4. Soparkar CN, Patrinely JR, Cuaycong MJ, et al. The silent sinus syndrome. A cause of spontaneous enophthalmos. Ophthalmology 1994;101(4):772–778
5. Kass ES, Salman S, Rubin PA, Weber AL, Montgomery WW. Chronic maxillary atelectasis. Ann Otol Rhinol Laryngol 1997;106(2):109–116
6. Brandt MG, Wright ED. The silent sinus syndrome is a form of chronic maxillary atelectasis: a systematic review of all reported cases. Am J Rhinol 2008;22(1):68–73
7. Facon F, Eloy P, Brasseur P, Collet S, Bertrand B. The silent sinus syndrome. Eur Arch Otorhinolaryngol 2006;263(6):567–571
8. Hourany R, Aygun N, Della Santina CC, Zinreich SJ. Silent sinus syndrome: an acquired condition. AJNR Am J Neuroradiol 2005;26(9):2390–2392
9. Vander Meer JB, Harris G, Toohill RJ, Smith TL. The silent sinus syndrome: a case series and literature review. Laryngoscope 2001;111(6):975–978
10. Annino DJ Jr, Goguen LA. Silent sinus syndrome. Curr Opin Otolaryngol Head Neck Surg 2008;16(1):22–25
11. Davidson JK, Soparkar CN, Williams JB, Patrinely JR. Negative sinus pressure and normal predisease imaging in silent sinus syndrome. Arch Ophthalmol 1999;117(12):1653–1654
12. Numa WA, Desai U, Gold DR, Heher KL, Annino DJ. Silent sinus syndrome: a case presentation and comprehensive review of all 84 reported cases. Ann Otol Rhinol Laryngol 2005;114(9):688–694
13. Scharf KE, Lawson W, Shapiro JM, Gannon PJ. Pressure measurements in the normal and occluded rabbit maxillary sinus. Laryngoscope 1995;105(6):570–574

14. Kass ES, Salman S, Montgomery WW. Manometric study of complete ostial occlusion in chronic maxillary atelectasis. Laryngoscope 1996;106(10):1255–1258
15. Illner A, Davidson HC, Harnsberger HR, Hoffman J. The silent sinus syndrome: clinical and radiographic findings. AJR Am J Roentgenol 2002;178(2):503–506
16. Rose GE, Sandy C, Hallberg L, Moseley I. Clinical and radiologic characteristics of the imploding antrum, or "silent sinus," syndrome. Ophthalmology 2003;110(4):811–818
17. Burroughs JR, Hernández Cospín JR, Soparkar CN, Patrinely JR. Misdiagnosis of silent sinus syndrome. Ophthal Plast Reconstr Surg 2003;19(6):449–454
18. Hamedani M, Pournaras JA, Goldblum D. Diagnosis and management of enophthalmos. Surv Ophthalmol 2007;52(5):457–473
19. Habibi A, Sedaghat MR, Habibi M, Mellati E. Silent sinus syndrome: report of a case. Oral Surg Oral Med Oral Pathol Oral Radiol Endod 2008;105(3):e32–e35
20. Kass ES, Salman S, Montgomery WW. Chronic maxillary atelectasis in a child. Ann Otol Rhinol Laryngol 1998;107(7):623–625
21. Yip CC, McCulley TJ, Kersten RC, Tami TA, Kulwin DR. Silent sinus syndrome as a cause of diplopia in a child. J Pediatr Ophthalmol Strabismus 2003;40(5):309–311
22. Hwang PH, Irwin SB, Griest SE, Caro JE, Nesbit GM. Radiologic correlates of symptom-based diagnostic criteria for chronic rhinosinusitis. Otolaryngol Head Neck Surg 2003;128(4):489–496
23. Thomas RD, Graham SM, Carter KD, Nerad JA. Management of the orbital floor in silent sinus syndrome. Am J Rhinol 2003;17(2):97–100
24. Blackwell KE, Goldberg RA, Calcaterra TC. Atelectasis of the maxillary sinus with enophthalmos and midface depression. Ann Otol Rhinol Laryngol 1993;102(6):429–432
25. Sciarretta V, Pasquini E, Tesei F, Modugno GC, Farneti G. Endoscopic sinus surgery for the treatment of maxillary sinus atelectasis and silent sinus syndrome. J Otolaryngol 2006;35(1):60–64

11 Primary Endoscopic Surgery of the Maxillary Sinus

Amir Minovi and Wolfgang Draf

More complex endonasal surgery of the paranasal sinuses was first performed at the beginning of the 20th century.[1,2] Catastrophic complications during endonasal surgery, however, caused by primitive surgical conditions (e.g., using head lights and naked eyes) led to issues such as skull base injuries followed by meningitis, brain abscess, and/or encephalitis during that preantibiotic era. Early in the 20th century, Mosher therefore described endonasal ethmoid surgery as the most dangerous operation in all of surgery.[3] Thus for many decades most surgeons favored the external approach for paranasal sinus surgery because it presented a lower risk for most dangerous complications.

Cowper (1707) and Ziem (1886) were the first surgeons who treated the maxillary sinus through an opened alveole.[4] Jourdain (1761) and Hartmann (1883) used the natural ostium of the maxillary sinus opening.[5] The middle meatal antrostomy was first described by Siebenmann (1899).[4] Lamorier (1743) and Desault (1789) published the canine fossa approach to the maxillary sinus. Claoué (1902), Lothrop (1898), and Mikulicz (1886) can be seen as the founders of the endonasal fenestration of the maxillary sinus.[4,5] Caldwell (1893)[6] and Luc (1897)[7] described a large fenestration of the maxillary sinus through the canine fossa in combination with a drainage through the inferior nasal meatus. Denker (1905)[8] developed a radical addition to the Caldwell–Luc procedure by resection of the piriform crest via a nasolabial incision.

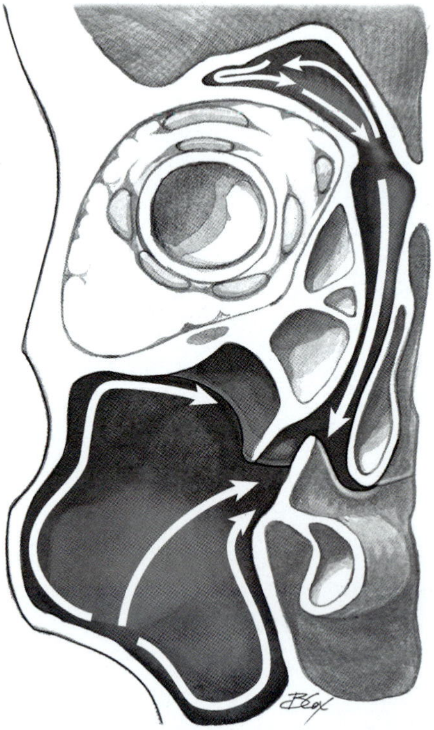

Fig. 11.1 Drawing of the ostiomeatal complex (OMC): physiologic secretion transport from frontal and maxillary sinus into the middle nasal meatus.

A new era in sinus surgery began in the early 1970s with the development of different angled endoscopes based on the Hopkins rod lens technology and its use in the evaluation of the paranasal sinuses.[9,10] Unlike Messerklinger, who investigated the anatomy and pathophysiology of the nose and its relationship to chronic sinusitis, Draf examined the different sinuses systematically. He was the first person to perform endoscopy of the frontal and the sphenoid sinus. Primarily, his goal was to develop solid indications for sinus surgery, thereby avoiding unnecessary, radical operations, especially because the imaging techniques were still poor at that time, offering only plain x-ray and at times, conventional tomography. Soon after, like Messerklinger he started to perform endoscopic treatment of inflammatory diseases. Nasal endoscopy with rigid instruments and computerized tomography (CT) of the paranasal sinuses enabled the surgeon to approach the ostiomeatal complex (OMC) more precisely. Based on Messerklinger's studies, Stammberger and later Kennedy introduced a conservative type of sinus surgery to restore normal mucociliary flow in the region of the OMC, which they named functional endoscopic sinus surgery (FESS) (**Fig. 11.1**).[11,12]

Indications and Contraindications

Primary endoscopic maxillary sinus surgery (PEMSS) has many advantages over surgery using an external approach. PEMSS allows for

- Intranasal incisions, which help to avoid vestibular fistula
- Minimal intranasal and intrasinus trauma
- Preservation of the bony framework and mucous membrane needed for restoration of normal mucociliary clearance

The most common indications are

- Chronic and/or recurrent maxillary sinusitis, unresponsive to prior medical treatment
- Complicated acute maxillary sinusitis
- Fungal maxillary sinusitis with formation of mycetoma
- Antrochoanal polyp
- Mucocele
- Control of epistaxis
- Resection of small benign tumors, especially inverted papillomas
- Resection of selected malignant tumors

Relative contraindications are

- High-risk patients not suitable for general anesthesia (e.g., those with immunosuppressive conditions, advanced coronal heart disease, coagulopathy)
- Extended tumors with involvement of the lateral and/or anteroinferior regions of the maxillary sinus
- Untreated dentogenic maxillary sinusitis

Preoperative Evaluation

The Patient's History

The most important aim of any surgical procedure is to relieve the patient's symptoms. Not all symptoms of chronic sinusitis can be eliminated with surgical treatment. It is, therefore, vital to take the time to listen to the patient and to establish his or her main problems. A discussion is then required to make clear to the patient what can be achieved with surgery, and which symptoms are likely to be improved. It is important to remember that sinus surgery is not about treating a CT scan, but is part of the treatment regimen of a well-informed patient. In general, the history taken should include the following aspects.

Symptoms of the Present Illness

Patients frequently present their diagnosis to the surgeon, instead of describing their symptoms. Detailed questioning about the patient's symptoms is required with concentration on the duration, time of onset, and any symptom-free intervals. The patients also should be asked if they suffer from the most common symptoms of chronic sinusitis. These include

- Nasal obstruction
- Hyposmia
- Headache and location of pain
- Recurrent facial swelling
- Postnasal drip
- Facial pressure

Past Medical and Surgical History

Most patients who are referred for sinus surgery have been treated medically in the past. Many of them have received several antibiotic treatments in conjunction with systemic and/or topical corticosteroids. It is mandatory to ask all patients about any previous sinus surgery. The following questions require particular attention.

- Has the patient undergone any antibiotic therapy? What were the effects?
- Has the patient had local/systemic corticosteroid treatment? Was it in conjunction with antibiotic treatment? What was the duration of the treatment?
- Is the patient on any other medication, particularly agents that can cause mucosal swelling as a side effect such as antihypertensive drugs?
- Has the patient undergone any previous surgery? When?
- Was the previous surgery successful and were there symptom-free intervals after the surgery?
- Does the patient have Samter's triad (polyps, asthma, aspirin intolerance)?

Physical Examination and Endoscopy

Routine physical examination includes anterior rhinoscopy and rigid/flexible endoscopy. The anterior rhinoscopy, possibly with the examination microscope, gives the surgeon a first impression of the sinonasal condition. The following features should be noted from this examination.

- Septal deviation
- Color, texture, and turgor of the mucosa
- Size and shape of the turbinates

Endoscopic examination of the nasal cavity with rigid and flexible endoscopes is now the gold standard in the preoperative evaluation of chronic sinusitis. In our hospital, we prefer the flexible endoscope as it is well tolerated, even in children, and most patients do not even require local anesthesia. A zero- or 30-degree angled rigid endoscope also can be used to examine the nasal cavity. Before using a rigid endoscope, a mixture of topical anesthetic and a vasoconstrictor should be applied to the nasal mucosa. By displaying the endoscopic image on a television monitor, it is possible to demonstrate any pathology to the patient. The following anatomic structures should be evaluated routinely.

- Relationship between the middle turbinate and the nasal septum
- Paradoxical middle turbinate (a medially rather than laterally concave middle turbinate)
- The presence of a concha bullosa (an air-filled, pneumatized middle turbinate) (**Fig. 11.2**)
- The extent and size of any polyps (**Fig. 11.3**)

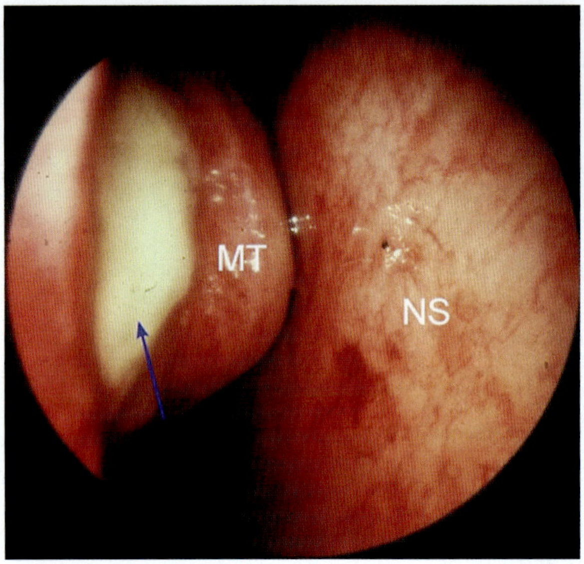

Fig. 11.2 Endoscopic view of a pyocele (*blue arrow*) in a concha bullosa. NS, nasal septum; MT, middle turbinate.

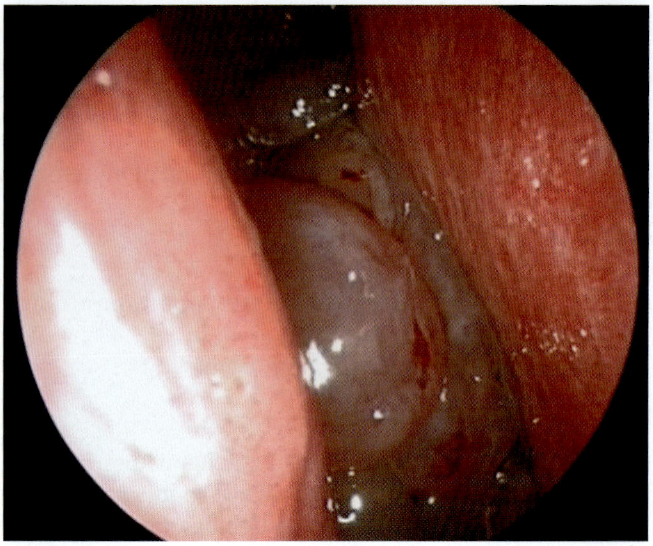

Fig. 11.3 Extended polyposis with complete obstruction of the middle nasal meatus.

The evaluation of olfaction preoperatively is mandatory. Up to 45% of patients with chronic sinusitis complain of olfactory dysfunction.[13,14] Acoustic rhinometry is a noninvasive technique to measure the cross-sectional area of regions of the nasal airway. It has become more and more popular because it is rapid, noninvasive, and requires minimal cooperation from the subject. In case the patient does not feel improvement of airflow postoperatively, this investigation may be repeated as objective documentation. It is interesting to note that a patient's subjective feeling about nasal airflow and the objective measurement do not always correlate. Rhinomanometry is an objective technique, in which changes in air pressure and the speed of air flow through the nasal cavities are measured during breathing. This allows the nasal resistance to airflow to be calculated.

Imaging

Computerized tomography (CT) is absolutely essential in planning endoscopic sinus surgery. In the event of a postoperative complication, a surgeon has little medicolegal defense if a preoperative CT scan was not performed. Scanning is best performed in the axial plane with additional coronal and sagittal reconstructed images. This minimizes any artifacts caused by dental fillings. Sagittal planes are very helpful in determining the extension of the frontal and sphenoid sinuses. Ideally, a CT scan should be done when the disease is quiescent and there is no acute inflammation of the sinuses. The extent of mucosal disease found at the time of surgery may differ from what is shown on the CT scan. In the majority of the cases, the findings are underestimated based on the CT scans.[15] With the help of CT, the surgeon should evaluate extension and distribution of the disease and analyze important anatomic landmarks, variants, and any surgically hazardous anatomy. CT scans should be shown to the patients before surgery to explain the proposed surgery, and must be present in the operating room for the surgeon to review during surgery. Several authors have suggested a preoperative checklist for CT evaluation in functional endoscopic sinus surgery.[16] For maxillary sinus surgery, we recommend the following CT work-up, ideally done with the radiologist on the day of surgery.

- General overview of the paranasal sinuses in the coronal planes (**Fig. 11.4**)

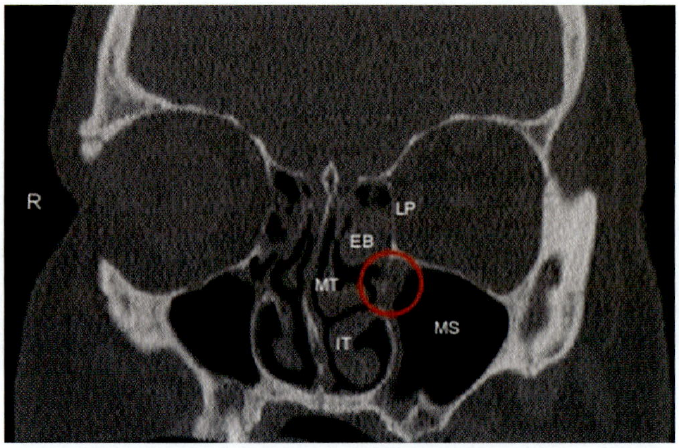

Fig. 11.4 Coronal computed tomography (CT) scan shows mild opacification of the OMC (*red circle*). MS, maxillary sinus; LP, lamina papyracea; EB, ethmoid bulla; MT, middle turbinate; IT, inferior turbinate.

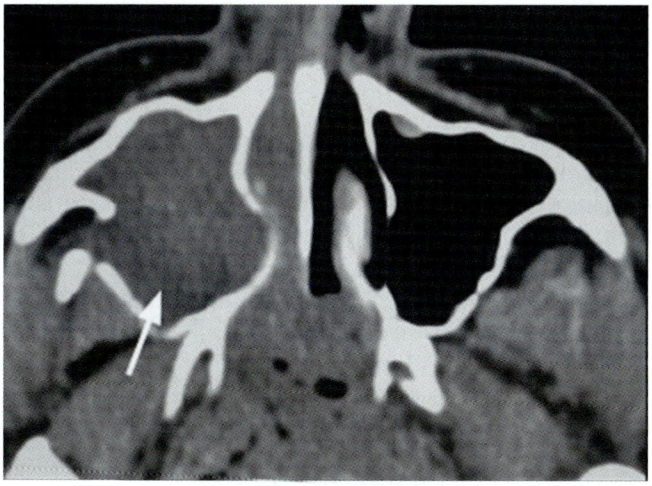

Fig. 11.5 Unilateral total opacification of the right maxillary sinus (*arrow*) in an inverted papilloma (axial computed tomography scan).

- Are the sides (right and left) correctly labeled?
- Assess the ostiomeatal complex
- Any unilateral maxillary sinus opacification? (**Fig. 11.5**)
- Evaluation of important anatomic landmarks (axial and coronal planes)
  - o Uncinate process: shape, course, and site of insertion
  - o Lamina papyracea: possible dehiscent areas (**Fig. 11.6**)
  - o Middle turbinate: degree of pneumatization, presence of a concha bullosa, extension of resection in previous surgery

In unilateral maxillary sinus opacification, a dentogenic sinusitis should be ruled out by a maxillofacial surgeon. If there is suspicion of an inverted papilloma, magnetic resonance imaging (MRI) is very helpful for further surgical planning (**Fig. 11.7**).

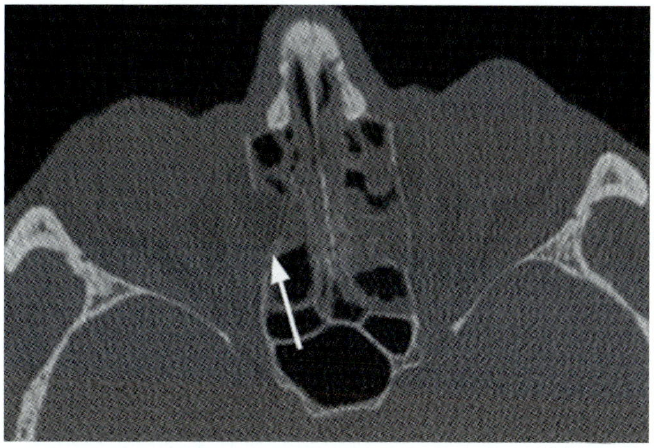

Fig. 11.6 Axial computed tomography (CT) scan showing partial dehiscence of the lamina papyracea (*arrow*).

Informed Patient Consent

Before surgery the patient should be informed about the advantages and possible complications of the surgery. It is mandatory also to mention possible catastrophic complications. The following points should be included in the preoperative conversation with the patient:

- Failure, revision surgery
- Alternative forms of treatment
- Bleeding, infection, wound-healing disturbances
- Injury to the optic nerve with possible reduced vision or blindness

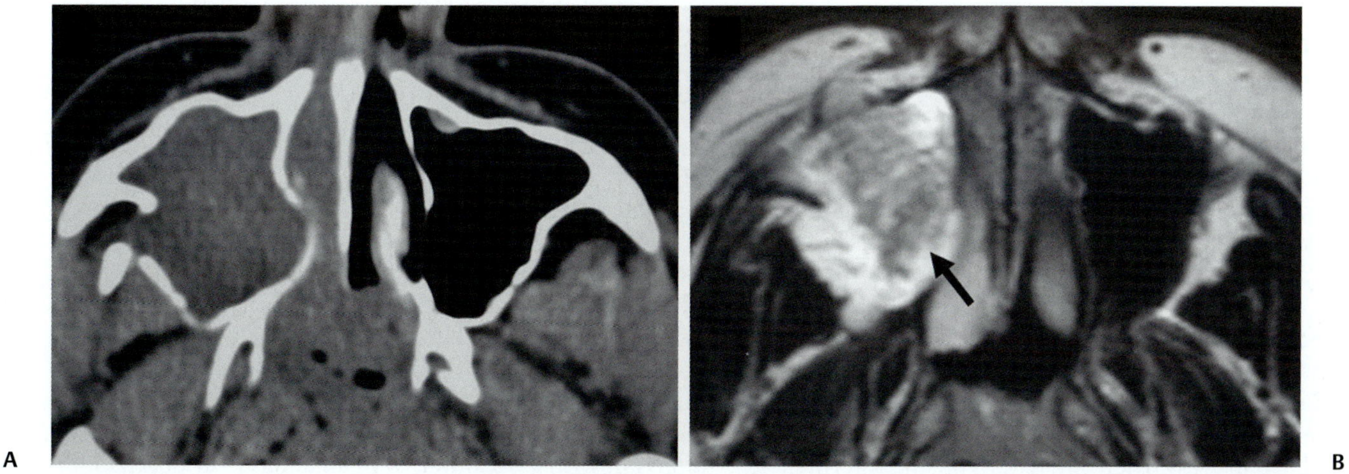

Fig. 11.7 Inverted papilloma. **(A)** Axial computed tomography (CT) scan shows total opacification of the right maxillary sinus with involvement of the middle meatus and nasal cavity. In a CT scan, an inverted papilloma is not distinguishable from chronic sinusitis. **(B)** Axial T1-weighted magnetic resonance image (MRI) proves the existence of heterogeneous tumor tissue in the maxillary sinus (*arrow*), which is very specific for inverted papilloma.

- Injury to the ocular muscles with possible permanent double vision
- Injury of the dura with cerebrospinal fluid leaks, meningitis, encephalitis
- Epiphora
- Olfactory disturbances
- Hypesthesia in the palate, teeth, or face
- Burns to the upper lip in case of contact with a hot drill, although extremely rare

It has been shown that the better the patient is informed regarding the necessary surgical steps, limitations, possible failures and complications, the more he or she will trust the surgeon even if the result is below his or her expectations. Meticulous postoperative care adds to this significantly.

Instrumentation

In endoscopic maxillary sinus surgery, the rigid fiberoptic nasal telescope provides superb visualization of the operative field.[12,17] The zero-degree, 4-mm rigid telescope is used for the major part of the surgery. In children, one can use the 2.7-mm rigid endoscope. Most of the surgical field can be visualized with the zero-degree scope. In particular, beginners of endoscopic sinus surgery should perform almost the whole surgery with the zero-degree scope. As the angle of the telescope rises, so does the risk of disorientation. Therefore, the 30-, 45-, and 70-degree telescopes are only used for work in areas "around the corner" of the maxillary sinus. With a 30-degree endoscope, one is able to get an orientation over the middle meatal antrostomy, whereas the 45-degree endoscope is a very helpful instrument for judging the inferior region of the maxillary sinus. A camera is usually attached to the eyepiece of the endoscope and the endoscopic view is transmitted to a monitor. The surgeon can perform the surgery while looking through the endoscope or at the monitor, or a combination of both. Most surgeons nowadays look at the monitor, which allows for a more relaxed working position.

Most commonly, a Freer elevator is used to medialize the middle turbinate and gain a better view of the uncinate process and ethmoid bulla. One also can use it for incision and removal of the uncinate process. Most surgeons prefer the sickle knife for this part of procedure. Blakesley forceps is suitable to remove mobilized polyps or tissue; the straight forceps is appropriate for removing the loose parts of the bone from the surgical area. Different types of curved suctions are used in the maxillary sinus. The backbiters (Rhinoforce Stammberger antrum Punch; Karl Storz Endoscopy-America, Inc., El Segundo, CA) are best for removal of the uncinate process. There are left, right, and intermediate backbiters. A major advantage is that one can take about three bites with these instruments before they need to be cleaned. They also can be used to widen the middle antrostomy in an anterior direction.

Surgical Techniques

Anesthesia

PEMSS today is performed usually under general anesthesia in combination with local vasoconstrictor medications. As a local anesthetic, a combination of lidocaine 1% and 1/100,000 to 1/200,000 epinephrine is injected into the agger nasi and the uncinate process area. Furthermore, better vasoconstriction is achieved by additional placing of cotton swabs soaked in naphazolinhydrochlorid and cocaine 10% (maximal single dose rate of 2 mL) in the nasal cavity for 10 minutes. Time is spared if the injection is performed before the surgeon scrubs and the patient is sterile wrapped. Bleeding is a major concern during endonasal sinus surgery. In many cases, bleeding can be minimized with the support of specific anesthetic techniques. The anesthesiologist should be informed continuously about the actual bleeding condition, and should follow the surgery on a monitor. Intraoperative communication between the ear, nose, and throat (ENT) surgeon and the anesthesiologist is essential.

If the comorbidities of the patient provides no contraindication, the anesthesiologist should intraoperatively aim at a mean arterial pressure of 60 mm Hg and a heartbeat rate of 50 to 60/min. Arterial hypotension will minimize hemodynamic causes for bleeding and, if required, can be achieved by intravenous administration of β-blockade or arterial vasodilators. The influence of various anesthetics on bleeding is under discussion. A total intravenous technique may have advantages with regard to bleeding on the microcirculatory level. If anesthetic techniques fail to provide a clear view of the surgical field, temporary application of cotton plugs soaked with adrenaline 1:1000 is useful.[18] The risk of adrenaline-induced cardiac arrhythmias nowadays is almost negligible, when a total intravenous technique is used and the volatile anesthetic halothane is avoided.

Endoscopic Uncinectomy

As described above the surgeon should first analyze the superior attachment and the anatomic variations of the uncinate process.[19] In 70% of cases, the uncinate process is inserted into the lamina papyracea. In 30% of cases, it is attached to the skull base or to the middle turbinate (**Fig. 11.8**). Using a zero-degree scope, the uncinectomy or infundibulotomy is started by gentle medialization of the middle turbinate (**Fig. 11.9**). The next step consists of resection of the uncinate process and exposure of the ethmoid bulla. The uncinectomy can be performed in a posterior-to-anterior direction with a backbiter, or in an anterior-to-posterior direction with a sickle knife (**Figs. 11.10A-F**) or Freer elevator. The most cranial part of the uncinate process should be left intact preventing any mucosa damage and scar tissue formation around the frontal recess. The uncinate process is

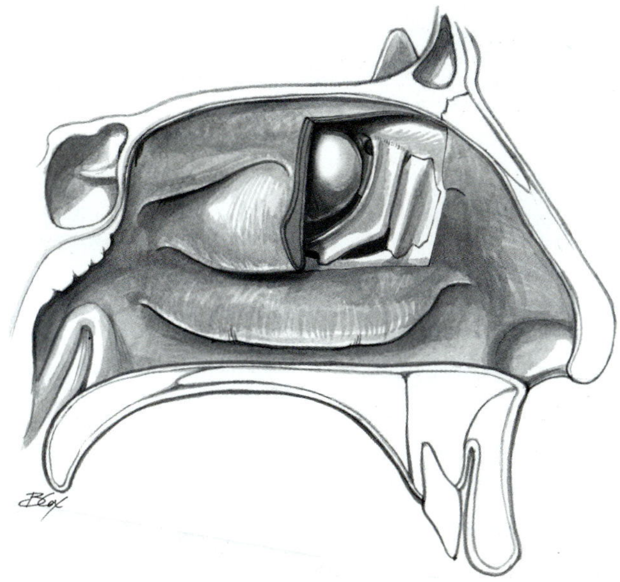

A

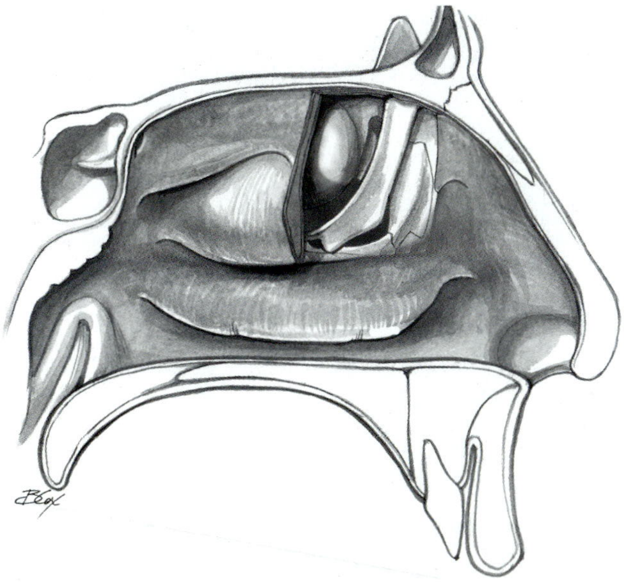

B

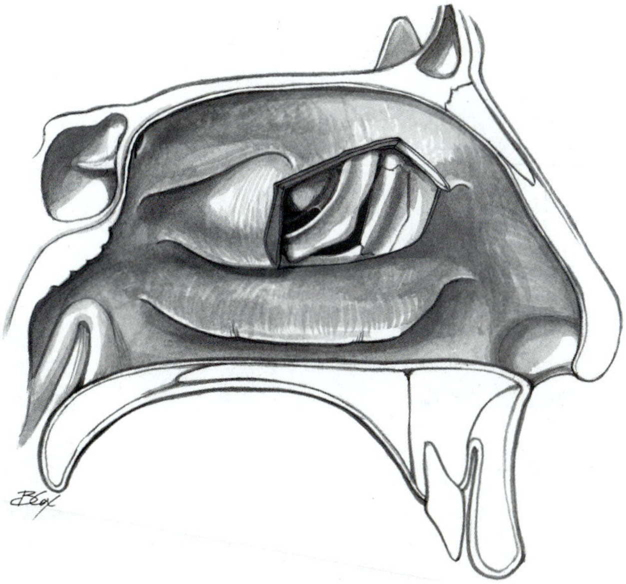

C

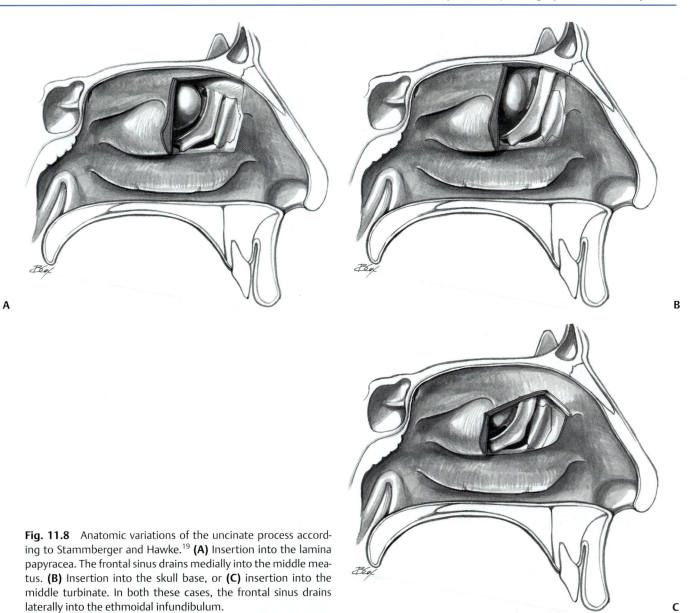

Fig. 11.8 Anatomic variations of the uncinate process according to Stammberger and Hawke.[19] **(A)** Insertion into the lamina papyracea. The frontal sinus drains medially into the middle meatus. **(B)** Insertion into the skull base, or **(C)** insertion into the middle turbinate. In both these cases, the frontal sinus drains laterally into the ethmoidal infundibulum.

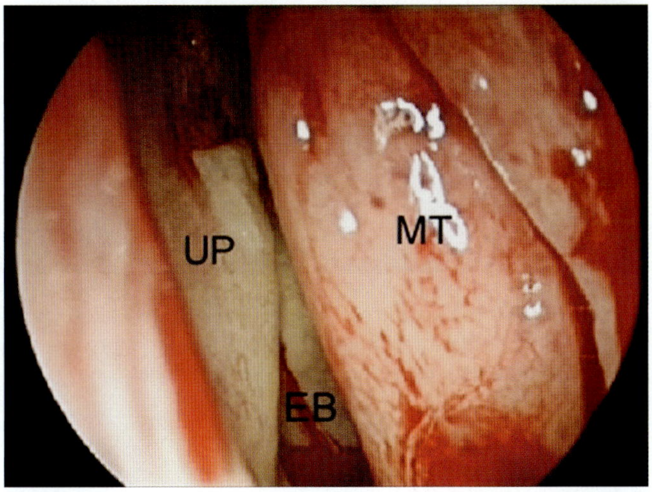

Fig. 11.9 Intraoperative view with a 45-degree endoscope after medialization of the middle turbinate (MT). EB, ethmoid bulla; UP, uncinate process.

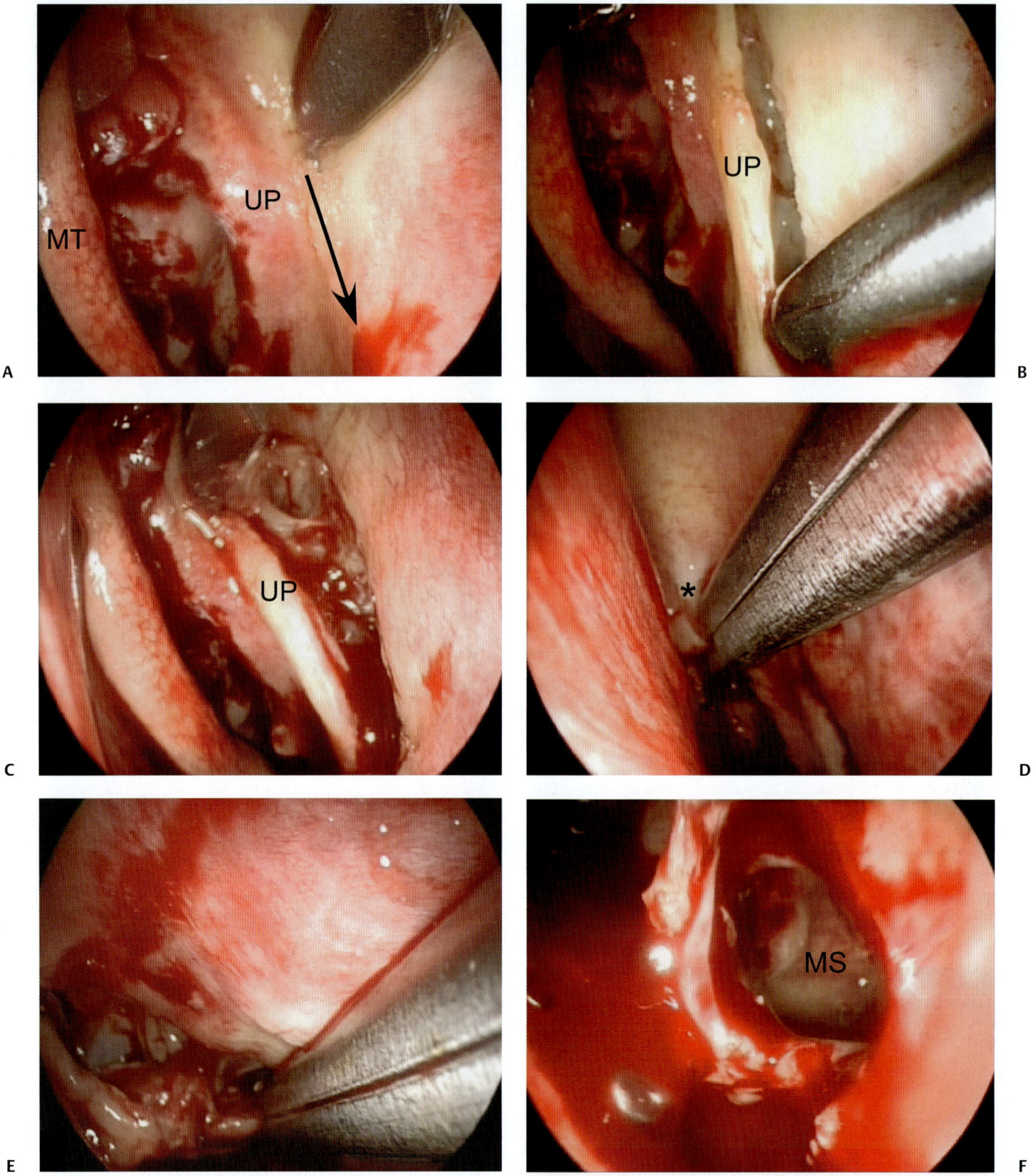

Fig. 11.10 Endoscopic uncinectomy using a 45-degree angled telescope on the left side. **(A,B)** Incision of the uncinate process (UP) with a sickle knife in anterior to posterior technique (*arrow*). **(C)** Medialization of the uncinate process with a sickle knife. **(D,E)** Resection of cranial (*) and caudal attachment. **(F)** Endoscopic view into the maxillary sinus (MS) after uncinectomy. MT, middle turbinate.

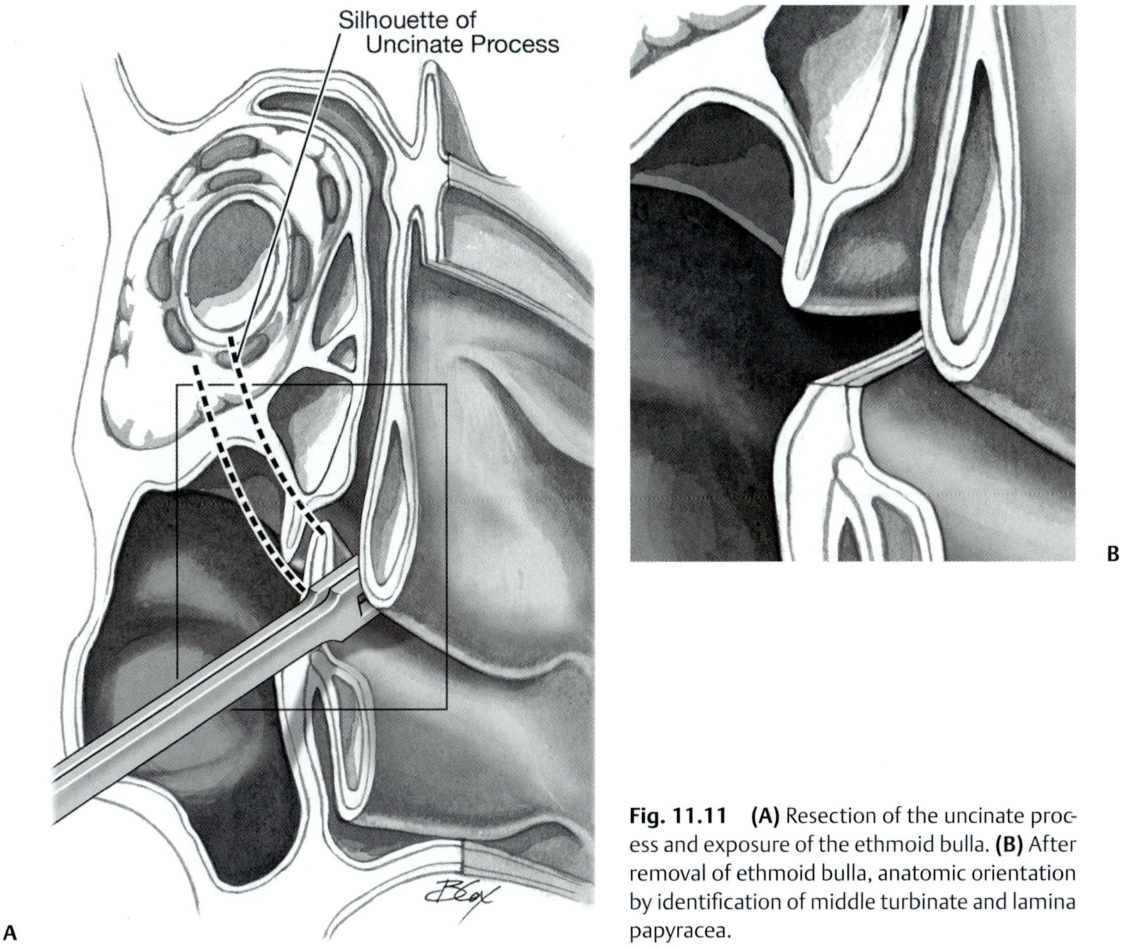

Fig. 11.11 **(A)** Resection of the uncinate process and exposure of the ethmoid bulla. **(B)** After removal of ethmoid bulla, anatomic orientation by identification of middle turbinate and lamina papyracea.

very thin and its incision should not be deeper than 1 mm to avoid any damage to the lamina papyracea. Once the uncinate process is incised and mobile (**Figs. 11.10A,B,C**), it can be removed with a straight forceps by a rotating and pulling maneuver at its upper and lower insertion (**Figs. 11.10D,E**). Remnants of the uncinate process can be removed with a backbiter anteriorly until the thick lacrimal crest is approached. Unlike the uncinate process, this bone usually is thick and there is a remarkable resistance. At this point, one should not go further anteriorly to avoid damage to the nasolacrimal duct **(see Videos 11.1 and 11.2)**. Overall, the uncinectomy can be regarded as the first step for exposure of the ethmoid bulla and the ethmoid sinuses (**Fig. 11.11**).

In the case of concha bullosa, the head of the middle turbinate is incised with a sickle knife and the lateral portion removed with a through-cutting straight forceps. One should definitely preserve the medial portion and the superior attachment of the middle turbinate to prevent a floppy middle turbinate. In cases of septal deviation with limited access to the ostiomeatal complex (OMC), we first perform a septoplasty. If the middle nasal meatus is filled with polyps, we first remove the polyps to expose the uncinate process. This step can be performed with soft tissue shavers. In experienced hands, the uncinectomy can also be done with the shaver. Oscillation of the blade is realized by continuous suction, which permanently removes soft tissue, blood, and debris from the operative area. The soft tissue shavers are available in various sizes and shapes and have an oscillate speed of at least 1000 rpm.

Endoscopic Middle Meatal Antrostomy

The maxillary sinus ostium can usually be visualized after the uncinate process has been removed. The ostium can be identified with a thin curved suction cannula. For further steps the 45-degree telescope is preferred. Enlargement of the natural ostium is managed posteriorly and inferiorly by extending its border to the posterior fontanel (**Fig. 11.12**). This step can be performed with a through-cutting and side-biting punch forceps. Dissections extended too far posteriorly may lead to arterial bleeding from the branches of the sphenopalatine artery. This bleeding can be managed with electrocautery. Extending dissections too far anteriorly should be avoided because this may cause damage to the nasolacrimal duct.[20] Although its advantage has not been

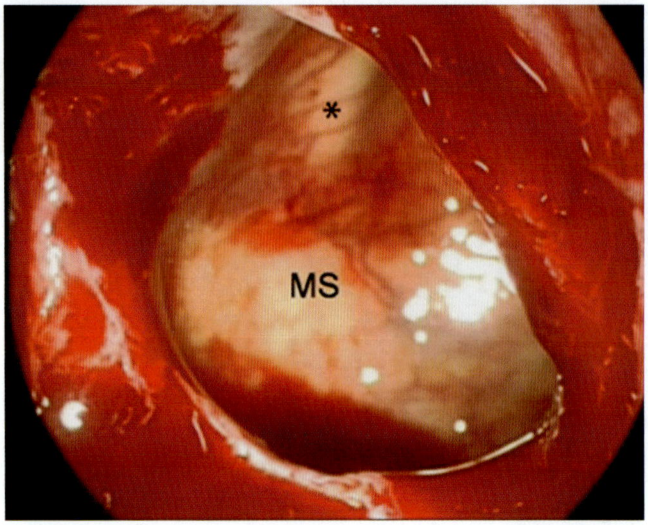

Fig. 11.12 View into the left maxillary sinus (MS) with a 45-degree angled endoscope (* = infraorbital nerve) after uncinectomy and enlargement of the natural ostium.

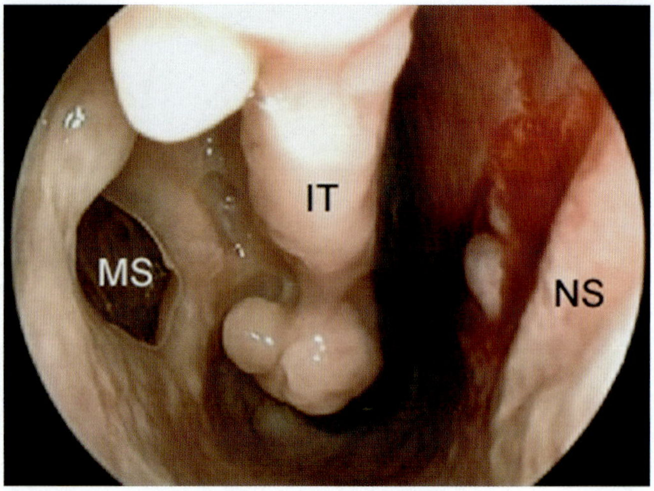

Fig. 11.13 Situs after inferior meatal antrostomy combined with conchotomy. IT, inferior turbinate; MS, maxillary sinus; NS, nasal septum.

established, surgical connection of accessory ostia with the natural ostium is routinely performed to prevent circular transportation of secretions. With the help of the 45- and 70-degree telescope the maxillary sinus is examined and treated, when necessary. For removal of polyps in the inferior or lateral region of the maxillary sinus, we use the 90-degree curved Blakesley and/or the curved forceps after Heuwieser. In cases of huge polyposis of the maxillary sinus, we prefer to remove polyps with a curved soft tissue shaver. In case of intense bleeding with poor visualization of the operative field, the middle meatus is temporarily packed with cotton plugs as described above. With the help of the 70-degree telescope, the inferior and far lateral areas of the sinus can be inspected.

Also, endoscopic maxillary sinus surgery is performed usually as the first step in different pansinus operations. In cases of massive or recurrent polyposis with opacification of all sinuses (pansinusitis), we first perform a middle meatal antrostomy and proceed to a frontal sinus surgery type I, II, or III after Draf,[21,22] depending upon the pathology (**see Videos 11.3 and 11.4**).

Endoscopic Inferior Meatal Antrostomy

Nowadays the indication for inferior meatal antrostomy is rare. Usually, we first perform a gentle conchotomy, corresponding to the planed window in the inferior medial wall of the maxillary sinus. It is useful to incise the inferior turbinate with a septal scissor parallel to the inferior margin in a way that a posteriorly pedicled flap is created. The length of this flap depends on the length of the planed window. The pedicle is cut with a cutting snare to reduce the bleeding to a minimum. Bipolar coagulation helps to provide meticulous hemostasis. Doing so, the result achieved is similar to those designed already by Claoue. The inferior portion of the medial maxillary sinus wall is opened with a 90-degree curved Blakesley. This primary window can be enlarged with a backbiter anteriorly (**Fig. 11.13**). With the popularity of FESS, the indication for an inferior antrostomy has decreased considerably. In our opinion, this type of surgery is indicated only in persistent or recurrent isolated maxillary sinusitis with cysts, polyps, or mycetomas due to dental pathology in the alveolar recess of the maxillary sinus.

Endonasal Medial Maxillectomy

Endoscopic endonasal medial maxillectomy can be regarded as an extended endonasal approach to the maxillary sinus for resection of benign and, in special circumstances, malignant tumors. Details of this technique were published in 1910/1911 by Canfield in the United States[23] and at the same time by Sturmann[24] in Germany. It was later called the endonasal Denker operation. Interestingly enough, the nasolacrimal sac is not mentioned in either of the early publications. Recently, several authors reported on their experience with medial maxillectomy for removal of inverted papilloma (see below). The following areas may be resected in medial maxillectomy according to the patient's needs: medially the complete medial wall of the maxillary sinus and the inferior turbinate; the anterior and posterior fontanel and maxillary process of the maxillary bone including the inferior part of the nasolacrimal drainage system if necessary. If indicated, the posterior maxillary sinus wall also can be removed. Usually, we first perform a wide middle meatal antrostomy with removing the medial maxillary wall cranially up to the level of the orbital floor.

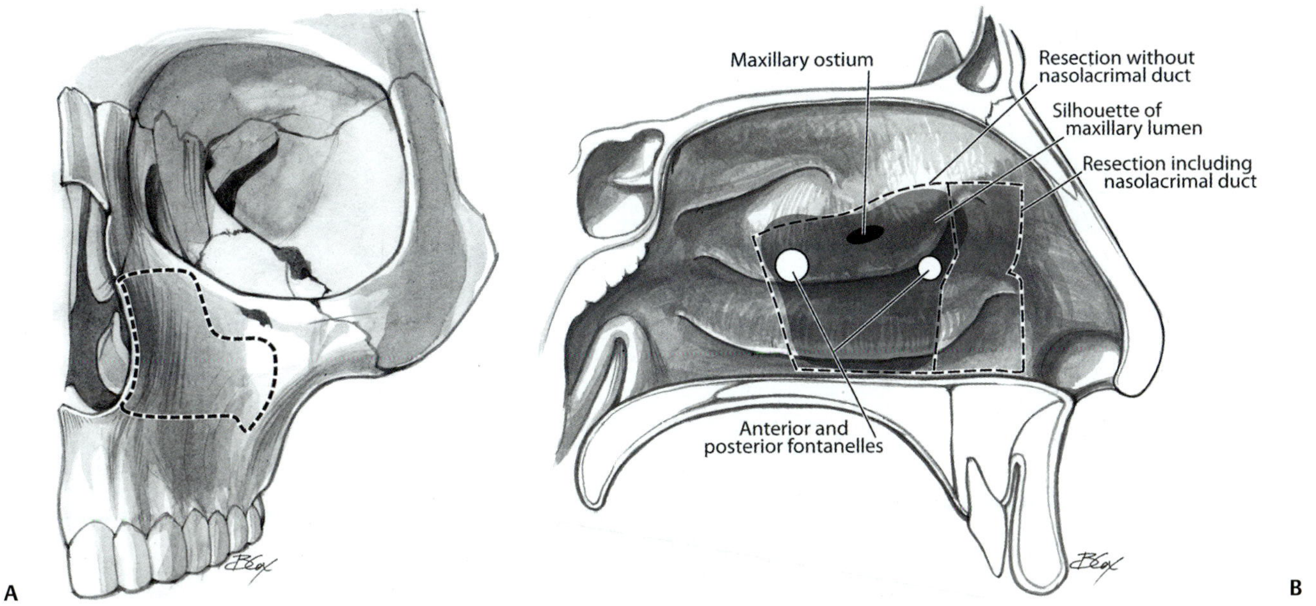

Fig. 11.14 **(A)** Extent of bony resection in endonasal Denker surgery with parts of piriform aperture, lacrimal bone, and anterior maxillary sinus wall. **(B)** Resection of the medial parts of the maxillary bone including the medial maxillary sinus wall and parts of the middle and inferior turbinate with preservation of the nasolacrimal duct. Resection can be widened including the nasolacrimal duct and a little area of the piriform aperture.

In the next step, depending on the tumor extension, the medial wall is resected until the posterior margin of the tumor is reached. Bleeding from branches of the sphenopalatine artery can be stopped with electrocautery. Then, the medial maxillary sinus wall is resected anteriorly. In large tumors, the anterior dissection includes the lacrimal bone with the nasolacrimal duct. In this case, an endonasal endoscopic dacryocystorhinostomy is performed at the end of the medial maxillectomy. With this extended approach, the tumor margins can be visualized sufficiently to achieve a total removal. Diseased bone should be freed of pathology with a diamond burr. Tumors involving the mucosa of the posterior and/or anterior wall of the maxillary sinus may require a wider exposure of the entire sinus. In this case, the medial maxillectomy is combined with the resection of the medial portion of the anterior wall including the piriform crest. An endonasal Denker operation[25] is the result. **Figure 11.14** shows the resection area in this case.

Application of Endoscopic Maxillary Sinus Surgery for Special Pathologies

Mucoceles

Mucoceles are slowly expanding epithelial-lined lesions containing mucus and have been found in all paranasal sinuses. They show an expanding behavior and can lead to pressure atrophy of the bone with extra sinonasal growth into the orbit and endocranium.[26–28] Mucoceles are mostly found in the frontal sinus; maxillary sinus mucoceles are relatively rare and account for ~10% of all paranasal sinus mucoceles.

Most cases of maxillary sinus mucoceles can be treated with an endonasal endoscopic approach. Usually the frontal wall of the mucocele sack is dissected and marsupialized (**see Video 11.5**). For mucoceles located too far lateral of the maxillary sinus, we prefer an osteoplastic maxillary sinus approach (**Fig. 11.15**).

In one of the largest studies, Bockmühl et al[29] analyzed the results of 290 mucoceles in 255 patients. Seventy-two patients had a mucocele of the maxillary sinus. In 42 mucoceles the etiology was previous surgery, most commonly a Caldwell–Luc operation. The majority of the mucoceles (69.3% n = 57) could be operated through an endonasal approach. The long-term results of this and other studies show that endonasal endoscopic surgery is an effective and safe approach for the majority of this type of pathology.[27,30–32]

Inverted Papilloma

Inverted papilloma (IP) accounts for ~70% of all sinonasal papillomas and from 0.5 to 4% of all neoplasms of the sinonasal tract.[33] They are characterized by a high recurrence rate, a tendency for malignant transformation, and multicentric involvement. Traditionally, lateral rhinotomy or midfacial degloving with en bloc tumor resection in combination with medial maxillectomy were used and are standard ap-

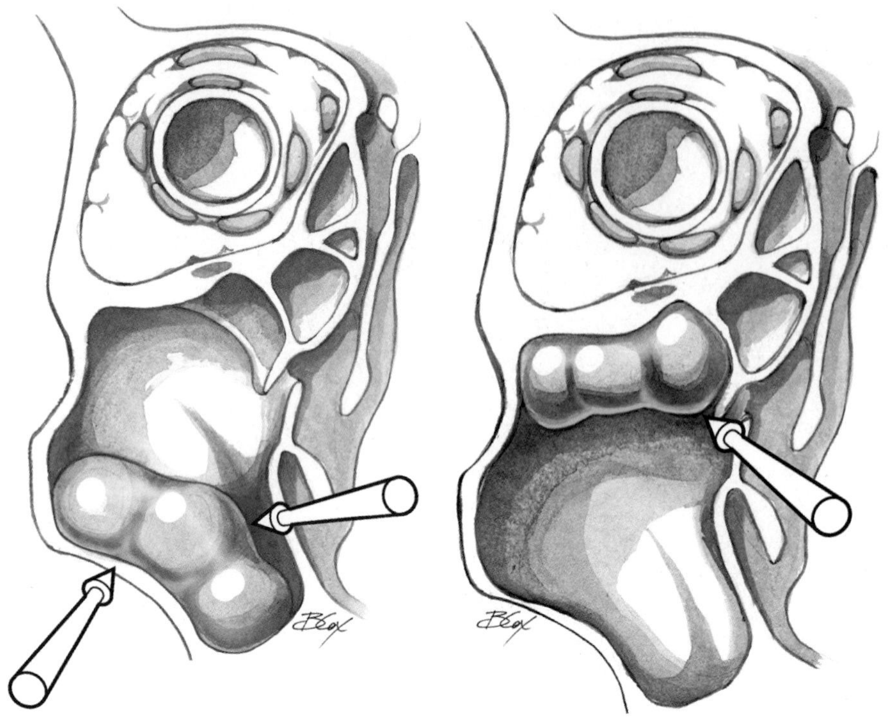

A,B

Fig. 11.15 **(A)** Far laterally located maxillary sinus mucoceles might be contraindications for an exclusively endonasal endoscopic approach in contrast to **(B)** medial mucoceles.

proaches today.[34–37] However, there is currently a growing body of evidence to support endonasal endoscopic surgery in the resection of these tumors showing comparable rates of recurrence to an external approach.[38–41] When properly indicated and planned, endonasal procedures can favorably compete with traditional external techniques in the surgical treatment of IP.

For IP of the maxillary sinus, the kind of operation varies in relation to the site of origin and the extent of the lesion. To choose the best surgical approach (i.e., to assess the endonasal endoscopic respectability), preoperative imaging is inalienable. Patient's symptoms are more or less unspecific, and at the time of clinical examination it is almost impossible to distinguish IP from inflammatory polyps, even in unilateral distribution of nasal polyps. In the assessment of sinonasal expansile lesions, CT scan is generally considered the examination of choice. However, CT scanning cannot differentiate between retained secretion of inflamed mucosa and IP. According to Ojiri et al,[42] this limitation can be overcome by using MRI, which, apart from differentiating neoplastic tissue from inflammatory changes, identifies a convoluted cerebriform pattern suggestive for IP on T2-weighted or enhanced T1-weighted sequences in ~80% of cases. In unilateral maxillary sinus opacification, preoperative MRI can be very helpful for further surgical planning and better informed consent (**Fig. 11.7**).

Basically, we use a completely endonasal endoscopic resection or an endonasal procedure combined with an osteoplastic maxillary sinus (OMS) technique as described by Feldmann.[43] In general, like mucoceles whenever the lesion originates far laterally in the maxillary sinus (**Fig. 11.15**), we tend to perform a combined procedure. All medially localized tumors are resected via an endonasal endoscopic procedure, which includes the medial maxillectomy or enlarged maxillary sinus technique indicated as an endonasal Denker operation.[25] IPs that originate from the posterolateral, anterior, or inferior wall of the maxillary sinus are managed by a combined procedure of endoscopic and osteoplastic maxillary sinus operation (**see Video 11.6**). The OMS is started with a typical horizontal and slightly curved incision (~3 cm) at the canine fossa (**Fig. 11.16**). In the next step, the soft tissue is prepared in the subperiosteal plane and the anterior wall of maxillary sinus exposed. The infraorbital nerve is identified to prevent its damage during the bone dissection work. After that, the bone window is created with a special saw[43] through the osteoplastic approach. An 8-hole plate, which is lightly curved, is put in place for drilling the burr holes. After this, the bony graft is removed and the lateral region of the maxillary sinus is bluntly freed from tumor using a surgical pad. The dissection work is continued until all tumor parts are removed from the maxillary sinus. In the final step, the bone graft that was temporarily taken out is replaced and fixed with two screws.

If feasible, lesions are removed en bloc, but in large tumors the nasal portion of the mass is first debulked to focus subsequently on the most critical lateral areas, where dissection is always performed in the subperiosteal plane. Then drilling of the diseased-underlying bone is accomplished and frozen sections from surgical bed margins are taken to ensure surgical radicality and complete tumor removal. In a few cases, the additional use of the microscope can be helpful (**see Video 11.7**). During the last years, several series

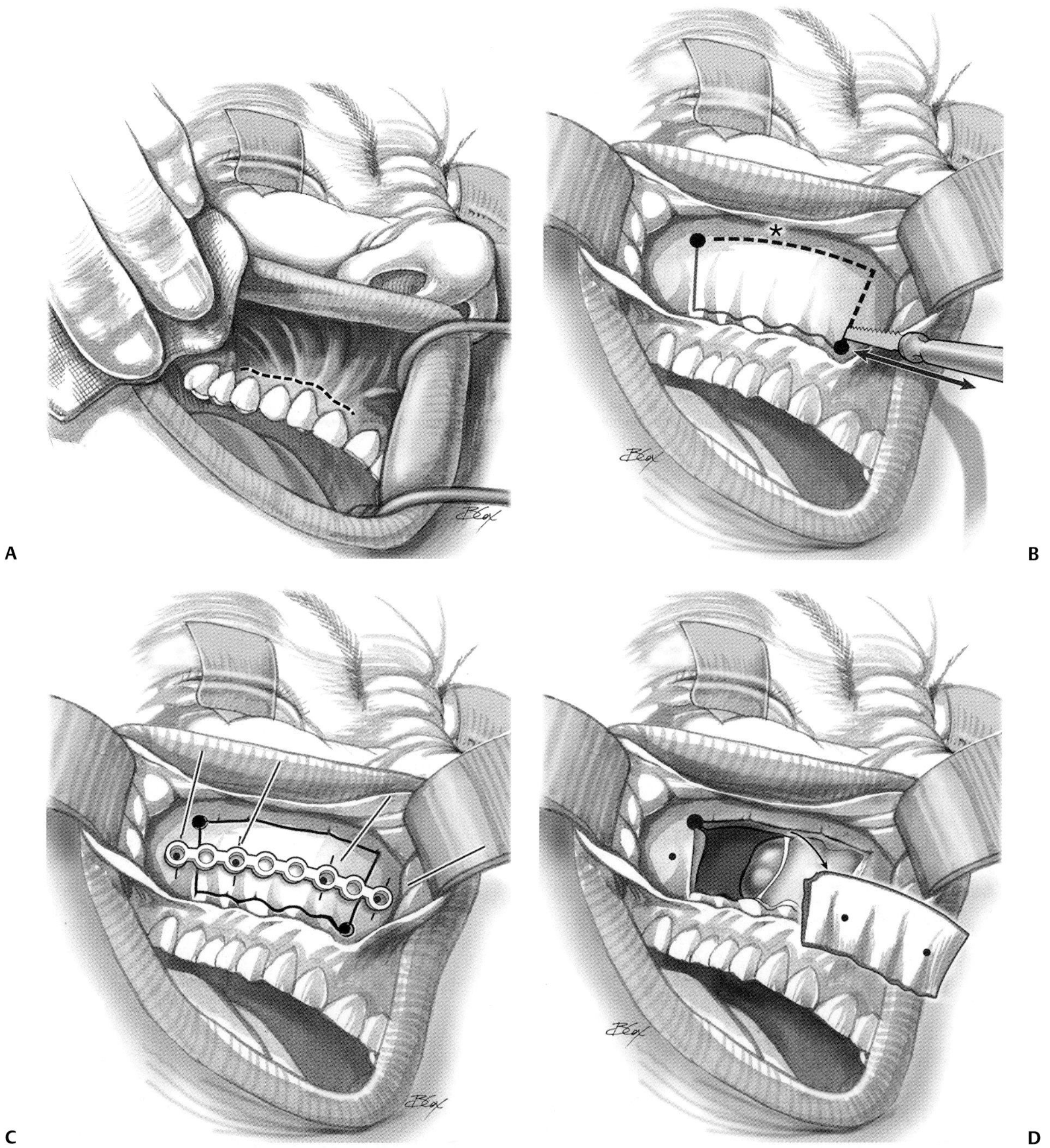

Fig. 11.16 Osteoplastic maxillary sinus approach for resection of inverted papilloma with extension into far lateral regions of the maxillary sinus. **(A)** Horizontal incision in the canine fossa. **(B)** Subperiosteal dissection, identification of the infraorbital nerve (*) and creation of a bony window by circumcising a bone graft with a jigsaw. **(C)** Fixation of a curved eight-hole plate to the bony window and marking of outer burr holes for later reattachment. **(D)** Temporary removal of the bone graft. (*continued*)

have been published reporting on the endonasal endoscopic management of IP; increasingly, this has been accepted as the surgical modality of choice for most IP.[38–41,44–46] Our own study[44] reported on 45 IPs of the maxillary sinus, which were treated by an endonasal and/or osteoplastic maxillary sinus approach. Fifty-three percent of the IPs could be removed via an endonasal approach. The remainder were resected either by combined ($n = 16$) or exclusively osteoplastic ($n = 6$) procedures (**Fig. 11.17**). During the follow-up period, ranging from 12 to 175 months (median 74 months) four recurrences (8.8%) were observed. Three tumors had been reoperated via a combined approach with one endonasal surgery. Hence, the recurrence rate for endonasal surgery was 2.2% compared with 6.6% after combined approach. The mean recurrence interval after endonasal surgery was 24 months in contrast to 101 months after combined approach.

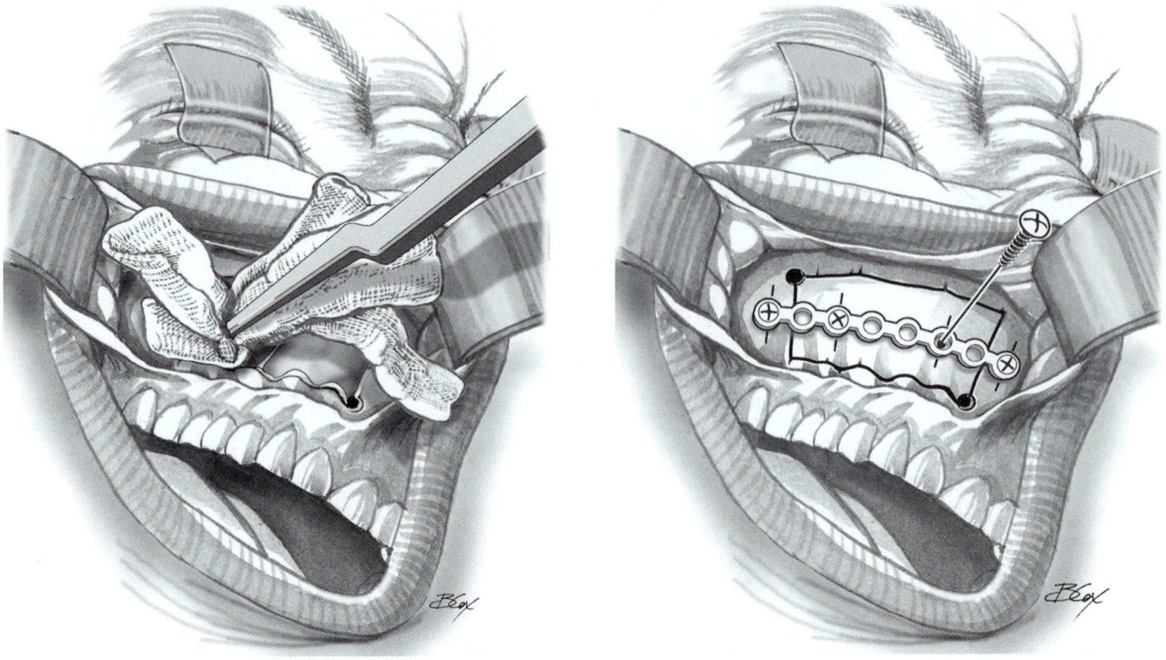

E F

Fig. 11.16 (*continued*) Bone graft and blunt dissection **(E)** of the tumor with a surgical pad. **(F)** Refixation of the bone graft with two outer screws.

Antrochoanal Polyp

Antrochoanal polyps (ACP) are benign lesions that are most commonly seen in children. This isolated polyp has its origin from the mucosa of the maxillary sinus and grows through the natural or accessory maxillary sinus ostium into the nasal cavity and can extend into choana and nasopharynx (**Fig. 11.18**). The major symptom is a unilateral nasal obstruction. Treatment of choice is primary endoscopic removal with resection of the basis in the maxillary sinus (**see Video 11.8**). Complete removal of the polyp's base is mandatory to prevent a recurrence.

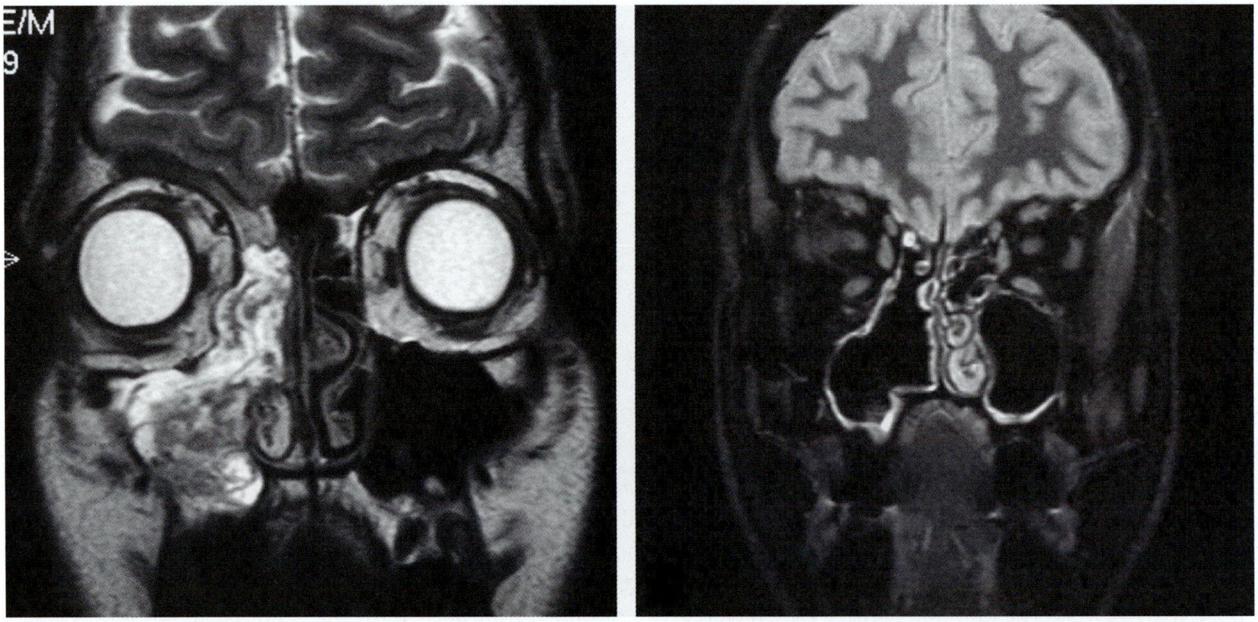

A B

Fig. 11.17 **(A)** Preoperative T2-weighted coronal magnetic resonance image presenting a large inverted papilloma that originated from the anterior lateral wall of the right maxillary sinus as well as the ethmoid. **(B)** Postoperative short tau inversion recovery (STIR) sequences after tumor resection via a combined technique including an osteoplastic maxillary sinus approach and endonasal medial maxillectomy (6 years postoperatively). No sign of recurrence.

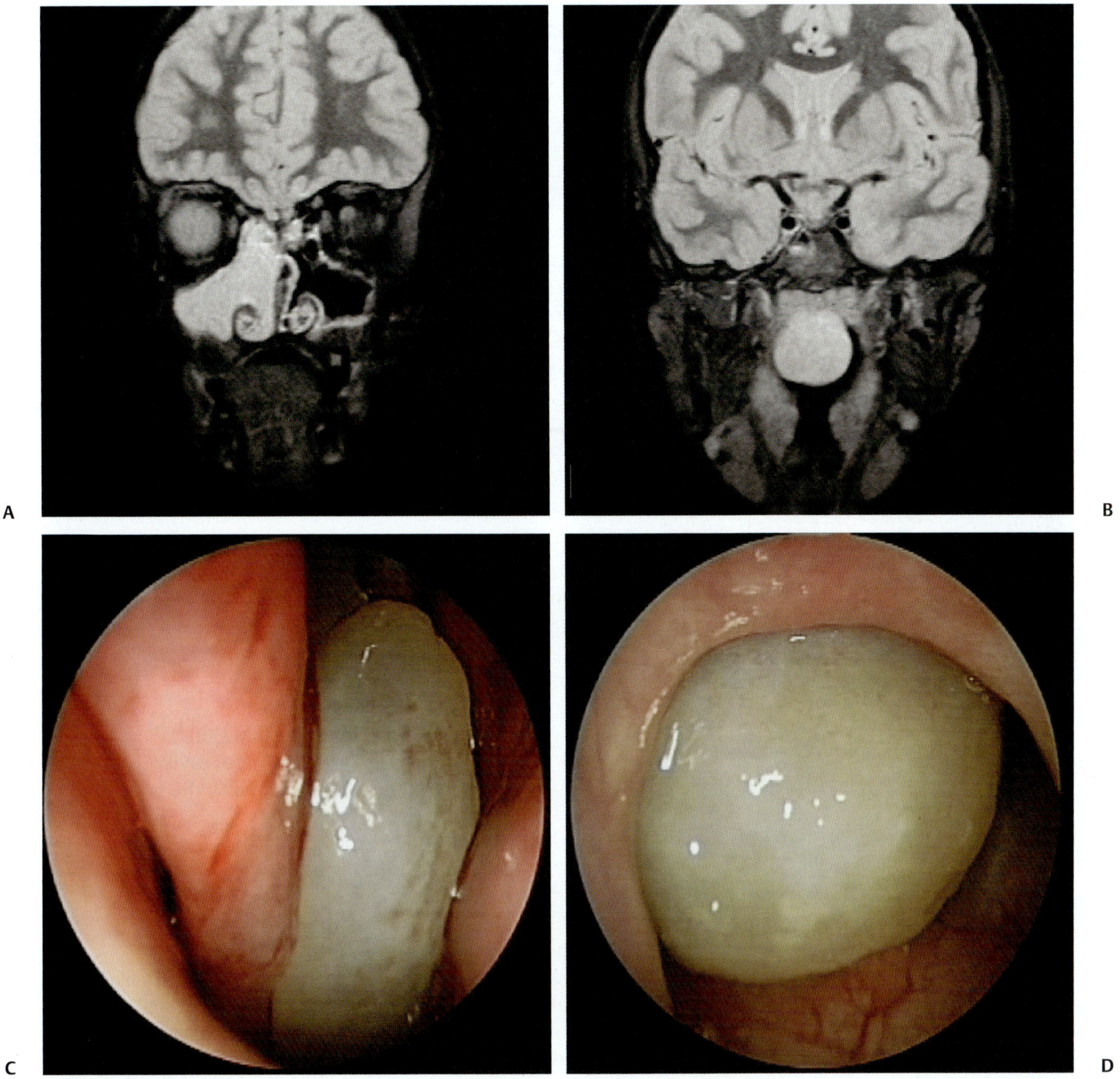

Fig. 11.18 Antrochoanal polyp. **(A,B)** Coronal T2-weighted magnetic resonance imaging (MRI) scan shows complete opacification of the right maxillary sinus and the middle meatus with extension into the nasopharynx. The polyp is hyperintense on T2-weighted MRI scans. **(C)** Endoscopic view of an antrochoanal polyp as a single large polyp in the middle meatus with **(D)** extension into the nasopharynx as seen transorally.

Complications

The paranasal sinuses present a complex anatomy surrounded by important structures. Despite extensive surgical experience, complications still happen. In endoscopic maxillary sinus surgery, minor and rarely major complications as mentioned above may occur. For prevention of disastrous complications, the surgeon should follow certain guidelines and be aware of high-risk areas. Fracture or perforation of the lamina papyracea during sinus surgery can lead to periorbital emphysema and ecchymosis. Injury of the periorbit usually occurs during uncinectomy or during middle meatal antrostomy. In most cases, careful analysis of the CT scans can prevent this complication. It is mandatory to distinguish emphysema from retrobulbar hematoma because the first is observed, but the second frequently needs immediate in-

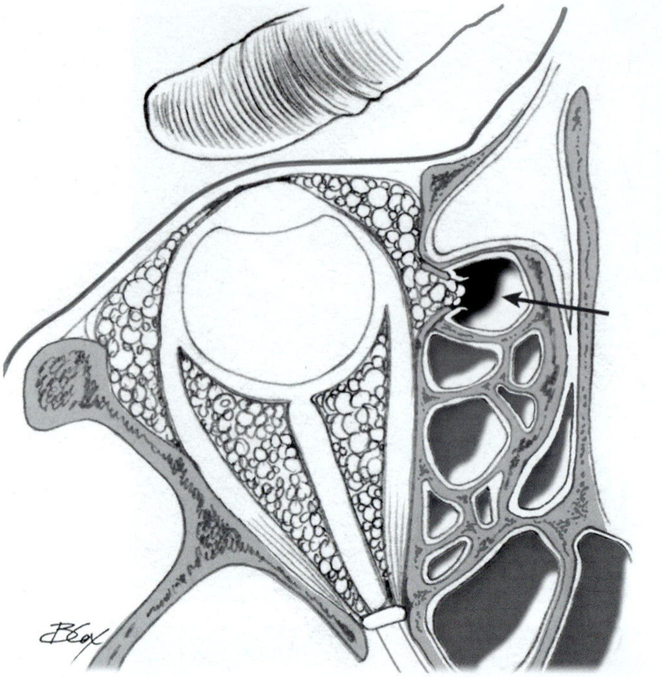

Fig. 11.19 Bulb-pressing test: gentle pressure of the eye and simultaneous endonasal observation can be helpful to identify the lamina papyracea and possible injuries. In this case, orbital fat (*arrow*) can be identified intranasally by bulb pressing maneuver.

tervention. In this case, a lateral canthotomy should be performed immediately to decrease the intraorbital pressure (**see Video 11.9**).

Here is a summary of surgical recommendations to reduce complications in endoscopic maxillary sinus surgery:

- Early identification of lamina papyracea and middle turbinate as the most important anatomic landmarks
- Careful observation of the eye bulb throughout surgery by the surgeon and the assisting nurse
- Bulb-pressing test after Draf and Stankiewicz[47,48] can be helpful when there is suspicion of injury to the lamina papyracea (**Fig. 11.19**).
- Always dissect laterally to the middle turbinate, never medially and superiorly
- The middle meatal antrostomy should be performed just above the inferior turbinate and should not go further anteriorly than the head end of the middle turbinate
- Identification of the infraorbital nerve before dissection of the bony window in osteoplastic maxillary sinus approach

Postoperative Care

No standardized recommendations concerning postoperative care exist in the literature. The following general recommendations for postoperative treatment may be useful. Local aftercare of the surgical area by the ENT surgeon:

Pearls

- The most common indication of primary endoscopic maxillary sinus surgery is chronic rhinosinusitis unresponsive to conservative treatment.
- The main aim of surgery is removing the pathology and maintaining the physiologic drainage of the sinuses into the ostiomeatal complex
- Meticulous preoperative analysis of CT scans and individual anatomy is essential for adequate surgery.
- Complete uncinectomy is mandatory to prevent recurrent maxillary sinusitis.
- Early intraoperative identification of important anatomic landmarks is mandatory.
- Endonasal endoscopic approach can be combined with osteoplastic technique for resection of tumors and other pathologies like mucoceles in the lateral area of the maxillary sinus.

- Daily, in the first postoperative days and with a continuously expanding interval based on each individual patient for about 3 months
- Regular endoscopic control of the surgical area
- Local aftercare should consist of
  - o Removal of fibrin clots and crusts
  - o Separation of synechiae and adhesions
  - o Suction of secretion from the nasal cavity
- Daily local care of the operative area by the patient:
  - o Application of topical steroids
  - o Inhalation and irrigation of the nose
  - o Application of ointments
  - o Minimum of 3 months

Acknowledgment

The authors would like to thank Mo Motamedi, Ph.D., Department of Cell Biology, Harvard Medical School, and Marc Pearson, M.D., Department of Otorhinolaryngology, Ruhr University Bochum, for their kind cooperation.

References

1. Halle M. Externe und interne operation der nasennebenhoehleneiterungen. Berl Klein Wschr. 1906;43:1369–1372
2. Spiess G. Die endonasale chirurgie des sinus frontalis. Arch Laryngol 1899;9:285–291
3. Mosher H. The surgical anatomy of the ethmoid labyrinth. Ann Otol Rhinol Laryngol 1929;38:870–891
4. Draf W. Surgical treatment of the inflammatory diseases of the paranasal sinuses. Indication, surgical technique, risks, mismanagement and complications, revision surgery. Denecke, JH, ed. Otorhinolaryngol 1982;235(1):133–305
5. Denecke HJ. Die oto-rhino-laryngologischen Operationen. 2nd ed. Berlin: Springer; 1953:209
6. Caldwell GW. Diseases of the accessory sinuses of the nose and an improved method of treatment for suppuration of the maxillary antrum. NY State J Med 1893;58:526–528

7. Luc H. Une nouvelle méthode opératoire pour la cure radicale et rapide de l'empyème chronique du sinus maxillaire. Arch Laryngol (Paris) 1897;10:273–285
8. Denker A. Zur radikaloperation des chronischen kieferhöhlenempyems. Arch Laryngol Rhinol. 1905;17:221–232
9. Draf W. Die Endoskopie der Nasennebenhöhlen. Berlin/Heidelberg/New York: Springer; 1978
10. Messerklinger W. Endoscopy of the Nose. Baltimore:Urban und Schwarzenberg; 1978
11. Kennedy DW. Functional endoscopic sinus surgery. Technique. Arch Otolaryngol 1985;111(10):643–649
12. Stammberger H. Endoscopic endonasal surgery—concepts in treatment of recurring rhinosinusitis. Part I. Anatomic and pathophysiologic considerations. Otolaryngol Head Neck Surg 1986;94(2):143–147
13. Minovi A, Hummel T, Ural A, Draf W, Bockmuhl U. Predictors of the outcome of nasal surgery in terms of olfactory function. Eur Arch Otorhinolaryngol 2008;265(1):57–61
14. Pade J, Hummel T. Olfactory function following nasal surgery. Laryngoscope 2008;118(7):1260–1264
15. Mann WJ, Amedee RG, Iemma M. An assessment of radiologic discrepancies in patients with paranasal sinus disease. Am J Rhinol 1992;6:211–213
16. Simmen D, Jones N. Manual of Endoscopic Sinus Surgery and Its Extended Applications. Stuttgart/New York: Thieme Medical Publishing; 2005
17. Kennedy DW, Zinreich SJ, Shaalan H, Kuhn F, Nuclear R, Loch E. Endoscopic middle meatal antrostomy: theory, technique, and patency. Laryngoscope 1987; 97(8 Pt 3, Suppl 43)1–9
18. Anderhuber W, Walch C, Nemeth E, et al. Plasma adrenaline concentrations during functional endoscopic sinus surgery. Laryngoscope 1999; 109(2 Pt 1, 2 Pt 1)204–207
19. Stammberger H, Hawke M. Essentials of Functional Endoscopic Sinus Surgery. St. Louis:Mosby; 1993
20. Schauss F, Weber R, Draf W, Keerl R. Surgery of the lacrimal system. Acta Otorhinolaryngol Belg 1996;50(2):143–146
21. Draf W. Endonasal micro-endoscopic frontal sinus surgery. The Fulda concept. Oper Tech Otolaryngol—Head Neck Surg 1991;2:234–240
22. Draf W. Endonasal frontal sinus drainage type I–III according to Draf. In: Kountakis S, Senior B, Draf W, eds., The Frontal Sinus. Berlin/Heidelberg/New York: Springer; 2005:219–232
23. Canfield RB. The submucous resection of the lateral nasal wall in chronic empyema of the antrum, ethmoid and sphenoid. JAMA 1908;51:1136–1141
24. Sturmann D. Die intranasale Eröffnung der Kieferhöhle. Berl Klin Wochenschr. 1908;27:1273–1274
25. Brors D, Draf W. The treatment of inverted papilloma. Curr Opin Otolaryngol Head Neck Surg 1999;7:33–38
26. Delfini R, Missori P, Iannetti G, Ciappetta P, Cantore G. Mucoceles of the paranasal sinuses with intracranial and intraorbital extension: report of 28 cases. Neurosurgery 1993;32(6):901–906, discussion 906
27. Lund VJ. Endoscopic management of paranasal sinus mucocoeles. J Laryngol Otol 1998;112(1):36–40
28. Natvig K, Larsen TE. Mucocele of the paranasal sinuses. A retrospective clinical and histological study. J Laryngol Otol 1978;92(12):1075–1082
29. Bockmühl U, Kratzsch B, Benda K, Draf W. Surgery for paranasal sinus mucocoeles: efficacy of endonasal micro-endoscopic management and long-term results of 185 patients. Rhinology 2006;44(1):62–67
30. Har-El G. Endoscopic management of 108 sinus mucoceles. Laryngoscope 2001;111(12):2131–2134
31. Khong JJ, Malhotra R, Selva D, Wormald PJ. Efficacy of endoscopic sinus surgery for paranasal sinus mucocele including modified endoscopic Lothrop procedure for frontal sinus mucocele. J Laryngol Otol 2004;118(5):352–356
32. Serrano E, Klossek JM, Percodani J, Yardeni E, Dufour X. Surgical management of paranasal sinus mucoceles: a long-term study of 60 cases. Otolaryngol Head Neck Surg 2004;131(1):133–140
33. Hyams VJ. Papillomas of the nasal cavity and paranasal sinuses. A clinicopathological study of 315 cases. Ann Otol Rhinol Laryngol 1971;80(2):192–206
34. Lawson W, Kaufman MR, Biller HF. Treatment outcomes in the management of inverted papilloma: an analysis of 160 cases. Laryngoscope 2003;113(9):1548–1556
35. Phillips PP, Gustafson RO, Facer GW. The clinical behavior of inverting papilloma of the nose and paranasal sinuses: report of 112 cases and review of the literature. Laryngoscope 1990;100(5):463–469
36. Raveh E, Feinmesser R, Shpitzer T, Yaniv E, Segal K. Inverted papilloma of the nose and paranasal sinuses: a study of 56 cases and review of the literature. Isr J Med Sci 1996;32(12):1163–1167
37. Thorp MA, Oyarzabal-Amigo MF, du Plessis JH, Sellars SL. Inverted papilloma: a review of 53 cases. Laryngoscope 2001;111(8):1401–1405
38. Kraft M, Simmen D, Kaufmann T, Holzmann D. Long-term results of endonasal sinus surgery in sinonasal papillomas. Laryngoscope 2003;113(9):1541–1547
39. Lund VJ. Optimum management of inverted papilloma. J Laryngol Otol 2000;114(3):194–197
40. Tomenzoli D, Castelnuovo P, Pagella F, et al. Different endoscopic surgical strategies in the management of inverted papilloma of the sinonasal tract: experience with 47 patients. Laryngoscope 2004;114(2):193–200
41. Wormald PJ, Ooi E, van Hasselt CA, Nair S. Endoscopic removal of sinonasal inverted papilloma including endoscopic medial maxillectomy. Laryngoscope 2003;113(5):867–873
42. Ojiri H, Ujita M, Tada S, Fukuda K. Potentially distinctive features of sinonasal inverted papilloma on MR imaging. AJR Am J Roentgenol 2000;175(2):465–468
43. Feldmann H. [Osteoplastic operation of maxillary sinus (author's transl)]. Laryngol Rhinol Otol (Stuttg) 1978;57(5):373–378
44. Minovi A, Kollert M, Draf W, Bockmühl U. Inverted papilloma: feasibility of endonasal surgery and long-term results of 87 cases. Rhinology 2006;44(3):205–210
45. Winter M, Rauer RA, Göde U, Waitz G, Wigand ME. [Inverted papilloma of the nose and paranasal sinuses. Long-term outcome of endoscopic endonasal resection]. HNO 2000;48(8):568–572
46. Woodworth BA, Bhargave GA, Palmer JN, et al. Clinical outcomes of endoscopic and endoscopic-assisted resection of inverted papillomas: a 15-year experience. Am J Rhinol 2007;21(5):591–600
47. Draf W. Complications of micro-endoscopic sinus surgery. In: Course of Endonasal Micro-Endoscopic Sinus Surgery. Fulda, Germany: Fulda Academic Teaching Hospital; 1986
48. Stankiewicz JA. Complications of endoscopic sinus surgery. Otolaryngol Clin North Am 1989;22(4):749–758

12 Revision Maxillary Sinus Surgery including Canine Fossa Trephination

Marc A. Tewfik, Simon Robinson, and Peter-John Wormald

One of the keys to achieving successful outcomes from functional endoscopic sinus surgery (FESS) is controlling disease within the maxillary sinus. Depending on the disease process present, different approaches are required to achieve this. However, what is essential is to provide adequate ventilation and optimize the natural drainage pathway for the maxillary sinus. Additionally, it is important to reduce the disease load within the maxillary sinus to optimize the chance of the sinus mucosa returning to a healthy state.

Even if initial management of the maxillary sinus is optimal, there are several potential reasons for persistent disease within the sinus requiring further surgical intervention. Revision surgery may play a role in the continuum of management of the patient's disease condition; however, different care may be required at different time points and the underlying factors contributing to sinus disease must be sought and addressed. In this chapter, we provide an overview of the indications and the options for surgical treatment in the management of previously operated maxillary sinus, including the canine fossa trephination techniques.

■ Causes of Failed Maxillary Sinus Surgery

The potential causes for failed surgery are numerous. Several series have looked at the causes of postsurgical persistent or recurrent disease, and provide information regarding the frequency of various anatomic findings, many of which pertain to the maxillary sinus. Chu et al[1] evaluated 153 patients requiring revision endoscopic sinus surgery, and found the most common surgical alteration associated with recurrent sinus disease was middle meatal scarring and lateralization of the middle turbinate. This was usually the result of partial middle turbinectomy during the initial surgery. Lateralization of the middle turbinate was also reported by Musy and Kountakis[2] as the most common postsurgical finding associated with primary surgery failure. Other findings included incomplete anterior ethmoidectomy (64%), scarred frontal recess (50%), retained agger nasi cell (49%), incomplete posterior ethmoidectomy (41%), retained uncinate process (37%), middle meatal antrostomy stenosis (39%), and recurrent polyposis (37%). Ramadan[3] reviewed 52 cases and found that the most common cause of failure was residual air cells and adhesions in the ethmoid area (31%), followed by maxillary sinus ostial stenosis (27%), frontal sinus ostial stenosis (25%), and a separate maxillary sinus ostium stenosis (15%).

Focusing more specifically on the maxillary sinus, Richtsmeier[4] reviewed 85 patients presenting with persistent maxillary sinus symptoms after endoscopic sinus surgery and identified 10 categories of reasons for failure. These included obstructed natural ostia, disease in the anterior ethmoid or frontal sinus, resistant organisms, intrasinus foreign body, incurable mucosal disease, noncompliant patient, wrong primary diagnosis, maxillary osteitis, mucus maltransport, and immunodeficiency. Cohen and Kennedy[5] simplified this by clustering the above into six large categories of local problems: recirculation, infection draining into the maxillary sinus from elsewhere, retained foreign material (including infected dental work), failure of mucociliary transport, scar separation of the sinus from the nasal cavity, and local osteitis.

Recirculation

The recirculation phenomenon may be caused by a retained or partially resected uncinate process with an iatrogenic posterior fontanelle antrostomy. Less frequently, it can be caused by scarring at the anterior aspect of the antrostomy. The "missed ostium sequence," as described by Parsons et al,[6] occurs when there is incomplete removal of the most anterior portion of the uncinate process, obscuring the position of the natural maxillary sinus ostium. This prevents the middle meatal antrostomy from communicating with the natural ostium, resulting in a recirculation phenomenon (**Fig. 12.1**). In this instance, mucociliary flow causes mucous to reenter the sinus causing a functional obstruction of the maxillary sinus and continued sinus disease (**Fig. 12.2**). The treatment at surgery is to resect the intervening tissue; this removes the bridge generating the recirculation. A 70-degree scope is ideally suited to examine these regions and to ensure that there is no residual uncinate or scarring present.

Infection Draining into the Maxillary Sinus from Elsewhere

A common cause of persistent disease in the maxillary sinus is mucous and/or mucopus draining into it. Infected secre-

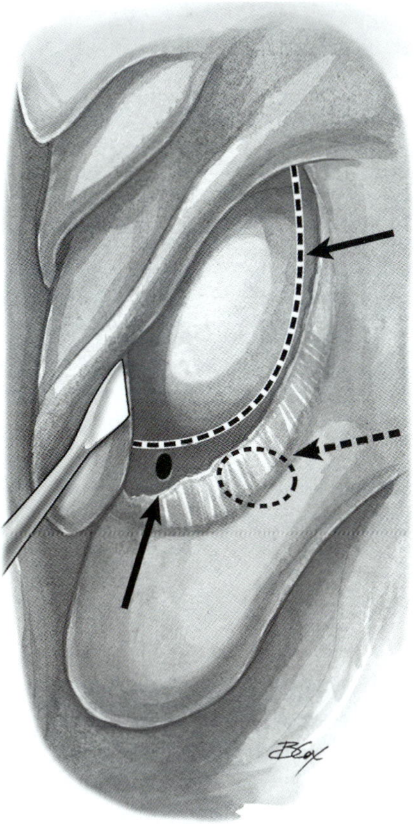

Fig. 12.1 The "missed ostium sequence": after the uncinectomy has been performed, 2 to 3 mm of residual uncinate remains (*solid black arrow*), obscuring the natural maxillary sinus ostium (*broken black arrow*). This may not be recognized by the surgeon, and can result in a posterior fontanelle ostium being created. This can subsequently result in a mucus recirculation phenomenon. The position of the original edge of the uncinate process is illustrated by the dotted line.

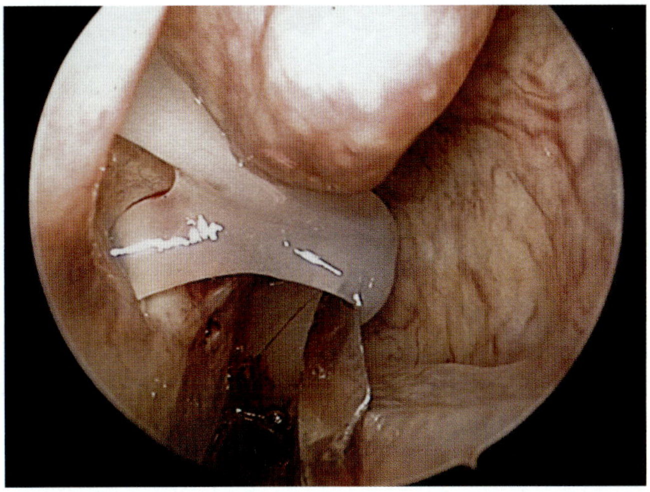

Fig. 12.2 Intraoperative picture of mucus recirculation; a sickle knife is used to demonstrate a stream of mucus originating from the natural maxillary sinus ostium, and partly flowing back into the sinus through an accessory ostium in the posterior fontanelle.

tions may also originate either from disease in the frontal sinus, frontal recess, and/or the anterior ethmoid cells, and these areas can usually be identified easily on a computed tomography (CT) scan (**Figs. 12.3A,B**). It is essential to localize accurately the origin of the infected material and to target treatment toward these areas; in most cases, this will lead to resolution of the maxillary disease. Even after managing this frontal or ethmoidal disease, however, there may be a requirement to control and eradicate disease within the maxillary sinus that may have arisen because of the persistent infected load seeping into the maxillary sinus.

A
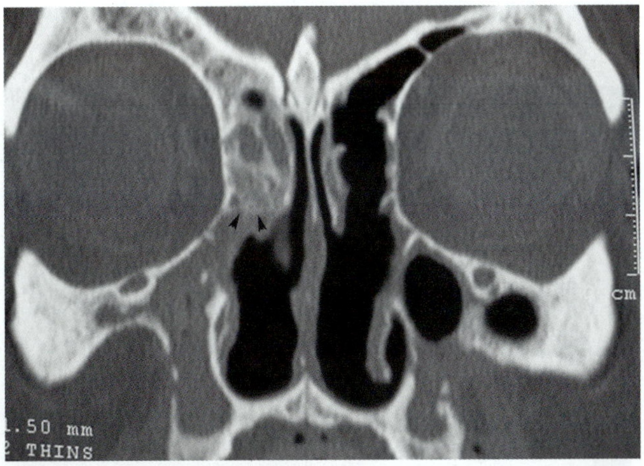

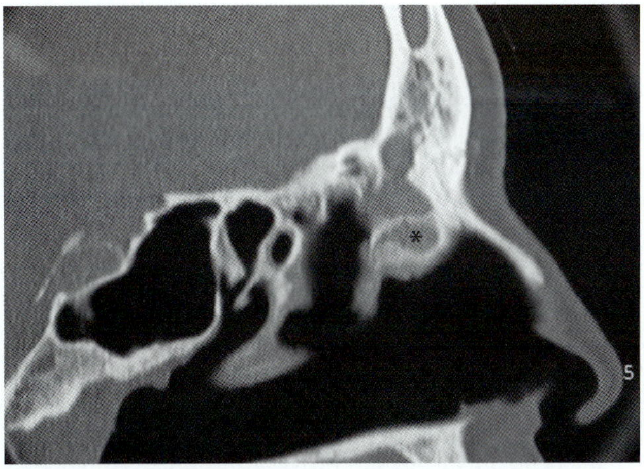
B

Fig. 12.3 **(A)** Coronal computed tomography (CT) scan of the sinuses, bone window, demonstrating diseased residual right ethmoids cells with significant osteitis and new bone formation (*arrowheads*), representing a source for mucus draining into the diseased right maxillary sinus ostium. **(B)** Parasagittal CT scan of the sinuses, bone window, in the same patient showing disease in a retained agger nasi cell (*asterisk*) and frontal sinus.

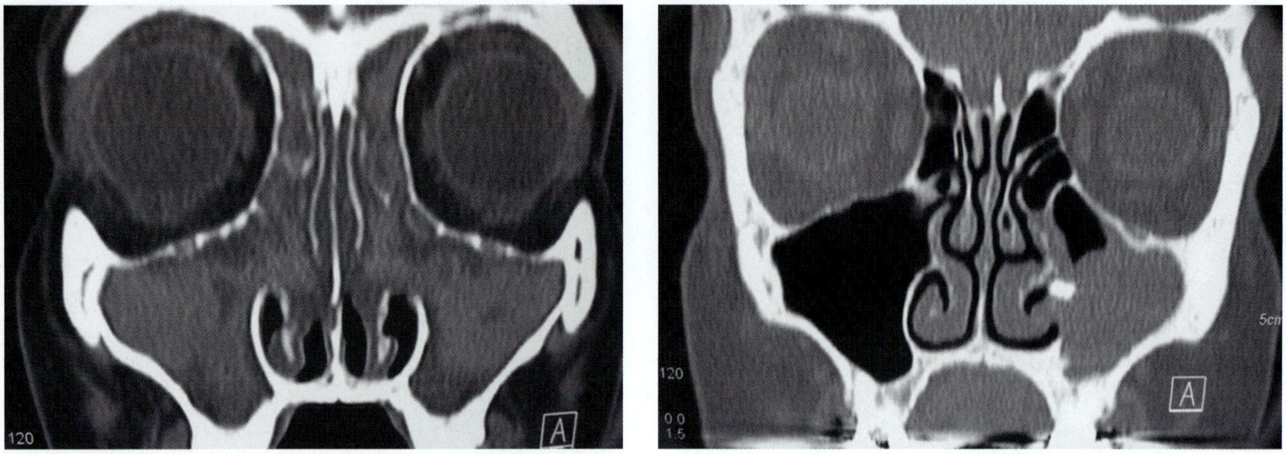

A B

Fig. 12.4 **(A)** Coronal computed tomography (CT) scan of the sinuses, soft tissue window, demonstrating diffuse fungal rhinosinusitis, with complete opacification of bilateral maxillary sinuses and typical double-densities. **(B)** Coronal CT scan of the sinuses, soft tissue window, showing partial opacification of the left maxillary sinus, and a metal density representing dislodged dental amalgam.

Retained Disease or Foreign Material

Careful attention should be given to the possibility of retained foreign bodies on the sinus floor, including inspissated concretions, dental filling material, or bone chips. These may be manifested on preoperative CT imaging by partial to complete opacification, double densities (**Fig. 12.4A**), calcifications, or metal artifact (**Fig. 12.4B**). However, the diagnosis can only be confirmed by endoscopic examination using angled scopes during surgery. This is achieved by first performing an uncinectomy and middle meatal antrostomy, followed by inspection with a 70-degree endoscope.

Polyps and thick tenacious mucous in the floor and anterior regions of the sinus require removal. In patients with severe and aggressive disease, such as allergic fungal rhinosinusitis, as well as the nonallergic eosinophilic rhinosinusitis variants, leaving eosinophilic mucin within the sinus may contribute to a rapid recurrence of disease.[7] This may be due to ongoing exposure to fungus within the mucin, or toxic substances such as major basic protein released by the eosinophils.

Figure 12.5 demonstrates ointment left within the maxillary sinus during prior surgery. It must be emphasized that no ointment should ever be left within the sinonasal cavity, as the petroleum component within the ointment cannot be absorbed or cleared by the body and remains as a foreign body. Occasionally, a unique reaction known as myospherulosis occurs, which was so named due to its histopathologic pattern once mistakenly thought to represent endosporulating fungus. Patients who develop myospherulosis appear more likely to form postoperative adhesions, which may hasten the need for revision surgery.[8]

Instances when maxillary disease is inaccessible through a wide middle meatal antrostomy may require a sublabial approach via canine fossa trephination. This permits the inspection and debridement of the entirety of the sinus cavity. If inspissated material, such as eosinophilic mucin is evident on the floor of the sinus, the offending material can either be lifted up using the tip of the trocar as a spoon to where it can be accessed by a curved suction through the middle meatal antrostomy, or simply removed using the microdebrider. In a study of patients with severely diseased maxillary sinuses, those who underwent canine fossa trephination and clearance of the sinuses had significantly improved long-term outcomes with regard to disease recurrence and symptom scores as compared with patients who did not have the procedure performed.[7]

Failure of Mucociliary Transport

Failure of mucociliary transport often results from systemic disease, such as cystic fibrosis or Kartagener syndrome.

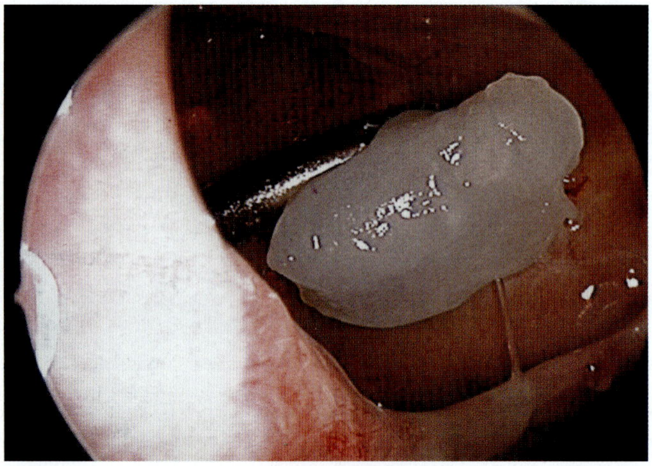

Fig. 12.5 Endoscopic view of antibiotic ointment left within the maxillary sinus during a previous surgery.

These entities are identified by careful history, laboratory studies, and light as well as electron microscopy. In these situations, a "megaostium" (i.e., one that encompasses most of the medial wall of the maxillary sinus) should be created to allow for copious nasal irrigation with concomitant appropriate head positioning and gravity drainage.

Scar Formation

Complications of prior endoscopic sinus surgery include the formation of synechiae causing obstruction of the nasal passage or sinus outflow tract, osteitis with significant bony hypertrophy, or even mucocele formation. A condition predisposing to scar formation and ostial stenosis is the creation of circumferential mucosal trauma during surgery, particularly if the antrostomy produced is not large.

The maxillary sinus is infrequently the site of mucocele formation, accounting for less than 10% of all paranasal sinus mucoceles.[9,10] However, the most common situation leading to the development of mucoceles in this area is following Caldwell–Luc procedures, where the mucosa has been stripped. This process can be suspected on CT when there is smooth, round enlargement of a completely opacified sinus with associated bony remodeling and thinning (**Fig. 12.6**).

Osteitis

Both the employment of through-cutting instruments and the judicious use of a powered microdebrider are helpful in preventing excessive mucosal stripping during FESS. This, in turn, minimizes the exposure of bone, which leads to osteitis, persistent inflammation, and perhaps further scarring and bony hypertrophy. Unopened infraorbital ethmoid (Haller) cells can directly obstruct maxillary sinus outflow (**Fig. 12.7**). Alternatively, even when opened, a diseased residual Haller cell may have osteitic partitions creating persistent localized mucosal hypertrophy. These partitions can be a focus for residual inflammation, if not totally resected.[11]

Biofilms

A biofilm is a multicellular community of bacteria that is embedded in a self-produced exopolysaccharide matrix and irreversibly attached to a surface. The existence of biofilms on the sinus mucosa of patients with chronic rhinosinusitis (CRS) is well described, and there is increasing evidence that biofilms affect the postoperative evolution of these patients. In an initial study, Bendouah et al[12] cultured 31 bacterial strains from post-ESS patients, of which 22 were significant biofilm producers. They found a correlation between the in vitro biofilm-producing capacity of *Pseudomonas aeruginosa* and *Staphylococcus aureus* and unfavorable evolution after ESS, as determined by questionnaire and endoscopy. In a retrospective analysis of 40 sinus surgical patients conducted in our department, bacterial biofilms were detected in 50% of these.[13] This subset of patients had significantly worse preoperative radiologic scores, as well as statistically worse postoperative symptoms and mucosal outcomes. The only other factor that was statistically related to an unfavorable outcome was the presence of fungus at the time of surgery. In this study the presence of polyps, eosinophilic mucin, or pus was not related to poor outcome. This provides evidence that biofilms indeed may play an active role in perpetuating inflammation in CRS patients, and may explain the recurrent and resistant nature of this disease.

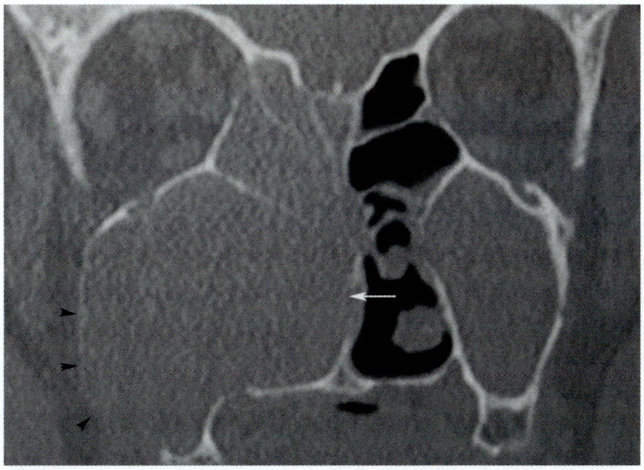

Fig. 12.6 Coronal computed tomography (CT) scan of the sinuses, bone window, demonstrating a right maxillary sinus mucocele arising after previous Caldwell–Luc procedure; note the smooth, rounded enlargement of the completely opacified right maxillary sinus, with associated thinning of the lateral (*arrowheads*) and medial walls (*white arrow*) of the sinus.

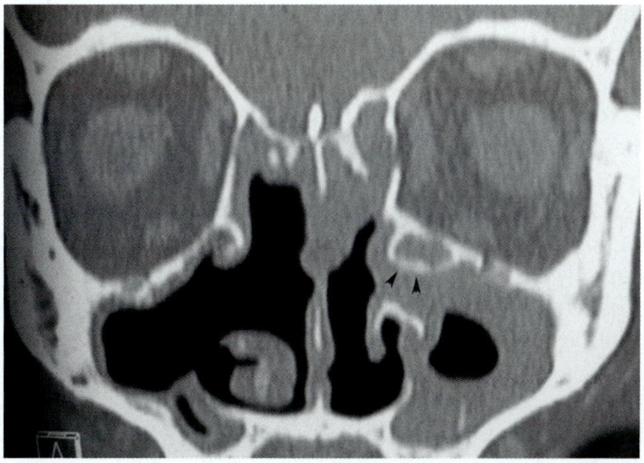

Fig. 12.7 Coronal computed tomography (CT) scan of the sinuses, demonstrating an infraorbital ethmoid cell (*arrowheads*), or Haller cell, contributing to outflow obstruction of the left maxillary sinus, which is partially opacified.

Given that biofilms present on sinus mucosa are difficult to eradicate with conventional antibiotic therapy, our department has investigated the usefulness of topical antibiotics via nasal irrigation. This was done with the aim of delivering high concentrations of antibiofilm agents with potentially low systemic absorption and side effects. Mupirocin was capable of reducing biofilm mass in vitro by greater than 90% at concentrations of 125 µg/mL or less, in all *S. aureus* isolates investigated.[14] Ciprofloxacin and vancomycin were largely ineffective within safe dosage ranges. To examine the efficacy and tolerability of topical mupirocin in the clinical setting, a prospective open-label pilot study was performed.[15] Sixteen patients with surgically recalcitrant CRS, who had positive nasendoscopically guided cultures for *S. aureus*, were treated with a 3-week course of 0.05% mupirocin in lactated ringers nasal lavages given twice daily. Fifteen of the 16 patients had improved nasendoscopic findings after treatment; 12 patients noted overall symptom improvement based on the sinonasal outcome test (SNOT-20) and visual analogue scale (VAS) questionnaires; and 15 patients had negative swab results for *S. aureus* after treatment. Only minimal adverse effects were experienced. Thus, the topical application of mupirocin via nasal irrigation may be useful in eliminating *S. aureus* biofilms present on the sinus mucosa of patients with CRS, and may offer an additional treatment to patients with recalcitrant sinusitis.

Other Causes

Cigarette smoking has been associated with statistically worse outcomes after ESS based on disease-specific quality of life measures.[16] Exposure to cigarette smoke adversely affects mucosal ciliary function,[17] as well as sinus cilia regeneration following functional endoscopic sinus surgery.[18] A history of smoking should be elicited for all patients presenting with postoperative sinonasal complaints and smoking cessation encouraged, with an emphasis on the detrimental effects of cigarette smoke on nasal and sinus health.

In patients with post-ESS symptoms where no origin for their symptoms can be identified, other causes of sinonasal symptoms should be considered. In the case of facial pain, neuralgia, migraine-equivalent (midfacial headache), or dental problems may be responsible. Axial CT should be used to carefully assess the possibility of a small periapical abscess producing pain. In individuals with a history of migraine or multiple surgeries, a trial of amitriptyline may be warranted.

Preoperative Management

Clinical Assessment

The clinician should attempt to elicit the patient's symptoms and classify them according to severity. The total severity can be classified by having patients answer the following question using a VAS graded on a 10-cm scale, "How troublesome are your symptoms of rhinosinusitis?" A VAS score of ≤ 3 corresponds to mild, >3 to 7 corresponds to moderate, and >7 corresponds to severe.[19]

The goal of the medical work-up is to identify mucosal, systemic, and environmental factors responsible for poor outcome. A history of underlying immune deficiency, connective tissue disorder, cigarette smoking, malignancies, or genetic disorder such as cystic fibrosis or primary ciliary dyskinesia should be sought. A complete immune work-up, and possibly a vaccine response, should be ordered to rule out immune deficiency if suspected. Blood work is also helpful to rule out other systemic disorders such as Wegener granulomatosis and sarcoidosis. Defects in functional immune response not evident in static testing have been identified in certain patients who have refractory CRS. In the absence of response to all other therapies, a 6-month trial of intravenous high-dose immunoglobulin (IVIG) may be warranted.[20]

Sinonasal endoscopy, preferably rigid, is essential in evaluating persistent disease. It may help identify structural anomalies, masses, or secretions not seen on anterior rhinoscopy. The presence of a posterior fontanelle ostium and circular flow of mucus should be sought. This can often be seen with a 30-degree endoscope.

The bacteriology of CRS may vary in an individual patient over time. Obtaining endoscopically guided cultures from the middle meatus or the sphenoethmoid recess (not the nasal cavity) will help in the selection of antibiotic therapy, particularly in cases unresponsive to empiric therapy. Care must be taken to avoid contact with the nasal wall or vestibule to minimize contamination, and to sample directly within purulent secretions when present, rather than adjacent areas.

Imaging Studies

CT of the sinuses is essential for completing the assessment of the patient with persistent post-ESS complaints. Preferably, the patient should undergo a high-definition helical multislice CT scan of the sinuses, with cuts measuring 0.5 to 1 mm in the axial plane, and reconstructed in the coronal and parasagittal planes. CT may be used to assess disease load or to identify technical factors that may not be revealed on endoscopy such as the presence of a natural or accessory ostium, residual ethmoid cells, Haller cells, persistent frontal recess and frontal sinus disease, obstructions to sinus drainage, or mucocele formation. Disease load can be determined from identifying the number of sinuses involved with disease and the extent of their involvement. The Lund–Mackay staging system is an effective method of standardizing reporting of radiologic severity of disease.[21,22]

In patients selected to undergo revision maxillary sinus surgery, particular attention must be paid to the preopera-

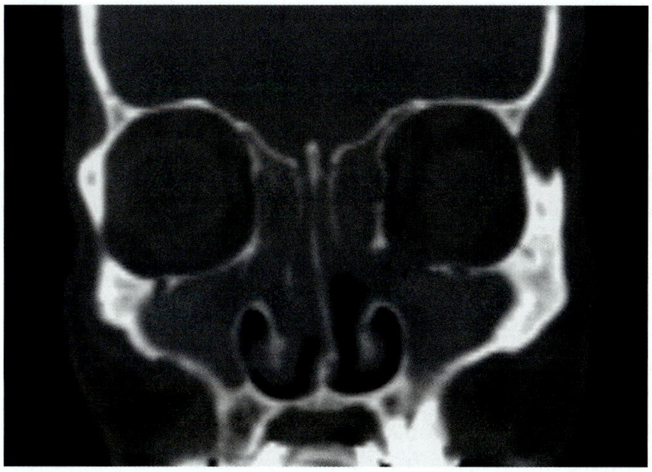

Fig. 12.8 Coronal computed tomography (CT) scan of the sinuses, bone window, demonstrating a sizable bony defect (*arrowheads*) in the lamina papyracea of the left orbit.

tive CT scan specifically to determine the level of integrity of the lamina papyracea. Areas of dehiscence—which may be due to the previous surgery, exuberant disease, or underlying patient anatomic variations—can be present and can be of significant size (**Fig. 12.8**) (**see Video 12.1**). For this reason, it is prudent practice always to verify the integrity of the lamina papyracea prior to clearing disease from this area. This is done by applying gentle pressure to the globe of the eye, while inspecting for transmitted movement of the lamina under endoscopic visualization. Cases of dehiscence of the lamina papyracea after previous endoscopic sinus surgery are often the result of forcing instruments, such as a curved suction, into the area of the natural maxillary sinus ostium under poor visualization, in the setting of severe mucosal disease and edema. The most common area for dehiscence in the lamina papyracea is just posterior to the frontal process of the maxilla, where the bone is thinnest. Recognition of this situation is of utmost importance for patients who will undergo a canine fossa puncture or trephination, as the use of the microdebrider to clear disease overlying the dehiscence could result in orbital penetration with disastrous consequences. In this instance, polyps should be carefully cleared using cold steel instruments, such as through-biting Blakesley forceps.

Finally, it must be emphasized that in the presence of unilateral disease, bony expansion, or destruction, or exuberant local disease out of proportion to the rest of the sinus cavities, it is essential to exclude the possible diagnosis of neoplasm (either benign or malignant). Magnetic resonance imaging (MRI) scans should be obtained in patients suspected of having a nasal mass, to better delineate the tumor size and differentiate it from pooled sinus secretions.

The Role of Image-guided Surgery

It is uncommon for image guidance to play a role in revision surgery to the maxillary sinus. There may be a place in situations where disease is extending beyond the confines of the maxillary sinus (i.e., into the infratemporal fossa or orbit).

Medical Management

A detailed discussion of the medical management of refractory maxillary sinus disease is beyond the scope of this chapter, and is covered elsewhere in this book. However, it must be stressed that an adequate trial of maximal medical therapy should be given preoperatively and documented in the chart. Systemic steroids may be beneficial in the preoperative period to reduce the size and vascularity of polyps in patients with significant nasal polyposis. A preliminary study recently published found that 30 mg of prednisone administered daily for 5 days preoperatively resulted in a significantly improved surgical field grading score during endoscopic sinus surgery.[23] Empiric treatment regimes range from 30 to 50 mg of prednisone daily for between 5 and 7 days preoperatively. However, further studies are necessary to clarify the optimal dose of steroids, length of treatment, and groups of patients that would benefit from this treatment.

Surgery

Indications for Revision Surgery

The role of revision surgery is principally to improve medical management and surgery should be planned and executed to optimize this. This is achieved by reducing disease load, by removing recurrent nasal polyps or hypertrophic sinonasal mucosa, and/or by improving access for continuing medical care in the form of topical solutions. Wide antrostomies are necessary in certain patients for problem sinuses to provide better access for irrigating solutions. The patient can never truly be deemed a failure of therapy until all obstructions to drainage and ventilation (or irrigation) have been corrected. Continued postoperative medical therapy is essential and can be considered an integral part of surgery.

The decision to reoperate a patient with maxillary sinus disease is centered principally on the demonstration of a symptomatic obstruction to sinus drainage or the presence of significant disease load in the sinuses. This must be tempered by the clinician's judgment, experience, and comfort level. Given the nature of endoscopic sinus surgery and the close proximity of numerous critical structures, special care must be taken to avoid serious intraoperative complications from damage to adjacent structures.[24–26] Preoperative sinus imaging and a precise understanding of the patient's anatomy are thus of paramount importance.

Indications for revision sinus surgery can be grossly divided into four main categories:

A. Incomplete previous surgery

- Persistence of symptoms and signs of CRS with or without nasal polyposis or recurrent acute sinusitis with retained uncinate process or persistent ethmoid cells on CT
- Unrepaired septal deviation, persistent concha bullosa, or Haller cell impairing maxillary sinus drainage (**see Videos 12.2, 12.3, and 12.4** for demonstrations of the surgical approach to each of these problems)
- Missed ostium sequence with recirculation of mucus (**see Video 12.5** demonstrating the uncinectomy and middle meatal antrostomy in the presence of an accessory mallary ostium)

B. Complications of previous surgery

- Synechia formation causing obstruction of nasal passage or sinus outflow
- Lateralization of the middle turbinate with or without adhesions between the middle turbinate and lateral nasal wall
- Significantly denuded bone, with subsequent osteitis and bony hypertrophy impairing sinus outflow
- Suspected mucocele formation

C. Recurrent sinus disease

- Recurrent nasal polyps refractory to maximal medical management
- Persistent isolated sinusitis that is symptomatic
- Recurrent allergic fungal rhinosinusitis
- Concurrent nasal polyposis and an intolerance or contraindication to oral cortisone

D. Histologic evidence of neoplasia
- Unexpected diagnosis of neoplasia on pathologic analysis with subtotal resection
- Localized severe disease suspicious for neoplasia such as inverted papilloma

Revision Uncinectomy and Maxillary Antrostomy

Prior to performing revision uncinectomy or maxillary antrostomies, it is essential to manage any adhesions in the region. Any simple adhesions between the middle turbinate and lateral nasal wall can be divided with through-cutting instruments. A decision must be made as to the position of the middle turbinate. If the middle turbinate is in a lateralized position, then it may be important to fix it in a more midline position. Our preferred method is to suture the middle turbinate to the septum with a 4–0 Vicryl (Ethicon, Somerville, NJ) suture running from one middle turbinate, through the septum, then the contralateral middle turbinate. The stitch is then run forward and tied just inside the nasal vestibule.

The swing-door technique of uncinectomy was created with the aim of achieving a complete removal of the mid-portion of the uncinate process and exposing the natural ostium of the maxillary sinus. This technique is ideally performed during the initial surgical attempt. However, if there is an indication for revision maxillary sinus surgery and a retained uncinate process is one of the contributing reasons, then elements of this technique can be applied as needed. A sickle knife is used to cut the uncinate horizontally just under the axilla of the middle turbinate (**Figs. 12.9, 12.10**). The tip of the sickle knife should go through all three layers (mucosa–bone–mucosa) and will then be felt to strike the hard bone of the frontal process of the maxilla. Risk of penetration of the orbit is extremely small as the uncinate attaches to the frontal process on the maxilla in this region and not onto the lacrimal bone as it does above the inferior turbinate insertion. Next, the pediatric backbiter is introduced into the middle meatus and the free edge of the uncinate mobilized with the tooth of the backbiter (**Fig. 12.11**). This allows the tooth to be slid into the hiatus semilunaris and the uncinate engaged. Usually, three bites of the back-

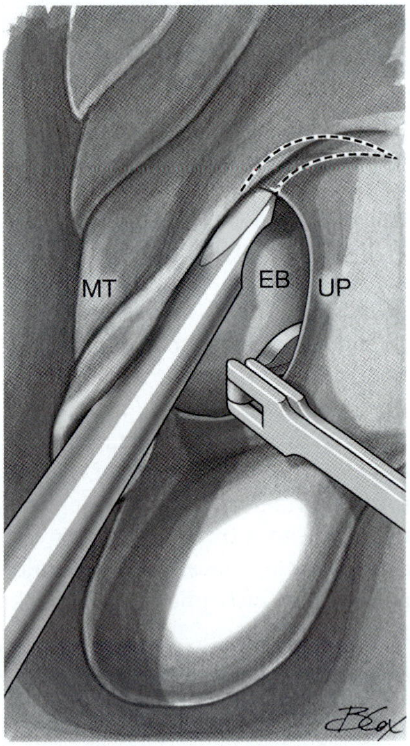

Fig. 12.9 In this diagram, the sickle knife makes the upper cut directly under the axilla of the middle turbinate. A pediatric backbiter is introduced at the vertical and horizontal portions of the uncinate process and the lower cut is made. EB, ethmoid bulla; UP, uncinate process; MT, middle turbinate.

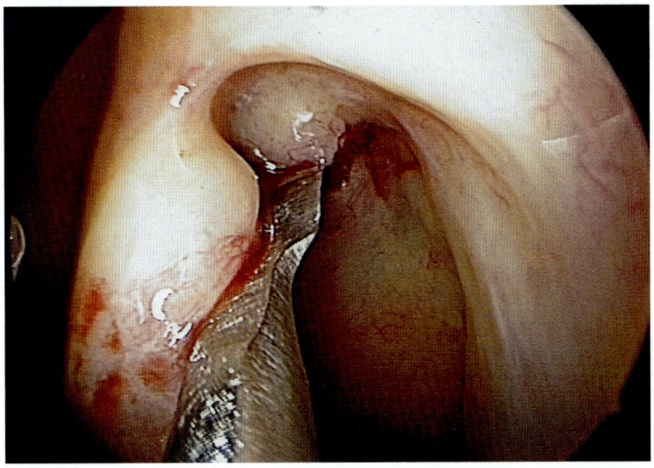

Figs. 12.10 Intraoperative photo of the sickle knife making the upper horizontal cut in the uncinate process directly under the axilla of the left middle turbinate.

biter are necessary before the frontal process is reached, but this may vary from patient to patient and be considerably less in patients with a retrocurved uncinate (**Fig. 12.12**) or who have had previous surgery. With the third bite, the backbiter is rotated from horizontal until it is angled at 45 degrees so that the tooth when closed should pass medial to the nasolacrimal duct. The risk of injury to the nasolacrimal duct is reduced with this maneuver. The right-angled ball probe is placed through the inferior cut behind the uncinate process and the midportion of the uncinate process is fractured anteriorly (**Fig. 12.13**). Next, an upturned 45-degree through-biting Blakesley forceps is used to cut the uncinate flush with the lateral nasal wall (**Figs. 12.14A,B**). The midportion of the uncinate can now be removed in one piece (**Fig. 12.14C**).

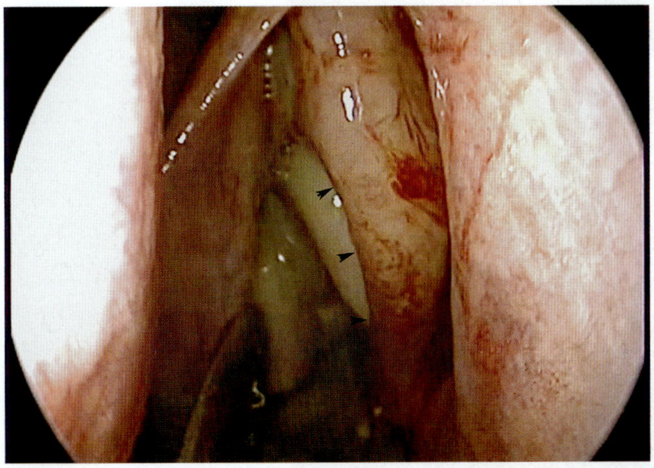

Fig. 12.12 Endoscopic view inside the left middle meatus demonstrating a retrocurved uncinate process; the free edge is indicated (*arrowheads*).

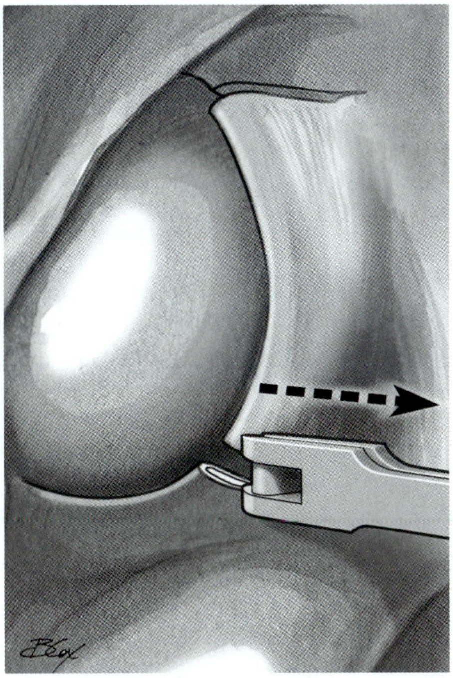

Fig. 12.11 Illustration of the pediatric backbiter making the lower horizontal cut at the transition between the middle portion and the horizontal portion of the uncinate process.

It is important to note that we discourage the use of the microdebrider for removal of the midportion of the uncinate. To remove the uncinate flush with the frontal process of the maxilla, the microdebrider blade needs to be pushed firmly against the orbital wall. This significantly increases the risk of orbital penetration and damage to the medial rectus muscle. If the microdebrider blade is used only very gently against the frontal process, inevitably, a variable amount of uncinate will remain and this will make identification of the natural ostium more difficult. In addition, even gentle use of the microdebrider blade on this portion of the lamina papyracea may be sufficient to penetrate the orbit. The thinnest and therefore the most dangerous region of the lamina papyracea is the region directly behind the frontal process of the maxilla and may, in fact, be dehiscent in some patients. We therefore recommend that microdebriders should be avoided in this area. Removal of the midportion of the uncinate is easily and cleanly achieved with cold steel instruments without significant risk to the orbit and is therefore the recommended technique. Removal or trimming of the horizontal section of the uncinate is often performed with the microdebrider as the direction of the blade in inferior and away for the lamina papyracea therefore not putting this area at risk. This is described below.

Before any attempt is made to visualize the natural ostium, the zero-degree endoscope should be changed to the 30-degree endoscope. This allows better visualization of the middle meatus and greater precision in the dissection.

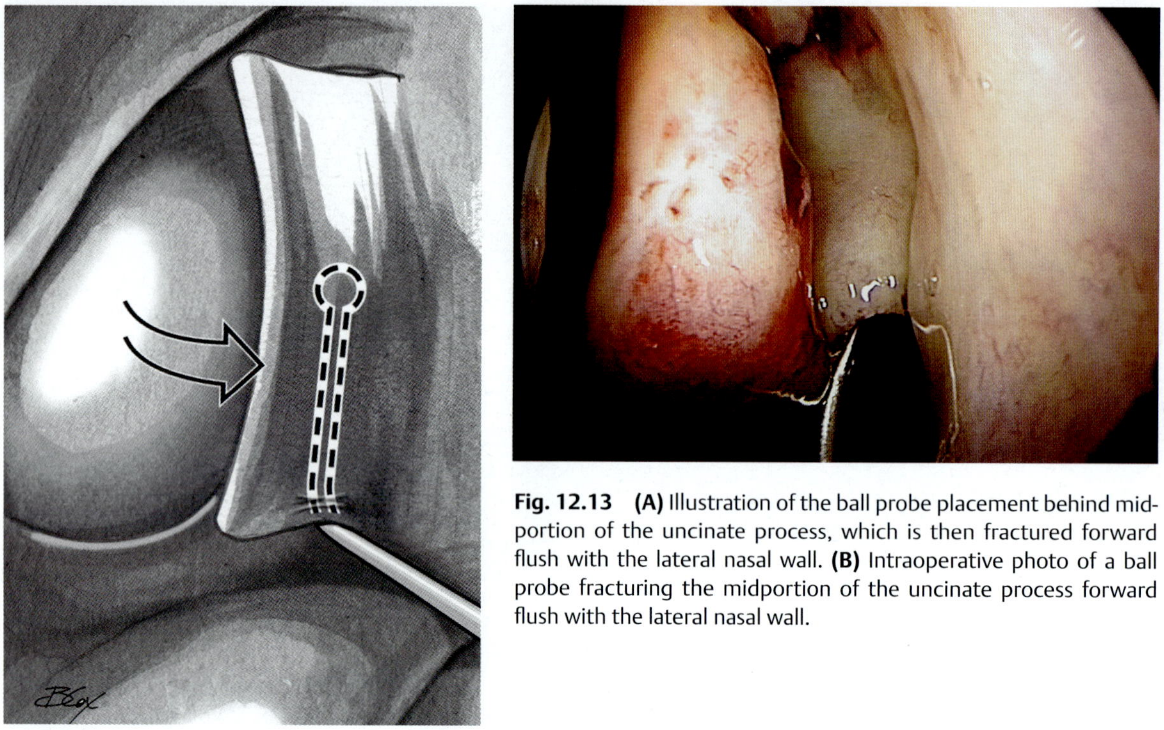

A

B

Fig. 12.13 **(A)** Illustration of the ball probe placement behind midportion of the uncinate process, which is then fractured forward flush with the lateral nasal wall. **(B)** Intraoperative photo of a ball probe fracturing the midportion of the uncinate process forward flush with the lateral nasal wall.

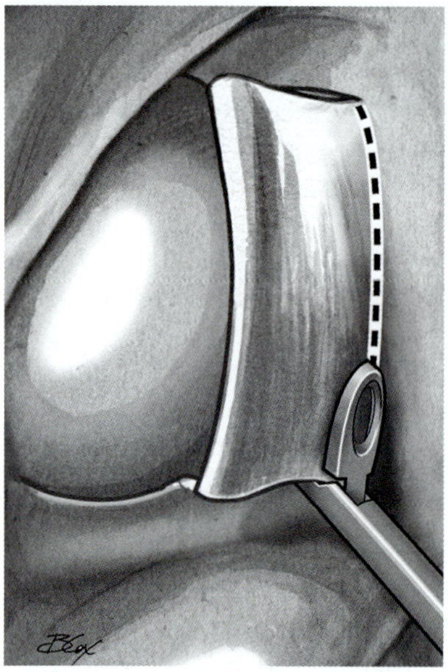

A

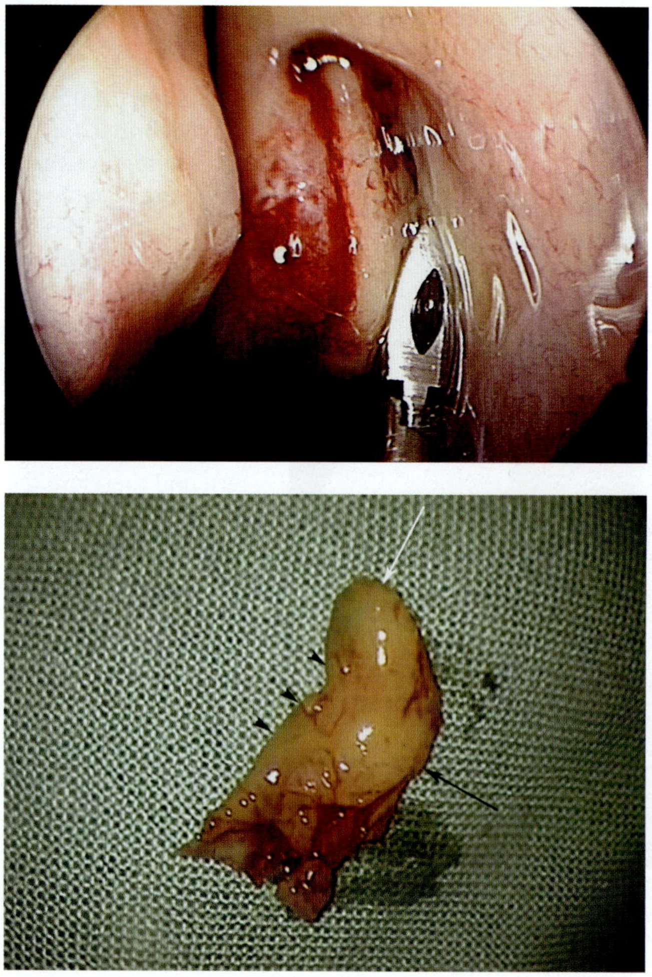

B

C

Fig. 12.14 **(A)** The 45-degree through-biting Blakesley is used to cut the uncinate process flush with the lateral nasal wall. **(B)** Intraoperative photo of the 45-degree through-biting Blakesley cutting the uncinate process flush with the lateral nasal wall. **(C)** The removed middle portion of the uncinate process, with the superior portion (*white arrow*), anterior cut edge (*black arrow*), and posterior free edge (*arrowheads*) indicated.

The natural ostium is found by placing the tip of the ball probe directly over the cut edge of the horizontal portion of the uncinate. If possible, any residual horizontal portion of uncinate bone should be dissected free from between its two mucosal layers. The double right-angled ball probe is used to elevate the mucosa off the medial side of the uncinate (**Fig. 12.15**). The bone is then fractured medially and the mucosa on the lateral side is elevated. The bone can then be removed using a straight Blakesley forceps (**Fig. 12.15**), leaving only the mucosal layers, which are then delicately trimmed with the microdebrider. This allows the edges of the mucosa to be closely applied resulting in first intention healing. Failure to remove the bone from the horizontal portion of the uncinate can leave exposed bone between the mucosal layers resulting in granulation and scar tissue formation. Once the mucosal edges of the horizontal uncinate are trimmed, this will expose the natural ostium of the maxillary sinus with no trauma to the superior and posterior regions of the natural ostium.

It may be necessary to enlarge the meatal antrostomy to examine the sinus with an angled scope accurately, and to instrument the sinus in case of diseased material requiring removal. This is done by removing the posterior fontanelle using a straight through-biting Blakesley forceps or microdebrider. An antrostomy diameter of ~10 × 10 mm is usually sufficient to perform these tasks. Furthermore, in cases of accessory or iatrogenic sinus ostia located in the area of the posterior fontanelle (**Fig. 12.16**), or in the missed ostium sequence as described above, it is necessary to join surgically the posterior ostium to the natural maxillary sinus ostium. This is done to prevent the recirculation phenomenon, which may account for recurrent sinusitis symptoms after ESS. This can be done by inserting a backbiter into the accessory ostium and coming forward to the natural ostium (**see Video 12.5**); any excessive tissue edges can be carefully microdebrided thereafter.

It is currently unclear whether creating a wide meatal antrostomy is detrimental to the long-term health of the maxillary sinus. A study in our department showed that there was a significant decrease in nitric oxide (NO) concentration in the maxillary sinuses and nasal cavities of patients with large maxillary sinus ostia (greater than 5 × 5 mm).[27] NO is produced by nitric oxide synthase (NOS) type II in the mucosa of the sinuses,[28,29] and its production is induced by bacterial inflammation.[30] It is known to stimulate ciliary motility, and is believed to play an important role in

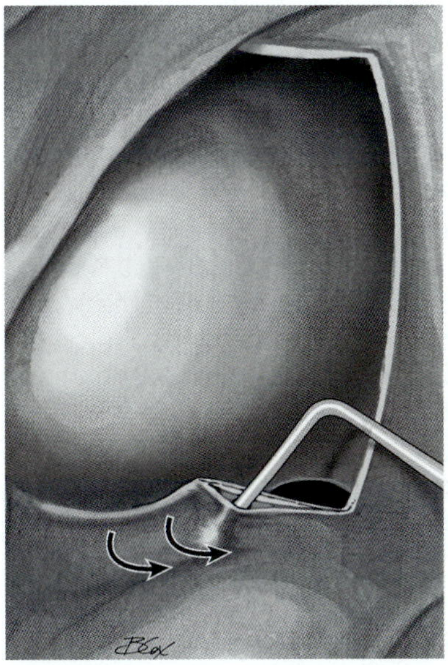

A

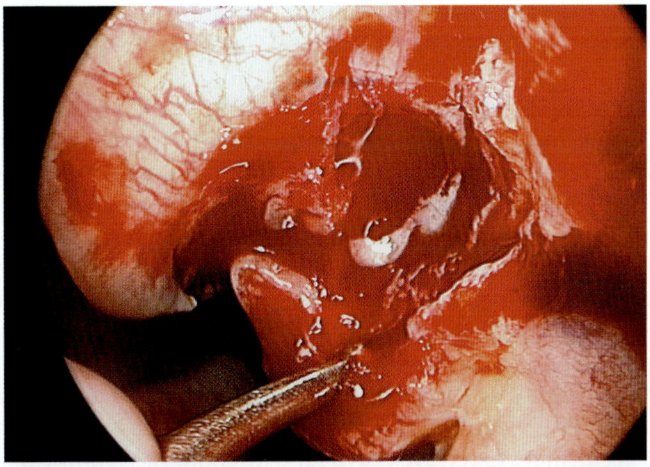

B

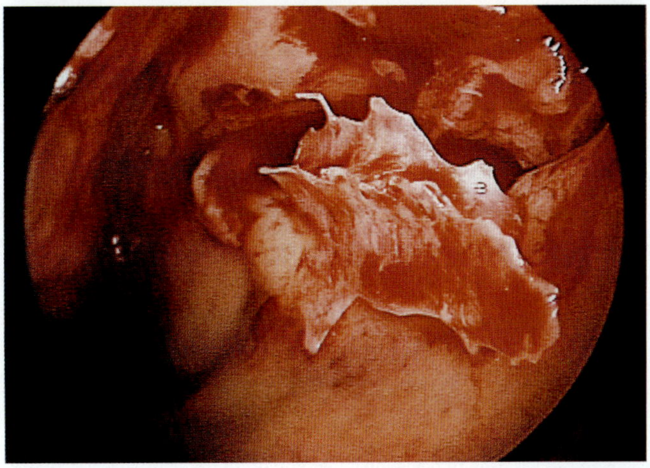

C

Fig. 12.15 **(A)** Diagram illustrating the double right-angle ball probe dissecting the bone of the horizontal portion of the uncinate process. **(B)** Intraoperative photo of the ball probe dissecting the bone away from the mucosa of the horizontal portion of the uncinate process. **(C)** Bone of the horizontal portion of the uncinate process removed from between the two layers of mucosa.

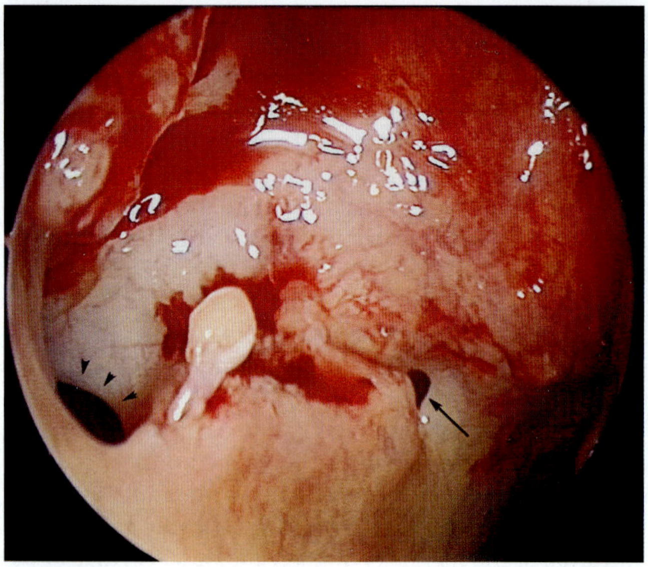

Fig. 12.16 Endoscopic view of the right natural maxillary ostium anteriorly (*arrowheads*), as well as an accessory ostium in the posterior fontanelle (*black arrow*), using a 30-degree endoscope.

the innate immune defenses of the nasal mucosa to bacteria, viruses, and fungi.[31] However, it is not known whether a lower concentration of NO in the nasal cavity and sinuses actually predisposes to recurrent infections; this association still needs to be studied.

Another consequence of removal of the posterior fontanelle during enlargement of the maxillary meatal antrostomy may be the drainage of secretions from the frontal and anterior ethmoid sinuses into the maxillary sinus. The natural drainage pathway of the former two sinuses begins above the natural maxillary sinus ostium, and runs along the base of the ethmoid bulla, then across the posterior fontanelle and under the eustachian tube to the nasopharynx.

For the aforementioned reasons, enlargement of the maxillary sinus ostium into the posterior fontanelle is not performed in all patients, but rather is reserved for those with more severe disease. This includes extensive polyp formation within the maxillary sinus, or large amounts of thick and viscid secretion, such as fungal mucous. Additionally, patients with Samter's triad and cystic fibrosis should have a wide meatal antrostomy to allow copious sinus irrigation and delivery of topical therapy.

Following the uncinectomy, it is useful to grade the extent of disease affecting the maxillary sinus at the time of surgery. This will aid in the intraoperative decision-making process. A 70-degree endoscope is used to visualize the maxillary sinus contents through the natural ostium, and the level of disease is graded according to **Table 12.1**. Grade 1 (**Fig. 12.17A**) and grade 2 (**Fig. 12.17B**) are reversible with adequate clearance of mucus and aeration of the maxillary sinus, but grade 3 disease is irreversible (**Fig. 12.17C**). Therefore, the polyps, and especially the thick eosinophilic mucus should be cleared before reepithelialization and reciliation occur.

Anterior Approaches to the Maxillary Sinus including Canine Fossa Trephination

Extensive maxillary sinus disease can be a difficult problem to tackle endoscopically, especially in the anterior and inferior regions of the antrum. Access by way of the natural ostium of the maxillary sinus will only allow the posterior lateral wall, the posterior region of the roof, and the posterior wall of the maxillary sinus to be cleared of pus, fungal debris, and polyps. As we have stressed, it is essential to remove as much of the disease burden as possible to allow for resolution of symptoms. Access to these areas has been aided by the recent introduction of 90- and 120-degree cutting blades. Alternatively, an inferior meatal approach may be used, but once again, access to the anterior half of the maxillary sinus is compromised. This is due to the two fulcrums that the microdebrider and instruments must pass to reach the sinus cavity (**Fig. 12.18**). Therefore, in many patients with extensive maxillary sinus disease, complete removal of all polyps and debris requires access through the anterior maxillary wall of the maxillary sinus. With this access the

Table 12.1 Endoscopic Grading of the Diseased Maxillary Sinus with Associated CT Finding and Suggested Management

Grade	Endoscopic Findings	CT Findings	Suggested Surgery
1	Normal or slightly edematous mucosa	Minimal mucosal thickening and ostiomeatal complex obstruction	Uncinectomy alone with visualization of the natural ostium
2	Edematous mucosa with small polyps, without significant eosinophilic mucus	Moderate mucosal edema and/or opacification (uniform consistency, air bubbles or fluid levels)	Enlargement of the maxillary ostium to ~1 × 1 cm, with suction clearance of the sinus
3	Extensive polyps and tenacious mucus	Double densities and complete maxillary opacification*	Canine fossa trephination with complete clearance of polyps and mucus, and creation of a large antrostomy

*Not all completely opacified maxillary sinuses will need trephination if the contents of the sinus are easily removed with suction.

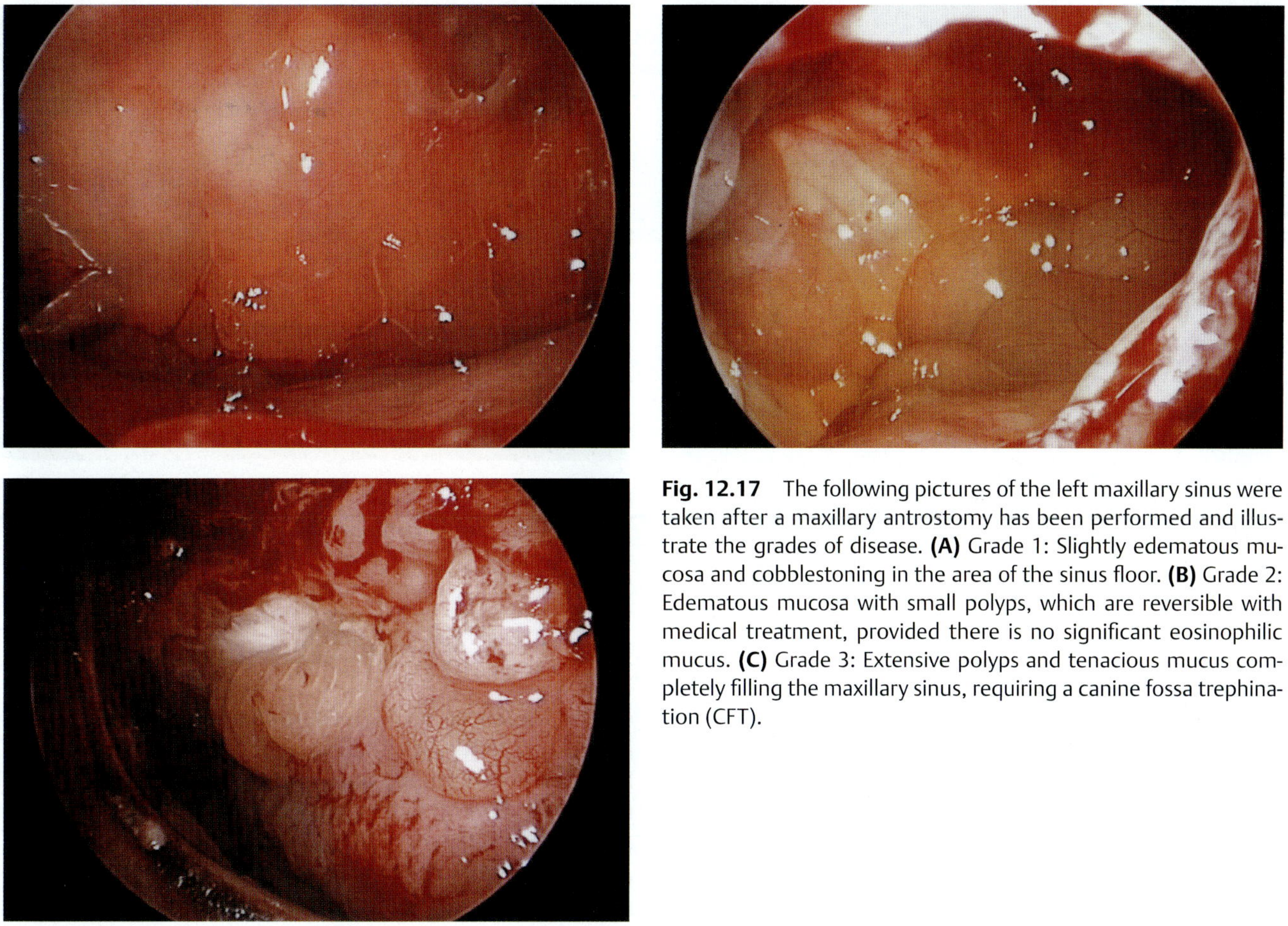

A B C

Fig. 12.17 The following pictures of the left maxillary sinus were taken after a maxillary antrostomy has been performed and illustrate the grades of disease. **(A)** Grade 1: Slightly edematous mucosa and cobblestoning in the area of the sinus floor. **(B)** Grade 2: Edematous mucosa with small polyps, which are reversible with medical treatment, provided there is no significant eosinophilic mucus. **(C)** Grade 3: Extensive polyps and tenacious mucus completely filling the maxillary sinus, requiring a canine fossa trephination (CFT).

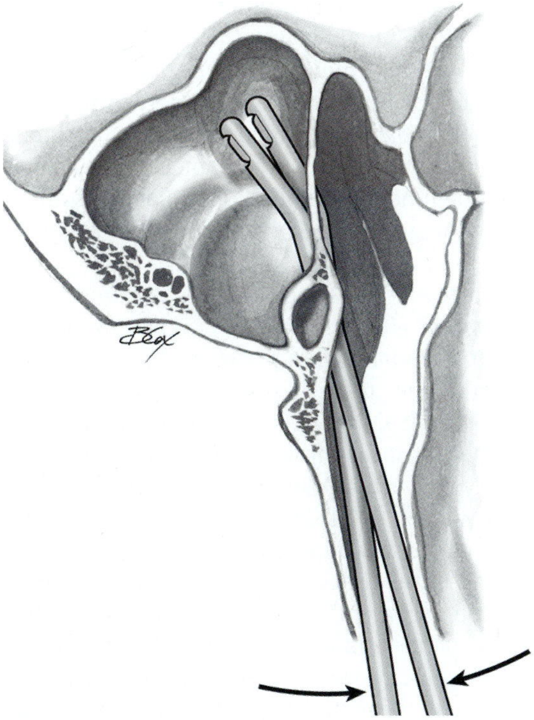

Fig. 12.18 Axial section through the maxillary sinus demonstrating the microdebrider blade being passed through an inferior meatal antrostomy. Due to the anterior fulcrum at the nasal vestibule and the posterior fulcrum at the antrostomy, only the posteromedial region of the sinus can be effectively cleared.

blade or instrument has only one fulcrum, and so a much greater range of motion within the sinus can be achieved (**Fig. 12.19**). One such method is the traditional Caldwell–Luc approach performed through the anterior wall of the maxillary sinus. This is, however, associated with significant morbidity such as facial numbness or paresthesia (9%), oroantral fistulas (1%), gingivolabial wound dehiscences (1.5%), and dacryocystitis (2.5%).[7] Canine fossa puncture (CFP) was initially proposed as an alternative method of obtaining access to the maxillary antrum.

A description of this standard technique is as follows:[32] the lip of the patient is elevated and the canine tooth identified. The root of this tooth is traced superiorly with the finger until the canine fossa is palpated. A small volume of

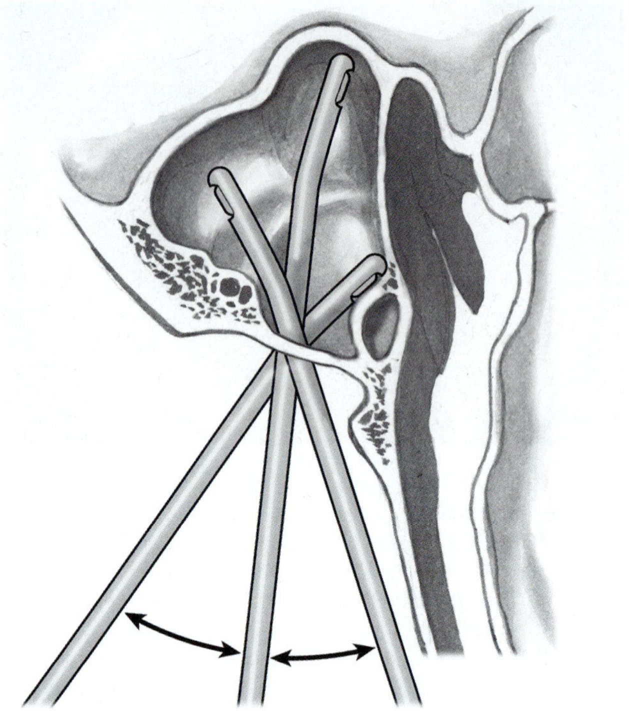

Fig. 12.19 Axial section through the maxillary sinus demonstrating the microdebrider blade being passed through a canine fossa puncture. As a result of the single fulcrum at the anterior face of the maxilla, the entire sinus can be accessed by the microdebrider.

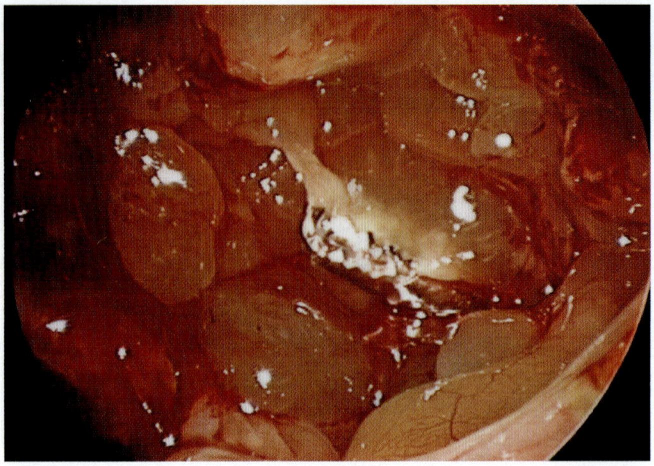

Fig. 12.20 Endoscopic view through a right maxillary antrostomy, using a 70-degree endoscope, illustrating the microdebrider blade which has been passed though the canine fossa trephination (CFT) site in the anterior face of the maxilla.

2% lidocaine with 1:80,000 of adrenalin is infiltrated into this region. A small incision is made in the gingivobuccal sulcus above and slightly lateral to the apex of the canine tooth, and the soft tissue is dissected off the anterior face of the maxilla. A canine fossa trocar (Karl Storz, Tuttlingen, Germany) is placed in the fossa and directed posteriorly. Using a rotating forward motion, a round 4-mm opening is created, which allows insertion of a straight or a curved 4-mm microdebrider blade. When the bone is too thick, a couple of firm taps with the palm of the hand is usually sufficient to drive the trocar through the bone. However, occasionally tapping with a mallet is necessary. This sublabial mucosal incision is small enough to close spontaneously and is not sutured. After the tip of the trocar is felt to fully penetrate the sinus, it is withdrawn and the microdebrider is introduced into the puncture with its blade kept closed to prevent soft tissues from being aspirated in during this step. Once inside the sinus, the 70-degree telescope is introduced into the nasal cavity to look through the antrostomy. At this point, the gate of the blade is opened, which helps to remove most of the blood from within the sinus and allows visualization of the blade within the maxillary sinus (**Fig. 12.20**). This step is important to confirm the position of the microdebrider in the sinus, and not in the orbit or soft tissues. The blade can then be used to remove polyps under direct vision.

The incidence of complications with the old CFP technique was 75%.[32] In a review of 37 CFPs in 21 patients, the most common complaint was of cheek swelling in 38% of the sides, followed by facial pain (32%), facial numbness (30%), cheek pain (27%), dental numbness (27%), gingival complications (24%), and facial tingling (16%). Most of these (75.5%) resolved within the first month after surgery; however, 28% had persistent complications with facial tingling, numbness, or continued pain. These longer-term complications are thought to be a result of injury to branches of the infraorbital nerve. Thus, the anatomy of the nerve as it exits the infraorbital foramen and divides into the anterior superior alveolar nerve (ASAN) and middle superior alveolar nerve (MSAN) is of particular importance when performing this procedure. Cadaver research conducted in our department had determined that the safest entry point for the canine fossa trocar was the junction of the midpupillary line and a horizontal line running along the base of the pyriform aperture (**Fig. 12.21**).[33]

One of the shortcomings of the canine fossa puncture is that it is performed in a blind manner. Even though the soft tissues anterior to the maxilla are dissected off, the precise area through which the trocar is placed is not visualized, and the ASAN or the MSAN could thus be injured. Additionally, the use of the trocar may fracture the thin bone of the anterior maxillary wall around the puncture site. The edges of the trocar are meant to act as a drill, cutting the bone with a rotating motion and minimal pressure. If significant pressure is applied to the trocar, a fracture of the surrounding bone will often occur, enlarging the area of trauma and increasing the risk of nerve injury. And even if the trocar creates a sharp 4-mm puncture in the bone, the 4-mm debrider blade fits very snugly through this opening and manipula-

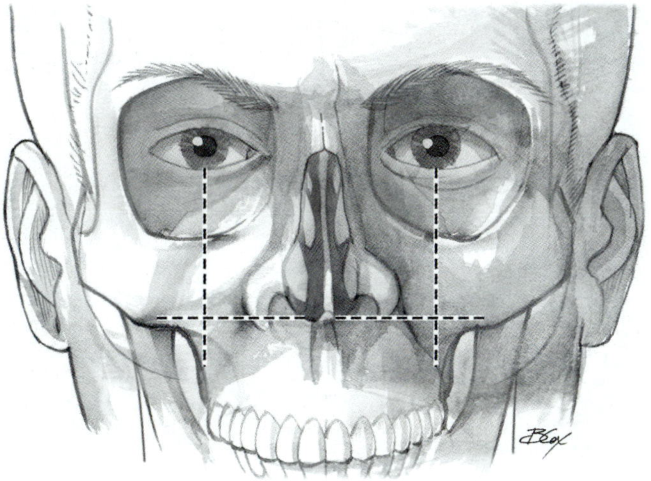

Fig. 12.21 The landmarks for the canine fossa puncture/trephine are the intersection between a vertical line through the pupil and a horizontal line through the floor of the nose.

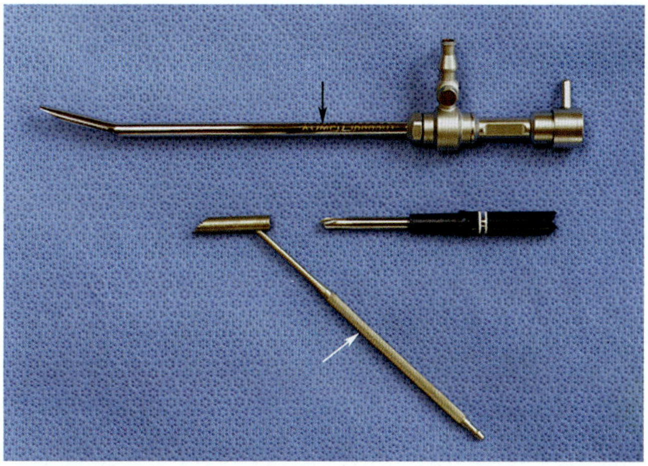

Fig. 12.22 The canine fossa trephination kit (Medtronic ENT, Jacksonville, FL) consisting of an endoscope sheath (*black arrow*) with a protruding blade, which allows retraction of soft tissues during dissection on the anterior face of the maxilla; a reusable drill guide (*white arrow*), and 5-mm reusable drill bit that fits the microdebrider handpiece.

tion of the blade within the sinus may itself cause fracture of the surrounding bone, with the potential of neurologic injury. Furthermore, devitalized bone fragments may act as a nidus of persistent inflammation and granulation within the maxillary sinus. To overcome all of these problems, a new technique, referred to as canine fossa trephination, was devised to improve the bony penetration through the anterior face of the maxillary sinus.

Canine fossa trephination (CFT) is now our procedure of choice for anterior approaches to the maxillary sinus (**see Video 12.6**). The essential difference between CFT and CFP is that a 5-mm hole is accurately drilled through the anterior maxillary face under direct visualization rather than using a trocar. To enable us to do this, new instrumentation

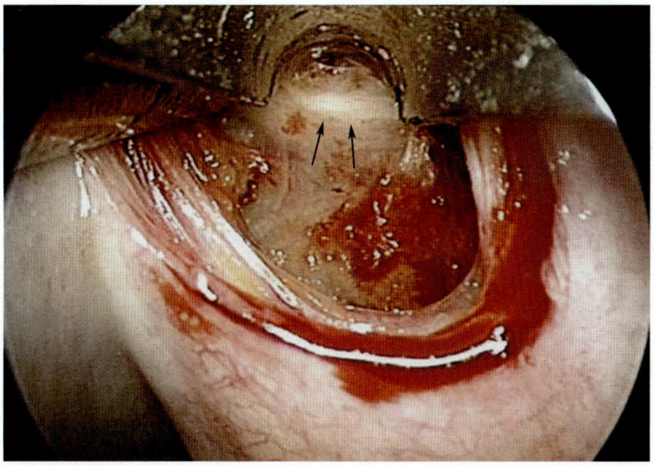

Fig. 12.23 A branch of the anterior-superior alveolar nerve is seen on the anterior face of the maxilla (*black arrows*); the dissection is therefore carried a little further to avoid injury to the nerve.

has been developed to aid in the accurate placement of the drill hole. The canine fossa trephination kit (**Fig. 12.22**) consists of an endoscope sheath with a protruding blade, which allows retraction of soft tissues during dissection on the anterior face of the maxilla. In addition, the kit contains a reusable drill guide and 5-mm reusable drill bit that fits the microdebrider handpiece. The endoscope sheath is placed on a zero-degree scope, the lip is held up and gingivobuccal sulcus infiltrated with lidocaine and adrenalin. An angled 6-mm incision is made in the gingivobuccal sulcus using a 15-blade or Colorado diathermy needle. A suction Freer elevator is used to elevate the soft tissues off the anterior face of the maxilla in a subperiosteal plane. Once this is achieved, the extension on the endoscope sheath is used to hold away soft tissues allowing clear visualization of the subperiosteal plane on the anterior face of the maxilla. The dissection is then continued in a superior and lateral direction, to expose the area located at the intersection of the midpupillary line and a horizontal line running along the lower border of the nasal alae. It is not uncommon to visualize one of the branches of the anterior-superior alveolar nerve on the anterior face of the maxilla (**Fig. 12.23**). If a branch is seen, the dissection is carried a little further to avoid injury to the nerve (**see Video 12.7**).

The canine fossa drill guide (Medtronic ENT, Jacksonville, FL) is then placed on the anterior face of the maxilla at the junction of the two lines described above. The canine fossa drill (Medtronic ENT) is attached to the microdebrider handpiece and irrigation is attached to the back of the drill guide, allowing irrigation of the burr during drilling. The burr is used at 12,000 rpm for best results. Note that the drill should be maneuvered so that it is perpendicular to the anterior

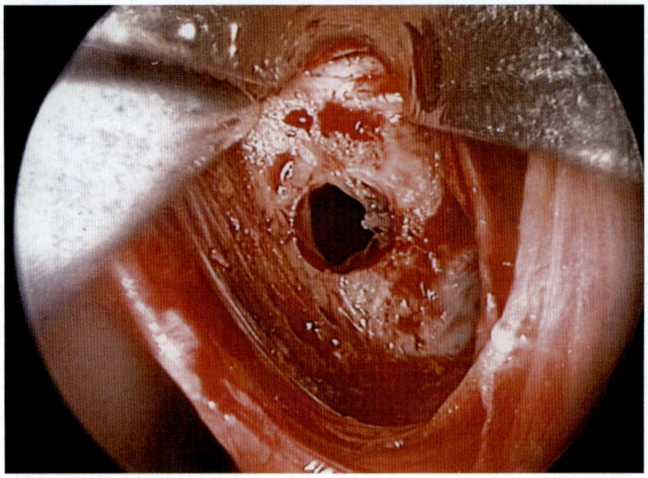

Fig. 12.24 A 5-mm hole is drilled into the anterior face of the maxilla.

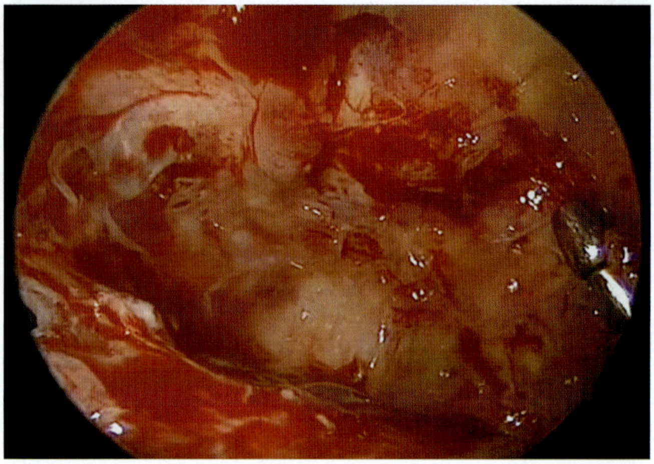

Fig. 12.25 View through the middle meatal antrostomy using a 70-degree endoscope, showing an angled suction passed via the trephination in the anterior face of the maxilla and used to clean the inferior, lateral, and retrolacrimal recesses of the maxillary sinus.

face of the maxilla and not angled tangentially to the maxilla. A 5-mm diameter hole is drilled through the bone (**Fig. 12.24**), and a Frazier suction is used to remove any bone dust from the hole and surrounding soft tissues. The 4-mm microdebrider blade is then placed through the trephine into the maxillary sinus in the closed position, and a 70-degree endoscope is passed transnasally to the maxillary antrostomy. At this point, the gate of the blade is opened to remove the blood from within the sinus and to allow visualization of the blade within the maxillary sinus. This confirms the position of the microdebrider, and this step is important to avoid inadvertent injury to the orbit or soft tissues. The first step is to enlarge the maxillary antrostomy as this provides improved visualization into the sinus with the 70-degree scope. The blade is used to enlarge the maxillary sinus antrostomy, removing any residual uncinate process and posterior fontanelle up to the posterior wall of the maxillary sinus. This affords the widest possible view through the antrostomy, and the surgeon can then remove polyps and thick mucous from the sinus under direct vision. Angled suctions are used for the lateral recesses and anterior face of the maxillary sinus (**Fig. 12.25**). The endoscope can also be placed through the trephine into the sinus to inspect and ensure the complete removal of disease material. It is important to note that only polypoid tissue and mucin are removed, and the denuding of bone is avoided. This helps to ensure a speedy reepithelialization and reciliation in the postoperative period.

As for the middle portion of the uncinate process, care is taken not to microdebride tissues based superiorly in the area of the lamina papyracea because of the risk of orbital penetration. If this needs to be performed due to a significant amount of polypoid tissue narrowing the antrostomy, the scrub nurse should be asked to gently push on the eye while the surgeon inspects the lamina for transmitted movement, indicating a bony dehiscence (**see Video 12.1**). If movement is seen, it is recommended not to use powered instrumentation for this area, but rather to clear the polyps using through-biting Blakesley forceps.

To assess whether the new technique reduced the incidence and severity of complications, a clinical study of 63 patients was undertaken, including 36 bilateral procedures giving a total number of 99 anatomically directed canine fossa punctures (aCFP; without the trephination kit) and trephines (CFT; with trephination kit).[34] The overall frequency of adverse events was significantly reduced to 45%, compared with the previously reported 75% with the traditional blind technique. The number of patients complaining of persisting adverse effects was reduced from 28% to 5%. The 67 CFT procedures had a significantly lower frequency of adverse events (40%) than the 32 aCFP procedures (53%). This again emphasizes the need to visualize the anterior face of the maxilla before placing the trephine and also emphasizes the increased risk of nerve injury if a trocar rather than trephination set is used.

We have focused on the use of CFT and its applications in revision maxillary sinus surgery. However, it must be recognized that the principles promoted in revision surgery are often applicable in primary surgery, and CFT is a very useful tool in the management of many disease processes within the maxillary sinus. In patients with extensive polyposis and/or eosinophilic mucin, mucopyoceles, antrochoanal polyps, foreign bodies, and other situations where access to parts of the maxillary sinus not attainable through a maxillary antrum is required, then CFT is the approach of choice.

Postoperative Care

Patients who have undergone either the canine fossa puncture or trephination usually do not require suturing of their gingivobuccal incisions. They are advised to rinse their mouths with saline after meals during the first few postoperative days, until the incisions have sealed. Nasal saline irrigation is begun on the day after surgery, and all patients receive 5 to 10 days of broad-spectrum antibiotics. The first postoperative visit and debridement is performed at 2 weeks.

Conclusion

Even if initial management of the maxillary sinus is optimal, there are several potential reasons for persistent disease within the sinus requiring further surgical intervention. The causes of persistent maxillary sinus symptoms after endoscopic sinus surgery can be categorized into recirculation, infection draining into the maxillary sinus from elsewhere, retained foreign material, failure of mucociliary transport, scarring, and local osteitis. The goal of the clinical evaluation and diagnostic imaging studies is to determine the underlying factors contributing to sinus disease.

Revision maxillary sinus surgery seeks to improve medical management by reducing disease load and improving the maxillary sinus drainage pathway, providing access for topical medications. This is done by removing recurrent nasal polyps or hypertrophic sinonasal mucosa from the maxillary sinus disease and ensuring an adequate maxillary antrostomy. To achieve this, depending on the technical factors identified, revision uncinectomy, scar division, middle turbinate medialization or enlarging the antrum posteriorly into the fontanelle, may be performed. The canine fossa trephination technique is a highly effective way to reduce disease load in the severely diseased maxillary sinus, whether in revision surgery or in the primary setting. Recent modifications to this technique have been successful in reducing the rate of associated complications.

Pearls

- The goal of assessment of the patient with symptoms suggesting persistent or recurrent sinus disease is to identify the presence of technical, mucosal, and systemic factors contributing to poor outcome by using the appropriate tests.
- Know that medical management will be required after surgery. Protocols should be in place to manage recurrent or recalcitrant bacterial or fungal colonization of the maxillary sinus.
- The goal of surgery is to provide a well-ventilated, epithelialized, and disease-free maxillary sinus. It should be noted that in some situations, medical management may be required to further treat those patients with severe mucosal disease.
- Causes of persistent maxillary sinus symptoms after ESS can be clustered into six large categories: recirculation, infection draining into the maxillary sinus from elsewhere, retained foreign material, failure of mucociliary transport, scar formation, and local osteitis.
- Indications for revision endoscopic sinus surgery can be broadly categorized as follows: (1) incomplete previous surgery, (2) complications of previous surgery, (3) recurrent or persistent sinus disease, and (4) histologic evidence of neoplasia. These criteria are not absolute and the decision to reoperate is most often based on clinician judgment and experience.
- Surgery is aimed at either improving the natural maxillary sinus drainage pathway (i.e., uncinectomy, scar division, middle turbinate medialization, or changes to the antrum) or through removal of persistent and significant maxillary sinus disease via the canine fossa trephine approach.

References

1. Chu CT, Lebowitz RA, Jacobs JB. An analysis of sites of disease in revision endoscopic sinus surgery. Am J Rhinol 1997;11(4):287–291
2. Musy PY, Kountakis SE. Anatomic findings in patients undergoing revision endoscopic sinus surgery. Am J Otolaryngol 2004;25(6):418–422
3. Ramadan HH. Surgical causes of failure in endoscopic sinus surgery. Laryngoscope 1999;109(1):27–29
4. Richtsmeier WJ. Top 10 reasons for endoscopic maxillary sinus surgery failure. Laryngoscope 2001;111(11 Pt 1):1952–1956
5. Cohen NA, Kennedy DW. Revision endoscopic sinus surgery. Otolaryngol Clin North Am 2006;39(3):417–435, vii vii.
6. Parsons DS, Stivers FE, Talbot AR. The missed ostium sequence and the surgical approach to revision functional endoscopic sinus surgery. Otolaryngol Clin North Am 1996;29(1):169–183
7. Sathananthar S, Nagaonkar S, Paleri V, Le T, Robinson S, Wormald PJ. Canine fossa puncture and clearance of the maxillary sinus for the severely diseased maxillary sinus. Laryngoscope 2005;115(6):1026–1029
8. Sindwani R, Cohen JT, Pilch BZ, Metson RB. Myospherulosis following sinus surgery: pathological curiosity or important clinical entity? Laryngoscope 2003;113(7):1123–1127
9. Caylakli F, Yavuz H, Cagici AC, Ozluoglu LN. Endoscopic sinus surgery for maxillary sinus mucoceles. Head Face Med 2006;2:29
10. Har-El G. Endoscopic management of 108 sinus mucoceles. Laryngoscope 2001;111(12):2131–2134
11. Perloff JR, Gannon FH, Bolger WE, Montone KT, Orlandi R, Kennedy DW. Bone involvement in sinusitis: an apparent pathway for the spread of disease. Laryngoscope 2000;110(12):2095–2099
12. Bendouah Z, Barbeau J, Hamad WA, Desrosiers M. Biofilm formation by *Staphylococcus aureus* and *Pseudomonas aeruginosa* is associated with an unfavorable evolution after surgery for chronic sinusitis and nasal polyposis. Otolaryngol Head Neck Surg 2006;134(6):991–996
13. Psaltis AJ, Weitzel EK, Ha KR, Wormald PJ. The effect of bacterial biofilms on post-sinus surgical outcomes. Am J Rhinol 2008;22(1):1–6
14. Ha KR, Psaltis AJ, Butcher AR, Wormald PJ, Tan LW. In vitro activity of mupirocin on clinical isolates of *Staphylococcus aureus* and

its potential implications in chronic rhinosinusitis. Laryngoscope 2008;118(3):535–540
15. Uren B, Psaltis A, Wormald PJ. Nasal lavage with mupirocin for the treatment of surgically recalcitrant chronic rhinosinusitis. Laryngoscope 2008;118(9):1677–1680
16. Briggs RD, Wright ST, Cordes S, Calhoun KH. Smoking in chronic rhinosinusitis: a predictor of poor long-term outcome after endoscopic sinus surgery. Laryngoscope 2004;114(1):126–128
17. Agius AM, Smallman LA, Pahor AL. Age, smoking and nasal ciliary beat frequency. Clin Otolaryngol Allied Sci 1998;23(3):227–230
18. Atef A, Zeid IA, Qotb M, El Rab EG. Effect of passive smoking on ciliary regeneration of nasal mucosa after functional endoscopic sinus surgery in children. J Laryngol Otol 2009;123(1):75–79
19. Fokkens W, Lund V, Mullol J; European Position Paper on Rhinosinusitis and Nasal Polyps Group. EP3OS 2007: European position paper on rhinosinusitis and nasal polyps 2007. A summary for otorhinolaryngologists. Rhinology 2007;45(2):97–101
20. Chee L, Graham SM, Carothers DG, Ballas ZK. Immune dysfunction in refractory sinusitis in a tertiary care setting. Laryngoscope 2001;111(2):233–235
21. Bhattacharyya N. Computed tomographic staging and the fate of the dependent sinuses in revision endoscopic sinus surgery. Arch Otolaryngol Head Neck Surg 1999;125(9):994–999
22. Kountakis SE, Bradley DT. Effect of asthma on sinus computed tomography grade and symptom scores in patients undergoing revision functional endoscopic sinus surgery. Am J Rhinol 2003;17(4):215–219
23. Sieskiewicz A, Olszewska E, Rogowski M, Grycz E. Preoperative corticosteroid oral therapy and intraoperative bleeding during functional endoscopic sinus surgery in patients with severe nasal polyposis: a preliminary investigation. Ann Otol Rhinol Laryngol 2006;115(7):490–494
24. Dessi P, Castro F, Triglia JM, Zanaret M, Cannoni M. Major complications of sinus surgery: a review of 1192 procedures. J Laryngol Otol 1994;108(3):212–215
25. Maniglia AJ. Fatal and other major complications of endoscopic sinus surgery. Laryngoscope 1991;101(4 Pt 1):349–354
26. Stankiewicz JA. Complications of endoscopic sinus surgery. Otolaryngol Clin North Am 1989;22(4):749–758
27. Kirihene RK, Rees G, Wormald PJ. The influence of the size of the maxillary sinus ostium on the nasal and sinus nitric oxide levels. Am J Rhinol 2002;16(5):261–264
28. Moncada S, Palmer RM, Higgs EA. Nitric oxide: physiology, pathophysiology, and pharmacology. Pharmacol Rev 1991;43(2):109–142
29. Nathan CF, Hibbs JB Jr. Role of nitric oxide synthesis in macrophage antimicrobial activity. Curr Opin Immunol 1991;3(1):65–70
30. Nakane M, Schmidt HH, Pollock JS, Förstermann U, Murad F. Cloned human brain nitric oxide synthase is highly expressed in skeletal muscle. FEBS Lett 1993;316(2):175–180
31. Schlosser RJ, Spotnitz WD, Peters EJ, Fang K, Gaston B, Gross CW. Elevated nitric oxide metabolite levels in chronic sinusitis. Otolaryngol Head Neck Surg 2000;123(4):357–362
32. Robinson SR, Baird R, Le T, Wormald PJ. The incidence of complications after canine fossa puncture performed during endoscopic sinus surgery. Am J Rhinol 2005;19(2):203–206
33. Robinson S, Wormald PJ. Patterns of innervation of the anterior maxilla: a cadaver study with relevance to canine fossa puncture of the maxillary sinus. Laryngoscope 2005;115(10):1785–1788
34. Singhal D, Douglas R, Robinson S, Wormald PJ. The incidence of complications using new landmarks and a modified technique of canine fossa puncture. Am J Rhinol 2007;21(3):316–319

13 The Minimally Invasive Sinus Technique for the Maxillary Sinus

Peter J. Catalano

Since its introduction in the mid-1980s, functional endoscopic sinus surgery (FESS) has become the standard surgical intervention for patients with chronic sinusitis refractory to medical therapy. Unlike prior sinus procedures such as the Lothrop or Caldwell–Luc, FESS represented a targeted intervention, aimed at restoring normal sinus mucosal physiology. FESS was the first surgical model for the treatment of chronic sinusitis to address the underlying pathophysiologic mechanisms of sinusitis as first described by Messerklinger in 1978.[1]

Through his endoscopic examination of the nose, Messerklinger made several important discoveries. In his book entitled *Endoscopy of the Nose*, he describes a pattern of shifting light reflexes seen on the mucosal surface of the sinuses representing mucociliary movement that we now recognize as mucociliary transport or clearance. Using endoscopy in conjunction with time-lapse photography, he examined the direction of mucus movement and found that clearance was directed from the larger sinuses to their respective ostia. He also noted that contact between mucosal surfaces leads to disruption of mucociliary movement thereby causing retention of secretions with subsequent obstruction of the subordinate maxillary, frontal, and anterior ethmoid sinuses. Furthermore, he recognized that contact is most likely to occur in the narrow transition spaces (i.e., ethmoidal infundibulum, hiatus semilunaris superior, and retroagger space/nasofrontal recess). Although contact may be due to several causes, such as inflammation from environmental irritants, allergic rhinitis, viral infection, or anatomic distortions, these factors are most influential to the disruption of sinus physiology and development of sinusitis when they directly affect the aforementioned transition spaces. The theory that transition spaces represent the primary physiologic/anatomic bottleneck for the development of sinusitis is further supported by the high frequency with which both computed tomography (CT) and clinical exam findings demonstrate inflammation limited to the maxillary, frontal, and anterior ethmoid sinuses (the posterior ethmoid and sphenoid sinuses do not drain into transition spaces).

Another crucial principle introduced with FESS was that mucosal damage and mucociliary dysfunction is often a reversible process. Prior to Messerklinger, most rhinologists believed that the mucosal damage associated with chronic sinusitis was irreversible; therefore, procedures such as the Caldwell–Luc involved stripping of this "diseased" sinus mucosa. In his clinical experience with more than 2500 patients, Stammberger showed that once the transition spaces are cleared of disease, the larger sinuses usually heal without being touched even if mucosal damage seemed "almost irreversible."[2] Recent studies examining mucociliary clearance have shown that patients with chronic sinusitis have impaired mucociliary movement and that FESS is capable of correcting mucociliary dysfunction in these patients, thus demonstrating the reversibility of disease.[3–6] Moreover, others have shown that mechanical damage to nasal mucosal epithelium results in loss of cilia and decreased mucociliary transport.[7,8] To create optimal conditions for the reversal of disease to occur, surgical intervention should avoid destruction of cilia and emphasize mucosal preservation.

Following the discoveries of mucociliary clearance, the reversibility of mucosal damage in chronic sinusitis, and the role of transition spaces as a nidus for sinusitis, FESS was a logical advancement. The technique, based on conservatism, served as a targeted intervention addressing the narrowed transition spaces and reestablishing drainage through *primary birth* ostia while avoiding direct manipulation of the larger sinuses themselves. Kennedy demonstrated the favorable long-term results of FESS with 98.4% of 72 patients reporting improvement compared with before surgery over an average 7.8-year follow-up period.[9] Although there was a steep initial learning curve, many studies have since highlighted the relative paucity of complications associated with the procedure. In a study of 250 patients undergoing FESS, Levine reported that 8.3% of patients developed minor complications whereas only 0.7% developed major complications.[10] In comparison, a study of 670 patients undergoing the Caldwell–Luc procedure, the previous gold standard intervention for chronic maxillary sinusitis, Penttillä reported a 19% rate of major complications as a result of the operation.[11] Finally, because FESS is based on a minimally invasive approach compared with conventional sinus surgery, there was less overall postoperative discomfort and shorter hospital stays.

Although FESS initially established itself as a less invasive, more targeted, and more effective technique than its predecessors, conventional FESS has evolved beyond this description. Originally, proponents emphasized that FESS provides a conservative and effective surgical intervention, rarely requiring a middle meatal antrostomy or stripping of diseased nasal mucosa. Over time, however, there has been a departure from these conservative principles with a tendency toward more aggressive intervention. As a result, surgeons have excessive freedoms in the nose, and sinus procedures are not standardized. There is no longer a systematic reproducible surgical model called FESS, and the surgical intervention and decision-making varies widely depending on the surgeon. Routine resection of middle turbinates, creation of large maxillary antrostomies, removal of all ethmoid bone, and manipulation of normally functioning sinus ostia are common examples of an aggressive surgical trend that has evolved over time without validation. One would hope and expect that procedures and treatment philosophies would and should be modified over time. However, we should also expect that there be reasonable scientific proof in support of such change. The departure from FESS principles will be discussed at length in a subsequent section.

Although endoscopy offered a window for more precise visualization of nasal pathology, advances in other sinus instrumentation lagged. The original instruments used in FESS offered minimal precision, were associated with shear damage to normal mucosal tissue, and caused inadvertent stripping of mucus membranes. Technologic breakthroughs, coupled with a surgical model based on Messerklinger's principles, led to the next major advance in rhinology—powered instrumentation and MIST.

The Philosophy of the Minimally Invasive Sinus Technique

The minimally invasive sinus technique (MIST) is a targeted endoscopic intervention, introduced by Reuben Setliff, M.D., in 1994, with virtually identical goals to those originally reported for FESS. However, unlike *conventional* FESS, MIST strictly upholds Messerklinger's functional concepts so that the surgeon performs a very targeted initial intervention. Although sinus ostia are rarely enlarged, MIST is much more than *not* performing a middle meatal antrostomy. The procedure, as outlined in the following section, is the only stepwise intranasal intervention with a defined beginning and end for all patients regardless of disease severity, thereby standardizing the procedure for surgeons and patients alike. By starting at the most medial aspect of the lateral nasal wall and moving laterally, the surgeon minimizes risk to the lamina papyracea. Furthermore, the procedure still allows for extension into the less involved posterior ethmoid and/or sphenoid cavities while maintaining an anatomic-based progression. This elegant, reproducible technique avoids unnecessary disruption of normal mucosa while restoring mucociliary clearance through the primary birth ostia.

Although not specific to MIST, endoscopically guided powered instrumentation was first introduced with this procedure and is now routinely employed. In comparison to the early handheld instruments used in FESS, powered instruments provide through-cutting blades for improved precision and preservation of nondiseased mucosa, a key element to the restoration of normal mucociliary function. In one study, a powered microdebrider termed the *hummer* (Stryker Corp., Kalamazoo, MI), was shown by Setliff et al to be associated with accelerated healing and reduced synechiae formation.[12] Real-time continuous suctioning at the tip of the instrument obviates the need for frequent instrument removal for cleaning, thereby reducing mucosal trauma and decreasing operating time. Continuous real-time suction also improves intraoperative visibility with the potential for reduced operative morbidity. Finally, because MIST markedly reduces nasal trauma, eliminates exposed sinus bone, and decreases blood loss, the healing burden placed on the nose is minimal and the need for uncomfortable nasal packing eliminated.

MIST clearly offers several advantages over traditional methods employed in FESS. Although proponents of MIST recognize FESS as an effective surgical option for patients with chronic sinusitis, they question the need for departure from Messerklinger's functional concepts. MIST is a true embodiment of these principles and improves upon FESS by providing an anatomically based reproducible approach to sinus surgery, invokes powered instrumentation with real-time suctioning, preservation of mucosa and turbinate tissue, leaves the primary birth ostia undisturbed in most patients (see below), and decreases operative morbidity.

Turbinate tissue is critical to proper nasal and sinus physiology. Routine resection of the middle turbinate often leads to edema and/or stenosis of the nasofrontal duct, and can produce compensatory glandular hypertrophy of the remaining nasal tissue. Powered shaving (i.e., thinning) of the lateral aspect of the middle turbinate and powered resection of the lateral wall of concha bullosa can each improve middle meatal airflow without incurring the risks associated with turbinate resection. Turbinate surgery should always be coupled with the use of absorbable middle meatal stents to minimize the risk of middle meatal synechia.

Creation of a middle meatal antrostomy (MMA) is occasionally required. Absolute indications include the biopsy of an antral mass, to correct maxillary sinus recirculation due to a MMA that is *not* connected to or involving the primary birth ostium, resection of a maxillary sinus fungal ball or inverted papilloma, and to allow for the application of topical medications or repeated outpatient antral lavage in select cases or end-stage hyperplastic sinusitis. The concern with creation of an MMA is not whether it works, but whether it is necessary as a routine procedure in all patients. There is no study to date that demonstrates the routine need for or the proper size of an MMA. However, in 2004, Albu and Tomescu reported their study in which every surgical candidate with chronic rhinosinusitis (CRS) had an MMA on only one maxillary sinus, but not the other.[13] After a 19-month follow-up period, the results showed no difference in the postsurgical control of maxillary sinus symptoms or disease between the two sides. Thus, the potential risks of increased middle meatal scarring, interruption of mucociliary clearance and improper ostial function, development of maxillary recirculation by not including the natural ostia in the MMA, and the likely need for revision maxillary surgery preclude the routine creation of an MMA.

■ MIST: The Surgical Model

Preoperative Preparation

In the holding area, patients receive a series of nasal sprays with the aim of causing vasoconstriction, and thus greater operative visibility with decreased bleeding. Two sprays of oxymetazoline (0.05%) solution are administered in each nostril. Three such doses are delivered at 5-minute intervals. Following these three doses of oxymetazoline, a cocaine/epinephrine solution is delivered via an atomizer containing 8 mL cocaine (10%) and 0.16 mL of 1:100,000 epinephrine (diluted 1:50,000). Two sprays of this solution are administered every 5 minutes for the 15 minutes prior to surgery (three doses). Of note, the oxymetazoline sprays must be taken before and not concurrently with the cocaine/epinephrine solution as the former plays a role in limiting the systemic absorption, and potential toxicity of the cocaine solution.

Intraoperative Procedure

General anesthesia is preferentially achieved via a laryngeal mask technique (LMA). Three injections of lidocaine 1% with epinephrine 1:100,000 are given. The first is injected into the anterior and lateral attachment of the middle turbinate to the lateral nasal wall. The subsequent two injections are placed directly into the body of the middle turbinate (**Fig. 13.1**). If the surgeon plans to operate on the contralateral nasal cavity as well, then preinjection should be avoided because more bleeding may result from a rebound effect of the injections.

After the injections, a zero-degree endoscope is introduced and the middle turbinate gently medialized with a Freer elevator. Surgery then progresses anatomically in a step-wise manner, beginning with identification of the uncinate process at the hiatus semilunaris. The transition space located behind the uncinate associated with this landmark is the ethmoidal infundibulum. A pediatric backbiter is used, via a retrograde approach described by Parsons,[14] to incise the uncinate process from the hiatus semilunaris toward the nasolacrimal duct (posterior to anterior) (**Fig. 13.2**). This technique provides an added measure of safety by starting the uncinectomy at the furthest point from the lamina papyracea. The uncinectomy should be inspected to ensure that all three layers of the uncinate have been transected and the lamina papyracea has not been violated. Powered instruments can then be employed to extend the uncinate resection superiorly to uncover the agger nasi cells, as well as anterior and inferior to uncover the primary maxillary sinus ostium (**Fig. 13.3**). These steps serve to open the transition space of the maxillary sinus, agger nasi cells (anterior ethmoid), and frontal recess (**Fig. 13.4**).

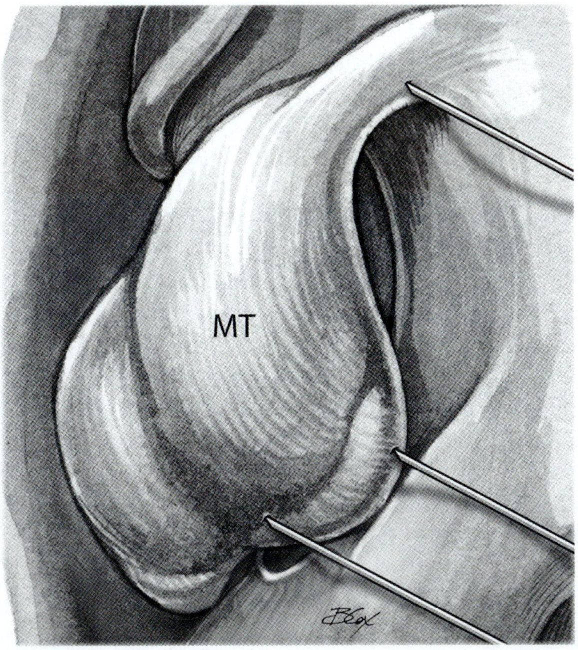

Fig. 13.1 Injections are made in the left lateral nasal wall and middle turbinate (MT).

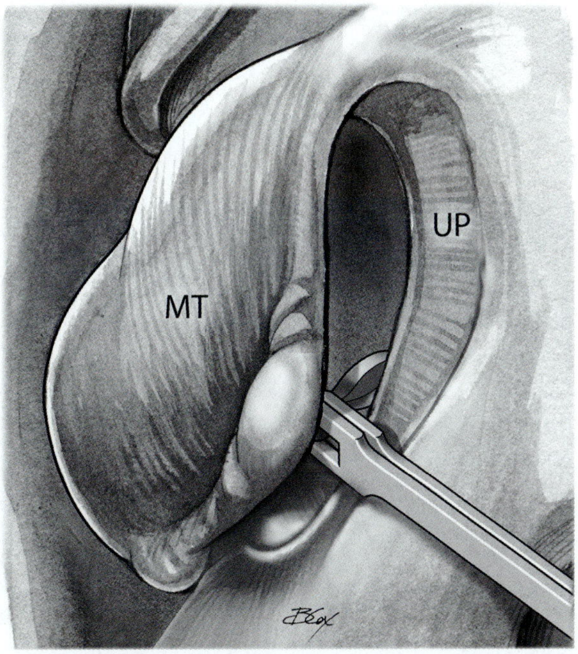

Fig. 13.2 A pediatric backbiter is used to perform a left retrograde uncinectomy. UP, uncinate process; MT, middle turbinate.

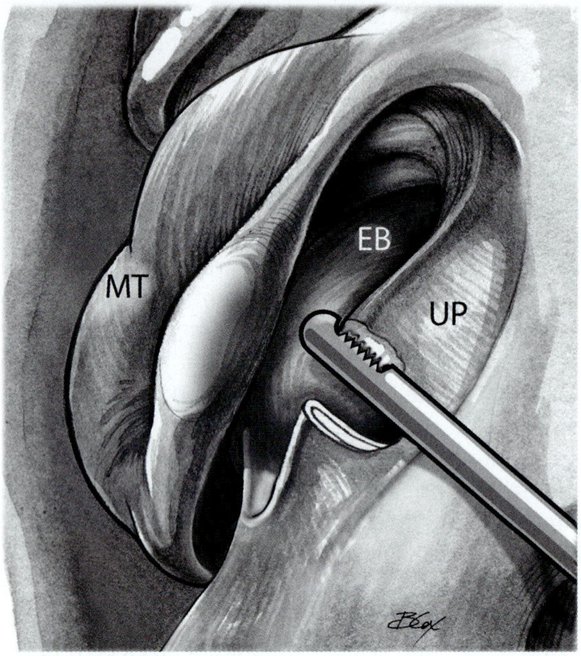

Fig. 13.3 The uncinectomy is completed superiorly and inferiorly using a microdebrider. EB, ethmoid bulla; UP, uncinate process; MT, middle turbinate.

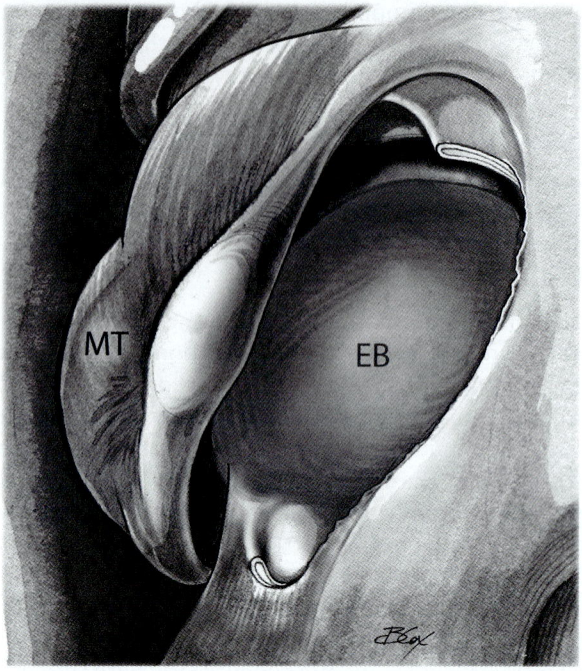

Fig. 13.4 The uncinectomy is complete exposing the maxillary os anterior and inferior in the ethmoidal infundibulum. The ethmoid bulla is also fully uncovered. EB, ethmoid bulla.

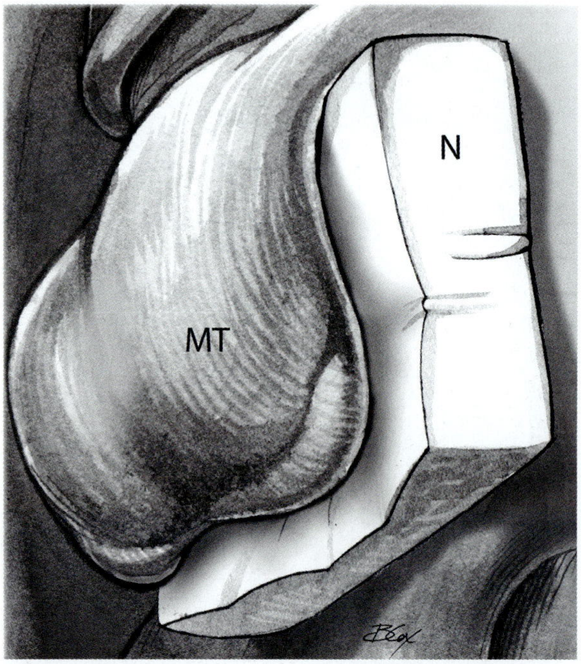

Fig. 13.5 Nasopore (Stryker Corp., Kalamazoo, MI) is placed as an absorbable middle meatal dressing to help with hemostasis, middle turbinate (MT) position, and reepithelization.

If multiple ostia are uncovered or identified in the lateral nasal wall, they are left undisturbed. Recent experience suggests that recirculation is uncommon in such cases as the mucociliary flow is already programmed *around* the additional ostia. This is in marked distinction to recirculation that occurs due to an MMA that is created in the posterior fontanelle that has no connection to the primary birth ostium. The latter case requires connection of the two ostia to correct the recirculation phenomenon.

Once the standard MIST procedure is complete, all patients receive a 1-cm wide by 2-cm long piece of Nasopore (Stryker Corp., Kalamazoo, MI) into the middle meatus[15] to prevent synechia (**Fig. 13.5**). Nasopore is a synthetic polyurethane resorbable sponge-like material that is biologically inert and functions well as a middle meatal spacer to aid in local hemostasis, medialization of the middle turbinate, and the prevention of synechia. No other nasal packing is placed. The nasopharynx, oropharynx, and hypopharynx are suctioned free of blood and debris that might have accumulated. The patient can then be safely reversed from anesthesia. Use of the laryngeal mask airway reduces the risk of coughing and/or bucking and the associated nasal hemorrhage during emergence (**see Videos 13.1, 13.2, and 13.3**).

Postoperative Care

All patients are prescribed an oral antibiotic for the first 5 days after surgery. Nasal saline irrigations are begun within

24 hours of surgery and maintained for a minimum of 4 weeks. Middle meatal debridement is rarely required postoperatively. Most patients are able to return to work or school in 24 to 48 hours following the procedure regardless of the extent of surgery. Thus, MIST is not minimal surgery; however, it is *minimally invasive* surgery. There are no diet or activity limitations for most patients. Pain is usually minimal and well controlled with acetaminophen. Antihistamines and nasal steroid sprays are avoided for the first month following surgery to avoid excessive mucosal dryness and reduced ciliary flow.

Outcome Studies

Since its introduction in the literature in 1996,[12,14] MIST has grown in popularity worldwide. However, it was not until January 2002 that a formal outcome study was published comparing MIST to FESS.[15] This study used the Chronic Sinusitis Survey (CSS) as the quality of life outcome instrument to assess improvement following MIST. The CSS was chosen because it has been proven a reliable, sensitive, and easily administered test to evaluate patient disability from chronic sinusitis. The CSS has also been used in previous outcome reports on FESS, allowing a direct comparison of the two techniques (**see Video 13.4**). To summarize: outcome from MIST as measured by the CSS medication, CSS symptom, and CSS total subscales either equaled or surpassed those after FESS. Compared with FESS, many more patients after MIST were improved to a level that was better than the normative symptom data for healthy individuals in the general population. The follow-up period for the MIST study was twice as long (23 months compared with 12 months) as the FESS study, yet still demonstrated improvement; and the surgical revision rate following MIST was 5.9% compared with an average of 10% following FESS. Furthermore, the results seen following MIST were consistent across the spectrum of disease severity (using CT grades I through IV), disproving the opinion that the procedure was only effective for minimal disease.

These findings strongly support the recommendation that MIST be considered the initial surgical intervention for the treatment of chronic sinusitis. It strongly suggests that an excellent quality of life for chronic sinus sufferers could be achieved with targeted surgical manipulation of the nose and sinuses, it validates Messerklinger's transition space theory and the reversibility of diseased nasal membranes, and it contradicts the rationale for the routine creation of a middle meatal antrostomy.

Another, less formal outcome study on MIST entitled "Minimally Invasive Sinus Surgery in the Geriatric Patient" was published in 2001.[16] The study used a geriatric population (ages 65–93) of 100 patients undergoing MIST for chronic sinusitis, to assess whether, due to their age, they had a greater potential for intra- or postoperative complications. Quality of life outcome following surgery was also assessed subjectively 6 months after surgery by the study patients. Eighty-four percent of patients reported feeling significantly better, 10% somewhat better, and 6% unchanged. In comparison, another study of 119 patients with chronic sinusitis reported that 80.2% of patients experienced relief after FESS.[10] Interestingly, 8 of 10 patients who reported feeling "somewhat better" after MIST, and two of six patients who experienced no improvement, had previously undergone aggressive FESS elsewhere. This supports the opinion that aggressive FESS may have "irreversible adverse effects on nasal and sinus function."

The study also assessed whether there was any exacerbation of preexisting medical conditions, or an increase in surgical morbidity after MIST. The 100 patients presented a spectrum of preexisting medical conditions including hypertension, coronary disease, gastrointestinal disorders, diabetes, bronchitis and asthma, thyroid disorders, gout, stroke, renal disease, prostate disease, dysrhythmias, and others. Early medical complications (within 96 hours of surgery) following MIST included 12 patients with headache, 6 with postoperative sinusitis, 4 had nausea and vomiting, 3 had fatigue, and 1 each with ataxia, hyposmia, syncope, incontinence, and hypoxia. The ataxia and syncope were self-limited and appropriate evaluation was obtained. The nausea, vomiting, incontinence, and hypoxia all occurred in the recovery area following surgery and were self-limited. In addition to verifying the efficacy of MIST for the treatment of chronic sinusitis, the results highlight the fact that minimal medical/surgical morbidity is experienced by geriatric patients following MIST, making the procedure equally safe for the oldest and potentially most frail portion of the population.

The findings of these studies are significant because they introduce several new concepts:

- Due to a combination of minimally invasive mucosal-sparing surgery, and biocompatible, biodegradable middle meatal stents, synechia following MIST are rare.[17]
- Because MIST does not manipulate the primary maxillary sinus ostium, the latter remains in the oblique or horizontal plane making it less likely to be obstructed by a lateralized middle turbinate, whereas the final position of an MMA is in the parasagittal plane, making it much more vulnerable to obstruction by a lateralized middle turbinate.
- Outcomes data has shown clinical equivalence, if not superiority, from MIST when compared with conventional FESS, thus excellent outcomes across the spectrum of disease can be achieved with *less invasive* surgery, and for the maxillary sinus, this means no antrostomy.

The results of these peer-reviewed articles validate MIST as an effective surgical treatment option for chronic sinusitis. We advocate that MIST should be considered as the initial procedure for patients undergoing ESS for chronic sinus disease. This would minimize the number of patients who receive more surgery (i.e., an MMA) than is required. In our experience,[15] the overall MIST revision rate is 6%, thus 94% of patients had appropriate surgery, with only 6% needing additional intervention, and this rarely included the need to perform an MMA.

Adjunctive Technologies—Sinuplasty

As in other medical fields, sinus surgery has evolved from open to less invasive surgical techniques. As recently as the 1970s, sinus surgery required external facial incisions and resulted in extensive removal of tissue and mucosa. It was hypothesized that diseased mucosa was the primary cause of the condition and should be removed.

With the advent of first FESS, and then MIST, treatment of chronic sinusitis took an evolutionary leap forward. These procedures pioneered the use of endoscopes and powered surgical instruments allowing sinus surgery to be performed through the nostrils. One of the goals of FESS and MIST is to uncover the primary sinus ostia to improve sinus ventilation and drainage while preserving the natural birth membrane sinuses and their ostia. During contemporary FESS, the sinus ostia are enlarged with metal surgical instruments, which pose a risk to the mucosal cilia lining the sinus ostia. During MIST, the ostia are uncovered or exposed by marsupializing the transition space to a given sinus, but the ostia remain untouched. Enter sinuplasty, a new technology based on balloon catheter dilatation of the sinus transition space and its ostia with the ability to preserve birth membranes.

To gain initial sinus access, the preshaped sinus guide catheter is introduced to the exit of the transition space of the target sinus under endoscopic visualization. A flexible sinus guide wire is introduced through the sinus guide catheter and gently advanced into the target sinus under fluoroscopic guidance. The sinus balloon catheter tracks smoothly over the guide wire and is positioned across the blocked ostium. Using fluoroscopy, or using sinus transillumination with a lighted guide wire, the position of the sinus balloon catheter is confirmed. It is gradually inflated to between 8 and 10 atmospheres of pressure to gently restructure and enlarge the blocked ostium. The balloon diameters range from 3.5 to 7 mm. The balloon is then deflated and removed, having enlarged the transition space and ostium to allow the return of normal sinus drainage and function. There is little to no disruption to the mucosal lining.

This technology has been first evaluated in eight human cadavers revealing micro fractures of the bony framework of the sinus ostium, with no visible damage to the skull base or corresponding neurovascular anatomy. In a subsequent study of 125 patients (the CLEAR study), the technology was again shown to be safe with 90% of the treated ostia remaining patent at 6-month follow-up, with longer-term follow-up providing consistent results at 1 and 2 years postsurgery. Personal experience to date in 500 patients has demonstrated safety and similar effectiveness.

Pearls

- Always evaluate the preoperative CT for Haller cells, location and position of the uncinate process, size of the infundibular space, secondary ostia, osteoneogenesis, and bone erosion.
- Always enter the infundibulum from the most inferior aspect of the hiatus semilunaris, what is called the "common final outflow pathway." Note this entry point is usually *lower* than the position of the maxillary os itself, and so the path of your uncinectomy should be angled slightly superior as you move from posterior to anterior along the uncinate process with your backbiter.
- Always follow your uncinate process as far anterior as you can to expose the maxillary os, which is usually located anterior and lateral along the floor of the infundibulum. However, be cautious *not* to extend your uncinectomy anterior to the anterior tip of the middle turbinate, or past the breakpoint on the lateral nasal wall to avoid orbital entry via the lamina. On occasion, the origin of the uncinate process *is* anterior to the origin of the middle turbinate; however, this is rare and is best addressed carefully with use of a 30-degree telescope to help assess this possibility.
- If multiple natural ostia are encountered, leave them alone! The only time recirculation is clinically significant is when it occurs after a man-made antrostomy in the posterior fontanelle and is not connected to the primary os. Naturally occurring secondary os are not problematic as the ciliary flow has already been established around these openings, thus avoiding recirculation.
- Remove as much uncinate process as possible, including superiorly to uncover the agger nasi cell. Inferiorly, you should be able to visualize the maxillary os with a zero- or 30-degree endoscope in all cases. Use of a short ball-tipped probe/seeker can be useful if the mucosa is polypoid and the os not immediately visible. Gentle probing of the os is acceptable with the seeker; however, routine use of a curved suction as a seeker with probing of the os is usually not advisable. If the os seems stenotic (which is rare), a balloon catheter can be used to dilate it to 5 mm.
- Allow polypoid tissue to recover as reversibility is common in this area once the uncinate is removed and the physiologic and anatomic "bottleneck" is corrected.
- Begin twice daily nasal saline irrigations the day after surgery and continue for 1 month. Nasal debridements are unnecessary in >98% of patients.

References

1. Messerklinger W. Endoscopy of the Nose. Baltimore: Urban and Schwarzenberg; 1978
2. Stammberger H. Endoscopic endonasal surgery—concepts in treatment of recurring rhinosinusitis. Part II. Surgical technique. Otolaryngol Head Neck Surg 1986;94(2):147–156
3. Ikeda K, Oshima T, Furukawa M, et al. Restoration of the mucociliary clearance of the maxillary sinus after endoscopic sinus surgery. J Allergy Clin Immunol 1997;99(1 Pt 1):48–52
4. Asai K, Haruna S, Otori N, Yanagi K, Fukami M, Moriyama H. Saccharin test of maxillary sinus mucociliary function after endoscopic sinus surgery. Laryngoscope 2000;110(1):117–122
5. Elwany S, Hisham M, Gamaee R. The effect of endoscopic sinus surgery on mucociliary clearance in patients with chronic sinusitis. Eur Arch Otorhinolaryngol 1998;255(10):511–514
6. Min YG, Yun YS, Song BH, Cho YS, Lee KS. Recovery of nasal physiology after functional endoscopic sinus surgery: olfaction and mucociliary transport. ORL J Otorhinolaryngol Relat Spec 1995;57(5):264–268
7. Yang TQ, Majima Y, Guo Y, Harada T, Shimizu T, Takeuchi K. Mucociliary transport function and damage of ciliated epithelium. Am J Rhinol 2002;16(4):215–219
8. Melgarejo Moreno PJ, Hellín Meseguer D, Alpay F. [Disturbances in mucociliary clearance after maxillary sinus surgery. Experimental study]. Acta Otorrinolaringol Esp 1997;48(2):105–108
9. Senior BA, Kennedy DW, Tanabodee J, Kroger H, Hassab M, Lanza D. Long-term results of functional endoscopic sinus surgery. Laryngoscope 1998;108(2):151–157
10. Levine HL. Functional endoscopic sinus surgery: evaluation, surgery, and follow-up of 250 patients. Laryngoscope 1990;100(1):79–84
11. Penttilä MA, Rautiainen MEP, Pukander JS, Karma PH. Endoscopic versus Caldwell-Luc approach in chronic maxillary sinusitis: comparison of symptoms at one-year follow-up. Rhinology 1994;32(4):161–165
12. Setliff RC III, Parsons DS. The "Hummer": new instrumentation for functional endoscopic sinus surgery. Am J Rhinol 1994;8:275–278
13. Albu S, Tomescu E. Small and large middle meatus antrostomies in the treatment of chronic maxillary sinusitis. Otolaryngol Head Neck Surg 2004;131(4):542–547
14. Setliff RC III. Minimally invasive sinus surgery: the rationale and the technique. Otolaryngol Clin North Am 1996;29(1):115–124
15. Catalano PJ, Roffman E. Outcome in patients with chronic sinusitis after the minimally invasive sinus technique. Am J Rhinol 2003;17(1):17–22
16. Catalano PJ, Setliff RC III, Catalano LA. Minimally invasive sinus surgery in the geriatric patient. Oper Tech Otolaryngol Head Neck Surg 2001;12(2):85–90
17. Catalano PJ, Roffman EJ. Evaluation of middle meatal stenting after minimally invasive sinus techniques (MIST). Otolaryngol Head Neck Surg 2003;128(6):875–881

14 Balloon Sinuplasty for the Maxillary Sinus

Winston C. Vaughan and Roy F. Thomas

Chronic rhinosinusitis affects 31 million adults in the United States each year, resulting in direct annual health care costs reaching $5.8 billion, with indirect costs higher due to lost productivity.[1,2] Current treatment options include medical therapy and management of allergies, with surgery reserved for those who fail medical treatment. Candidates for surgery are determined based on clinical and endoscopic exam findings, symptoms, and evidence of obstruction of the sinus on computed tomography (CT) scans.

Although an estimated 500,000 sinus procedures are performed annually,[3] many other patients decline surgery due to risks and morbidity involved, or are deemed to be poor surgical candidates owing to comorbid conditions. The goal of modern endoscopic surgery is to open the ostium of the sinus and to restore normal mucociliary clearance. When considering the maxillary sinus, this commonly involves removal of the uncinate process and creation of an antrostomy, which includes the natural ostium of the sinus. Of course, tissue removal introduces bleeding and potential for scarring, as well as recirculation phenomenon if the maxillary ostium is not included in the antrostomy. Recently, new techniques have been introduced that may have less morbidity than traditional dissection methods. This technology uses dilatational balloon catheter systems similar to those used in the fields of interventional cardiology, gastroenterology, vascular and urologic surgery. Two sets of Food and Drug Administration- (FDA-) approved devices utilize balloon catheter technology to access the natural ostium of the maxillary sinus and dilate it without removal of tissue. This may result in a functional ostium without some of the morbidities encountered with traditional dissection. Balloon catheter technology may be used alone or in combination with standard dissection, as a hybrid technique. We describe the technique for maxillary sinuplasty with the Relieva sinus balloon catheter (Acclarent, Menlo Park, CA) and briefly review the FinESS sinus treatment (Entellus Medical, Maple Grove, MN).

Indications and Contraindications for Sinus Balloon Dilation

Sinus balloon dilation is indicated for many of the similar indications for FESS.[4] We currently consider these devices in patients meeting the following criteria:

- History of chronic or recurrent sinusitis *and*
  - Failure of extended medical therapy to include oral and topical steroids, as well as evaluation and treatment of allergic conditions
  - A persistently abnormal CT scan, after at least 4 weeks of appropriate (preferably culture-directed) antibiotic therapy
  - Four or more documented episodes (data: symptoms with positive CT or endoscopic exam) of acute maxillary rhinosinusitis yearly

Balloon dilation may be contraindicated in patients with:

- Sinonasal polyps involving the maxillary sinus or the middle meatus
- Allergic fungal sinusitis
- Sinonasal tumors
- Extensive osteoneogenesis
- Previous history of facial trauma involving the maxillary sinus
- Mucopyocele

Instruments

Standard sinus surgery instrumentation including angled endoscopes (we routinely use 30 and 70 degree) are recommended to survey the lateral nasal wall during and after the procedure, to ensure cannulation and dilatation of the maxillary sinus ostium. In addition to standard instruments, maxillary sinuplasty requires guide catheters, flexible guide wires, balloon catheters, and an inflation device with manometer (**Fig. 14.1**). Guide catheters are available with multiple angulations, and balloon catheters are available in 3.5-mm, 5-mm (standard), 6-mm, and 7-mm sizes. Attachments are available to permit use with image guidance and have been found to be useful by some surgeons.[5] Sinus lavage catheters are also available for use after dilatation.

The balloon catheter dilation system is prepared according to the manufacturer's instructions. If fluoroscopy is to be used to confirm placement of the guide wire and balloon, then contrast medium diluted in sterile saline/water is used to inflate the balloon so as to be visible across the ostium. The anteroposterior (AP) view is recommended during cannulation of the maxillary sinuses. In some states in the United States, use of the C-arm requires specialized training, testing, and licensing to allow its use. Maxillary sinu-

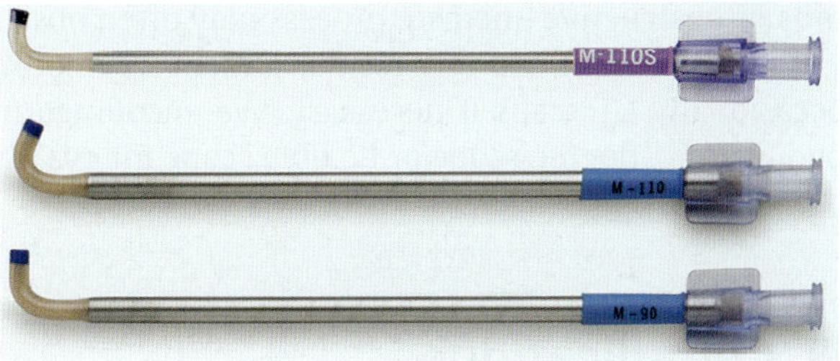

A

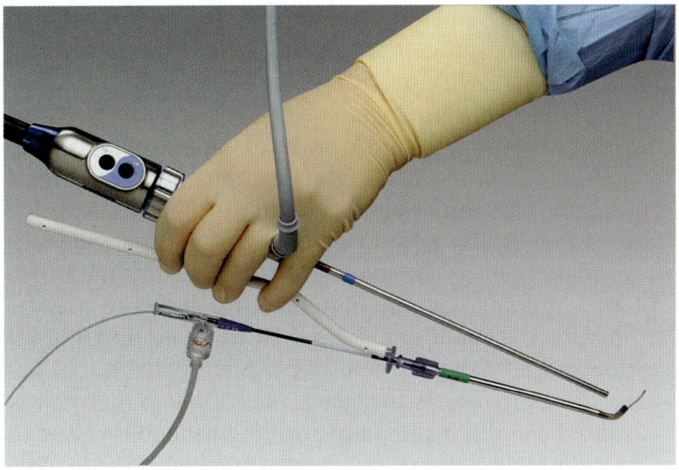

B

Fig. 14.1 **(A)** Balloon sinuplasty (Acclarent, Inc., Menlo Park, CA) guide catheters for the maxillary sinus are available in 90- and 110-degree configurations with smaller guide size designated "s." **(B)** Direct visualization system shown with guide catheter, guide wire, balloon, guide catheter handle, high pressure extension tubing and endoscope. Not shown: balloon inflation device. (Courtesy of Acclarent Inc., Menlo Park, CA)

plasty may also be performed without use of the C-arm by means of an illuminated guide wire (Luma; Acclarent, Menlo Park, CA). This guide wire utilizes fiberoptic light transmission to allow confirmation of placement in the targeted sinus through sinus transillumination. In the event that the transillumination method is used, contrast medium is unnecessary and sterile saline or water is used. The maximum recommended pressure is 16 atmospheres (1.6 megapascal), although in practice, we have found that between 8 and 12 atmospheres (800–1200 kilopascal) is typically sufficient. The 90- and 110-degree guide catheters are recommended for dilatation of the maxillary sinus.

Surgical Technique

Surgical technique is demonstrated in **Videos 14.1 and 14.2**. The sinuplasty equipment is prepared and tested prior to use. The nasal cavity is then prepped for endoscopic sinus surgery. Oxymetazoline 0.05% is applied to the nasal cavities on cottonoid pledgets. After appropriate time for vasoconstriction, the nasal cavities are surveyed endoscopically. Local injections may be made with 1% xylocaine with 1:100,000 epinephrine at the axilla of the middle turbinate and uncinate process. We have found, however, that with sinuplasty for the maxillary sinus local

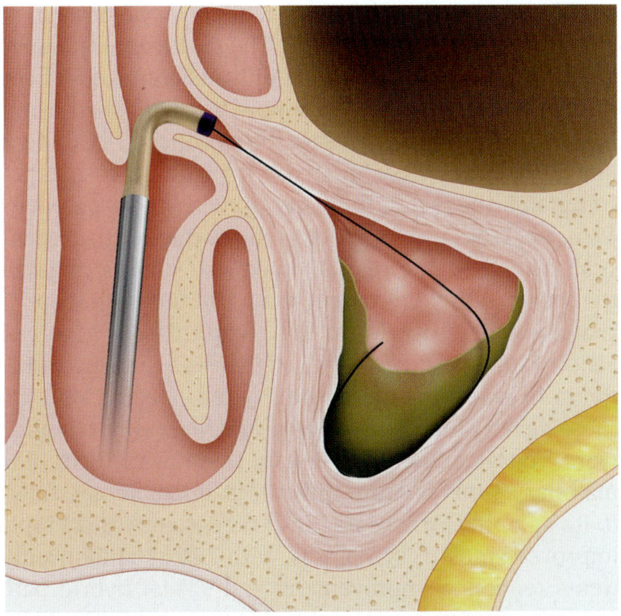

A

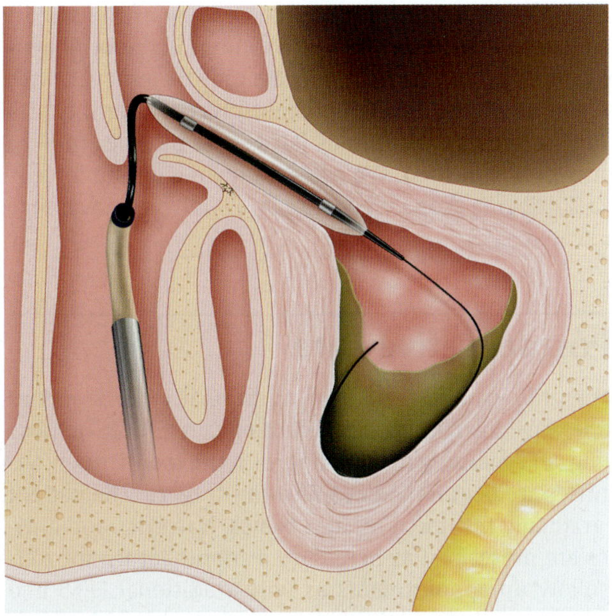

B

Fig. 14.2 **(A)** The guide catheter is placed at the maxillary ostium and the guide wire is advanced into the sinus. **(B)** The balloon is positioned across the ostium and inflated to dilate the sinus. (Courtesy of Acclarent Inc., Menlo Park, CA)

injections are frequently not necessary. The 90- or 110-degree guiding catheter with guide wire is then advanced into the nasal cavity under endoscopic visualization, and passed posterior to the uncinate process. It is then rotated downward to the expected location of the maxillary ostium at approximately the level of the junction of the lower third and upper two thirds of the middle turbinate. The guide wire is then gently advanced under fluoroscopic guidance until placement in the maxillary sinus is confirmed (**Fig. 14.2A**). Alternatively, the illuminated guide wire may be used with the room lights dimmed to allow transillumination of the maxillary sinus. The guide wire should not meet resistance as it is advanced. The balloon is then gently advanced over the guide wire until the balloon is centered across the sinus ostium. Radiopaque markers at the leading and trailing ends of the balloon assure that the balloon is completely deployed and may be visualized endoscopically and radiographically.

After confirmation of correct placement of the balloon, the assistant slowly inflates the balloon while reading off the pressures to the surgeon (**Fig. 14.2B**). Pressures of 8 to 12 atmospheres (800–1200 kilopascal) are usually adequate. The uncinate process will be noted to be displaced anteriorly during inflation. Following dilation of the maxillary sinus ostium, the contrast medium or saline is slowly withdrawn into the device and the balloon is removed from the nasal cavity. Angled endoscopes are then used to view the lateral nasal wall and maxillary sinus. We recommend use of both the 30- and 70-degree scopes for this purpose to assure that the true ostium has been dilated and an accessory ostium has not been created. If this is the case, it should be joined to the natural ostium with standard endoscopic instrumentation, such as a seeker, 90-degree forceps or backbiter. If the uncinate process precludes endoscopic view of the maxillary sinus and dilation of the true ostium is in doubt, the inferior portion of the uncinate process may be removed with backbiting or angled through-cutting forceps. After the dilation has been performed, sinus lavage and biopsies may be performed as indicated. We use a 90-degree giraffe forceps with a 70-degree scope when biopsy or polyp removal may be indicated.

Postoperative Care

Postoperative care is similar to traditional FESS. Standard postoperative instructions include no heavy lifting, no nose blowing, and sneezing or coughing with the mouth open. Saline rinses are begun the day following surgery. The patient may gradually resume normal routines. Narcotics and antibiotics are prescribed as necessary. Patients return for routine follow-up appointments as with traditional FESS and the middle meatus is debrided as needed, although this is frequently unnecessary. The maxillary ostium is visualized with an angled endoscope if possible, although an edematous or obstructive uncinate process may often obstruct the view. In this case, we rely on the patient's symptoms and occasionally CT scans if necessary. We encourage use of a pediatric 70-degree scope or flexible scope for evaluation of the postdilation ostia.

Complications

Potential complications for ostial dilation are similar to FESS. These include adhesions, stenosis of ostia, orbital, lacrimal, neurovascular, and intracranial injuries.[6] Performing dilation, as with FESS, the surgeon must preoperatively review the patient's CT scans, utilize his/her knowledge of paranasal sinus anatomy during surgery and be prepared to deal with complications if they arise. In practice, however, we have found dilatation of the maxillary sinus to be a very safe technique. The most common pitfall encountered is creation of an accessory ostium rather than dilating the natural ostium of the maxillary sinus. This is due to the location of the ostium and the need to pass the guide wire behind the uncinate, then anteroinferior and laterally to access the sinus. This is why we feel it is crucial to visualize the true ostium with angled endoscopes prior to termination of the procedure. In addition, inflation of the balloon may destabilize the uncinate process as it is displaced anteriorly. If the uncinate is felt to be at risk for scarring to the middle turbinate, it may be partially removed.

Outcomes

Initial outcome data are now available for balloon dilation, confirming that it is a safe and effective technique, in selected patients (**Figs. 14.3A,B**). The multicenter prospective CLEAR (Clinical Evaluation to Confirm Safety and Efficacy in the Paranasal Sinuses) Study now has published 6-month, 1-, and 2-year follow-up data for its cohort.[7–9] Of 142 maxillary ostia that were dilated with balloon catheters, 124 completed the 6-month follow-up with a 91% patency rate, 1% nonpatent, and 8% indeterminate due to inadequate visualization.[7] At one year, 92 maxillary sinuses remained in the study: 90% were patent with 10% indeterminate.[8] At 2 years, patency rates were not recapitulated; however, revision rates were reviewed, with seven sinuses in 65 patients followed for the entire 2 years needing revision. Of these seven sinuses, five were maxillary sinuses and two were frontal sinuses. These data seem to confirm that the maxillary sinus is more difficult to dilate successfully due to its anatomy. At 2 years, 51 of 60 patients (85%) reported improved sinusitis symptoms, with 77% of balloon-only patients reporting improvement, and 93% of hybrid patients reporting improvement. Lund–Mackay and SNOT-20 scores showed significant improvement in both sets of patients at 2 years as well.[9]

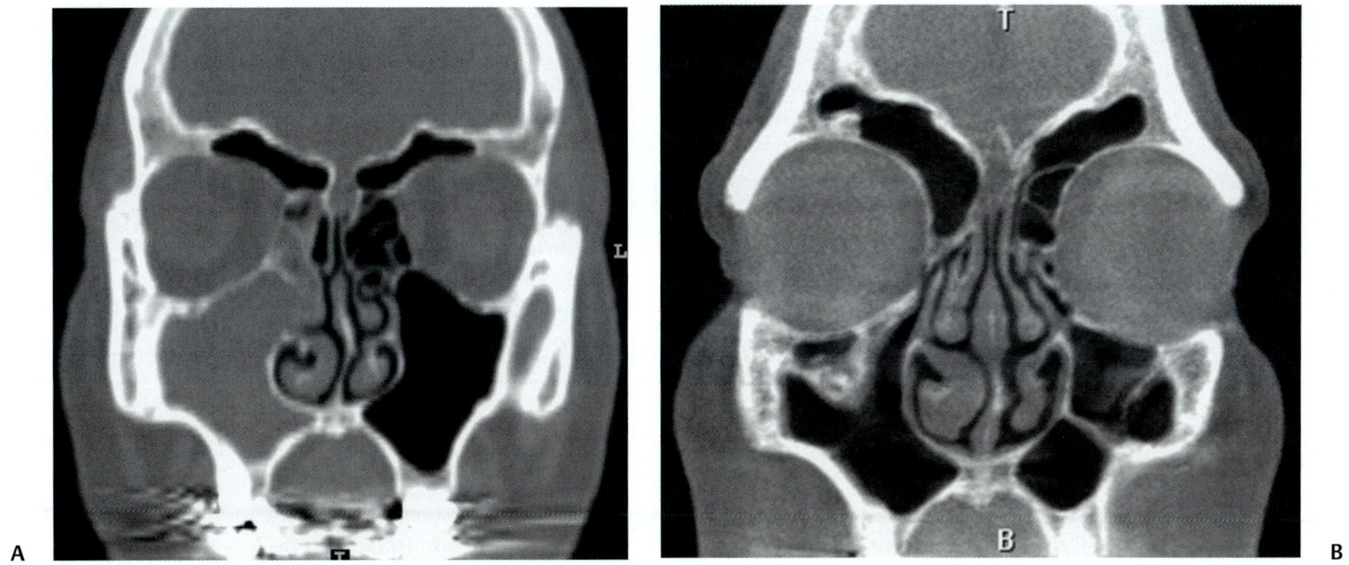

Fig. 14.3 **(A)** Preoperative computed tomography (CT) scan showing obstruction of the right maxillary sinus with anterior ethmoid disease. **(B)** Postoperative CT scan 2 years following dilation showing long-term patency of the maxillary sinus and resolution of the ethmoid disease.

Other Available Technology

The FinESS sinus treatment (Entellus Medical, Maple Grove, MN) was approved for human use by the FDA in April 2008 (**Fig. 14.4**). This sinus treatment accesses the maxillary sinus via an antral puncture. A dual lumen catheter is then passed into the maxillary sinus. The double lumen allows use of a microendoscope to visualize the ostiomeatal complex while a balloon catheter is passed into the ostium. This is then inflated to dilate the ostium and ethmoid infundibulum. This procedure can be performed under local anesthesia. The BREATHE I clinical study is collecting long-term follow-up data, which may help establish its effectiveness and allow comparison with other sinus dilation techniques and standard FESS.

Conclusion

Balloon catheter dilatation of the maxillary sinus is a safe, effective, and minimally invasive technique available to the sinus surgeon for a selected subset of patients. The surgeon must always be willing to convert to a traditional approach if so indicated. Due to the position of the maxillary ostium, it is recommended that it be viewed with angled endoscopes to ensure that an accessory ostium is not created that could lead to mucus recirculation. If visualization is not possible, the lower portion of the uncinate may be removed for this purpose.

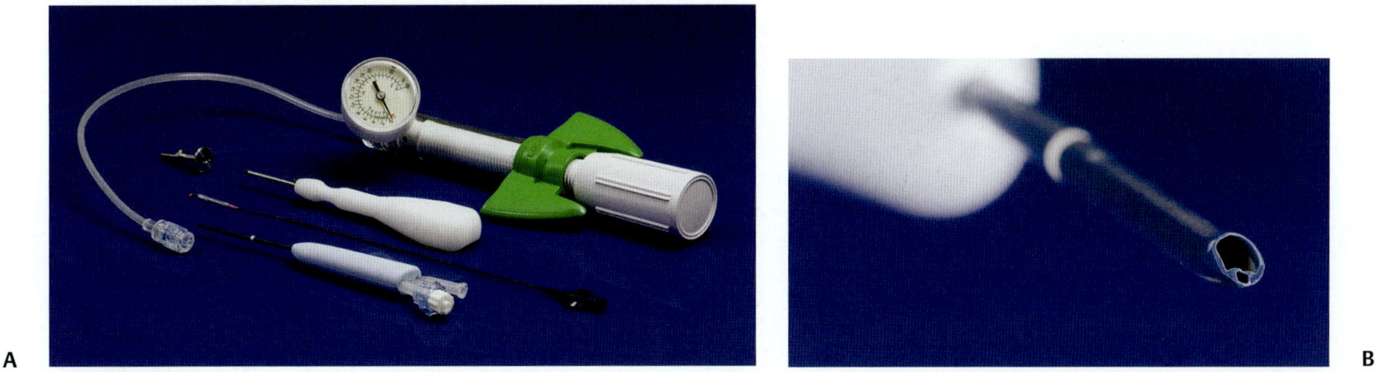

Fig. 14.4 **(A)** FinESS (Entellus Medical, Maple Grove, MN) sinus treatment system includes trocar, dual lumen cannula, balloon inflation device, and balloon catheter. **(B)** Dual lumen cannula allows visualization of placement of balloon catheter with a microendoscope across the maxillary sinus ostium prior to inflation. (Courtesy of Entellus Medical, Maple Grove, MN)

Pearls

- Patients with isolated maxillary sinus disease with failure of medical management may be candidates for balloon dilatation.
- Patients with comorbid conditions may benefit from a less invasive procedure such as balloon catheter dilation.
- Dilation of the maxillary sinus may be technically challenging due to the position of the ostium and uncinate process.
- Correct placement of the guide wire may be confirmed either fluoroscopically or via transillumination.
- Confirmation of dilation of the true maxillary sinus ostium is recommended through use of angled endoscopes, preferably 30 and 70 degree.
- Balloon catheter dilatation may be combined with traditional FESS techniques.
- A portion of the uncinate process may be removed to help with access in the office and surveillance.
- Potential complications are similar to FESS.
- Long-term patency is similar to FESS.

References

1. Lethbridge-Cejku M, Rose D, Vickerie J. Summary health statistics for U.S. adults: National Health Interview Survey, 2004. National Center for Health Statistics. Vital Health Stat 2006;10(228):19–22
2. Anand VK. Epidemiology and economic impact of rhinosinusitis. Ann Otol Rhinol Laryngol Suppl 2004;193:3–5
3. Owings MF, Kozak LJ. Ambulatory and inpatient procedures in the United States 1996. National Center for Health Statistics. Vital Health Stat 1998;13(139):25
4. Clinical Indicators. Endoscopic sinus surgery, adult. In: Clinical Indicators for Otolaryngology–Head and Neck Surgery. Alexandria, VA: American Academy of Otolaryngology- Head and Neck Surgery; 2000
5. Leventhal D, Heffelfinger R, Rosen M. Using image guidance tracking during balloon catheter dilation of sinus ostia. Otolaryngol Head Neck Surg 2007;137(2):341–342
6. Stankiewicz JA. Complications of endoscopic sinus surgery. Otolaryngol Clin North Am 1989;22(4):749–758
7. Bolger WE, Brown CL, Church CA, et al. Safety and outcomes of balloon catheter sinusotomy: a multicenter 24-week analysis in 115 patients. Otolaryngol Head Neck Surg 2007;137(1):10–20
8. Kuhn FA, Church CA, Goldberg AN, et al. Balloon catheter sinusotomy: one-year follow-up—outcomes and role in functional endoscopic sinus surgery. Otolaryngol Head Neck Surg 2008; 139(3, Suppl 3)S27–S37
9. Weiss RL, Church CA, Kuhn FA, Levine HL, Sillers MJ, Vaughan WC. Long-term outcome analysis of balloon catheter sinusotomy: two-year follow-up. Otolaryngol Head Neck Surg 2008; 139(3, Suppl 3) S38–S46

15 The View in Support of Middle Turbinate Preservation and Medialization

John Lee, Jayakar V. Nayak, and James N. Palmer

The middle turbinate (MT), also known as the middle concha, has always been regarded as a key landmark in endoscopic sinus surgery (ESS). Its location, forming the medial boundary of the ostiomeatal complex, places it at the center of much of the effort to restore functional mucociliary clearance, particularly in the maxillary sinus. Determining the appropriate surgical approach to the MT has been a controversial topic for as long as intranasal surgery has been performed.[1] Arguments in favor of MT resection have included easier endoscopic access, prevention of MT lateralization and synechia formation, increased maxillary antrostomy patency rates, as well as inflammatory changes to the MT itself.[2–6] However, the MT is a normal anatomic structure within the nasal cavity whose physiologic properties contribute to the overall milieu of the paranasal sinuses. Keeping this in mind, the debate on MT preservation or resection should revolve around whether this structure is, in fact, involved in the disease process itself. In the setting of a normal MT, we believe that the MT can and should be preserved in the majority of cases regarding maxillary sinus surgery. In this chapter, we aim to address the reasons for preservation of the MT as well as describe techniques to preserve this structure in various clinical situations.

Physiologic Reasons for Preservation

The MT plays a wide variety of physiologic roles within the nasal cavity. Some of the most accepted critical functions include the following:[1,7–10]

- Directing and maintaining laminar airflow
- Humidifying and warming inspired air
- Particulate filtration to protect the maxillary and ethmoid cavities from the drying effects of inspired air, which may disrupt mucociliary clearance
- Participation in the nasal cycle
- Participation in olfaction

Given these functions, it would seem detrimental to routinely resect the MT in all cases of sinus surgery. The continued presence of unfiltered, cold, dry air flowing in a turbulent fashion may potentially lead to chronic mucosal dryness, squamous metaplasia, and even atrophy of the nasal mucosa. Although difficult to quantify, one study has tried to evaluate the changes in the nasal cavity environment following turbinate resection. In a selection of patients undergoing middle and inferior turbinate resection for inverted papilloma removal via a midfacial degloving approach, the authors found a significant decrease in nasopharyngeal humidity and temperature when compared with the nonoperated side.[11] Although this study involves a much more extensive procedure than partial middle turbinectomy alone, the results suggest possible problems that may be encountered with loss of turbinate tissue. Along this same spectrum is the risk of atrophic rhinitis. Similar to other authors, we have noticed certain patients who develop chronic drying and crusting within the maxillary sinus following MT sacrifice.[12,13] One final concern is the development of empty nose syndrome (ENS). Although this entity of paradoxical nasal obstruction in the presence of a widely patent nasal cavity is more commonly associated with inferior turbinate resection, there has been a recent case report of ENS associated with MT resection alone.[14] Clearly then, although the full role of MT function remains incompletely understood, there is enough potential for unforeseen physiologic problems that may arise with unjustified MT sacrifice.

Anatomic Reasons for Preservation

Perhaps the most important reason for MT preservation is that the turbinate represents a consistent bony landmark in ESS. Arising from the third ethmoturbinal in the nasal cavity, the MT has three distinct planes and attachments. The anterior one-third of the MT sits in the parasagittal plane and attaches superiorly at the skull base at the lateral edge of the lamina cribrosa. The middle one-third lies in the coronal plane and turns laterally to insert into the lamina papyracea. And finally, the posterior one-third lies in the axial plane and attaches to both the lamina papyracea and the medial wall of the maxillary sinus.[15] This three-dimensional attachment provides significant stability to the MT. In addition, the MT provides a bony structural boundary to many of paranasal sinus drainage pathways:

- The MT forms the medial boundary of the ostiomeatal complex (OMC), the functional drainage pathway of the frontal, maxillary, and anterior ethmoid sinuses
- The basal lamella of the MT provides the boundary between the anterior and posterior ethmoids
- The anterior, superior portion of the MT provides the medial boundary of the frontal recess (when the

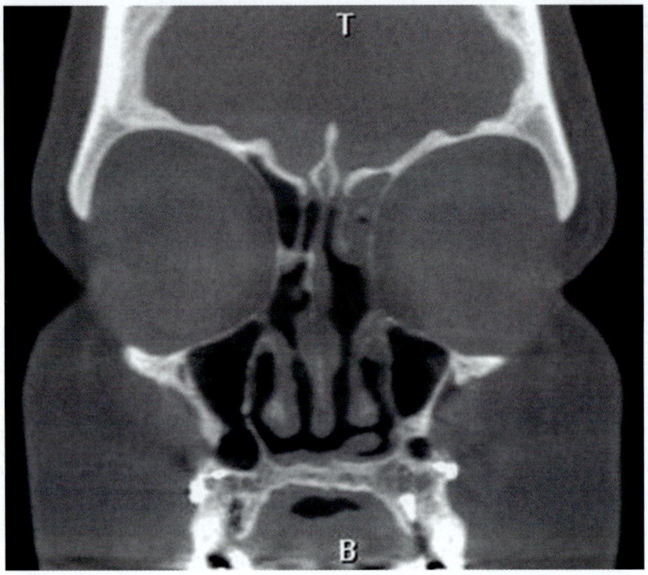

Fig. 15.1 Partially resected middle turbinate causing left frontal recess obstruction.

uncinate inserts into the lamina papyracea) and is a consistent landmark for the thinnest portion of the skull base at the lateral lamella of the cribriform plate

With such an important anatomic role in ESS, it is no surprise that most surgeons believe that MT sacrifice contributes to the disorientation and the surgical challenge of revision cases. In fact, in a study specifically analyzing the complications of ESS, Vleming et al has shown a significantly higher complication rate for revision ESS in the scenario of previous MT resection. These complications included injury to the lamina papyracea, orbital hematoma, and cerebrospinal fluid leakage.[16]

For those who argue that partial anterior, inferior MT resection avoids the loss of a bony landmark, the concern then becomes iatrogenic frontal sinus disease. The denuded mucosa of the partially resected and weakened MT is often seen adherent to the lateral nasal wall, which can obstruct the frontal sinus outflow tract (**Fig. 15.1**).[8,17] In a study of patients who were referred for revision ESS, Swanson et al found a statistically significant higher incidence of frontal sinusitis (75%) in patients who had previous MT resection during their initial procedure.[18] With the risk of increased surgical complications as well as iatrogenic frontal sinusitis, we certainly feel that MT resection should not be routinely performed in all cases of ESS.

The Preservation versus Resection Debate

The historical background of MT preservation during ESS dates back to the original description of the surgery itself. Messerklinger (cited in Kennedy) advocated a meticulous mucosal sparing technique with all attempts made to preserve the MT.[19] This is in contrast to the Wigand technique, which included a partial MT resection during routine ESS.[20] Undoubtedly, these two schools of thought surrounding the MT helped create the long running debate of MT preservation versus resection. The most commonly used reasons for resection include the following:[2–6]

- Easier endoscopic access
- Prevention of MT lateralization and synechiae formation
- Higher maxillary antrostomy patency rates
- Inflammation and polypoid degeneration of the MT

With the exception of the last reason, we feel that routine MT resection is not justified and that current endoscopic technique and skill will overcome many of the concerns regarding MT preservation. Indeed, if the disease process involves the MT with significant inflammation or polypoid change, preservation of this structure may not be indicated. A recent study has shown that nasal polyposis recurrence rates were much lower in patients who had MT resection in conjunction with ESS.[21] However, a normal MT in the setting of chronic rhinosinusitis deserves a different approach. The large variety of zero-degree and angled endoscopes that are available in 4-mm and 2.7-mm diameters provide the endoscopic surgeon numerous options to navigate and operate in the middle meatus region. With respect to the maxillary sinus, the advent of curved instrumentation in both adult and pediatric sizing allows for unhindered surgery with minimal mucosal trauma to the MT. Endoscopic access is clearly no longer a viable reason for routine MT resection.

Perhaps the most cited justification for MT sacrifice is the concern for postoperative lateralization of the MT, resulting in synechiae formation and occlusion of the maxillary and ethmoid sinuses.[22] In fact, this is regarded to be the most common complication after ESS with rates as high as 43%.[23] In an effort to avoid this complication, the practice of MT resection was introduced. Although reports of high antrostomy rates (96.5%) and low synechiae rates (3%) have been reported with partial MT resection, these findings have been inconsistent in the medical literature.[2,5,24] Studies by Ramadan et al and Kinsella et al have shown no statistical difference in lateral synechiae formation between patients who had MT preservation versus resection.[25,26] An important point to mention, however, is that none of these studies were randomized controlled trials. In 1998, Stewart concluded that a properly conducted trial comparing MT resection and preservation would require a minimum of 420 patients per treatment group to detect a 5% difference in synechiae formation.[3] To date, no such study has been performed and until that time, arguments in favor of either approach are largely influenced by surgeon bias. Given the fact that the reasons for routine MT sacrifice are not fully substantiated in the medical literature, we feel that a conservative approach to this normal, physiologic, and consistent landmark in the nasal cavity is both prudent and appropriate.

Middle Turbinate Preservation and Medialization Techniques

As endoscopic skill and experience were developed, an alternative to MT sacrifice was introduced. Techniques of MT preservation and medialization appear to satisfy both camps of the MT debate. In addition to addressing concerns of MT lateralization and synechia formation, endoscopic surgeons can now preserve a critical bony landmark in the nasal cavity. We describe some of the most commonly employed techniques below.

Controlled Synechiae with Abrasion Techniques

In 1999, Bolger et al described a technique of controlled synechia formation between the medial MT and nasal septum using a sickle knife blade. This procedure involved making four 0.5-cm cuts on each surface and placing Gelfilm (Pfizer Pharmaceuticals, New York, NY) or Merocel (Medtronic, Mystic, CT) lateral to the turbinate to allow for medial synechia formation.[27] This would then prevent the MT from lateralizing and the subsequent concerns of synechiae formation would be eliminated. In 2000, a modification of this technique was described by Friedman et al and is currently our preferred abrasion method. Instead of a sickle knife, the microdebrider was employed to form a limited and controlled synechia just posterior to the medial MT caudal edge and the adjacent nasal septum (**see Video 15.1**). Friedman et al used Telfa (Covidian, Mansfield, MA) lateral to the turbinate for 24 to 48 hours postsurgery and achieved a 92% medialization rate and 88% lateral synechiae-free rate in their series.[17] In our institution, we prefer to use a Merocel pack placed in a latex-free glove finger as our standard middle meatal spacer, which is removed at one week. We feel that the glove finger prevents the mucosal abrasion, which can occur with Telfa or many of the middle meatal sponges.

Suturing Technique

Our preferred method of medializing the MT after ESS involves a technique that was described by Thorton in 1996. A 4–0 Vicryl (Ethicon, Somerville, NJ) suture is passed through the MT and nasal septum on both sides and then brought back through to the original side, in the manner of a horizontal mattress suture, and then tied down. In a series of 31 patients treated with this transseptal suturing technique, a 96.7% lateral synechiae-free rate was achieved.[7] This method of preserving and medializing the MT has been employed with good success at other institutions.[28,29]

At our institution, we prefer to use a purple-dyed 4–0 Vicryl suture on a tapered needle. We then relax the curve of the needle before loading it on the needle driver. The suturing technique is then performed much the same as was originally described by Thornton (**see Video 15.2**). This modification was described by Bradley F. Marple (via personal correspondence) and allows for easier manipulation of the needle within the nasal cavity itself. The senior author has employed this method for several years with excellent success of medializing the MT. The dyed suture also allows for easier identification in the postoperative period should the suture need to be removed after medialization has occurred.

Concerns about Preservation and Medialization

One of the concerns that arose after the advent of MT medialization techniques is the potential for obstruction of airflow to the olfactory mucosa in the superior nasal vestibule. To address this concern, Friedman et al measured subjective and objective olfactory function in patients following microdebrider-mediated synechiae formation. In a series of 50 patients, there was no subjective change in olfactory function after surgery and objective scores actually improved, although this did not reach statistical significance.[30] With these findings, the risk of airflow limitation to the olfactory fossa following MT medialization remains theoretical at best. Nonetheless, as further study continues in olfactory function, the advantage of the suturing technique is the ability to remove the suture in the postoperative period. Risks of olfactory dysfunction following MT resection do not employ the same reversibility.

Partial Resection and Preservation

Early proponents of MT resection cited anatomic variants such as a concha bullosa or a paradoxical MT as absolute indications to remove the MT.[3] In the setting of a paradoxical MT, we certainly agree that partial MT resection may be necessary for definitive endoscopic access both during surgery and in the postoperative period. However, our preferred method of dealing with a concha bullosa is to resect only the lateral half of the turbinate using a combination of a sickle knife and endoscopic scissors (**see Video 15.3**). The remaining medial half of the MT can then be medialized with the abrasion or suturing technique, and a middle meatal spacer is placed to prevent lateral synechiae formation. This technique will thus allow for preservation of the medial half of the MT, which continues to serve as a consistent landmark in ESS.

Conclusion

In conclusion, the question of what constitutes the best approach to the middle turbinate in endoscopic sinus surgery has long been a controversial one. However, the development and success of MT medialization techniques allows for preservation of normal nasal structure and function without compromising mucociliary clearance. Given the availability of this option and the concern of MT resection causing frontal sinusitis, loss of normal physiologic balance and increased difficulty in revision cases, preservation and medialization of the middle turbinate appears to be the most prudent approach in the vast majority of endoscopic sinus surgery.

Pearls

- The MT plays important roles in normal nasal physiology including temperature, humidification, filtration, and olfaction.
- The MT is a key anatomic landmark in understanding and performing ESS.
- MT resection has been associated with higher complication rates in revision endoscopic sinus surgery as well as a higher incidence of iatrogenic frontal sinusitis.
- There have been no randomized controlled studies comparing MT resection and preservation in ESS.
- MT medialization techniques allow for preservation of a normal physiologic structure while addressing the concerns for postoperative lateralization.

References

1. Morgenstein KM, Krieger MK. Experiences in middle turbinectomy. Laryngoscope 1980;90(10 Pt 1):1596–1603
2. Davis WE, Templer JW, Lamear WR, Davis WE Jr, Craig SB. Middle meatus antrostomy: patency rates and risk factors. Otolaryngol Head Neck Surg 1991;104(4):467–472
3. Stewart MG. Middle turbinate resection. Arch Otolaryngol Head Neck Surg 1998;124(1):104–106
4. Rice DH. Middle turbinate resection: weighing the decision. Arch Otolaryngol Head Neck Surg 1998;124(1):106
5. Toffel PH. Secure endoscopic sinus surgery with partial middle turbinate modification: a 16-year long-term outcome report and literature review. Curr Opin Otolaryngol Head Neck Surg 2003;11(1):13–18
6. Shih C, Chin G, Rice DH. Middle turbinate resection: impact on outcomes in endoscopic sinus surgery. Ear Nose Throat J 2003;82(10): 796–797
7. Thornton RS. Middle turbinate stabilization technique in endoscopic sinus surgery. Arch Otolaryngol Head Neck Surg 1996;122(8):869–872
8. Kennedy DW. Middle turbinate resection: evaluating the issues—should we resect normal middle turbinates? Arch Otolaryngol Head Neck Surg 1998;124(1):107
9. LaMear WR, Davis WE, Templer JW, McKinsey JP, Del Porto H. Partial endoscopic middle turbinectomy augmenting functional endoscopic sinus surgery. Otolaryngol Head Neck Surg 1992;107(3): 382–389
10. Moore GF, Freeman TJ, Ogren FP, Yonkers AJ. Extended follow-up of total inferior turbinate resection for relief of chronic nasal obstruction. Laryngoscope 1985;95(9 Pt 1):1095–1099
11. Lindemann J, Leiacker R, Sikora T, Rettinger G, Keck T. Impact of unilateral sinus surgery with resection of the turbinates by means of midfacial degloving on nasal air conditioning. Laryngoscope 2002;112(11):2062–2066
12. Friedman WH, Katsantonis GP. The role of standard technique in modern sinus surgery. Otolaryngol Clin North Am 1989;22(4):759–775
13. Wigand ME. Endoscopic Surgery of the Paranasal Sinuses and Anterior Skull Base. 1st ed. New York: Thieme Medical Publishing; 1990
14. Houser SM. Empty nose syndrome associated with middle turbinate resection. Otolaryngol Head Neck Surg 2006;135(6):972–973
15. Stammberger HR, Kennedy DW; The Anatomic Terminology Group. Paranasal sinuses:anatomic terminology and nomenclature. Ann Otol Rhinol Laryngol Suppl 1995;167:7–16
16. Vleming M, Middelweerd RJ, de Vries N. Complications of endoscopic sinus surgery. Arch Otolaryngol Head Neck Surg 1992;118(6):617–623
17. Friedman M, Landsberg R, Tanyeri H. Middle turbinate medialization and preservation in endoscopic sinus surgery. Otolaryngol Head Neck Surg 2000;123(1 Pt 1):76–80
18. Swanson P, Lanza D, Vining E, Kenedy D. The effect of middle turbinate resection upon the frontal sinus. Am J Rhinol 1995;9(4):191–195
19. Kennedy DW. Functional endoscopic sinus surgery. Technique. Arch Otolaryngol 1985;111(10):643–649
20. Wigand ME, Steiner W, Jaumann MP. Endonasal sinus surgery with endoscopical control: from radical operation to rehabilitation of the mucosa. Endoscopy 1978;10(4):255–260
21. Marchioni D, Alicandri-Ciufelli M, Mattioli F, et al. Middle turbinate preservation versus middle turbinate resection in endoscopic surgical treatment of nasal polyposis. Acta Otolaryngol 2008;128(9):1019–1026
22. Havas TE, Lowinger DS. Comparison of functional endonasal sinus surgery with and without partial middle turbinate resection. Ann Otol Rhinol Laryngol 2000;109(7):634–640
23. Lazar RH, Younis RT, Long TE, Gross CW. Revision functional endonasal sinus surgery. Ear Nose Throat J 1992;71(3):131–133
24. Biedlingmaier JF, Whelan P, Zoarski G, Rothman M. Histopathology and CT analysis of partially resected middle turbinates. Laryngoscope 1996;106(1 Pt 1):102–104
25. Ramadan HH, Allen GC. Complications of endoscopic sinus surgery in a residency training program. Laryngoscope 1995;105(4 Pt 1): 376–379
26. Kinsella JB, Calhoun KH, Bradfield JJ, Hokanson JA, Bailey BJ. Complications of endoscopic sinus surgery in a residency training program. Laryngoscope 1995;105(10):1029–1032
27. Bolger WE, Kuhn FA, Kennedy DW. Middle turbinate stabilization after functional endoscopic sinus surgery: the controlled synechiae technique. Laryngoscope 1999;109(11):1852–1853
28. Baluyot ST. Middle turbinate stabilization. Arch Otolaryngol Head Neck Surg 1997;123(1):117
29. Lindemann J, Keck T, Rettinger G. Septal-turbinate-suture in endonasal sinus surgery. Rhinology 2002;40(2):92–94
30. Friedman M, Tanyeri H, Landsberg R, Caldarelli D. Effects of middle turbinate medialization on olfaction. Laryngoscope 1999;109(9): 1442–1445

16 The View in Support of Middle Turbinate Resection

Leslie A. Nurse and James A. Duncavage

As was stated in Chapter 15, the middle turbinate (MT) is an important landmark in endoscopic sinus surgery (ESS). Resection of the middle turbinate remains a source of considerable debate and controversy in the surgical management of sinonasal disease. Despite the volume of literature both supporting and disparaging the removal of the MT, there is only sparse objective evidence for either. The current rhinology literature remains inconclusive regarding the best management of the middle turbinate during sinus surgery.

A great deal of controversy surrounding MT resection appears to be based on each surgeon's personal philosophy regarding nasal physiology and anatomy. The debate obviously divides those who preserve and those who propose varying degrees of turbinate excision, from partial to near-total removal. Historically, the practice of MT resection was condemned. Messerklinger felt that (with few exceptions) the MT should be preserved.[1] Partial removal was only to be reserved in cases of concha bullosa or paradoxical MT, and resection in these instances was always conservative. Conversely, Wigand and colleagues recommended partial or total MT resection as a routine step in virtually all ESS.[2] Both approaches to the middle turbinate yielded successful outcomes, thus supporting the use of either philosophy. Yet, even with the good results seen with either approach, surgeons who either routinely resect or those who routinely preserve the MT disavow the opposing method vehemently. Surgeons often cling to their respective positions on the issue quite passionately. Even in the face of such fervor, however, there are surprisingly very few studies that provide a hard scientific rationale in the approach to MT preservation or resection. In fact, virtually all of the literature that exists on the subject of MT resection is based on nonrandomized, retrospective data. In 2001, Clement and White[3] reviewed over 500 articles describing turbinate surgery over a period of 35 years and not one randomized controlled study was identified. Their conclusion is essentially the overarching theme regarding MT resection: there really is no conclusive evidence supporting or discrediting the procedure. For every study that appears to favor one approach, there are others that endorse the opposing view; thus management is largely based on personal surgical belief or anecdotal experience.

In the following section, we will review the relevant middle turbinate anatomy. The rational for its resection in sinus surgery will be discussed including some of the controversies and theoretical problems associated with removal of the middle turbinate, specifically addressing the validity or actual occurrence of complications of removal of the turbinate.

Anatomy of the Middle Turbinate

The MT is embryologically derived from the ethmoid bone. Structurally, the MT can be divided into three segments.[4] The anterior third attaches superiorly and vertically to the skull base at the horizontal plate of the ethmoid bone just lateral to the cribriform plate (**Fig. 16.1**). This attachment may be pneumatized in up to 12% of the population,[5] thus forming an aerated vertical segment of the MT, which may be referred to as the interlamellar cell (**Fig. 16.2**). This aerated segment is subject to the same inflammatory and infectious processes as other sinonasal mucosa, thereby resulting in obstruction of drainage from the ethmoid infundibulum. The middle segment of the MT, the ground or basal lamella, inserts laterally, attaching it to the lamina papyracea. This attachment divides the ethmoid sinus into anterior and posterior compartments. The posterior segment of the MT is attached inferiorly and oriented horizontally, inserting onto the perpendicular process of the palatine bone anterior to the sphenopalatine foramen.[4] The anterior-superior portion of the MT, an important surgical landmark, forms the medial boundary of the frontal recess. Therefore, lateralization of the MT can lead to structural narrowing of the frontal sinus outflow tract and frontal sinusitis.[6] Also to be considered is the variability in the shape of the MT wherein there may be paradoxical curvature or pneumatization. Pneumatization of the head of the middle turbinate, or concha bullosa, is also a variation of special consideration in patients where this may cause nasal obstruction or obstruction of the ostiomeatal unit (**Fig. 16.3**).

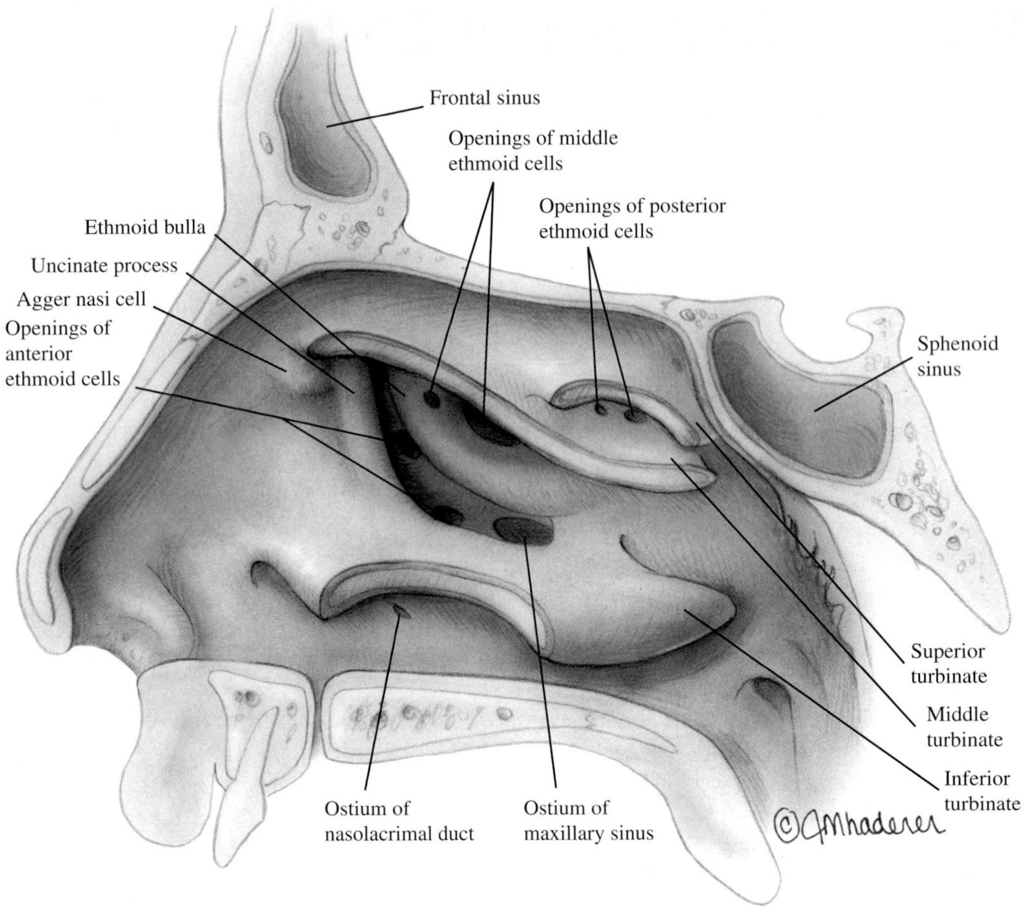

Fig. 16.1 The lateral nasal wall, showing the anatomy of the middle turbinate and surrounding structures. (From Levine HL, Clemente MP. Sinus Surgery: Endoscopic and Microscopic Approaches. New York: Thieme Medical Publishing; 2005:15. Reprinted with permission.)

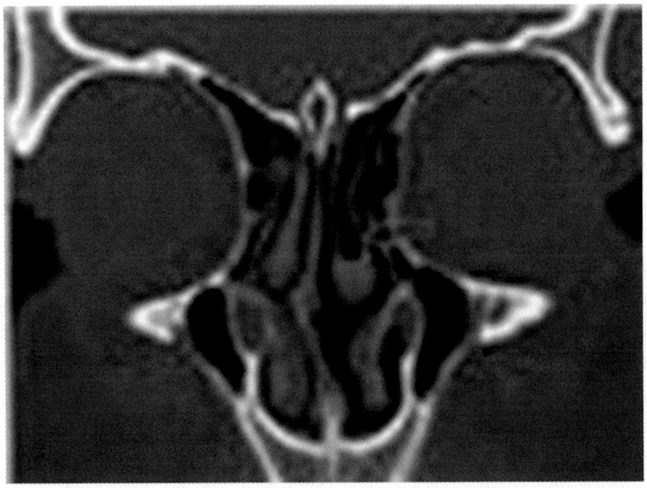

Fig. 16.2 Pneumatization of the vertical attachment of the middle turbinate or interlamellar cell.

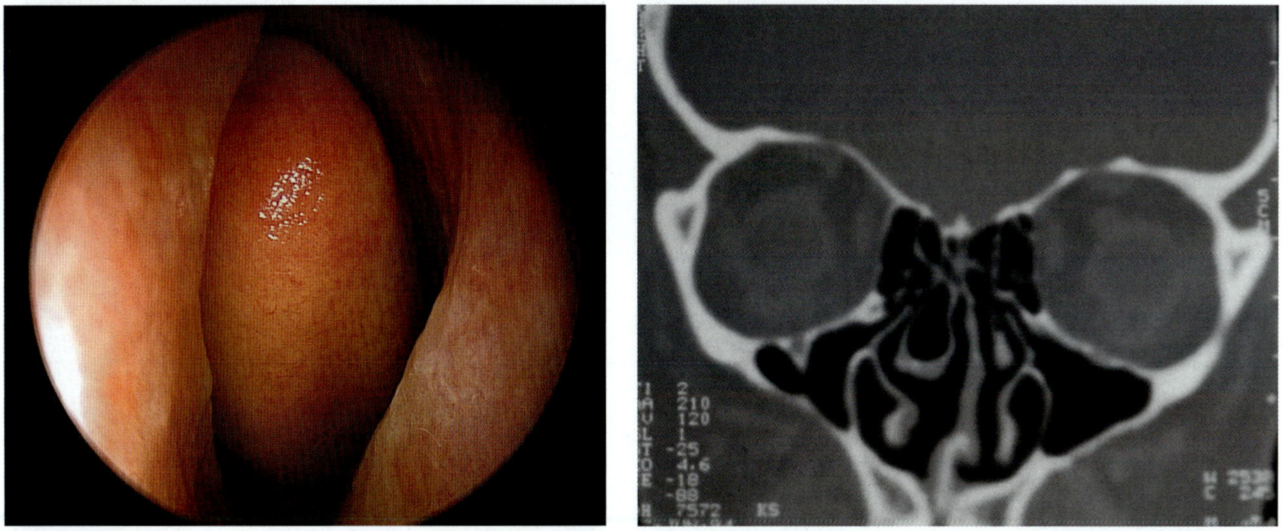

A B

Fig. 16.3 (A,B) Concha bullosa. **(A)** Endoscopic view of a large right concha bullosa cell with partial occlusion of the nasal airway. **(B)** Computed tomography (CT) scan of right concha bullosa cell.

The Resection versus Preservation Debate

The middle turbinate debate is largely centered on one crucial question: how much middle turbinate can one safely resect? The effect of MT resection on normal sinus and nasal physiology remains uncertain. The nasal turbinates are thought to function collectively to direct and assist in lamination of nasal airflow, humidify and warm inspired air, and provide a mechanical defense against particulate matter. As compared with the inferior turbinate, the MT is significantly smaller, contains less vascular and erectile tissue, accounts for a negligible portion of nasal airway resistance, and is believed to have less functional significance.

Despite this evidence, as well as literature supporting the safety of middle turbinectomy, the procedure continues to provoke a considerable amount of controversy, particularly regarding lateralization of the turbinate remnant as a factor promoting postoperative frontal sinusitis. Other concerns include loss of a significant surgical landmark, development of atrophic rhinitis, postoperative hemorrhage and anosmia. The controversy surrounding MT resection appears to be based on personal philosophy regarding nasal physiology and anatomy.

Middle Turbinate Resection Techniques

There are currently several indications for the removal of the MT in ESS that are more generally accepted. Some cited indications for middle turbinate resection include treatment of concha bullosa that participate in nasal obstruction and/or prevent access to the middle meatus in the "crowded nose,"[6] removal of disease involving the turbinate,[7] surgical access to the paranasal sinuses, and treatment of headache related to the middle turbinate syndrome where contact between an enlarged MT and either the septum or lateral nasal wall leads to stimulation of the sensory portion of the trigeminal nerve.[8]

The techniques for MT resection are also varied. Kennedy and Sinreich[9] describe a technique where the turbinate is split in the middle and only the lateral portion is removed, leaving the medial portion intact to function physiologically. Wigand describes resecting the posterior third of the middle turbinate when performing any retrograde sphenoethmoidectomy.[10] Morgenstein and Krieger describe a technique that involves cutting the superior attachment of the MT then snaring the anterior two-thirds.[11] Freedman and Kern describe resection of the middle turbinate to within 0.5 cm of the skull base as an integral part of all headlight intranasal sphenoethmoidectomies.[7] In the majority of patients, this maneuver addresses disease involving the turbinate (e.g., polyposis or osteitis); turbinate resection is advocated regardless of the amount of pathology involving the middle turbinate.

The technique of MT resection employed by the senior author is depicted in **Fig. 16.4**, as a modification of the techniques described by Wigand (**see Video 16.1**). It is performed with the use of a zero-degree 4-mm telescope. Initially, the middle turbinate is fractured medially toward the septum using a Freer elevator to expose its vertical, superior attachment (**Fig. 16.4A**). This attachment is incised with a straight turbinate scissor at its most anterior portion (**Figs. 16.4B,C**). The body of the turbinate is then grasped with straight Wilde forceps and pulled inferiorly and posteriorly, leaving at least 0.5 cm of the superior attachment

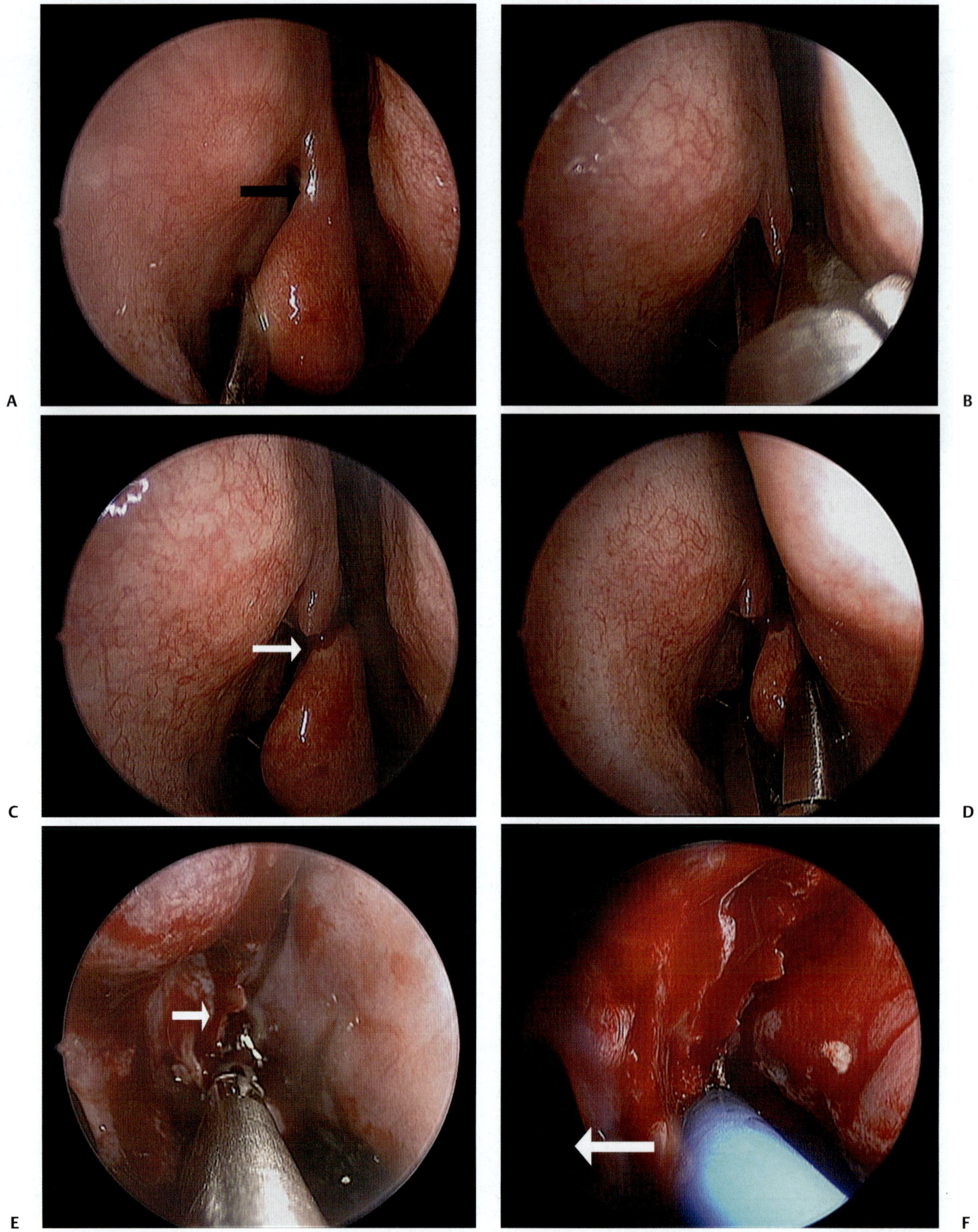

Fig. 16.4 (A–F) Technique of endoscopic right partial middle turbinectomy. **(A)** Middle turbinate being medially fractured to expose its vertical attachment (*black arrow*) superiorly. **(B)** Vertical attachment incised with straight turbinate scissors at its most anterior part. **(C)** After this incision of the anterior, superior attachment (*white arrow*). **(D)** The head of the turbinate is grasped and dissected inferiorly and posteriorly along the length of the turbinate back to the basal lamella. **(E)** Incision of the posterior turbinate attachment completes the partial resection. White arrow indicates remnants of the superior and basal lamella attachments being preserved as a landmark. **(F)** Suction cautery applied to the posterior attachment remnant to coagulate small branches of sphenopalatine artery. White arrow indicates maxillary sinus ostium.

and basal lamella to preserve as landmarks (**Figs. 16.4D,E**). The most posterior attachment of the MT is then incised using through-biting forceps thereby completing the partial resection. The remainder of the posterior attachment is then suction cauterized to coagulate small branches of the sphenopalatine artery, as prophylaxis against intraoperative or postoperative hemorrhage (**Fig. 16.4F**).

Concerns about Middle Turbinate Resection

Historically, the practice of MT resection has been condemned, largely due to theoretical and actual observed complications following removal. The most prominent of these concerns and complications include alteration in nasal function including air humidification, filtration, and airflow;[6] increased incidence of frontal sinusitis;[6] ethmoid scarring;[12] development of anosmia;[13] postoperative epistaxis;[14] loss of anatomic landmark for revision surgery;[6] and the development of atrophic rhinitis.[10]

Alteration in Nasal Function

If the turbinates play a role in the lamination of nasal airflow, it is quite possible that their removal may contribute to postoperative changes in nasal airflow resistance. Is there evidence of such an effect? Recently, Brescia et al[14] sought to define the effect of MT resection on nasal airflow. In this retrospective study, 23 patients with extensive sinonasal polyposis who had undergone partial resection of the middle turbinate ESS were compared with 25 polyp patients who had ESS with MT preservation. The outcomes examined included endoscopic scoring of polyposis and measurement of nasal airway resistance by computerized rhinomanometry performed at 3 months and 12 months after surgery. The findings of this study were improvement of endoscopic score and a statistically significant reduction of nasal airway resistance after both surgical techniques, with no statistically significant difference in the mean nasal airway resistance values before and after when comparing MT resection versus preservation.

Previously, prospective evaluation of the effect of MT resection on nasal airflow was performed by Cook et al.[15] They evaluated 31 consecutive patients who underwent ESS with partial middle turbinectomy performed as part of their surgery. They measured pre- and postoperative nasal airflow and nasal airway resistance using computerized rhinomanometry and found that all patients had significant improvement in nasal airflow ($p < 0.001$) and significant decrease in nasal resistance ($p < 0.001$) compared with preoperative measures. Obviously this study lacks a control group of patients who did not have turbinates removed; thus, the data should be considered with this in mind.

Anosmia

It has been shown that olfactory neuroepithelium exists within the superior portions of the middle turbinate. In the late 1890s and early 1900s, both von Brunn[16] and Read[17] independently performed histologic evaluations in animals and humans and used their findings to develop schemata demonstrating the distribution of the olfactory neuroepithelium. According to these schemata, there is olfactory neuroepithelium localized to a small portion of the superior parts of the middle turbinate. However, this is a relatively small amount of olfactory tissue compared with the entire distribution of surface area available for olfaction, thus one could conclude that MT resection should not significantly affect olfaction. However, in combination with age-related decrease in olfactory neuroepithelium, there may be a perceptible difference in older patients after MT resection or as younger patients get older. Clinically, this has not been the case. Beidlingmanger[13] reviewed the records of 110 patients undergoing 198 partial middle turbinate resections during endoscopic sinus surgery. The patients were evaluated for the complications of anosmia, bleeding, and crusting. Patients undergoing endoscopic sinus surgery with partial middle turbinate resections were evaluated by histopathologic and computed tomography (CT) analyses. In this review of 110 patients with 198 partial turbinate resections, there was only one patient who complained of anosmia. Also of note in this study, one patient required vessel ligation for bleeding, and no patients had excessive crusting. This 0.9% incidence of anosmia is comparable to the 0.8% incidence in Wigand's series of 220 patients who underwent ESS with turbinate preservation. Similarly, in two other large series of over 1000 patients each, Lawson[18] and Freedman and Kern[7] found no increased risk of anosmia or atrophic rhinitis in patients who underwent MT resections. Similarly, Toffel, who reported a large series of patients over 16 years who underwent partial middle turbinectomy, emphasizes the importance of preserving the superior rim of turbinate in which olfactory epithelium may reside to minimize the possibility of postoperative olfactory disturbance.[19]

Scarring and Frontal Sinusitis

Postoperative scarring can be a source of great disappointment after ESS. The incidence of scarring for all undergoing ESS ranges from 4 to 27% in the literature,[12] which may lead to recurrent symptoms and the need for further surgery. Reports of MT resection leading to lateral scarring of the MT to the nasal wall have been described.

Scarring of frontal sinus outflow secondary to middle turbinate resection is also an outcome that has been discussed in the literature. This scarring is thought to be related to the healing process after middle turbinectomy.[6] The proposed mechanism is that a middle turbinate cut near its anterior superior attachment becomes destabilized, and the lateral aspect of the MT remnant adheres to the surgical field. Granulation tissue in the ethmoid cavity gives way to scar and gradual traction on the turbinate remnant drawing it across the area of the frontal recess. The ensuing inadequate drainage and ventilation of the frontal sinus leads to sinusitis.

There is data both supporting and disproving that MT resection can cause frontal sinusitis in this manner. In 1995, Swanson et al[6] performed a retrospective review to determine if MT resection affected postoperative frontal sinus disease. They identified 110 consecutive patients with chronic or recurrent acute sinusitis, 69 of whom had previous middle turbinectomy and 41 patients with intact MTs after prior sinus surgery. In 42 patients, CT scans were scored and defined as having mild to moderate or severe disease. Frontal sinusitis seen on CT scan was present in 30 of 40 (75%) patients who had MT resection versus 9 of 20 (45%) patients who did not, and this difference was statistically significant ($p < 0.05$). They also considered the degree of MT resection in this study by using CT scans to determine the height of MT resection in the frontal recess area and found no statistical difference between patients with high and low resection.

The authors discussed several potential weaknesses of their study, including its retrospective nature, the lack of information on preoperative sinus disease, and the lack of standardization of operative indications or technique. Scar formation and maxillary antrostomy patency were not addressed in this study.

Conversely, in 1998, Fortune and Duncavage[20] retrospectively reviewed 155 consecutive patients undergoing partial MT resection for either sinusitis or nasal obstruction. Their findings revealed a 10% rate of frontal sinusitis after partial middle turbinectomy and found that the development of sinusitis in these patients was largely associated with preoperative comorbidities such as asthma, nasal polyps, and severe disease on CT or diseased middle turbinates.

Why Not Preservation?

In some instances, preservation of the MT can be a contributing factor to failure after ESS. Some propose that the MT may play a role in the pathogenesis of inflammatory nasosinusal disease secreting vasoactive sensory neuropeptides.[21] More likely, however the preserved MT may often be destabilized by its pathology or by inherent anatomic abnormalities like paradoxical curvature. In such instances, lateral scarring of the turbinate can lead to further obstruction of maxillary sinus drainage despite our most earnest surgical attempts to improve it. There is evidence to support a potentially higher rate of postoperative synechiae with MT preservation versus resection.[22] Examples of such scarring can be seen in **Fig. 16.5**. Additionally, visualization of the sphenoethmoidal region is aided by its absence allowing for the detection of scarring in this area, which may be easily addressed with office-based manipulation thus avoiding the need for revision surgery.

It is our practice to facilitate postoperative management by regular examinations of the sinus openings for early indications of scar formation. With the access afforded by

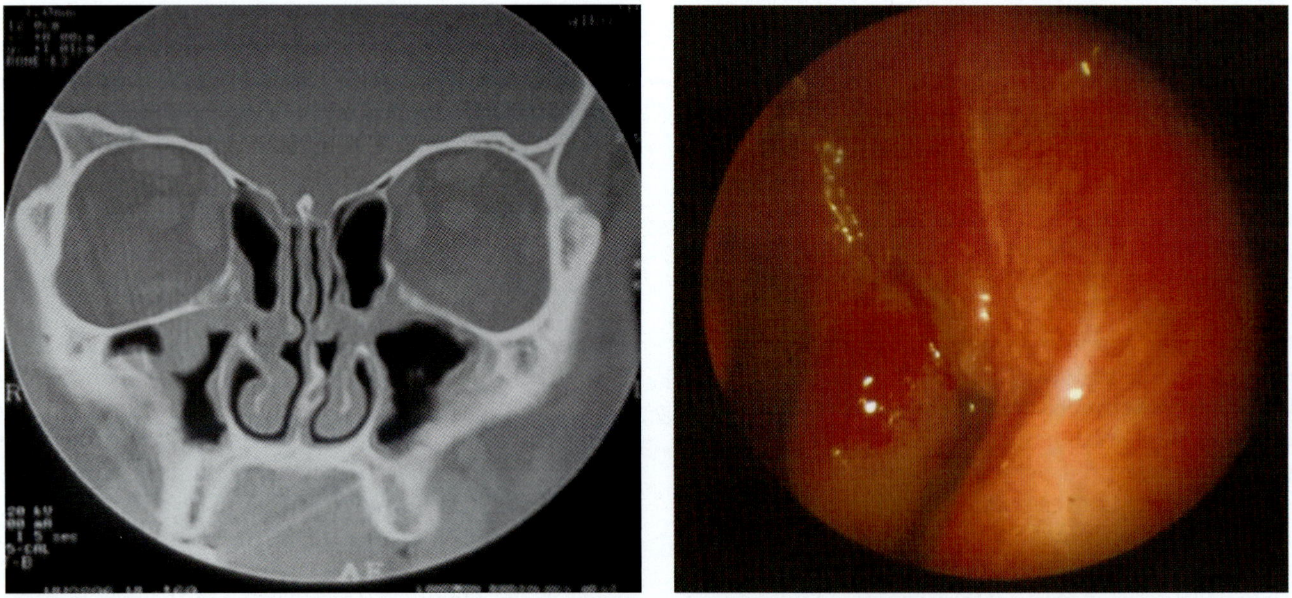

A B

Fig. 16.5 (A,B) Postoperatively, unresected middle turbinates have scarred laterally to cause maxillary outflow obstruction. In both cases, previous ethmoidectomy and maxillary antrostomies were performed.

partial MT resection, both visualization and manipulation of these openings are possible in the office using topical anesthesia.

A regular postoperative schedule of examinations allows for examination at times when such scar formation is anticipated to begin. With this in mind, patients are examined at 1, 2, 6, and 8 weeks after surgery, with additional examinations as needed based on each exam.

Conclusion

The role of middle turbinate resection in endoscopic sinus surgery, despite the myriad of studies and articles on the subject, remains uncertain. The degree to which MT resection may have deleterious effects on nasal airflow, postoperative scarring and future surgery, with the loss of surgical landmarks is emphasized in some studies and refuted in others. The one prevailing theme of these studies is that none meets the standard of prospective randomized controlled evidence from which one may extrapolate a conclusion about which approach is best. Thus, all we are left with are the studies of those in whose hands both methods seem to work quite well. There are some points that must be kept in mind when approaching the turbinates, regardless of which side of the fence one favors. Complete removal of the middle turbinate including its most superior attachment is neither recommended nor necessary in the absence of malignancy or other invasive disease. The most superior attachment, if left in place may serve as a landmark and may contain olfactory neuroepithelium whose preservation would prevent theoretical diminution in olfaction, either immediately or long-term. Care should be taken to address the possibility for hemorrhage from the posterior turbinate attachment. In the hands of those familiar with their respective techniques, both yield successful outcomes.

Pearls

- Despite the volume of literature both supporting and disparaging the removal of the MT, there still is sparse objective evidence for either. The current rhinology literature remains unclear regarding the best management of the middle turbinate during sinus surgery.
- The effect of middle turbinate resection on normal sinus and nasal physiology remains uncertain. Although the role of the inferior turbinates in nasal airflow has been demonstrated, the middle turbinate, which contains less vascular and erectile tissue, accounts for a negligible portion of nasal airway resistance, and is believed to have less functional significance.
- There are currently several indications for the removal of the middle turbinates in endoscopic sinus surgery that are generally accepted. These include concha bullosa that participate in nasal obstruction and/or prevent access to the middle meatus, removal of disease involving the turbinate, and treatment of headache related to the middle turbinate syndrome where contact between an enlarged MT and either the septum or lateral nasal wall leads to stimulation of the sensory portion of the trigeminal nerve.
- Techniques for MT resection are varied and include removal of only the lateral portion, resection of the posterior third, and resection along the length of the turbinate to within 0.5 cm of the skull base.
- Proposed problems associated with MT resection include alteration in nasal function, increased incidence of frontal sinusitis secondary to scarring, development of anosmia, bleeding, loss of an anatomic landmark for revision surgery, and the development of atrophic rhinitis.
- Complete removal of the middle turbinate including its most superior attachment is neither recommended nor necessary in the absence of malignancy or other invasive disease. The most superior attachment, if left in place, may serve as a landmark and may contain olfactory neuroepithelium whose preservation would prevent theoretical diminution in olfaction, either immediately or long-term.

References

1. Messerklinger W. Endoscopic diagnosis and surgery of recurrent sinusitis. In: Krajira Z, ed. Advances in Nose and Sinus Surgery. Zagreb: Zagreb University; 1985
2. Wigand ME, Steiner W, Jaumann MP. Endonasal sinus surgery with endoscopical control: from radical operation to rehabilitation of the mucosa. Endoscopy 1978;10(4):255–260
3. Clement WA, White PS. Trends in turbinate surgery literature: a 35-year review. Clin Otolaryngol Allied Sci 2001;26(2):124–128
4. Lang J. Clinical Anatomy of the Nose, Nasal Cavity, and Paranasal Sinuses. New York: Thieme Medical Publishing, 1989
5. Amedee RG, Miller AJ. Sinus anatomy and function. In: Bailey BJ et al, eds. Head and Neck Surgery–Otolaryngology. 3rd ed. Philadelphia: Lippincott-Raven; 2001: 321–328
6. Swanson PB, Lanza DC, Vining EM, Kennedy DW. The effect of middle turbinate resection upon the frontal sinus. Am J Rhinol 1995;9:191–195
7. Freedman HM, Kern EB. Complications of intranasal ethmoidectomy: a review of 1,000 consecutive operations. Laryngoscope 1979;89(3):421–434
8. Goldsmith AJ, Zahtz GD, Stegnjajic A, Shikowitz M. Middle turbinate headache syndrome. Am J Rhinol 1993;7(1):17–23
9. Kennedy DW, Sinreich SJ. Functional endoscopic approach to inflammatory sinus disease: current perspectives and technique modifications. Am J Rhinol 1988;2:89–96
10. Wigand ME. Endoscopic Surgery of the Paranasal Sinuses and Anterior Skull Base. New York: Thieme Medical Publishing; 1990:134–141

11. Morgenstein KM, Krieger MK. Experiences in middle turbinectomy. Laryngoscope 1980;90(10 Pt 1):1596–1603
12. Gaskins RE. Scarring in endoscopic ethmoidectomy. Am J Rhinol 1994;8:271–274
13. Biedlingmaier JF, Whelan P, Zoarski G, Rothman M. Histopathology and CT analysis of partially resected middle turbinates. Laryngoscope 1996;106(1 Pt 1):102–104
14. Brescia G, Pavin A, Giacomelli L, Boninsegna M, Florio A, Marioni G. Partial middle turbinectomy during endoscopic sinus surgery for extended sinonasal polyposis: short- and mid-term outcomes. Acta Otolaryngol 2008;128(1):73–77
15. Cook PR, Begegni A, Bryant WC, Davis WE. Effect of partial middle turbinectomy on nasal airflow and resistance. Otolaryngol Head Neck Surg 1995;113(4):413–419
16. Von Brunn A. Contributions to the microscopic anatomy of the human nose. Arch Micr Anat 1892;39:632–651
17. Read E. A contribution to the knowledge of the olfactory apparatus in dog, cat, and man. Am J Anat 1908;8:17–47
18. Lawson W. The intranasal ethmoidectomy: an experience with 1,077 procedures. Laryngoscope 1991;101(4 Pt 1):367–371
19. Toffel PH. Secure endoscopic sinus surgery with partial middle turbinate modification: a 16-year long-term outcome report and literature review. Curr Opin Otolaryngol Head Neck Surg 2003;11(1):13–18
20. Fortune DS, Duncavage JA. Incidence of frontal sinusitis following partial middle turbinectomy. Ann Otol Rhinol Laryngol 1998;107(6):447–453
21. Marchioni D, Alicandri-Ciufelli M, Mattioli F, et al. Middle turbinate preservation versus middle turbinate resection in endoscopic surgical treatment of nasal polyposis. Acta Otolaryngol 2008;128(9):1019–1026
22. Vleming M, Middelweerd RJ, de Vries N. Complications of endoscopic sinus surgery. Arch Otolaryngol Head Neck Surg 1992;118(6):617–623

17 Caldwell–Luc Surgery

Paul T. Russell and Samuel S. Becker

Before the advent of Caldwell–Luc surgery in the 1890s, maxillary sinus disease had been treated by antral washout through the alveolus after removal of a tooth, as described, for example, by William Cowper in 1707. Others described opening the sinus into the nasal passage; however, poor lighting and an incomplete understanding of the sinonasal anatomy led to failures and a decline in popularity of that method. A canine fossa approach to antral washout was used by Desault and Lamorier in the late 18th century. This same approach was advocated by Jansen in the late 19th century; however, he also described packing the sinus to stimulate granulation tissue formation. Still others—notably Lothrop, Claoue, Mikulicz, and Canfield—popularized the inferior meatal antrostomy for surgical management of maxillary sinus infection.

In the last decade of the 19th century, three surgeons working independently—George Caldwell of the USA, Scanes Spicer of England, and Henri Luc of France—described creation of an anterior antral window for surgical extirpation of diseased sinus mucosa, to be used in conjunction with an inferior meatal antrostomy. Caldwell–Luc surgery, as it became known, was the primary workhorse for maxillary sinus disease until the 1920s, when intranasal procedures gained in popularity. With the introduction of the nasal endoscope and the advent of functional endoscopic sinus surgery (FESS) in the 1980s, Caldwell–Luc surgery was pushed even further into the background, and today it is utilized only in patients with tumors, masses, or persistent maxillary sinus disease after other medical and surgical therapies have failed.

The Caldwell–Luc Approach and the Caldwell–Luc Procedure

Clarification should be made of some basic terminology. In the canine fossa puncture (described in detail in Chapter 12 of this book) the maxillary sinus is entered through a sublabial, anterior approach placed in a location designed to minimize complication and morbidity. The location of this puncture—traditionally just lateral to the canine fossa—is intended to minimize trauma to the branches of the infraorbital nerve and the anterior superior alveolar nerve that innervate this area. Endoscopes, powered instruments, and other tools may be placed through what is typically a 4 to 5 mm opening. In the *Caldwell–Luc approach*, this opening is enlarged with cutting instruments (typically Kerrison rongeurs) for improved anterior access to the maxillary sinus. In the *Caldwell–Luc procedure* (also known as transbuccal radical antrostomy), the maxillary sinus mucosal lining is removed—typically via a Caldwell–Luc approach—and a gravity drainage port is created with an inferior meatal antrostomy.

Indications for Caldwell–Luc Surgery

Morbidity from the Caldwell–Luc approach and procedure can be significant and long-lasting. It is for this reason that appropriate indications should be adhered to when considering Caldwell–Luc. Mucosal preserving techniques should always be tried prior to any attempt at mucosal extirpation. Advances in endoscopy and endonasal instrumentation designed specifically to reach into the recesses of the maxillary sinus have led to significantly increased possibilities via endoscopic endonasal approaches, and these less traumatic approaches should be given first consideration. On the other hand, tumors, foreign bodies, and fungal disease, or cases where extended access to the pterygopalatine fossa is required, are some instances where a Caldwell–Luc approach via anterior antral window is appropriate. Others have used this approach in the surgical repair of facial trauma, including orbital floor fractures.

The Caldwell–Luc procedure, involving mucosal extirpation, may be considered for cases of persistent maxillary sinusitis in the context of failed aggressive medical and surgical interventions, or in cases of tumor removal. Common anatomic reasons for surgical failure such as missed natural ostium sequence, recirculation, and retained uncinate process must be ruled out prior to performance of a Caldwell–Luc procedure for chronic rhinosinusitis.

Surgical Technique of the Caldwell–Luc Approach and Procedure

The Caldwell–Luc approach begins with a gingivolabial incision in the mucosa superior to the canine tooth. This incision

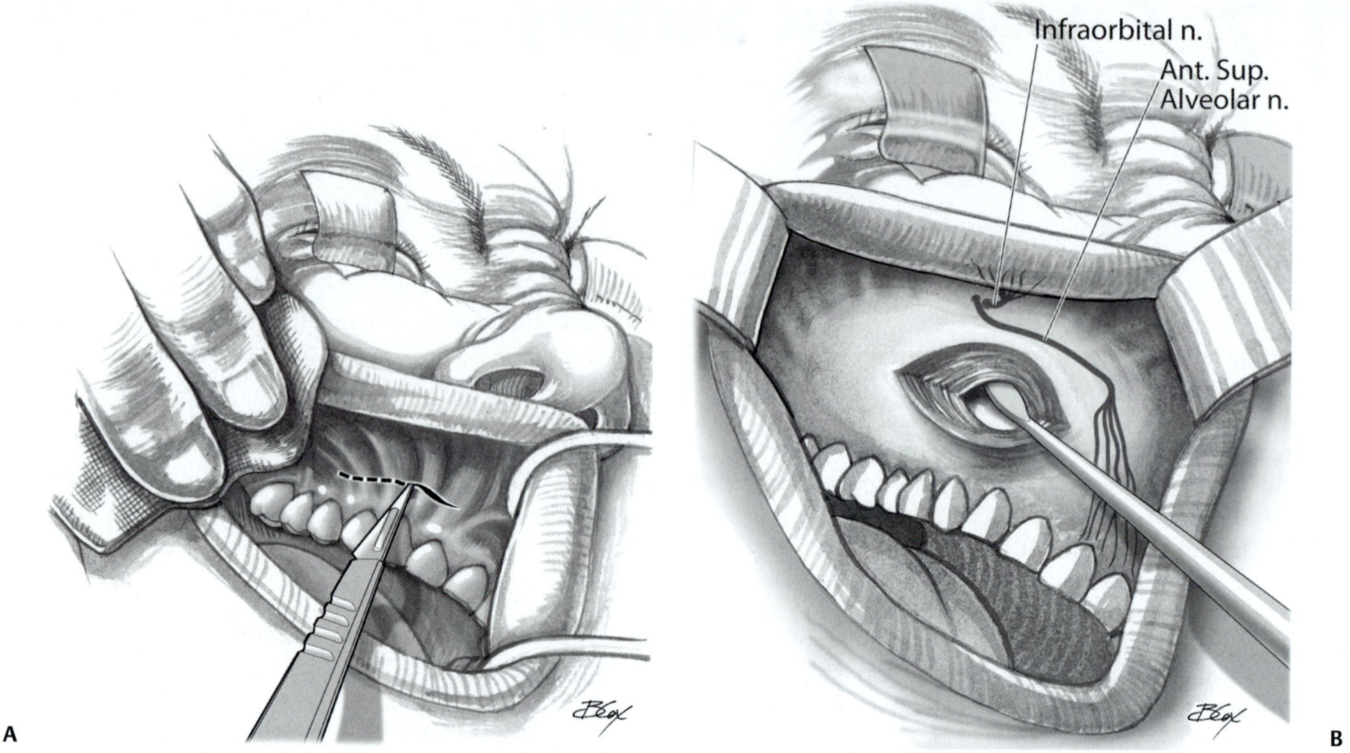

Fig. 17.1 (A,B) An incision has been made through the upper lip mucosa and down through the periosteum to expose the face of the antrum. Retractors are placed for increased exposure while a periosteal elevator is used to increase exposure over the face of the maxilla. Elevation is carried superiorly to the level of the infraorbital nerve.

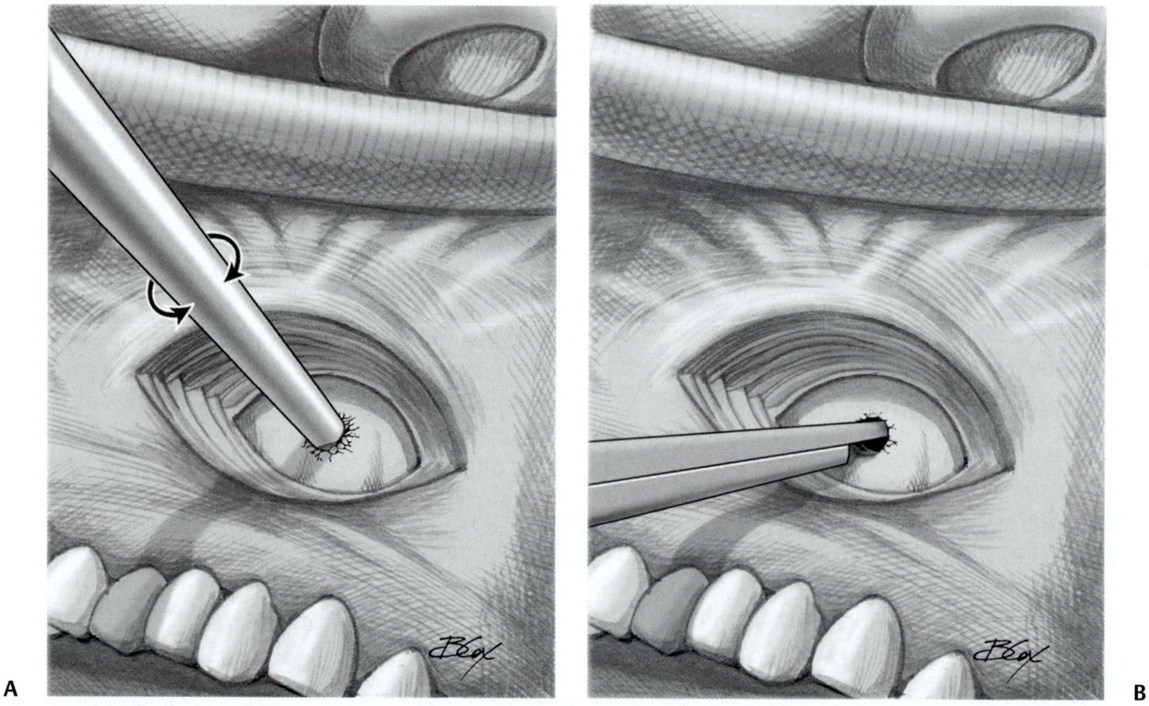

Fig. 17.2 (A) A small opening into the antrum is made using a trocar. Placement is performed in a location just superolateral to the canine fossa. **(B)** After opening into the maxillary sinus, the opening is enlarged using a Kerrison punch.

is carried laterally to the level of the first molar with care to maintain enough vertical height on the inferior mucosal cuff for adequate tension-free wound closure at the end of the procedure. The incision is made through the periosteum and wide subperiosteal elevation is performed widely over the face of the maxilla. Elevation is carried superiorly to the level of the infraorbital nerve. Attention should be paid to the infraorbital nerve and the anterior superior alveolar nerve. The nerves are protected while the sinus is entered through the anterior wall (**Fig. 17.1**).

The transantral opening is placed in a location just superolateral to the canine fossa to minimize trauma to branches of the infraorbital and anterior superior alveolar nerves. (Details of precise canine fossa placement are described in Chapter 12.) Various methods have been described to perform the anterior antrostomy. Traditionally, the opening has been created via a small puncture with a trocar aimed medially, followed by a Kerrison punch to enlarge the opening (**Fig. 17.2**). Others have supported the use of a high-speed drill as a less traumatic and more precise method of entering the sinus.

After entrance into the sinus, the contents are removed with grasping instruments. The sinus mucosa is then elevated and removed with curved Coakley curettes and grasping forceps (**Fig. 17.3**). An inferior meatus antrostomy is frequently performed to allow for nonphysiologic, gravitational drainage. In cases where an intranasal maxillary antrostomy has not previously been performed, one is created with standard endoscopic endonasal techniques. The anterior maxillary wall is left open, and the incision is closed in layers with absorbable suture (**see Video 17.1**).

Surgical Technique of the Endoscopic Endonasal Caldwell–Luc Procedure

In some situations where a Caldwell–Luc procedure is appropriate, we have begun to use a modified version, the endoscopic endonasal Caldwell–Luc procedure, which is performed in the following fashion. After endoscopic endonasal resection of the middle turbinate, a large maxillary antrostomy is created using traditional endoscopic techniques. Resection of the medial maxillary sinus wall is continued posteriorly to the junction of the medial and posterior sinus walls with the use of through-biting forceps and the powered instrumentation. Next, using a 70-degree endoscope in combination with angled forceps, meticulous removal of the mucosa from the posterior maxillary sinus wall is performed. Mucosal stripping is continued anteriorly with removal from the lateral, superior, and inferior maxillary sinus walls. Appropriate care is taken to avoid injury to the infraorbital nerve when working along the sinus roof. Frontal sinus instruments are used for optimal access to the mucosa of the lateral maxillary sinus wall. More recently, adjust-

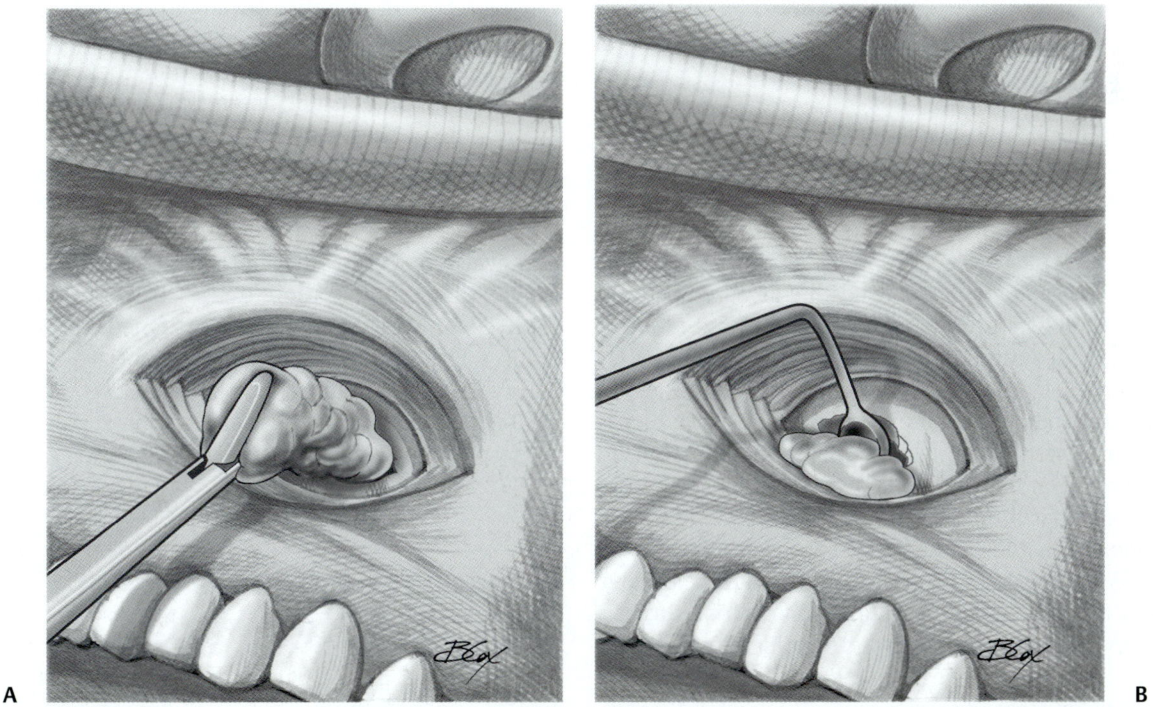

Fig. 17.3 (A,B) After entrance into the sinus, the contents are removed with grasping instruments. The sinus mucosa is then elevated and removed with curved Coakley curettes and grasping forceps.

able angled forceps have been introduced that can be used for this purpose. When the limit of anterior visualization is reached using the 70-degree endoscope, change to the 120-degree endoscope is made, allowing full visualization of the anterior maxillary sinus wall. It should be emphasized that with this approach the entire inner surface of the maxillary sinus can be visualized. Utilizing the 120-degree endoscope in this manner can be a significant technical challenge, and practice in a cadaver laboratory is recommended prior to use on a patient. Complete removal of the diseased mucosa is continued along the anterior wall using angled Coakley curettes until all bony maxillary sinus walls are exposed. An angled-tip burr may then be used to drill down any remaining bony abnormalities (**see Video 17.2**).

Postoperative Care

Frequent postoperative visits are vital to good results after Caldwell–Luc surgery. Because of the mucosal extirpation, frequent debridements are required in the early weeks to fully remove the blood and scabs, which are the products of surgery. Postoperative discomfort generally limits the amount of debridement that is possible with each visit, and extended visits may be required. In our experience, postoperative care will either lead to remucosalization or to scarring of the sinus. In fact, scarring may be preferable because it functions as a means of sinus auto-obliteration.

Complications of Caldwell–Luc Surgery

Compared with FESS, Caldwell–Luc surgery is associated with significantly more patient morbidity. It is for this reason that endoscopic, mucosal preserving approaches should always be preferred—when possible—to Caldwell–Luc surgery. Unlike the typical recovery time of several weeks after FESS, patients should be forewarned that healing from an external Caldwell–Luc procedure may take several months. Complications encountered with Caldwell–Luc include facial edema and pain, bleeding and hematoma, numbness in the infraorbital and anterior superior alveolar nerve distributions, dacryocystitis and persistent epiphora, devitalized teeth, and oroantral fistulae. Facial hypoesthesia is particularly common and its impact on patient quality of life should not be underestimated. Some of these symptoms may be encountered by upwards of 20% of patients. Mucoceles have been noted to occur many years after the initial surgery. More serious, though extremely rare, complications include inadvertent entrance into the orbit and damage to the ocular contents. It is likely that the endoscopic endonasal Caldwell–Luc procedure has significantly less morbidity than the conventional external approach; however, at this point in time there is not enough data to prove this statement.

Management Options after Failed Caldwell–Luc Surgery for Chronic Rhinosinusitis

Caldwell–Luc surgery should be a *last resort* for patients with chronic rhinosinusitis. Only when patients have failed aggressive medical and mucosa-preserving surgical intervention should Caldwell–Luc surgery be considered as a treatment option. When these guidelines are followed, the Caldwell–Luc approach and procedure has been shown to have success rates exceeding 90%. However, some patients have persistent disease after Caldwell–Luc surgery.

Treatment of recalcitrant sinus disease in these patients is difficult, but several options are available. First, it must be recognized—and patients must be forewarned—that unlike FESS, recovery after Caldwell–Luc surgery may take months, not weeks. For this reason, early reintervention is discouraged. In some patients, however, symptoms may persist or recur years after surgery.

Evaluation should involve careful examination of the sublabial area as well as the sinus with 30- and 70-degree endoscopes. Scars in the sublabial area should be palpated and examined for tenderness and discomfort. All corners of the sinus itself should be visualized endonasally in search of inflamed mucosa, necrotic debris, or pockets of infection. Dedicated sinus computed tomography (CT) is imperative to look for the presence of abscesses, which may have formed within the sinus itself—trapped in the scar tissue filling the sinus.

It should be recognized that patients who have had Caldwell–Luc surgery may get sinus infections once or twice per year, like every other patient with chronic rhinosinusitis. Because of the poor mucosal function, these infections may persist longer than usual, and in addition to standard medical treatment, they may require in-office debridements. In patients who fail medical treatment, revision surgery may be indicated. Some have advocated revision endoscopic mucosal-sparing surgery such as creation of a “mega-antrostomy” (removal of posterior-inferior turbinate with endoscopic medial maxillectomy) in these cases. Others support a revision Caldwell–Luc procedure for cases of failed Caldwell–Luc procedures. Either approach may be appropriate. The treatment, however, must be tailored to the disease: a focal abscess or loculated pocket of mucous must be marsupialized and will not respond to a “mucosal-preserving” surgery.

Evidence-based Review of Caldwell–Luc Surgery

The continued use of Caldwell–Luc surgery sparks a great deal of controversy in the otolaryngology–head and neck surgery community. Although most agree that Caldwell–Luc is reserved as a final effort for patients who have failed traditional surgery and whose disease is incompletely accessible to endoscopic approaches, some argue that it simply should never be used at all. Formal evaluation of the efficacy and complications of the Caldwell-Luc approach and procedure are uncommon, but some studies have been done.

In one study from 1997, 150 patients were randomized to FESS or Caldwell-Luc surgery. At 7-year follow-up, 20% of the FESS patients had undergone revision surgery compared with 18% of the Caldwell-Luc patients.[1] Another study from 1997 found a revision surgery rate of 18% in FESS patients versus 5% in the Caldwell-Luc group.[2] More recently, a 5-year retrospective study showed a 92% success rate after an average 2-year follow-up on 37 patients who underwent 50 Caldwell-Luc procedures.[3] These studies and others suggest that, when used appropriately, the Caldwell-Luc procedure can lead to positive outcomes.

Several authors have suggested an intermediate procedure for use in surgery of the severely diseased maxillary sinus. The canine fossa puncture as a means to remove diseased mucosa (while sparing the mucosal base) has been used with some success. A 2005 study by Wormald evaluated 42 severely diseased maxillary sinuses and found improved symptom control in patients who underwent combined maxillary antrostomy and mucosal clearance via canine fossa puncture versus those who had maxillary antrostomy alone.[4] A 2008 study found similarly superior results when comparing mega-antrostomy with mucosal clearance via canine fossa puncture to maxillary antrostomy alone in patients with severely diseased maxillary sinuses.[5] These results have been challenged by a 2008 study that found no advantage to canine fossa puncture and mucosal clearance when comparing 13 patients who underwent standard middle meatal antrostomy to 11 patients who underwent antrostomy with mucosal clearance via the canine fossa approach.[6]

It is, however, well known that Caldwell-Luc surgery has a high rate of complication and patient morbidity, and for this reason should be used only as a last resort. A 1988 review of 670 patients who underwent Caldwell-Luc surgery at a single institution found a 19% complication rate.[7] Facial numbness continues to be among the most common of these complications. Cadaver studies by Wormald and others have elucidated the distribution patterns of the infraorbital nerve and anterior-superior alveolar nerve that lead to these sensory deficits when traumatized.[8] In fact, the simple canine fossa puncture—theoretically less invasive than a Caldwell-Luc approach or procedure—has been noted to have a long-term incidence of postoperative facial numbness that approaches 10%.[9]

These studies highlight the lack of strong evidence-based medicine that could determine the decision over when to use a Caldwell-Luc approach or procedure or some modification thereof. Future studies will be needed to bring clarity and certainty to this decision. In the meantime, innovation will likely lead to other hybrid approaches such as the canine fossa puncture and the endoscopic endonasal Caldwell-Luc procedure.

Pearls

- The Caldwell-Luc approach provides access to the maxillary sinus via the anterior face of the maxilla.
- The Caldwell-Luc procedure involves exenteration of the maxillary sinus mucosa, traditionally through a Caldwell-Luc approach.
- The Caldwell-Luc procedure is a procedure of last resort, appropriate in the treatment of sinusitis for patients who have failed aggressive medical and surgical therapy.
- The Caldwell-Luc approach and procedure have significant associated morbidity and should be reserved for patients who have not responded to prior surgical intervention.
- When used in this manner, Caldwell-Luc surgery has been found to have good outcomes.
- Morbidity to facial sensation may be minimized by paying careful attention to the typical distribution patterns of the infraorbital nerve and anterior superior alveolar nerve.
- Hybrid approaches—maxillary antrostomy with canine fossa puncture and the endoscopic endonasal Caldwell-Luc procedure—have recently been described and may decrease morbidity without compromising efficacy.

References

1. Penttilä M, Rautiainen M, Pukander J, Kataja M. Functional vs. radical maxillary surgery. Failures after functional endoscopic sinus surgery. Acta Otolaryngol Suppl 1997;529:173–176
2. Närkiö-Mäkelä M, Qvarnberg Y. Endoscopic sinus surgery or Caldwell-Luc operation in the treatment of chronic and recurrent maxillary sinusitis. Acta Otolaryngol Suppl 1997;529:177–180
3. Cutler JL, Duncavage JA, Matheny K, Cross JL, Miman MC, Oh CK. Results of Caldwell-Luc after failed endoscopic middle meatus antrostomy in patients with chronic sinusitis. Laryngoscope 2003;113(12):2148–2150
4. Sathananthar S, Nagaonkar S, Paleri V, Le T, Robinson S, Wormald PJ. Canine fossa puncture and clearance of the maxillary sinus for the severely diseased maxillary sinus. Laryngoscope 2005;115(6):1026–1029
5. Abd el-Fattah H, Nour YA, el-Daly A. Endoscopic radical antrectomy: a permanent replacement for the Caldwell-Luc operation. J Laryngol Otol 2008;122(3):268–276
6. Lee JY, Lee SH, Hong HS, Lee JD, Cho SH. Is the canine fossa puncture approach really necessary for the severely diseased maxillary sinus during endoscopic sinus surgery? Laryngoscope 2008;118(6):1082–1087
7. DeFreitas J, Lucente FE. The Caldwell-Luc procedure: institutional review of 670 cases: 1975-1985. Laryngoscope 1988;98(12):1297–1300
8. Robinson S, Wormald PJ. Patterns of innervation of the anterior maxilla: a cadaver study with relevance to canine fossa puncture of the maxillary sinus. Laryngoscope 2005;115(10):1785–1788
9. Robinson SR, Baird R, Le T, Wormald PJ. The incidence of complications after canine fossa puncture performed during endoscopic sinus surgery. Am J Rhinol 2005;19(2):203–206

18 Endoscopic Maxillary Sinus Surgery: From Minimal to Maximal

Aldo C. Stamm, Ronaldo Nunes Toledo, João Flávio Nogueira, and Shirley S. N. Pignatari

The maxillary sinus is the largest of the paranasal sinuses; it is found in the body of the maxilla bone. It is bound medially by the lateral nasal wall, superiorly by the orbital floor, anteriorly by the canine fossa, and inferiorly by the alveolar process of the maxilla.[1,2] The normally sterile maxillary sinus is lined by ciliated pseudostratified columnar epithelium covered by a double-layered mucous blanket. The deep layer lubricates the cilia, whereas the superficial layer captures foreign particles, which are transported by the cilia to the sinus ostium. Ciliary dysfunction or alterations in mucus composition can contribute to mucus stasis and subsequent infections.[1,2]

According to the studies of Zuckerkandl in 1882, the maxillary sinus ostium is usually shaped like a narrow ellipse, ranging from 3 to 19 mm (average 5 mm). Endoscopic visualization of the natural maxillary sinus ostium is uncommon because the ostium is frequently hidden by the intact uncinate process. On the other hand, "accessory" maxillary sinus ostia can be identified endoscopically. These accessory orifices are found in ~10% of the population and are located in the posterior fontanelle.[1–4]

Because it was first described by Leonardo da Vinci, the physiology and diseases of the maxillary sinus have been objects of medical interest. From a storage space for grease to lubricate the eyes' movements, to the lightening of the weight of the skull, improving vocal resonance, absorbing shocks to the face or skull, to regulating intranasal pressure, the maxillary sinus has several functions. It also can be the cause of several illnesses, especially those closely related to the face, nose, and eyes.[1–3]

With advances in rhinology, the physiology and diseases of the maxillary sinus have been better described, and several surgical approaches have been proposed, both for the treatment of maxillary sinus diseases and for lesions involving the orbit, pterygoid, and infratemporal regions. Much has happened since the surgical approaches proposed by Caldwell and Luc to the era of the endoscopic surgery.

In this chapter, we will present the most common endoscopic surgical procedures and approaches to the maxillary sinus, including balloon sinuplasty, minimally invasive sinus treatment (MIST) (**see Video 18.1**), conventional maxillary sinus antrostomy, medial maxillectomy and pterygoid surgical approaches. We will also discuss briefly the most frequent surgical indications, imaging and instrumentation, surgical complications, postoperative care and follow-up.

Surgical Indications

The major indications for endoscopic maxillary sinus surgery are lesions that involve the maxillary sinus, the pterygoid and infratemporal regions, including maxillary cysts, antrochoanal polyps, barotrauma, mucocele, polyps, chronic rhinosinusitis, inverted papilloma, carcinoma, juvenile angiofibroma, tumors located into the pterygoid and infratemporal spaces, among others.[5]

Imaging

Specific chapters of this book address the anatomy and imaging of the maxillary sinus. In general, computerized tomography (CT) of the paranasal sinuses is the best way to evaluate the anatomic parameters and diseases of the maxillary sinus. Axial and coronal views permit the identification of the uncinate process, nasolacrimal duct, orbit, infraorbital nerve, and diseases within the maxillary sinus itself or its adjacencies (**Fig. 18.1**). Sagittal reconstruction promotes the identification of the pterygoid fossa and its relationship with the maxillary sinus.

Instrumentation

The endoscopic maxillary surgery is usually performed with zero- and 45-degree endoscopes, and, in some cases, an endoscope of 70 degrees may be necessary. Although conventional endoscopic surgical instrumentation can also be used, some of the surgical instruments should be curved, and for infratemporal approaches, longer and thinner, but just as strong or stronger.[6] Straight and curved suction cannulas should be available and we recommend a blunted edge cannula to avoid unnecessary trauma and mucosal bleeding. A micro-Kerrison punch is used to remove thin delicate bony plates.

Monopolar and bipolar electrocautery permit the surgeon to control and minimize the bleeding. Powered instrumentation (i.e., microdebriders) is also important. Although not necessary, these instruments, which have multiple functions including suction, cutting, and irrigation, can be very useful during endoscopic surgery by improving the quality and presentation of the surgical field. At the present, newer

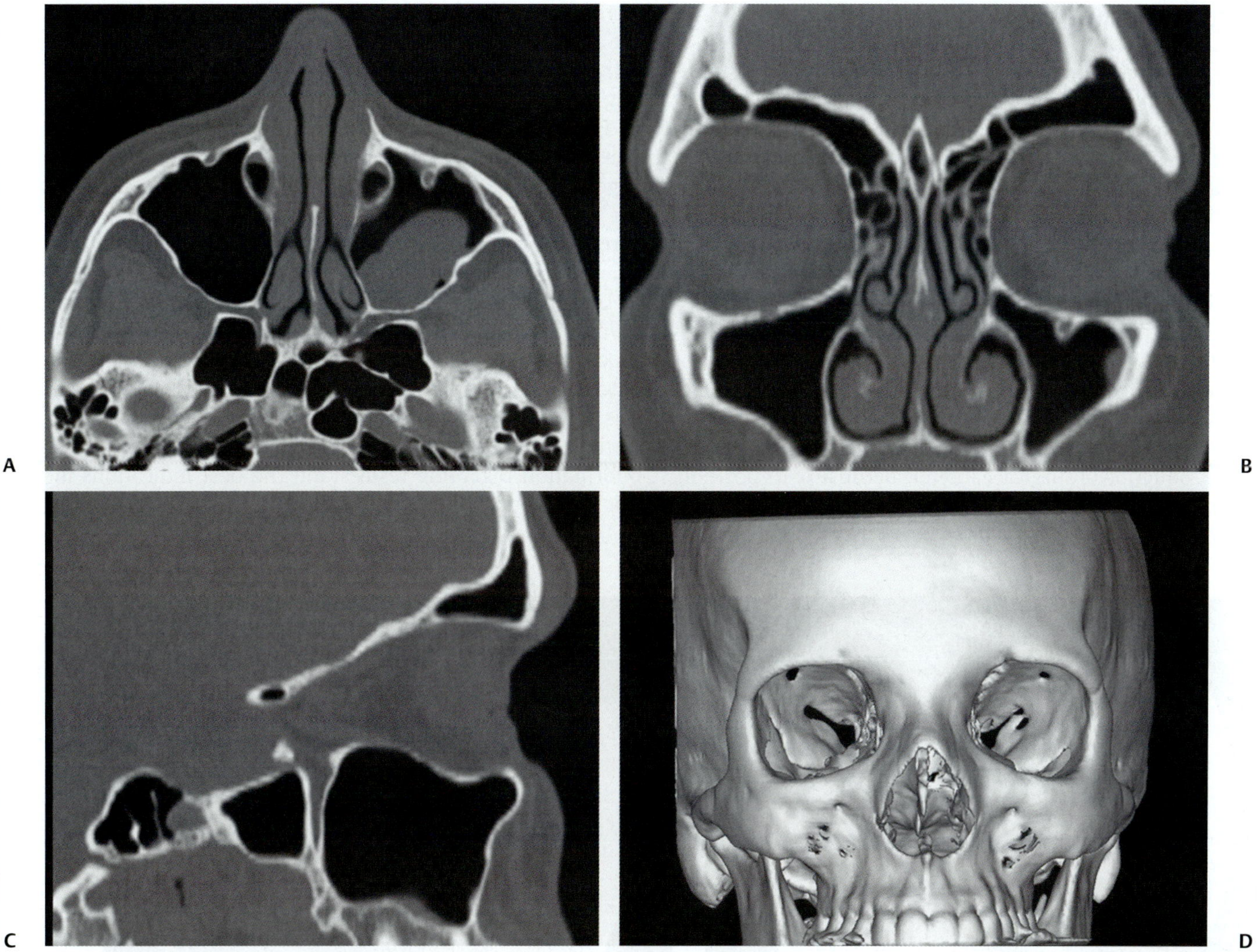

Fig. 18.1 **(A–D)** Paranasal sinus computer tomography (CT) scans. This is the best way to evaluate the maxillary sinus. **(A)** Axial cut to demonstrate the maxillary sinus relationships with the nasolacrimal duct and the pterygopalatine fossae. **(B)** Coronal view to evaluate the maxillary sinus relation to the orbit, infraorbital nerve, inferior turbinate, and uncinate process. **(C)** Sagittal reconstruction showing the pterygopalatine fossae. **(D)** Tridimensional reconstruction.

instruments with curved blades and burrs, able to remove bone and debulk some tumors are commercially available. The newest microdebriders also produce a more precise cut of the diseased tissue, avoiding mucosal stripping, and are accompanied by continuous irrigation, which improves visualization and diminishes the loss of blood. However, these instruments also require more attention from the surgeon. They can be potentially more dangerous to the tissues, and doctors should be acquainted with these powerful instruments before using them.

Image-guided systems are precise and have been very helpful. These systems of tridimensional navigation provide important information about the location of anatomic structures in the operative field and create an individual anatomic map generated from preoperative computerized tomography. These image-guided systems help to diminish the chances of surgical complications because they provide the surgeon with the exact location of every instrument in the surgical field.[6,7]

Surgical Techniques

The surgery is performed under hypotensive general anesthesia. The patient is placed in a supine position on the operating table, with the dorsum elevated 30 degrees and with the neck slightly flexed and the head extended and turned toward the surgeon. High concentration adrenaline-soaked cottonoids (1:1000) are placed into the nasal cavity for 10 minutes before the beginning of the surgical procedure.

Balloon Sinuplasty

Balloon catheter dilatation is a recently introduced minimally invasive tool in rhinology that works with the concept of remolding the anatomy of the paranasal sinus ostia without removing tissue or bone. Its use in patients has proven to be feasible, safe, and the most important indications include chronic rhinosinusitis, barotrauma, and trauma, among others. The system, composed of several guide-catheters, a pumping bomb, a guide wire, and a balloon, uses the same principles commonly used in other medical specialties such as vascular surgery, urology, cardiology, and gastroenterology. The introduction of balloon catheters under fluoroscopic guidance, followed by high pressure inflation, results in dilatation of the sinus ostium.[8–11]

The maxillary sinus ostium is known as the trickiest for the introduction of surgical catheters because of its position, which is hidden behind the uncinate process. The catheter introduction is usually accomplished by softly displacing the uncinate process with a 90-degree maxillary guiding catheter, under 45-degree, 4-mm endoscope visualization (**Fig. 18.2**).

The next step consists of fixing the position of the balloon. The balloon should be in contact with the entire circular edge of the maxillary sinus natural ostium. After positioning the balloon, it is inflated with ~8 to 10 atmospheres of pressure, resulting in dilation of the ostium. A catheter may also be used to provide suction and irrigation (**Fig. 18.2**).

Usually, there is no mucosal tearing or bone exposure; therefore, no nasal packing is needed after the surgical procedure and the patient can be discharged on the same day.[9–11] Balloon sinuplasty is a fairly new procedure and at this point, some controversies still exist. Further studies, complete with long-term follow-up should bring important information regarding results and the best indications for this surgical technique (**see Video 18.2**).

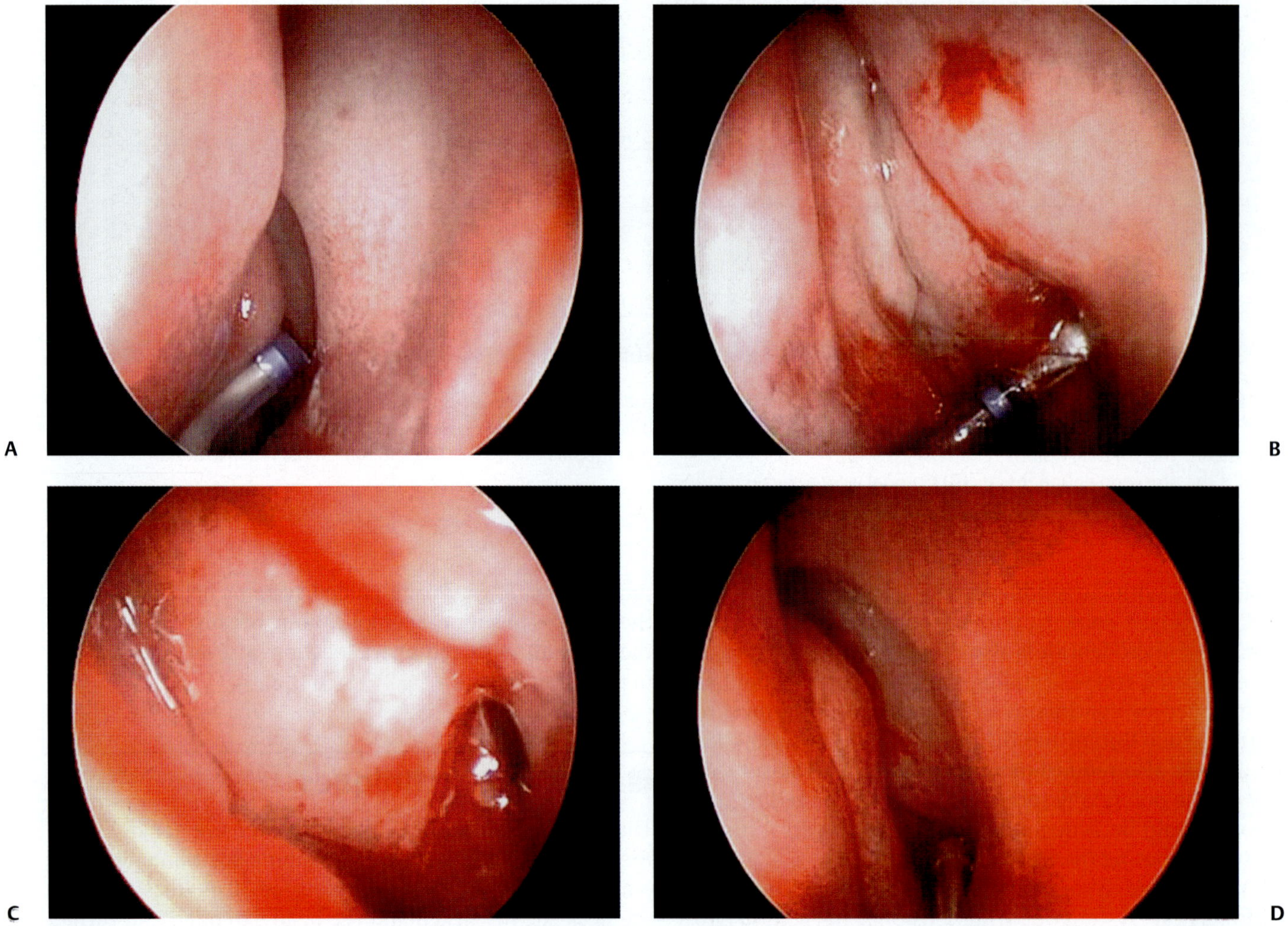

Fig. 18.2 **(A–D)** Balloon catheterization and dilatation of the maxillary sinus natural ostium. **(A)** Positioning of the catheter. **(B)** Positioning of the balloon at the maxillary sinus natural ostium. **(C)** Endoscopic visualization of a 45-degree endoscope of the dilated maxillary sinus natural ostium. **(D)** Endoscopic view of the middle meatus after the procedure.

Maxillary Antrostomy

This is probably the first and most important step in endonasal maxillary, ethmoid, and frontal endoscopic surgery. The uncinate process is removed to expose the anterior ethmoid and visualize the natural maxillary sinus ostium (**Fig. 18.3**). To ensure that this step is performed correctly and to prevent postoperative synechiae and iatrogenic complications, it is essential to understand the anatomy of the uncinate process.[12,13] The uncinate process is a hook-shaped structure composed of a thin bony plate that is covered by mucosa on both sides and lies in an approximately parasagittal plane. It is attached anteriorly to the posterior edge of the lacrimal bone and inferiorly to the superior edge of the inferior turbinate. It has a free posterior border. Yoon et al (cited in Wadwongthan et al) described eight types of the posteroinferior portion of the uncinate process during anatomic studies of the fontanelle and uncinate process.[14]

There is still some controversy about the upper insertion of the uncinate process. Some authors believe that it ascends isolated to the lacrimal bone, skull base, lamina papyracea, or middle turbinate superiorly. We conducted a study that shows multiple superior insertions of the uncinate process. This has important technical implications, especially for endoscopic frontal recess and sinus surgery. With correct removal of the uncinate process, the natural maxillary sinus ostium can be seen (**see Video 18.3**).[12–14]

The following points should be noted in an endoscopic maxillary antrostomy. A common error is failure to expose the natural maxillary sinus ostium, instead creating a separate antral fenestration in the posterior fontanelle. The presence of this fenestration may interfere with normal mucociliary clearance, causing mucus recirculation from the natural ostium through the fenestration back into the maxillary sinus, leading to recurrent complaints. As a general rule, the maxillary sinus can be endoscopically evaluated with a 45-degree endoscope following exposure of the natural ostium. If this cannot be done, the natural ostium can be enlarged in the inferior or posterior direction with suitable instruments. Indications for enlarging the natural maxillary sinus ostium include nasal polyposis in cystic fibrosis or aspirin intolerance, maxillary sinus aspergilloma, and tumors such as juvenile angiofibroma and inverted papilloma.

Endoscopic Medial Maxillectomy

Endoscopic medial maxillectomy (EMM) is a procedure that may be indicated in some cases of inverted papilloma resection or for malignant sinonasal neoplasms restricted to the lateral wall of the nasal cavity or medial maxillary sinus (**Fig. 18.4**). Initially, this procedure was described for the treatment of inverted papilloma and was characterized by en bloc resection of the lateral nasal wall, including the inferior turbinate and the nasolacrimal duct, beside the middle turbinate and the anterior and posterior ethmoid sinus.[15]

The procedure begins with resection of the middle turbinate attachment on the lateral nasal wall following the dissection of the ethmoid sinus of the lamina papyracea and the ethmoid fovea until the rostrum of the sphenoid sinus. If necessary, the ethmoid arteries are cauterized with a bipolar cautery. After the liberation of the ethmoid sinus, the incision of the nasal mucosa is made at the attachment of the middle turbinate to the inferior meatus, including the resection of all of the uncinate process, the lacrimal bone containing the nasolacrimal duct, and the inferior turbinate; for this, the incision should pass anteriorly to the head of the inferior turbinate. After the elevation of the nasal mucosa,

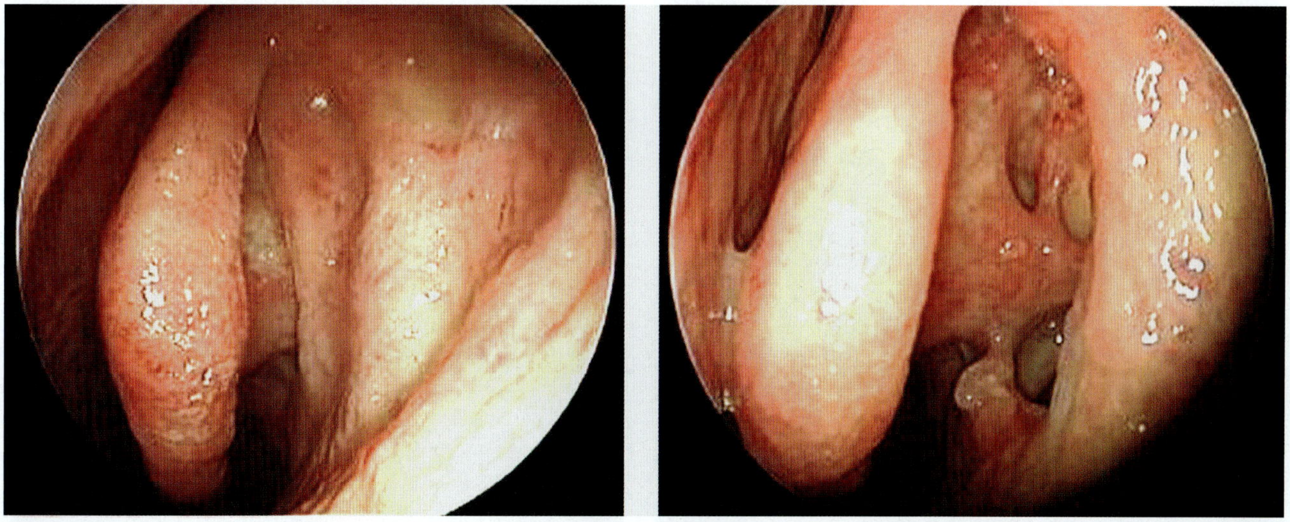

A B

Fig. 18.3 **(A)** Endoscopic view of the middle meatus. **(B)** Visualization of the maxillary sinus natural ostium, after the uncinate process removal. This is probably the most important step in this surgical procedure.

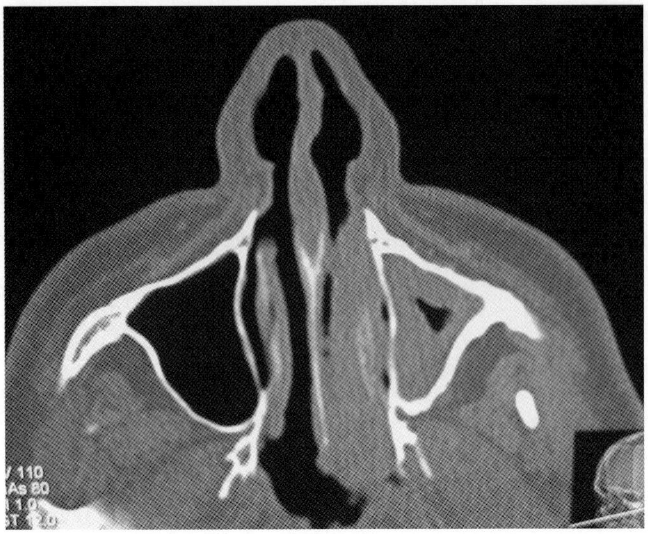

Fig. 18.4 Axial computer tomography (CT) scan of a paranasal sinus with nasal mucosa melanoma restricted to the lateral wall of the nasal cavity. Maxillar sinus with sinusitis due to occlusion of ostiomeatal complex.

using a drill or osteotome, an osteotomy is made on the lateral nasal wall until the inferior meatus reaches the floor of the nose. An osteotomy is then made at the inferior meatus junction of the nasal floor to the posterior wall of maxillary sinus (**Fig. 18.5**).

The nasal wall, along with the tumor, are both medially mobilized for the nasal cavity, with a dissection made inside the maxillary sinus. Posterior cuts separating the surgical piece of the posterior wall of the maxillary sinus are made, including cauterization of the sphenopalatine artery. The posterior attachment of the inferior turbinate is cut and the lateral wall along with the tumor is removed en bloc.[15]

Generally, the nasolacrimal duct is transected obliquely to avoid stenosis of the duct and epiphoras. The opening and the catheterization of the lacrimal sac during surgery is not necessary.

Currently, EMM is utilized for the removal of sinonasal neoplasms and has several variations, one of which is the extended endoscopic medial maxillectomy (EEMM). In these cases, the resection of the posterior wall of the maxillary sinus can be made, permitting access to pterygomaxillary and pterygopalatine fossas. Extension of the surgery for other paranasal sinuses, such as the sphenoid and frontal sinus, can be made. More recently, the resection of the pyriform aperture has been described in association with EMM; being an anterior form of EEMM.[16,17]

In the endoscopic resection of the pyriform aperture, an anterior cut of the attachment of the inferior turbinate head on the mucosa that covers the frontal process of the maxilla is made. From the incision, the mucosa is removed and the free margin of the pyriform aperture is exposed. The separation of the mucosa and the periosteum from the anterior wall of the maxillary sinus can be elevated until the emergence of the infraorbital nerve. The anterior wall of the maxillary sinus is opened with a drill or osteotome and the frontal process of the maxilla is resected. When the pyriform aperture is resected, access to the maxillary sinus is maximized and the tumoral lesions with small invasions of the anterior and medial wall can be seen.[16,17]

In the event of an inflammatory disease or a benign tumor with inverted papilloma, resection can be less extensive, generally with preservation of nasolacrimal duct or with partial resection of the inferior turbinate. The procedure is then called a modified endoscopic medial maxillectomy.[18]

Yet, the vision of the maxillary sinus is limited in this situation. Anatomic studies evaluating the volume of the maxillary sinus demonstrate that with medial maxillectomy, when the nasolacrimal duct and the inferior turbinate are preserved, vision to the maxillary sinus is extremely restricted: almost 70% of the volume of the sinus is covered by inferior turbinate and nasolacrimal duct attachment.[19] The

A

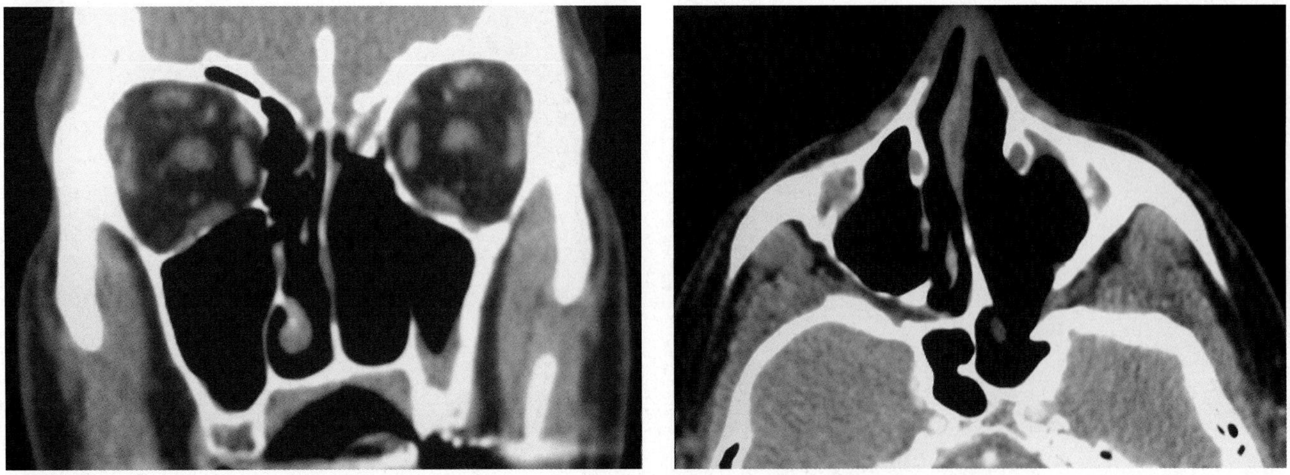

B

Fig. 18.5 **(A,B)** Paranasal sinus computer tomography (CT) scan after a medial maxillectomy. **(A)** Coronal view showing the limits of the resection. **(B)** Axial cut demonstrating the limits of the medial maxillectomy resection.

resection of the nasolacrimal duct and the inferior turbinate permits an adequate view of the lateral wall and of the nasal floor as well, in cases where the nasal wall is inferior to the nasal wall cavity.

Infratemporal Approach

The maxillary sinus has thin walls that face the lower nasal cavity medially, the orbit superiorly, the infratemporal fossa posterolaterally, the pterygopalatine fossa posteromedially, and the soft tissue of the cheek anterolaterally. The maxillary sinus provides a transantral avenue for extending a midline surgical approach for more extensive lateral exposure of the cavernous sinus and the infratemporal fossa.[20]

The transmaxillary approach is excellent for removing lesions that involve the medial portion of the maxillary sinus, and for larger lesions in the pterygopalatine, zygomatic, or infratemporal fossae such as angiofibromas (**see Video 18.4**). This approach can also be extended to gain exposure to the cavernous sinus.

The procedure begins with an anterior ethmoidectomy and continues with a wide middle meatus antrostomy to give maximal exposure of the posterior maxillary sinus wall. Sometimes it is necessary to remove the inferior turbinate, entirely resecting the medial wall of the maxillary sinus to obtain adequate exposure of the posterior and posterolateral wall of the sinus. During the removal of the inferior turbinate, special care must be taken to avoid injuring the terminal branches of the maxillary artery at the sphenopalatine foramen and the second division of the trigeminal nerve.[20–22]

The amount of posterior wall bone to be removed depends on the location and extent of the lesion as determined by preoperative image studies or by information from the image-guided system at the time of surgery. The posterior wall of the maxillary sinus can be opened by enlarging the sphenopalatine foramen with a micro-Kerrison punch and exposing the periosteum of the pterygopalatine, zygomatic fossae, and infratemporal fossae. It is important to try to preserve the integrity of the periosteum and avoid fat protrusion into the operative field. If fat does protrude into the sinus, it is reduced by bipolar electrocoagulation, which also is used to control any bleeding. This technique is particularly useful in removing angiofibroma when early identification of the feeding vessels is essential.

The transpterygoid and infratemporal accesses are extensions of the transmaxillary access. In the transpterygoid approach, lateral extensions of the sphenoid sinus (pterygoid recess) and lesions involving the pterygopalatine fossa and zygomatic fossa can be accessed. This may require removal of the medial and sometimes lateral pterygoid processes to achieve access to the lateral and pterygoid regions of the sphenoid sinus. A wide sphenoidotomy is also performed at the beginning or during the surgical operation. This access allows treatment of lesions involving the cavernous sinus that are lateral to the paraclival internal carotid artery.

The infratemporal access adds a medial endoscopic maxillectomy. In this surgical access, we resect the posterior wall and sometimes the lateral wall of the maxillary sinus, particularly in situations with lateral expansion of the lesion.

Conclusion

Endoscopic maxillary sinus surgery is currently considered the gold standard surgical approach for the treatment of many lesions involving the maxillary sinus and its adjacent structures. This surgical approach may vary from very minimal invasive procedures to large and extensive resections. The surgeon's final choice must be made based on the patient's disease, the surgeon's experience, and the availability of the necessary instrumentation.

Pearls

- The maxillary sinus is the largest of the paranasal sinuses.
- There are several surgical approaches to the maxillary sinus; the surgeon's choice should be based on experience, type and extension of the disease, and the availability of the necessary instrumentation.
- The maxillary sinus antrostomy is bounded by the nasolacrimal duct anteriorly, the orbital floor superiorly. This is important to remember when approaching the sinus surgically.
- Straight and angled endoscopes (30- or 45-degree) are paramount for any endoscopic maxillary sinus surgery.
- One of the most common causes for maxillary sinus revision surgery is the lack of inclusion of the natural ostium at the prior antrostomy.
- This principle is also valid for other minimal invasive endoscopic surgeries, such as balloon sinuplasty, MIST, and medial maxillectomy. A careful look at the natural ostium must always be a step in the procedure.

References

1. Lusk RP. Endoscopic approach to sinus disease. J Allergy Clin Immunol 1992;90(3 Pt 2):496–505
2. Navarro JAC. Surgical anatomy of the nose, paranasal sinuses, and pterygopalatine fossa. In: Stamm AC, Draf W, ed. Micro-endoscopic Surgery of the Paranasal Sinuses and the Skull Base. Heidelberg: Springer 2000;17–34
3. Nogueira JF Jr, Hermann DR, Américo RdosR, Barauna Filho IS, Stamm AE, Pignatari SS. A brief history of otorhinolaryngolgy: otology, laryngology and rhinology. Braz J Otorhinolaryngol 2007;73(5):693–703
4. Miller AJ, Amedee RG. Functional anatomy of the paranasal sinuses. J La State Med Soc 1997;149(3):85–90

5. Christmas DA, Yanagisawa E, Joe JK. Transnasal endoscopic identification of the natural ostium of the maxillary sinus: a retrograde approach. Ear Nose Throat J 1998;77(6):454–455
6. Lesserson JA, Schaefer SD. Instrumentation for endoscopic sinus surgery. Ear Nose Throat J 1994;73(8):522–524, 527, 531
7. Nogueira JF Jr, Stamm AC, Lyra M. Novel compact laptop-based image-guidance system: preliminary study. Laryngoscope 2009;119 (3):576–579
8. Vaughan WC. Review of balloon sinuplasty. Curr Opin Otolaryngol Head Neck Surg 2008;16(1):2–9
9. Christmas DA, Mirante JP, Yanagisawa E. Endoscopic view of balloon catheter dilation of sinus ostia (balloon sinuplasty). Ear Nose Throat J 2006;85(11):698–700, 700
10. Siow JK, Al Kadah B, Werner JA. Balloon sinuplasty: a current hot topic in rhinology. Eur Arch Otorhinolaryngol 2008;265(5):509–511
11. Bolger WE, Vaughan WC. Catheter-based dilation of the sinus ostia: initial safety and feasibility analysis in a cadaver model. Am J Rhinol 2006;20(3):290–294
12. Kennedy DW, Zinreich SJ, Shaalan H, Kuhn F, Naclerio R, Loch E. Endoscopic middle meatal antrostomy: theory, technique, and patency. Laryngoscope 1987; 97(8 Pt 3, Suppl 43)1–9
13. Albu S, Tomescu E. Small and large middle meatus antrostomies in the treatment of chronic maxillary sinusitis. Otolaryngol Head Neck Surg 2004;131(4):542–547
14. Wadwongtham W, Aeumjaturapat S. Large middle meatal antrostomy vs undisturbed maxillary ostium in the endoscopic sinus surgery of nasal polyposis. J Med Assoc Thai 2003;86(Suppl 2):S373–S378
15. Sadeghi N, Al-Dhahri S, Manoukian JJ. Transnasal endoscopic medial maxillectomy for inverting papilloma. Laryngoscope 2003; 113(4):749–753
16. Lim SC, Lee JK, Yoon TM. Extended endoscopic medial maxillectomy for sinonasal neoplasms. Otolaryngol Head Neck Surg 2008;139(2):310–312
17. Smith W, Lowe D, Leong P. Resection of pyriform aperture: a useful adjunct in nasal surgery. J Laryngol Otol 2009;123(1):123–125
18. Woodworth BA, Parker RO, Schlosser RJ. Modified endoscopic medial maxillectomy for chronic maxillary sinusitis. Am J Rhinol 2006;20(3):317–319
19. Tanna N, Edwards JD, Aghdam H, Sadeghi N. Transnasal endoscopic medial maxillectomy as the initial oncologic approach to sinonasal neoplasms: the anatomic basis. Arch Otolaryngol Head Neck Surg 2007;133(11):1139–1142
20. Stamm A, Pignatari SSN. Transnasal endoscopic-assisted surgery of the skull base. In: Cummings C, Flint P, Harker L, eds. Otolaryngology Head Neck Surgery. 4th ed. Philadelphia: Elsevier; 2005:3855–3876
21. Nogueira JF, Stamm AC, Lyra M, Balieiro FO, Leão FS. Building a real endoscopic sinus and skull-base surgery simulator. Otolaryngol Head Neck Surg 2008;139(5):727–728
22. Bossolesi P, Autelitano L, Brusati R, Castelnuovo P. The silent sinus syndrome: diagnosis and surgical treatment. Rhinology 2008;46(4):308–316

19 The Pterygopalatine Fossa

Belachew Tessema, Jean Anderson Eloy, and Roy R. Casiano

The pterygopalatine fossa (PPF) is a pyramidal space with incomplete osseous boundaries located among the maxillary, sphenoid, and palatine bones (**Fig. 19.1**). The PPF is bounded posteriorly by the pterygoid plates of the sphenoid bone, which fuses at the skull base into the pterygoid process. Medially, the perpendicular plate of the palatine bone constitute the wall of the PPF, which tapers inferiorly in a funnel-shaped space at the level of the attachment between maxillary bone and the pyramidal process of the palatine bone (**Fig. 19.2**). The maxillary tuberosity constitutes the anterior boundary of the PPF, which communicates with the orbital apex through the medial portion of the inferior orbital fissure. Through the pterygomaxillary fissure, the PPF merges laterally with the masticatory space of the infratemporal fossa. The pterygopalatine fossa communicates with the middle cranial fossa, orbit, nasal cavity, oral cavity, and the infratemporal fossa via rotundum and sphenopalatine foramina, the vidian and palatovaginal canals, and the greater and lesser palatine foramina.[1]

Topographically, the PPF can be divided into an anterior and posterior compartment. The anterior space is occupied by the third segment of the maxillary artery (MA) and its branches, whereas the posterior compartment is represented by the maxillary nerve and the sphenopalatine ganglion and its branches.[2] The pterygopalatine segment of the maxillary artery (third segment) runs on the anterior edge of the lateral pterygoid muscle and reaches the pterygopalatine fossa through the pterygomaxillary fissure (PMF). The MA passes horizontally deep to the mandibular ramus and gives off the buccal artery (BA), which supplies the buccinator muscle. It then turns medially through the PMF coursing in the anterior and superior direction to give off several branches. According to the order of branching in its course from the pterygomaxillary junction area, the posterosuperior alveolar artery (PSAA) and infraorbital artery (IOA) are located at the posterior wall of the maxilla and enter into the posterosuperior alveolar foramen and the infraorbital fissure, respectively (**Fig. 19.3**). Then, it divides into the descending palatine artery (DPA), which supplies the palate, the artery of the pterygoid canal (VA), which is located in the pterygoid canal, and the sphenopalatine artery (SPA).[3]

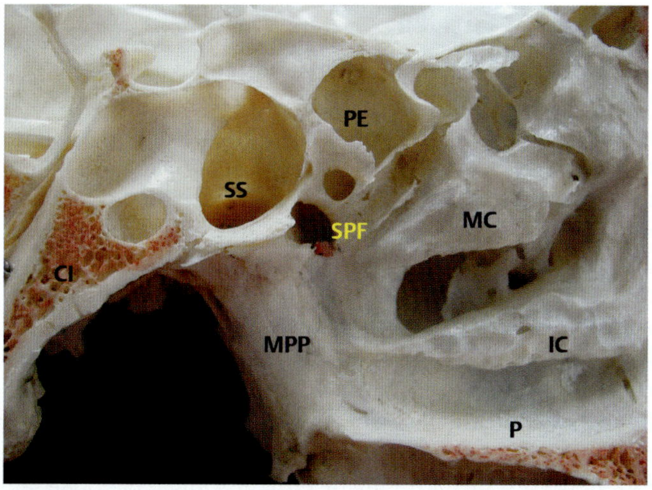

Fig. 19.1 Photomicrograph of a sagittal image of the bony medial boundaries of the left pterygopalatine fossa. SPF, sphenopalatine foramen; MPP, medial pterygoid plate; SS, sphenoid sinus; PE, posterior ethmoid cell; CI, clivus; MC, middle concha; IC, inferior concha; P, hard palate.

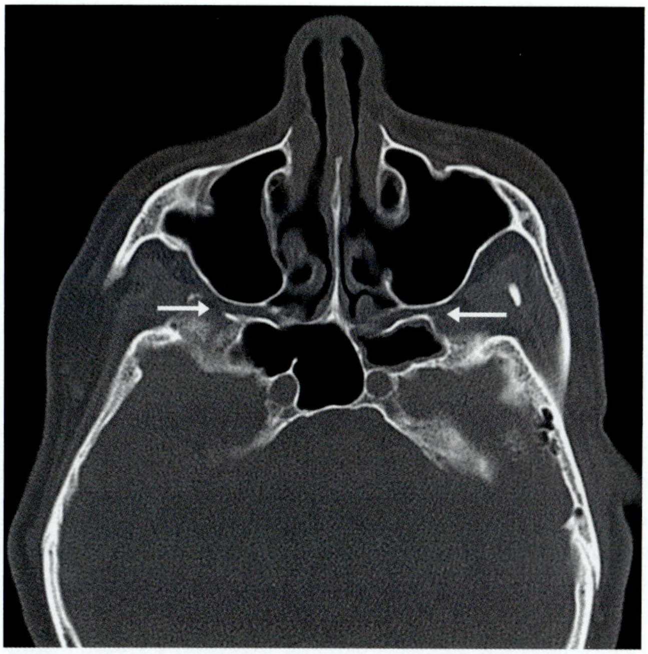

Fig. 19.2 Axial computed tomography (CT) scan showing the pterygopalatine fossa *(white arrows)*.

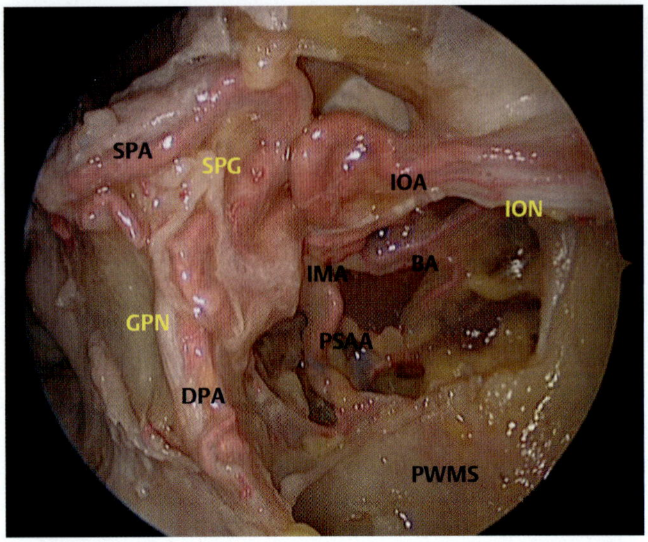

Fig. 19.3 Endoscopic view of the contents of the anterior compartment of the pterygomaxillary fossa. IMA, internal maxillary artery; BA, buccal artery; PSAA, posterior superior alveolar artery; SPA, sphenopalatine artery; IOA, infraorbital artery; DPA, descending palatine artery; SPG, sphenopalatine ganglion; GPN, greater palatine nerve; ION, infraorbital nerve; PWMS, posterior wall of maxillary sinus.

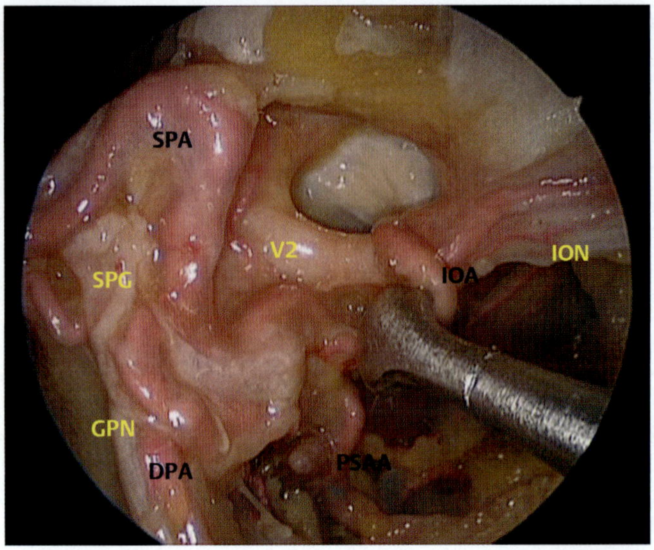

Fig. 19.4 Endoscopic view of the contents of the posterior compartment of the pterygomaxillary fossa. V2, maxillary division of trigeminal nerve internal; PSAA, posterior superior alveolar artery; SPA, sphenopalatine artery; IOA, infraorbital artery; DPA, descending palatine artery; SPG, sphenopalatine ganglion; GPN, greater palatine nerve; ION, infraorbital nerve.

Displacement of the vascular branches in the anterior compartment allows for visualization of the posterior compartment of the PPF (**Fig. 19.4**). The sphenopalatine ganglion (also known as the pterygopalatine ganglion) is naturally lodged into a niche of the posterior-inferior portion of the PPF just anterior to the pterygoid canal that conveys the vidian nerve. The maxillary nerve enters the PPF through the foramen rotundum and remains superolateral to the ganglion to give rise to its zygomatic branch while continuing to the infraorbital groove as the infraorbital nerve.[4] During its anterolateral course, the infraorbital nerve constitutes an important surgical landmark that defines the PPF (medial) from the infratemporal fossa (lateral). Neural rami of distribution from the sphenopalatine ganglion are divisible into few groups: ascending (or orbital), posterior (to the pharynx), internal (to the nose), and descending (to the palate). Communicating rami connect the maxillary nerve to the inferiorly located sphenopalatine ganglion.[5] These nerves, along with the presence of orbital rami, contribute to form the superior apex of the small ganglion conferring to it its characteristic macroscopic triangular-shaped appearance. The thin orbital rami carry parasympathetic neurons and erratically reach the nasal mucosa through the anterior or posterior ethmoidal canals. The sphenopalatine ganglion also receives sympathetic and parasympathetic fibers through the vidian nerve. This nerve, formed by the fusion of greater and deep petrosal nerves at the level of the lacerated foramen, enters the PPF through the pterygoid (vidian) canal along with the vidian branch of the maxillary artery. The greater and lesser palatine nerves (descending branches) arise from the inferior-posterior portion of the ganglion and through the palatine canals reach the oral cavity.

Endoscopic Endonasal Surgery of the Pterygopalatine Fossa

The endoscopic endonasal route allows exposure of the pterygopalatine fossa through its anteromedial surface (**see Video 19.1**). The medial wall of the maxillary sinus is enlarged by extending the maxillary antrostomy to create a mega antrostomy or by performing a modified medial maxillectomy (**Fig. 19.5**). The posterior-lateral attachment of the middle turbinate is removed to gain access to the sphenopalatine foramen. The foramen is formed by the sphenopalatine notch inferiorly against the lower surface of the body of the sphenoid (**Fig. 19.6**). The notch itself is formed anteriorly by the orbital process of the palatine bone, inferiorly and posteriorly by the upper edge of the vertical plate of the palatine bone and the sphenoid process, respectively. A small bony ridge, the ethmoid crest, usually points to the sphenopalatine foramen, with the latter laying either completely or partially above the crest (class I and II, respectively). Occasionally, the sphenopalatine foramen consists of two separate openings, a larger superior opening and a small inferior one (class III).

The orbital process of the palatine bone is removed and the sphenopalatine foramen is enlarged using a drill or a Kerrison rongeur (**Fig. 19.7**). The posterior wall of the maxillary sinus is then removed up to the vertical process of the pala-

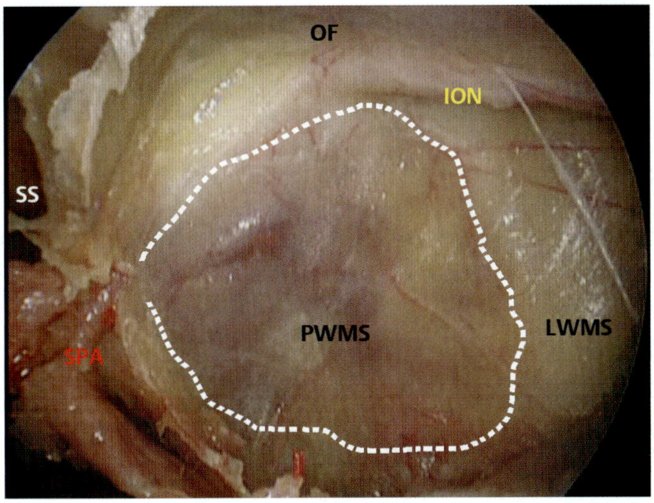

Fig. 19.5 Endoscopic view of the posterior wall of maxillary sinus with window into the pterygomaxillary fossa (PPF). SPA, sphenopalatine artery; PWMS, posterior wall of maxillary sinus; LWMS, lateral wall of maxillary sinus; SS, sphenoid sinus; OF, orbital floor; ION, infraorbital nerve. *Dashed white line* window to PPF.

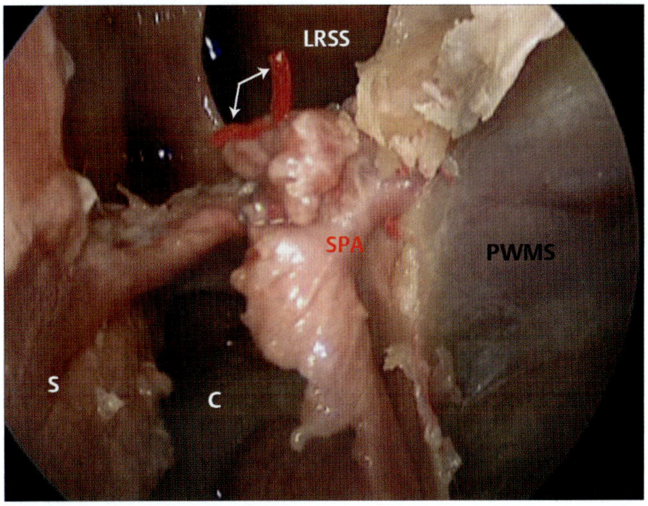

Fig. 19.6 Endoscopic image showing a direct view of the sphenopalatine foramen with a wide sphenoidotomy showing septal branch of the sphenopalatine artery. SPA, sphenopalatine artery; PWMS, posterior wall of maxillary sinus; LRSS, lateral recess of sphenoid sinus; S, septum; C, choanae. *White arrows* indicate the posterior septal branches of sphenoid sinus.

tine bone medially, and up to the angle between the lateral and posterior wall of the maxillary sinus to expose the pterygomaxillary fissure, which represents the communication between the pterygopalatine and the infratemporal fossa (**Fig. 19.8**). The pterygoid canal, the inferior part of the superior orbital fissure, the foramen rotundum, and the anterior surface of the pterygoid process can be identified and visualized. A wide sphenoid sinusotomy is then performed to determine the level of the sphenoid floor. The vidian foramen can be identified along the inferior bony face of the sphenoid sinus immediately posterior and perpendicular to the sphenopalatine foramen. The vidian nerve and artery can be identified in the pterygoid canal at the superior portion of the pterygopalatine fossa. Just medial to the vidian foramen, a small canal holding the pharyngeal or palatovaginal artery, which forms the sphenopalatine artery within the pterygomaxil-

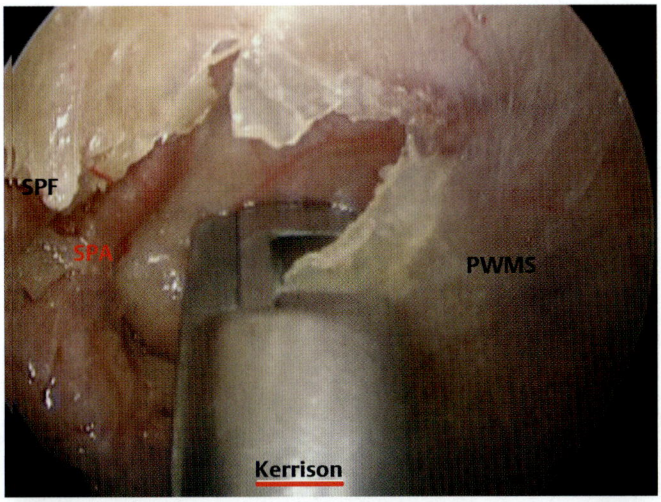

Fig. 19.7 Endoscopic resection of postwall of the left maxillary sinus with a Kerrison rongeur. SPA, sphenopalatine artery; SPF, sphenopalatine foramen; PWMS, posterior wall of maxillary sinus; Kerrison, Kerrison rongeur.

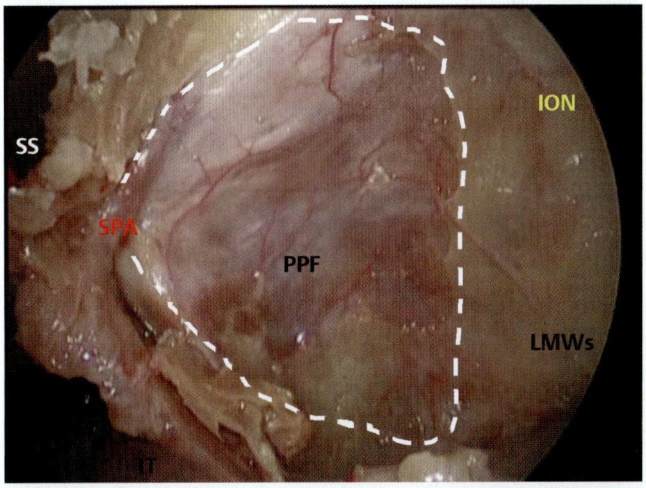

Fig. 19.8 View of the left maxillary sinus after endoscopic resection of the posterior maxillary wall for a window into the pterygomaxillary fossa (PPF). SPA, sphenopalatine artery; PWMS, posterior wall of maxillary sinus; LWMS, lateral wall of maxillary sinus; SS, sphenoid sinus; ION, infraorbital nerve; IT, inferior turbinate. *Dashed white line* window to PPF.

lary fossa, can be visualized. The vidian nerve is an important landmark for the identification of the foramen lacerum and for the intrapetrous carotid artery. Safe surgical dissection can be performed by drilling on the inferior and medial surface of the vidian canal. The inferior 180 degrees of the vidian canal should be drilled prior to proceeding to the superior 180 degrees to avoid inadvertent injury to the vessel.[1]

Through the foramen rotundum, the maxillary nerve travels from the cranial cavity into the pterygopalatine fossa. After piercing the foramen rotundum, this nerve passes through the pterygopalatine fossa and then reaches the inferior orbital fissure. The maxillary nerve is encountered during dissection within an area bounded superiorly by an oblique (or horizontal) line that connects the foramen rotundum and the infraorbital canal, inferiorly by a horizontal line at the level of the lower border of the sphenopalatine foramen, medially by a vertical line that passes through the foramen rotundum, and laterally by another vertical line at the posterior end of the infraorbital canal. In addition, the lower margin of the vidian canal can be used to depict the lowest level of the maxillary nerve more laterally. Before it becomes the infraorbital nerve, the maxillary nerve gives rise to the posterior alveolar nerve.[6] The infraorbital nerve is a consistent landmark that delineates the surgical boundaries between the pterygopalatine and the infratemporal fossa. The pterygopalatine fossa is located medially to it, whereas the infratemporal fossa is located laterally to it.

The identification of the vidian nerve and the maxillary nerve enable the surgeon to better define a surgical corridor between them that enables the exposure of the lateral wall of the sphenoid sinus (**Fig. 19.9**). The quadrangular area can have lesions arising in the pterygopalatine fossa, extending toward the middle cranial fossa and/or the cavernous sinus.[7] This quadrangular-shaped surgical corridor is delineated anteriorly by the pterygoid bone from the foramen rotundum to the pterygoid canal, posteriorly by the intrapetrous segment of the intracavernous carotid artery, superiorly by the maxillary nerve and inferiorly by the vidian nerve. The lateral extension of the dissection using this approach can destabilize the pterygoid process, and consequently, problems with mastication ensue due to malfunction of the lateral pterygoid muscle and the medial pterygoid muscle.[8]

Tumors of the Pterygopalatine Fossa

Tumors involving the pterygopalatine fossa can have multiple clinical presentations depending on the type and extent of tumor. Typical symptoms include unilateral nasal obstruction, epistaxis, V2 paresthesia, diplopia, and proptosis. Ocular symptoms with tumors involving the PPF can be secondary to affected pterygopalatine ganglion or cavernous sinus extension and subsequent abducens palsy. The differential diagnosis for lesions involving the PPF can be extensive including angiofibroma, carcinoma, lymphoma, melanoma, tumors of neural origin, and metastatic disease. It is important to note that imaging of tumors in the PPF usually identifies the extent of the tumor, but does not necessarily establish the diagnosis.

Juvenile nasopharyngeal angiofibroma (JNA) is the most frequent benign neoplasm of the nasopharynx (**Fig. 19.10**). JNA originates at the sphenopalatine foramen and extends into the nasal cavity, nasopharynx, paranasal sinuses, ptery-

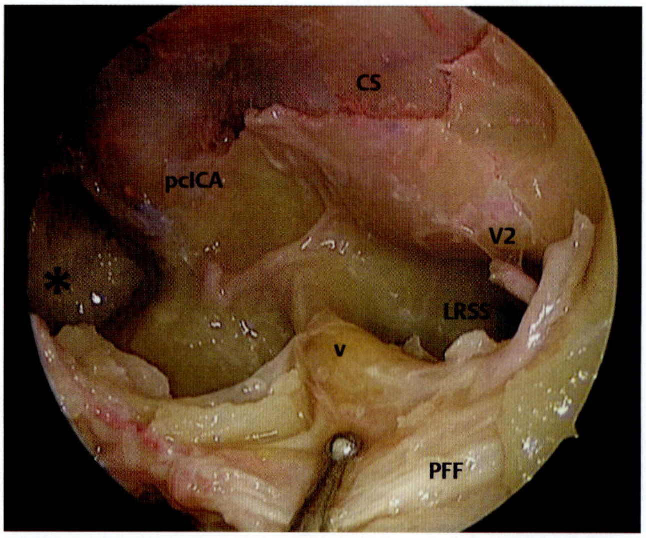

Fig. 19.9 Angled endoscopic view of the lateral recess of the sphenoid sinus with the vidian nerve coursing posteriorly toward the foramen lacerum and the intrapetrous carotid artery. pcICA, paraclival internal carotid artery; CS, dura of cavernous sinus; V2, maxillary division of trigeminal nerve; v, vidian nerve; PPF, pterygopalatine fossa; LRSS, lateral recess of sphenoid sinus. * indicates the clivus.

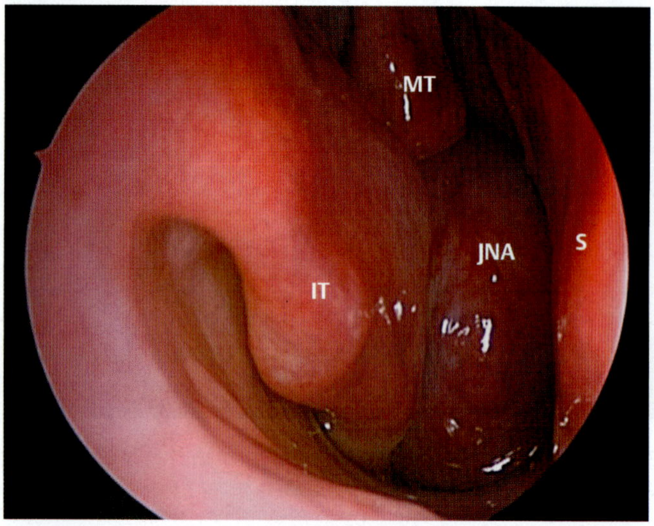

Fig. 19.10 Endoscopic view of a juvenile nasopharyngeal angiofibroma (JNA) in the right nasal cavity. IT, inferior turbinate; MT, middle turbinate; S, septum.

gopalatine fossa, infratemporal space and the cranial base. The main blood supply to the tumor is the internal maxillary artery; however, the tumor may receive secondary blood supply from branches of the internal carotid artery, temporal and facial arteries. The most common clinical presentation of patients with JNA is nasal obstruction followed by epistaxis. Contrast-enhanced high-resolution computed tomography (CT) with axial and coronal reconstruction is the method of choice for evaluating the location and extent of the angiofibroma. Magnetic resonance imaging (MRI) is useful for evaluation of intracranial extension and recurrence cases. Preoperative embolization 24 to 48 hours prior to resection is recommended to reduce perioperative blood loss. The resection of JNA has to be tailored to the extent of the tumor and experience of the surgeon. The most common surgical approaches used are endonasal endoscopic, midface degloving, lateral rhinotomy, transpalatal, midfacial translocation, and infratemporal.

Traditional approaches to the PPF via an anterior transmaxillary and transoral-transantral approaches have been associated with complications, such as facial edema, oroantral fistula, chronic maxillary sinusitis, vascular injury, injury of the infraorbital nerve, and dental injury. Therefore, lateral approaches especially for exposure and resection of malignant or invasive tumors have also been advocated. The endoscopic endonasal approach has been used for the surgical treatment of various neoplastic and inflammatory diseases of the PPF and its boundaries, as well as the lateral recess of the sphenoid sinus, which represents an extended pneumatization of the sphenoid bone just posterior to the PPF. In addition, this approach can be extended to reach the infratemporal fossa, cavernous sinus, middle cranial fossa, and nasopharynx. To perform a surgical access to or through the PPF a thorough knowledge and understanding of the intricate and complex neurovascular anatomy is necessary.[9] This surgical anatomy is further complicated by anatomic variations and protected positions that may be difficult to access especially when bleeding or space-occupying lesions obscure them. The use of the endoscopic approaches together with intraoperative image-guided navigation systems has allowed for further broadening of the indications of the extended endoscopic endonasal approaches to the pterygopalatine fossa safely.

Pearls

- Tumors involving the pterygopalatine fossa can have multiple clinical presentations depending on the type and extent of the tumors.
- PPF communicates with the orbital apex masticatory space, the infratemporal fossa, and the middle cranial fossa.
- Topographically, the PPF can be divided into an anterior and posterior compartment.
- The internal maxillary artery runs on the anterior edge of the lateral pterygoid muscle.
- The sphenopalatine foramen is formed by the orbital process of the palatine bone, the vertical plate of the palatine bone, and the sphenoid process.
- The vidian nerve can be identified at the superior portion of the pterygopalatine fossa. It is an important landmark for the identification of the foramen lacerum and for the intrapetrous carotid artery.
- The most common clinical presentation of patients with JNA is nasal obstruction followed by epistaxis.

References

1. Fortes FS, Sennes LU, Carrau RL, et al. Endoscopic anatomy of the pterygopalatine fossa and the transpterygoid approach: development of a surgical instruction model. Laryngoscope 2008;118(1):44–49
2. Isaacs SJ, Goyal P. Endoscopic anatomy of the pterygopalatine fossa. Am J Rhinol 2007;21(5):644–647
3. Prades JM, Asanau A, Timoshenko AP, Faye MB, Martin Ch. Surgical anatomy of the sphenopalatine foramen and its arterial content. Surg Radiol Anat 2008;30(7):583–587
4. Solari D, Magro F, Cappabianca P, et al. Anatomical study of the pterygopalatine fossa using an endoscopic endonasal approach: spatial relations and distances between surgical landmarks. J Neurosurg 2007;106(1):157–163
5. Rusu MC, Pop F, Curcă GC, Podoleanu L, Voinea LM. The pterygopalatine ganglion in humans: a morphological study. Ann Anat 2009;191(2):196–202
6. Herzallah IR, Elsheikh EM, Casiano RR. Endoscopic endonasal study of the maxillary nerve: a new orientation. Am J Rhinol 2007;21(5):637–643
7. Magro F, Solari D, Cavallo LM, et al. The endoscopic endonasal approach to the lateral recess of the sphenoid sinus via the pterygopalatine fossa: comparison of endoscopic and radiological landmarks. Neurosurgery 2006; 59(4, Suppl 2)ONS237–ONS242, discussion ONS242–ONS243
8. Cavallo LM, Messina A, Gardner P, et al. Extended endoscopic endonasal approach to the pterygopalatine fossa: anatomical study and clinical considerations. Neurosurg Focus 2005;19(1):E5
9. Kassam AB, Gardner P, Snyderman C, Mintz A, Carrau R. Expanded endonasal approach: fully endoscopic, completely transnasal approach to the middle third of the clivus, petrous bone, middle cranial fossa, and infratemporal fossa. Neurosurg Focus 2005;19(1):E6

20 The Maxillary Sinus and Surgical Treatment of Graves Orbitopathy

Man-Kit Leung and Ralph B. Metson

Graves disease is a systemic autoimmune disorder that can affect the thyroid, skin, and orbit. Although hyperthyroidism is the most common presenting manifestation, up to 80% of persons with Graves disease develop ocular findings, known as Graves orbitopathy.[1] Severe orbital disease poses a threat to vision in 3 to 5% of patients with Graves orbitopathy.[1,2]

The orbital symptoms associated with Graves disease represent an autoimmune process, although the exact mechanism is not completely understood. Accumulation of lymphocytes and deposition of mucopolysaccharides in orbital soft tissues lead to enlargement of extraocular muscles and orbital fat. In the restrictive confines of the bony orbit, the discrepancy between orbital volume and its expanded contents causes anterior displacement of the globe and posterior pressure on the orbital apex, which can result in exophthalmos and optic nerve compression. It is important to note, however, that the degree of proptosis does not correlate with the overall severity of disease because patients with poor compliance of the orbital septum may not exhibit significant proptosis, but can have severe compression at the orbital apex with optic neuropathy.

Clinical manifestations of Graves orbitopathy range from mild findings, such as tearing, photophobia, and conjunctival injection, to severe symptoms, such as disfiguring exophthalmos, diplopia, corneal ulceration from exposure keratopathy, and visual loss from optic neuropathy. The orbital manifestations of Graves disease follow a distinct and independent clinical course from the thyroid disease. The clinical course of Graves orbitopathy can be divided into acute and chronic phases. Whereas the acute phase is characterized by active inflammation and lasts 6 to 18 months, the chronic phase is characterized by stable fibrosis.[3] Medical treatment of Graves orbitopathy includes systemic corticosteroids and orbital radiation, which seem to be most effective during the acute phase of the disease. When medical treatments fail, however, surgical decompression of the orbit may be necessary and is preferably performed during the chronic phase when the orbitopathy has stabilized.

Surgical Treatment of Graves Orbitopathy

A variety of surgical techniques have been described to decompress the orbit by removing any combination of 1 to 4 bony walls.[4–7] In 1930 Oskar Hirsch was the first to report removal of the orbital floor for decompression of the orbit in a patient with exposure keratopathy due to Graves disease. The operation represented the first description of decompression of orbital contents into the maxillary sinus and resulted in resolution of corneal exposure.[4,5] In 1936 Edward Sewall developed an external ethmoidectomy approach to removal of the medial orbital wall.[6] This technique ultimately evolved into the transantral approach to orbital decompression with removal of the medial orbital wall and floor, introduced by Walsh and Ogura in 1957.[7]

The Walsh–Ogura technique was the mainstay of surgical treatment for Graves orbitopathy for many decades. This procedure enabled otolaryngologists to remove the orbital floor and medial wall through the familiar Caldwell–Luc approach, allowing for decompression of the enlarged orbital muscles and fat into the maxillary and ethmoid sinuses. Their technique involved a sublabial incision to expose and enter the maxillary antrum. A transantral ethmoidectomy was performed and the medial orbital wall was skeletonized. Bone of the lamina papyracea was removed up to the ethmoid roof, and bone along the orbital floor was removed, sparing the infraorbital nerve. Although effective decompression was achieved with this method, the incidence of postoperative diplopia was high. In 1993, Garrity et al reported on a series of 428 patients undergoing transantral orbital decompression for Graves orbitopathy and found a 64% incidence of new-onset postoperative diplopia.[8] Furthermore, patients undergoing unilateral decompression often developed hypoglobus with one eye appearing lower than the other. Other disadvantages of the Walsh–Ogura technique included paresthesia along the distribution of the infraorbital nerve and poor visualization of the skull base when performing the transantral ethmoidectomy.

Soon after the introduction of endoscopic instrumentation for the performance of sinus surgery in the mid-1980s, surgeons began to experiment with an entirely transnasal approach to treat diseases of the orbit, circumventing the need for external or sublabial incisions and reducing patient morbidity. Endoscopic orbital decompression was pioneered by Kennedy et al and Michel et al in the early 1990s.[9,10] Because high-resolution endoscopes provided improved visualization in key anatomic regions, including the orbital apex and skull base, this technique soon gained widespread acceptance for the treatment of patients with Graves disease, largely replacing the transantral approach.

Endoscopic Orbital Decompression

Patient Selection and Work-Up

Indications for endoscopic orbital decompression include severe exophthalmos, which may result in exposure keratopathy, corneal ulceration, or disfiguring proptosis; compressive optic neuropathy, which may present with color blindness, decreased visual fields, or decreased visual acuity; and diplopia in preparation for strabismus or eye muscle surgery. Surgery is best performed during the chronic phase of the disease when the orbitopathy has stabilized. In some cases, however, severe orbital symptoms may necessitate decompression during the active phase, such as for sight-threatening optic neuropathy that is refractory to medical treatment. The decision to operate must be a team decision involving both the ophthalmologist and the otolaryngologist.

Preoperative evaluation includes a complete head and neck examination, ophthalmologic evaluation, and computed tomography scans of the orbits and paranasal sinuses in coronal and axial planes. Ophthalmologic evaluation should include visual acuity, visual fields, conjunctival and corneal examination, Hertel exophthalmometry measurements, and extraocular motility testing. Preoperative and postoperative photography are recommended.

Surgical Technique

The patient is positioned in the supine position, and topical vasoconstriction is achieved with pledgets soaked in oxymetazoline or cocaine 4%. Draping is the same as with standard endoscopic sinus procedures, and the eyes are exposed in the surgical field, but protected with corneal shields. Image guidance systems may be used at the surgeon's discretion. Lidocaine 1% with epinephrine 1:100,000 is injected along the lateral nasal wall in the region of the maxillary line (a bony eminence that extends from the anterior attachment of the middle turbinate to the root of the inferior turbinate).

Surgery begins with an incision just posterior to the maxillary line through the uncinate process (**Fig. 20.1**) (**see Video 20.1**). The uncinate process is medialized and removed allowing for visualization of the natural ostium of the maxillary sinus. It is important to open the maxillary sinus widely to achieve good access to the orbital floor and prevent blockage of the ostium from orbital fat, which protrudes after decompression (**Fig. 20.2**). The ostium can be opened to the floor of the orbit superiorly, the back wall of the maxillary sinus posteriorly, the thick bone of the frontal process of the maxilla anteriorly, and the inferior turbinate inferiorly. A sufficiently widened antrostomy measures ~9

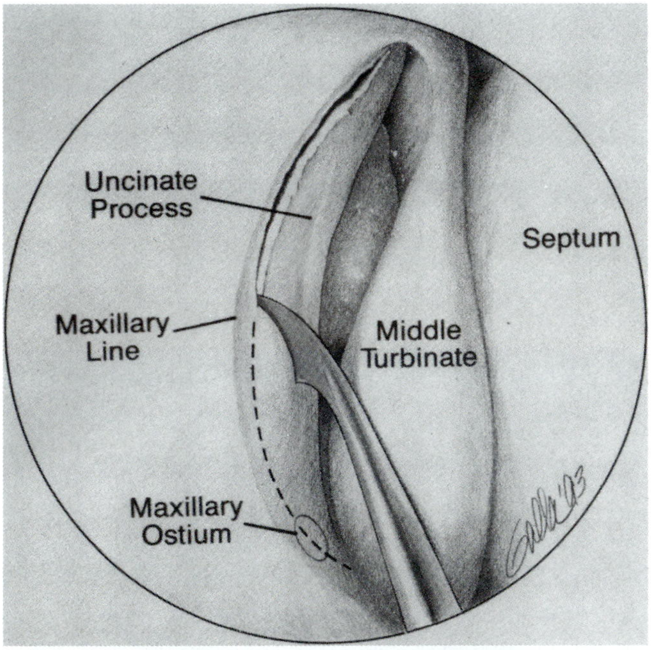

Fig. 20.1 View of the right nasal cavity at the start of decompression surgery. The uncinate process is incised just posterior to the maxillary line, an eminence that extends from the anterior attachment of the middle turbinate to the root of the inferior turbinate. (From Metson R, Dallow RL, Shore JW. Endoscopic orbital decompression. Laryngoscope 1994;104:952. Reprinted with permission.)

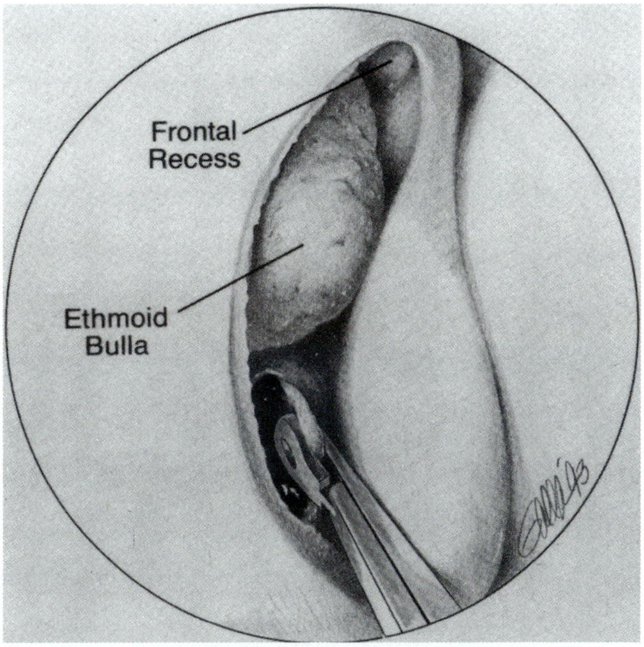

Fig. 20.2 The maxillary sinus ostium is enlarged superiorly to the floor of the orbit, posteriorly to the back wall of the maxillary sinus, anteriorly to the frontal process of the maxilla, and inferiorly to the inferior turbinate. A large maxillary antrostomy is necessary to optimize exposure and removal of the medial orbital floor. (From Metson R, Dallow RL, Shore JW. Endoscopic orbital decompression. Laryngoscope 1994;104:952. Reprinted with permission.)

to 16 mm in a well-pneumatized maxillary sinus. If the antrostomy is extended beyond the frontal process of the maxilla anteriorly, there is risk of damage to the nasolacrimal duct. Using a 30-degree endoscope, the wide antrostomy should allow easy visualization of the infraorbital nerve as it courses along the floor of the orbit.

We advocate removal of the middle turbinate during orbital decompression to optimize exposure of the medial orbital wall and facilitate postoperative cleanings. After a total sphenoethmoidectomy is completed, an image guidance system may be used to confirm removal of all ethmoid cells along the medial orbital wall.

A spoon curette is used to penetrate the thin bone of the lamina papyracea. This bone is elevated while preserving the underlying periorbita. Bone removal proceeds superiorly to the ethmoid roof, inferiorly to the orbital floor, and anteriorly to the maxillary line, and posteriorly to the face of the sphenoid sinus (**Fig. 20.3**). Bone is not removed in the region of the frontal recess to prevent herniation of orbital fat, which could lead to postoperative obstruction of the frontal sinus.

When removing the anterior portion of the lamina papyracea, it is not uncommon to remove fragments of the adjacent lacrimal bone. In this case, the thick white fascia of the underlying lacrimal sac may be uncovered, but should not be opened. Thick bone anterior to the maxillary line protects the majority of the lacrimal sac and need not be removed. As bone removal proceeds in a posterior direction, the underlying periorbita thickens and becomes white in appearance in the region of the orbital apex within 2 mm of the sphenoid face. This tissue corresponds to the annulus of Zinn, from which the extraocular muscles originate, and represents the posterior limit of decompression.

Removal of the orbital floor may be the most technically challenging portion of the procedure. Only the portion of the floor medial to the infraorbital nerve is removed. A spoon curette is used to engage the orbital floor at its medial extent and to down-fracture the bone (**Fig. 20.4**). The bone of the orbital floor is thicker than that of the medial orbital wall, and significant force may be required for this maneuver. If the spoon curette is not sturdy enough for this portion of the procedure, a more robust mastoid curette can be used. The floor may fracture in one large piece, typically with a natural cleavage plane along the infraorbital canal. More commonly, the floor fractures into several small pieces, in which case a 30-degree endoscopic and curved instrumentation may facilitate bone removal. The infraorbital canal is preserved as the lateral limit of dissection. No attempt is made to remove the dense bone lateral to the infraorbital canal, as it serves to support the globe and prevents postoperative hypoglobus.

Once the lamina papyracea and medial orbital floor have been removed, the periorbita is fully exposed. A sickle knife is typically used to incise the periorbita (**Fig. 20.5**). Care must be taken to avoid burying the tip of the knife, which

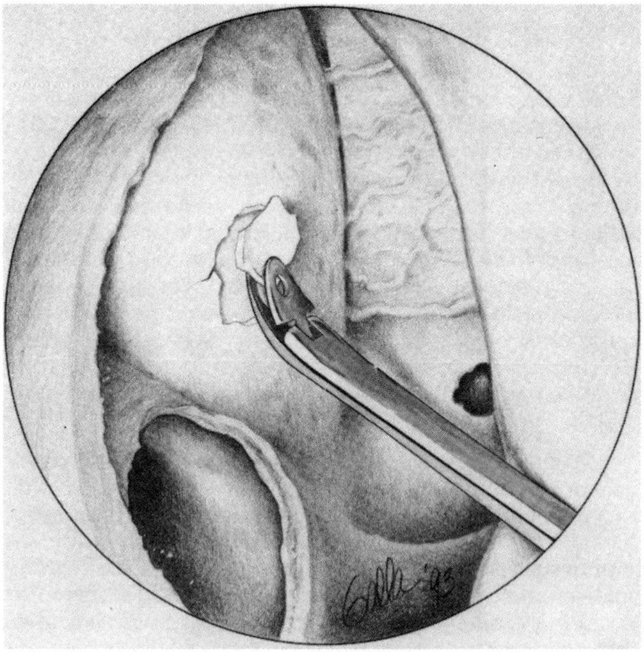

Fig. 20.3 A Blakesley forceps is used to remove bony fragments of the medial orbital wall and expose the underlying periorbita. (From Metson R, Dallow RL, Shore JW. Endoscopic orbital decompression. Laryngoscope 1994;104:952. Reprinted with permission.)

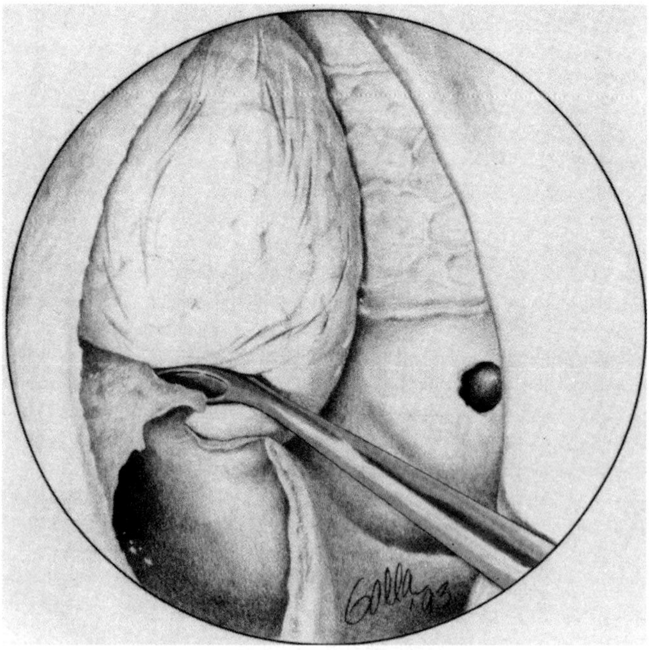

Fig. 20.4 A spoon or mastoid curette is used to down-fracture the medial portion of the orbital floor. Only bone that is medial to the infraorbital canal is removed. (From Metson R, Dallow RL, Shore JW. Endoscopic orbital decompression. Laryngoscope 1994;104:953. Reprinted with permission.)

could injure the underlying orbital contents, including the medial rectus muscle. The periorbital incision should be initiated at the posterior limit of decompression (just anterior to the sphenoid face) and brought anteriorly so that prolapsing fat does not obscure visualization. Parallel incisions are typically made adjacent to the ethmoid roof and orbital floor. To prevent prolapse of the medial rectus muscle and reduce the risk of postoperative diplopia, a sling of fascia overlying the medial rectus muscle may be preserved, while the remainder of the periorbita is removed using angled Blakesley forceps.[11] In patients with optic neuropathy, the fascial sling technique is not used to allow maximal decompression. A ball-tipped probe and sickle knife may be used to identify and divide any remaining fibrous bands, which often course superficially between lobules of orbital fat. On completion of the procedure, a generous prolapse of fat into the opened ethmoid and maxillary cavities should be observed (**Fig. 20.6**).

Depending on the clinical scenario and desired degree of decompression, a lateral decompression may be performed concurrently. When performed immediately after medial decompression, the orbital contents can be easily retracted in a medial direction allowing for excellent exposure of the lateral bony wall. If bilateral orbital decompressions are required, they may be performed concurrently or as staged procedures.

Nasal packing is not used to avoid compression of the exposed orbital contents and the optic nerve. The patient is discharged the morning after surgery with a prescription for antistaphylococcal oral antibiotics and instructions to begin twice-daily nasal saline irrigations. At the first postoperative visit one week after surgery, crusting is cleaned from the surgical site under endoscopic guidance.

For patients with severe comorbidities, a strong preference for local anesthesia, or in whom surgery is being performed on an only seeing eye, decompression may be accomplished under local anesthesia with sedation.[12] This approach allows the surgeon to monitor the patient's vision throughout the procedure. Sedation may be achieved with an intravenous bolus of propofol (0.4–0.8 mg/kg) before injection of local anesthesia, followed by an infusion of 75 to 95 µg/kg during the procedure. Local anesthesia is administered initially with 4% cocaine pledgets followed by injection of lidocaine 1% with epinephrine 1:100,000 as described for patients undergoing general anesthesia. Patients often report discomfort during incision of the periorbita. This sensation may be relieved by infiltration of a small amount of additional anesthetic solution into the medial orbit.

Results

The goals of orbital decompression vary depending on the indication for the procedure. In patients with compressive optic neuropathy, restoration of visual deficits is the key outcome, whereas in patients with corneal exposure

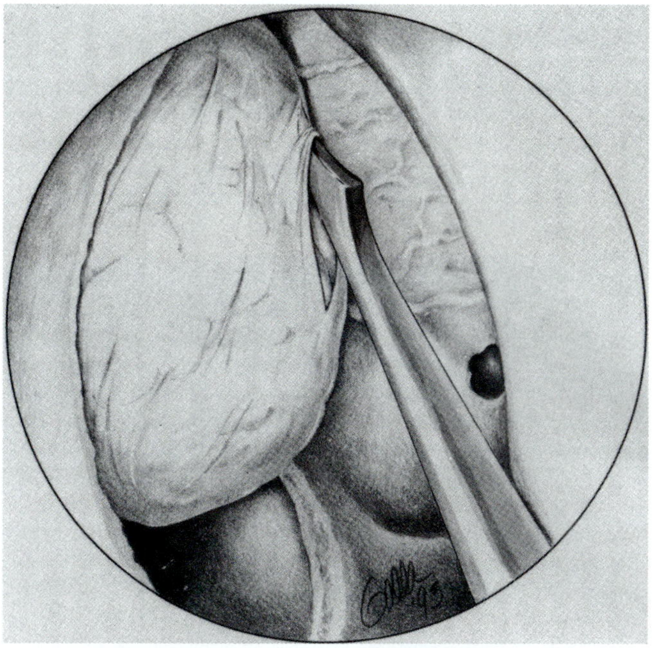

Fig. 20.5 The exposed layer of periorbital fascia is incised with a sickle knife and removed. (From Metson R, Dallow RL, Shore JW. Endoscopic orbital decompression. Laryngoscope 1994;104:953. Reprinted with permission.)

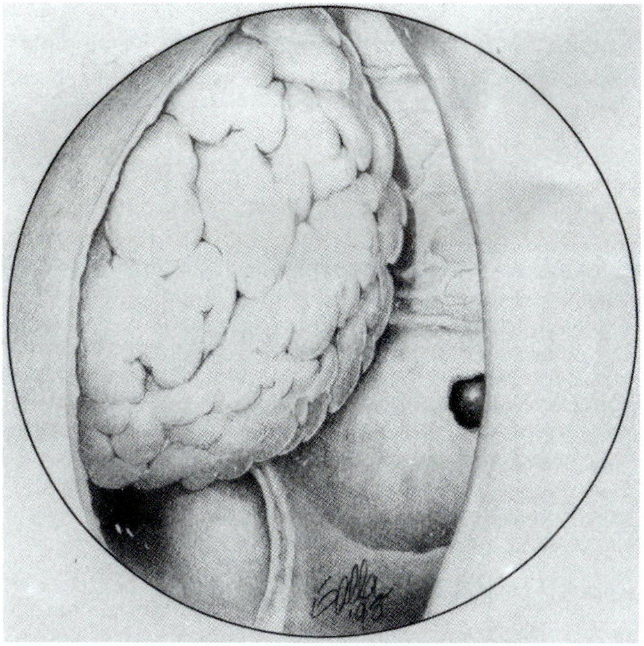

Fig. 20.6 Herniated orbital fat is seen bulging into the maxillary and ethmoid sinuses at the completion of the decompression. (From Metson R, Dallow RL, Shore JW. Endoscopic orbital decompression. Laryngoscope 1994;104:953. Reprinted with permission.)

or severe proptosis, ocular recession may be the primary endpoint. The rate of improvement after endoscopic orbital decompression for Graves orbitopathy ranges from 22 to 89%.[9,13–15] This wide variation in results reflects the diverse patient populations and definitions of improvement. Postoperative deterioration of visual acuity occurs in less than 5% of patients.[9,13–15] Ocular recession as a result of endoscopic decompression alone averages 3.5 mm (range 2–12 mm). The addition of concurrent lateral decompression to the endoscopic procedure provides an additional 2 mm of globe recession.[14]

Complications

Diplopia is a frequent complication of orbital decompression with 15 to 63% of postoperative patients reporting new-onset diplopia or worsening of preexisting symptoms.[8,10,14–17] This complication is believed to be a result of a change in the vector pull of the extraocular muscles. Decompressive surgery rarely alleviates preexisting diplopia. Patients who have diplopia after decompressive surgery frequently require strabismus surgery for correction. All patients should be informed of the possibility of postoperative double vision and the potential need for further surgical intervention.

Several methods to decrease postoperative diplopia have been reported. Multiple authors have described the preservation of a strut of inferomedial bone between the decompressed floor and medial wall.[13,18] When this strut is maintained, however, it is technically difficult to remove the orbital floor through a purely endoscopic approach. The maintenance of a fascial sling in the region of the medial rectus has been shown to decrease postoperative diplopia.[11] This technique provides similar support as the medial strut technique, but allows for endoscopic access to decompress the medial orbital floor. The concept of a balanced decompression (concurrent medial and lateral decompression) has also been shown to decrease postoperative diplopia.[15,19,20] When operating for compressive optic neuropathy, techniques designed to limit diplopia may also limit the extent of decompression, and postoperative diplopia often is accepted as a concession to improved vision.

Postoperative bleeding after decompression is best approached through endoscopic identification and direct cauterization of the bleeding site. Nasal packing generally is not used so as to avoid pressure on the exposed orbital apex and optic nerve. Postoperative infection is minimized through the use of postoperative antibiotics with staphylococcal coverage. A large maxillary antrostomy and limited bone removal in the frontal recess region minimize the risk of developing postoperative obstructive sinusitis. Epiphora may develop if the maxillary antrostomy is extended too far anteriorly with transection of the nasolacrimal duct. This complication may be treated with an endoscopic dacryocystorhinostomy. Leakage of cerebrospinal fluid, blindness, and hypesthesia along the infraorbital nerve distribution are rare complications that have been reported primarily after nonendoscopic decompression techniques.

Conclusion

During endoscopic orbital decompression for treatment of Graves orbitopathy, the maxillary sinus serves as the gateway to the orbital floor. Successful endoscopic decompression depends on the creation of a wide maxillary antrostomy, which provides adequate access for removal of the orbital floor and prevents postoperative sinusitis due to obstruction of the maxillary ostium.

Pearls

- A large maxillary antrostomy must be performed during endoscopic orbital decompression to allow for adequate exposure and access to the medial orbital floor. The wide maxillary antrostomy should allow visualization of the infraorbital canal with a 30-degree endoscope.
- A large maxillary antrostomy decreases the risk of postoperative sinusitis due to obstruction of the maxillary ostium by herniating fat.
- To obtain maximal orbital decompression, the medial orbital floor can be removed as far laterally as the infraorbital canal.
- Preservation of the lateral orbital floor during decompression allows for adequate support of the globe and prevents postoperative hypoglobus.
- Epiphora may occur following orbital decompression if the maxillary antrostomy is extended too far anteriorly with transection of the nasolacrimal duct. If this complication occurs, it can be treated with an endoscopic dacryocystorhinostomy.

References

1. Brent GA. Clinical practice. Graves' disease. N Engl J Med 2008;358(24):2594–2605
2. Bartalena L, Baldeschi L, Dickinson AJ, et al. Consensus statement of the European group on Graves' orbitopathy (EUGOGO) on management of Graves' orbitopathy. Thyroid 2008;18(3):333–346
3. Metson R, Pletcher SD. Endoscopic orbital and optic nerve decompression. Otolaryngol Clin North Am 2006;39(3):551–561, ix
4. Alper MG. Pioneers in the history of orbital decompression for Graves' ophthalmopathy. R.U. Kroenlein (1847-1910), O. Hirsch (1877-1965) and H.C. Naffziger (1884-1961). Doc Ophthalmol 1995;89(1-2):163–171
5. Hirsch O. Surgical decompression of exophthalmos. Arch Otolaryngol Head Neck Surg 1950;51:325–334
6. Sewall E. Operative control of progressive exophthalmos. Arch Otolaryngol Head Neck Surg 1936;24:621–624

7. Walsh TE, Ogura JH. Transantral orbital decompression for malignant exophthalmos. Laryngoscope 1957;67(6):544–568
8. Garrity JA, Fatourechi V, Bergstralh EJ, et al. Results of transantral orbital decompression in 428 patients with severe Graves' ophthalmopathy. Am J Ophthalmol 1993;116(5):533–547
9. Kennedy DW, Goodstein ML, Miller NR, Zinreich SJ. Endoscopic transnasal orbital decompression. Arch Otolaryngol Head Neck Surg 1990;116(3):275–282
10. Michel O, Bresgen K, Rüssmann W, Thumfart WF, Stennert E. [Endoscopically-controlled endonasal orbital decompression in malignant exophthalmos]. Laryngorhinootologie 1991;70(12):656–662
11. Metson R, Samaha M. Reduction of diplopia following endoscopic orbital decompression: the orbital sling technique. Laryngoscope 2002;112(10):1753–1757
12. Metson R, Shore JW, Gliklich RE, Dallow RL. Endoscopic orbital decompression under local anesthesia. Otolaryngol Head Neck Surg 1995;113(6):661–667
13. Schaefer SD, Soliemanzadeh P, Della Rocca DA, et al. Endoscopic and transconjunctival orbital decompression for thyroid-related orbital apex compression. Laryngoscope 2003;113(3):508–513
14. Metson R, Dallow RL, Shore JW. Endoscopic orbital decompression. Laryngoscope 1994; 104(8 Pt 1, 8 Pt 1)950–957
15. Shepard KG, Levin PS, Terris DJ. Balanced orbital decompression for Graves' ophthalmopathy. Laryngoscope 1998; 108(11 Pt 1, 11 Pt 1) 1648–1653
16. Wright ED, Davidson J, Codere F, Desrosiers M. Endoscopic orbital decompression with preservation of an inferomedial bony strut: minimization of postoperative diplopia. J Otolaryngol 1999;28(5):252–256
17. Eloy P, Trussart C, Jouzdani E, Collet S, Rombaux P, Bertrand B. Transnasal endoscopic orbital decompression and Graves' ophthalmopathy. Acta Otorhinolaryngol Belg 2000;54(2):165–174
18. Goldberg RA, Shorr N, Cohen MS. The medical orbital strut in the prevention of postdecompression dystopia in dysthyroid ophthalmopathy. Ophthal Plast Reconstr Surg 1992;8(1):32–34
19. Unal M, Leri F, Konuk O, Hasanreisoğlu B. Balanced orbital decompression combined with fat removal in Graves ophthalmopathy: do we really need to remove the third wall? Ophthal Plast Reconstr Surg 2003;19(2):112–118
20. Graham SM, Brown CL, Carter KD, Song A, Nerad JA. Medial and lateral orbital wall surgery for balanced decompression in thyroid eye disease. Laryngoscope 2003;113(7):1206–1209

21 Management of Persistent Maxillary Sinusitis: The View from India

Ramesh C. Deka and Venkatakarthikeyan Chokkalingam

Chronic rhinosinusitis (CRS) is defined as the mucosal inflammation of the nose and paranasal sinuses, persisting beyond a period of 12 weeks. Involvement of the maxillary sinus and ostiomeatal complex in CRS is a fairly common occurrence. During acute rhinosinusitis, in which there is generalized mucosal involvement of the nose and paranasal sinuses, the maxillary sinus is constantly soiled by the direct downpour of the inflammatory secretions from the frontal and anterior ethmoid sinuses. Due to its dependent position and mucociliary transport against gravity, acute inflammatory process within the maxillary sinus is more likely to become chronic and persistent if appropriate therapeutic intervention is not done. Although making a diagnosis of the patient with persistent maxillary sinusitis (PMS) is easy from its clinical symptoms and signs, endoscopic findings, and the radiologic images, the management of this condition is often difficult. In India, it is common to see patients presenting with PMS because of poverty and poor health care delivery. Despite multiple medical and surgical treatments being offered to them, patients with PMS show recurrences again owing to inadequacy of therapy and appropriate follow-up care. Diverse etiologic factors causing PMS also influence its poor results in India.

Etiopathogenesis of Persistent Maxillary Sinusitis

The pathophysiology of PMS is a diverse process: it includes both intrinsic and extrinsic factors such as infective bacteria, virus, fungus, coexisting allergy, systemic causes like diabetes, immunodeficiency, and mucociliary disorders. Autoimmune disorders like sarcoidosis and Wegener granulomatosis, and anatomic abnormalities also play an important role. Mucus stasis within the maxillary sinus due to ostiomeatal obstruction or mucociliary dysfunction is the common basis of PMS. Persistent obstruction results in decreased oxygen tension, reduced sinus pH, ciliary dysfunction, negative pressure within the sinus and all these lead to stasis and such a collection invites infection. Associated sneezing due to allergies and nose blowing promotes the entry of the infectious agents from the nasal cavity into maxillary sinus resulting in rhinosinusitis. The inflammatory role played by virus, bacteria, and fungi is of importance as it causes host inflammatory responses due to local (mucosal) production of chemical mediators like cytokines. It eventually leads to persistent maxillary sinusitis (PMS).

PMS has recently drawn a great deal of attention from both clinicians and basic researchers. The role of eosinophilic inflammation, biofilm formation, and superantigens needs special mention in the causation of persistent maxillary sinusitis. Studies[1,2] have shown that biofilms, which are a structural community of cells of bacteria (*Staphylococcus aureus* and *Pseudomonas aeruginosa*) or fungus enclosed in a self-produced matrix, play a significant role in CRS. In addition to biofilm formation, colonization in the nose and paranasal sinuses of toxigenic strains of bacteria like *S. aureus* may also yield exotoxins with super antigenic properties, which are capable of producing eosinophilic and lymphocytic local inflammatory responses. Allergy also plays a role in PMS and allergic stimulation results in the release of histamine, leukotrienes, tumor necrosis factor, and cytokines. These recruit inflammatory cells. A clinical association between asthma and CRS has long been recognized. Increased levels of leukotrienes have been observed in patients having associated asthma and nasal polyps.[3] In patients with PMS who receive antileukotriene therapy and experience improved outcomes suggests coexisting nasal allergy and/or asthma. Extra esophageal reflux diseases are also in the list of causative factors of refractory CRS.[4] Patients with a history of maxillofacial trauma may present with PMS due to anatomic disruption of the ostiomeatal drainage mechanism. In older patients, PMS unresponsive to medical therapy should raise the suspicion of presence of a neoplastic condition involving the maxillary sinus. Such a patient needs a detailed assessment including a computed tomography (CT) scan and endoscopic biopsy from the suspected area for a confirmation of the diagnosis.

Anatomic Considerations in the Pathophysiology of PMS

The anatomic aspect of paranasal sinuses including the maxillary sinuses influences the pathophysiology of persistent maxillary sinusitis and so it needs a consideration. The maxillary sinus is the largest of the paranasal sinuses and is surrounded on all its sides by the bony walls, except on the medial side where the natural ostium and accessory one (when present) provides communication to the nasal cavity.

The natural ostium is located in the superior aspect of the medial wall of the sinus, seen behind the lower attachment of uncinate process and above the superior portion of the inferior turbinate. The floor of the maxillary sinus is usually 4 to 5 mm below the floor of nasal cavity in adults and it explains the importance of mucociliary transport from the dependent portion of the sinus into the superiorly placed natural ostium and ethmoidal infundibulum. When the accessory ostium is present, it also plays an important role in the mucociliary transport and ventilation. The ethmoidal infundibulum is the common drainage point of the anterior group of sinuses: it is bound medially by the uncinate process, laterally by the lamina papyracea, and posteriorly by the anterior surface of ethmoidal bulla. It is obvious that anatomic abnormalities involving any of these structures like a bent or pneumatized uncinate process, prominent ethmoid bulla, and a Haller cell in the inferomedial aspect of orbit can compromise the drainage of the maxillary sinus. These abnormalities should be carefully looked into during endoscopic and radiologic assessment before making treatment plans in persistent maxillary sinusitis. Another anatomic consideration regarding the floor of the maxillary sinus is the close proximity of the root of the maxillary premolars and molars to the floor. Infection of the maxillary teeth, iatrogenic displacement of a maxillary tooth into the sinus, and injury to the sinus lining during extraction can also cause PMS of odontogenic origin.

Clinical Presentation of Persistent Maxillary Sinusitis

The most common symptoms are nasal congestion or blockage, purulent rhinorrhea, facial pain or pressure, discolored postnasal drainage, and anosmia or hyposmia. The other minor symptoms are headache, occasional fever, halitosis, fatigue, dental pain, dry cough, and ear pain/pressure/fullness. Maxillary sinusitis may also present with infraorbital pain and tenderness extending to the maxillary teeth. Children with PMS may not have the classical features and they may present with irritability as their only symptom. Persistent cough that is worse at night due to postnasal drip is another common feature seen in children.

Diagnosis

Intranasal examination with the help of nasal speculum and nasal endoscopic examination provides clinical evidence for the diagnosis of PMS. The status of the mucosal linings of the nose especially of the inferior and middle turbinates, middle meatus, presence of polyps and purulent secretions along the middle meatus help in diagnosing maxillary sinusitis (**Fig. 21.1**). Endoscopic examination also indicates the presence of anatomic abnormalities that may cause ostiomeatal blockage. In patients who have PMS after functional endoscopic sinus surgery (FESS), examination of the interior aspect of the maxillary sinus through the middle meatal antrostomy opening is important. It allows us to assess the condition of the mucosal lining of maxillary sinus, the presence of purulent secretions, and/or any residual/recurrent mucosal disease.

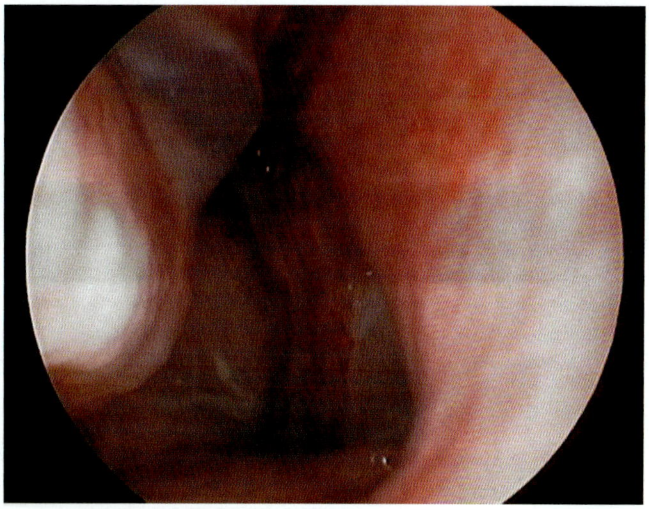

Fig. 21.1 Endoscopic evidence of persistent maxillary sinusitis–mucopurulent secretions in the middle meatus.

The Role of Nasal Swab, Sinus Aspiration, and Culture

Culture-directed therapy is important in patients with PMS who are unresponsive to empirical therapy. Cultures may be taken from the middle meatus with a swab stick during endoscopic examination. Despite precautions, cultures are more prone to contamination: sinus aspiration/puncture helps in identifying the pathologic organisms involved in PMS. It is done by a sublabial canine fossa approach in adults and an inferior meatal approach under general anesthesia in children. It is not routinely indicated in immunocompetent patients with uncomplicated PMS keeping in mind the rare but serious complications such as soft tissue emphysema, air embolism, vasovagal reaction, and injury to the orbit. Patients with PMS who are immunocompromised and have failed to respond to multiple courses of antimicrobial therapy need a sinus aspiration for a diagnosis.

Imaging in PMS: The Indian Experience

A noncontrast computed tomography (CT) scan of the paranasal sinuses (**Fig. 21.2**) with axial and coronal cuts is our preferred radiologic modality for assessing PMS. The plain

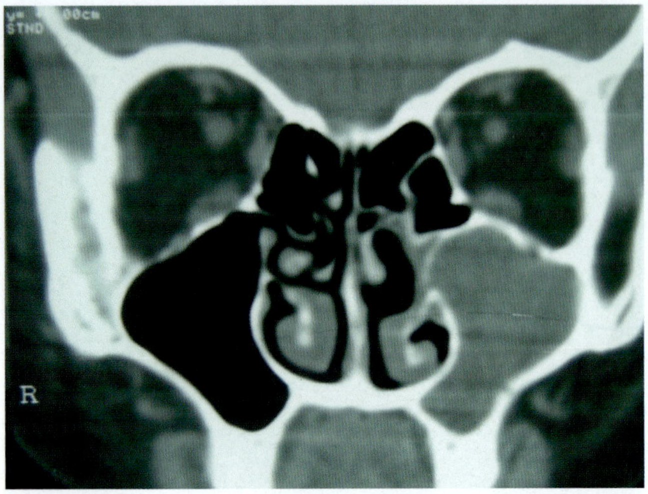

Fig. 21.2 Computed tomography (CT) coronal section showing complete opacification of the left maxillary sinus in persistent maxillary sinusitis.

radiographs lack the sensitivity, specificity and anatomic precision. MRI is not preferred due to its limited ability to display bony details. A CT scan helps in diagnosing changes within the maxillary sinus like focal or diffuse mucosal thickening, extensive polyps, anatomy of the ostiomeatal complex and anatomic abnormalities causing obstruction to the drainage pathway. It helps in assessing the response to treatment and also preoperative planning. It is very important to know whether symptoms of PMS correlate with the CT findings before determining the need for a surgical intervention. Studies have shown that there is CT evidence of asymptomatic paranasal sinus changes in patients without CRS,[5,6] and in such a situation therapy is controversial.

Treatment of PMS

PMS may present as three conditions with regard to its management: (1) PMS without polyp, (2) PMS with polyp, and (3) PMS after endoscopic sinus surgery. The treatment approach is different for each of these conditions.

Treatment of PMS without Polyp

These patients present with clinical symptoms of PMS persisting beyond a period of 12 weeks without any polyps in the middle meatus or nasal cavity on endoscopic examination. They present with characteristic endoscopic findings of rhinosinusitis (erythema, edema, nasal purulence) in the middle meatus and radiologic evidence of localized or diffuse mucosal thickening, partial opacification of maxillary sinus/ostiomeatal complex. Though all three factors (clinical symptoms, endoscopic examination, and radiologic examination) are assessed before therapy, treatment of these patients depends mainly on the clinical symptoms. If the symptoms are mild, intermittent with absence of nasal purulence, a short course of topical intranasal corticosteroid therapy for 8 weeks is indicated. The efficacy of treatment is assessed after 8 weeks by monitoring the improvement in symptoms and resolution of endoscopic findings. If there is good response to treatment, topical intranasal corticosteroids should be continued for at least 6 months as maintenance therapy.

If the patient with PMS has severe, frequent, and continuous symptoms or symptoms affecting the patient's daily activities, supported by endoscopic and radiologic findings, empiric therapy with broad-spectrum antibiotics should be given for 3 weeks. In ideal settings, culture-directed therapy is preferable over empiric treatment, as it targets the specific organism. Though culture-directed therapy may not be possible in all cases because of time constraints, it should be tried in patients in whom empiric antimicrobial therapy has failed and before contemplating FESS. Along with the antibiotics, topical intranasal corticosteroid therapy may be given for 6 to 8 weeks. A short course of oral steroids for 7 to 10 days before embarking on topical corticosteroid therapy is also recommended to treat the inflammatory component associated with PMS provided there are no contraindications. Saline spray/irrigation is helpful in the decongestion of the inflamed mucosa without causing rebound congestion like topical nasal decongestants. Saline irrigation also helps in washing away the inflammatory secretions and improves the mucociliary transport. If there is good response to this treatment, patients should be put on maintenance therapy with topical corticosteroid nasal spray for 6 months or longer as long as the symptoms warrant. If there is poor response, patients with PMS should be considered for FESS.

Treatment of PMS with Polyposis

Endoscopic and radiologic assessment helps in differentiating limited disease (polyps limited to the middle meatus or polyps beyond middle meatus but not obstructing nasal cavity) from extensive disease (polyps completely obstructing the nasal cavity). Patients with PMS with limited nasal polyposis and mild symptoms of CRS can be treated with topical corticosteroid nasal spray alone for 2 months, and if there is good response, they should be put on maintenance therapy for a further 6 months. For patients with moderate or severe symptoms affecting daily activities and extensive nasal polyposis, a 2-month course of topical corticosteroid and a 3-week course of antibiotics (especially for cases with symptoms and signs of infection, i.e., pain and nasal purulence on endoscopy) should be given. Initial treatment with oral steroids is of additional benefit. If there is a good response, they should be put on maintenance therapy with topical corticosteroid nasal spray for 6 months or longer to minimize recurrence of polyps. If there is poor response after 2 months of medical treatment, patients with PMS with polyposis should be considered for FESS.

The Indian Experience: Low-dose Macrolide Therapy and Topical Antifungal Nasal Lavage in PMS

In recent years, considerable evidence has emerged to suggest that macrolide antibiotics have an antiinflammatory effect[7] in addition to their well-established antibiotic effect. Macrolides accumulate in inflammatory cells at higher concentrations and have been shown to inhibit cytokines, increase inflammatory cell apoptosis, and inhibit the activation of the key proinflammatory transcription factor. The preliminary analysis of our ongoing study on the efficacy of low-dose, long-term macrolide therapy (roxithromycin 150 mg or clarithromycin 250 mg once daily for 3 months) in CRS has shown improvement in both subjective (nasal symptoms) and objective (endoscopic and CT findings) outcome measures.[8] Larger prospective randomized controlled trials are needed to know the efficacy of low-dose macrolide in PMS refractory to medical therapy and FESS.

Nasal lavage for the treatment of chronic rhinosinusitis has gained attention in the world literature in last decade. "Jal-Neti" (nasal water irrigation therapy) is an ancient yogic practice of cleaning the nostril with lukewarm water with a special utensil (lota). In India, it has been practiced for centuries and is recommended by medical practitioners, allied medical professionals, and yogic experts for the treatment of chronic rhinosinusitis. "Sutra-neti" (nasal cleaning with thread) is another ancient yogic technique of nasal cleansing wherein a length of string is inserted through the nose and into the mouth. The end is then pulled out of the mouth and while holding both ends at once the string is alternately pulled in and out of the nose and sinuses to clean the nasal passages. Though it is in practice, sutra-neti is not recommended by the medical professionals for the treatment of chronic rhinosinusitis in view of associated trauma to the already inflamed nasal mucosa.

It is assumed that intranasal application of the antifungal agent amphotericin B in the form of nasal lavage (20 mL of 100 µg/mL solution twice daily in each nostril) would reduce the fungal load by mechanical irrigation as well as reduce the immunologic changes produced by fungus in the nose and sinuses in patients with allergic fungal rhinosinusitis (AFRS). Topical antifungal nasal lavage when combined with the corticosteroid (fluticasone) nasal spray, which has antiinflammatory properties will have an additive effect in the treatment response. Although there is strong evidence to support the role of fungi in AFRS, there is a lot of controversy over the role of fungi in nonallergic CRS. Studies[9,10] have shown the presence of a fungal colony in the nose of normal volunteers and also in risk groups (such as patients with anatomic abnormalities like a deviated nasal septum, allergy to dust /pollens, house mites, etc.). In our experience, combination therapy of amphotericin B nasal lavage and topical corticosteroid nasal spray was found to be very effective in the treatment of AFRS with improvement in nasal symptoms, and endoscopic and radiologic findings.[11–14]

Endoscopic Sinus Surgery for PMS

Uncinectomy is the first and the most important step in FESS. If poorly performed, it results in surgical failure. The uncinate process can be seen as the union of three anatomic parts, upper or anterosuperior one-third, middle one-third, and posterior or horizontal one-third. In FESS, it is necessary to remove both the middle one-third to expose the natural ostium of maxillary sinus and the horizontal one-third of the uncinate process to allow the mucosa of ostium to be trimmed delicately and to heal by primary intention without scarring (**see Video 21.1**). The removal of the upper one-third of the uncinate process is not indicated in the surgery of maxillary sinus and the ostiomeatal complex unless there is associated disease in the frontal sinus.

The fontanelles (membranous areas in the medial wall of the maxillary sinus) are classified as anterior and posterior fontanelles in relation to the natural ostium. Failure of the surgeon to identify the natural ostium and the forceful insertion of angled instruments into the membranous part of the medial wall results in the creation of a posterior fontanelle ostium. It results in the circular flow of mucus and inflamed secretions between the unidentified natural ostium and the newly created posterior fontanelle ostium resulting in PMS after ESS.[15] This can be easily prevented by correct identification of the natural ostium after uncinectomy, the avoidance of blind instrumentation in the medial wall, and if an accessory ostium is found it has to be surgically joined with the natural ostium.

The studies in literature are not conclusive regarding the ideal size of the maxillary sinus ostium to be made in FESS.[16,17] For all practical purposes, if the maxillary sinus has minimal disease, uncinectomy and opening of the blocked natural ostium is sufficient for the long-term health of the sinus (**Fig. 21.3**). If there is extensive polyp formation with thick and viscid secretions, a large maxillary antrostomy is required.

Failure to remove the polyps attached to the anterior and inferomedial wall of the maxillary sinus is another cause for PMS after FESS. This may occur due to two reasons: (1) the inability to visualize the interiors of the maxillary sinus, and (2) the inability to remove the disease even after visualization. Better visualization can be achieved with angled endoscopes such as a 30-degree and 70-degree telescope. The removal of polyps from inaccessible areas can be achieved by angled forceps/microdebrider via the middle meatal antrostomies (**see Video 21.1**) or in difficult circum-

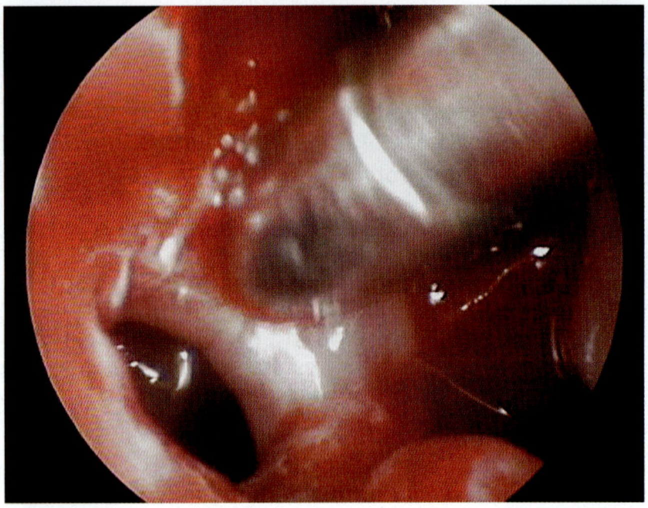

Fig. 21.3 Opening of blocked natural ostium during endoscopic sinus surgery.

stances by canine fossa puncture. Canine fossa puncture by a sublabial approach helps in the easy insertion of instruments/microdebrider via a small opening made in the canine fossa of the anterior wall of maxillary sinus for the removal of polyps.

Management of PMS after Functional Endoscopic Sinus Surgery (FESS)

Endoscopic examination and cleaning at regular intervals in the first 6 to 8 weeks after FESS is crucial for a good postoperative outcome. This helps in the healing process and improves the drainage and ventilation of the sinuses. If symptoms of sinusitis are persistent even after 8 weeks, endoscopic examination and radiologic assessment with CT scanning is required. Endoscopy helps in identification and treatment of causes of mechanical obstruction like crusts and synechiae formation. A CT scan helps to identify the residual/recurrent polyp within the sinus, mucocele formation, and anatomic factors causing obstruction to sinus drainage. Though anatomic factors causing obstruction and a mucocele has to be dealt by revision endoscopic sinus surgery, PMS with or without residual/recurrent polyps within the sinus can be treated with topical steroid spray and low-dose long-term macrolide therapy before embarking on FESS again. Topical instillation of antibiotics[18] (e.g., tobramycin) and irrigation with steroid solution are also helpful when there is evidence of continued inflammation, as these procedures allow the delivery of a higher concentration of medication to the affected sinus mucosa and minimizes the systemic side effects of medications.

In the management of patients with PMS who are refractory to medical or surgical treatment, it is important to consider the potential contribution of allergy to their symptoms. Allergy management should be included in the treatment protocol of PMS with or without polyp. Allergy management includes allergen reduction, avoidance, medications, and in extreme cases immunotherapy. It is also important to rule out systemic causes like immunodeficiency disorders and autoimmune diseases in patients with PMS who are refractory to treatment.

Conclusion

The management of persistent maxillary sinusitis continues to evolve. It is very important to understand the etiopathogenesis of this condition in a broad range and not focus on bacterial infection alone. The comprehensive management of PMS requires an understanding of the role of infective organisms with its characteristic biofilm formation and superantigen production, role of inflammatory process perpetuated by eosinophils, lymphocytes and their chemical mediators, the diverse etiological factors including anatomic abnormalities and the possible role of allergy. Treatment options include pharmacotherapy and surgery. The pharmacotherapy should be based on the etiopathogenesis and it includes antibiotics, topical/systemic steroids, topical antifungal therapy, and novel antiinflammatory therapies like antileukotrienes and low-dose macrolide therapy. Surgical treatment involves functional endoscopic sinus surgery with the aim to preserve function and provide ventilation to the affected sinus. Endoscopic sinus surgery should be contemplated for patients with moderate to severe disease with extensive polyps and patients with persistent maxillary sinusitis refractory to medical therapy.

Pearls

- The pathophysiology of PMS involves both intrinsic and extrinsic factors.
- The role of eosinophilic inflammation, biofilm formation, and superantigens needs special mention in PMS.
- Clinical symptomatology, endoscopic findings, and radiologic assessment are crucial in the diagnosis and management of PMS.
- Nasal swab/sinus aspiration and culture is indicated in patients with PMS who are immunocompromised and unresponsive to empirical therapy.
- Medical treatment for PMS includes antibiotics, topical/systemic steroids, antileukotrienes and low dose, long-term macrolide therapy.
- Functional endoscopic sinus surgery is indicated in patients with PMS refractory to medical therapy and in those with extensive polyps.

References

1. Mladina R, Poje G, Vuković K, Ristić M, Musić S. Biofilm in nasal polyps. Rhinology 2008;46(4):302–307
2. Galli J, Calò L, Ardito F, et al. Damage to ciliated epithelium in chronic rhinosinusitis: what is the role of bacterial biofilms? Ann Otol Rhinol Laryngol 2008;117(12):902–908
3. Parnes SM. The role of leukotriene inhibitors in patients with paranasal sinus disease. Curr Opin Otolaryngol Head Neck Surg 2003;11(3):184–191
4. DelGaudio JM. Direct nasopharyngeal reflux of gastric acid is a contributing factor in refractory chronic rhinosinusitis. Laryngoscope 2005;115(6):946–957
5. Bolger WE, Butzin CA, Parsons DS. Paranasal sinus bony anatomic variations and mucosal abnormalities: CT analysis for endoscopic sinus surgery. Laryngoscope 1991;101(1 Pt 1):56–64
6. Flinn J, Chapman ME, Wightman AJ, Maran AG. A prospective analysis of incidental paranasal sinus abnormalities on CT head scans. Clin Otolaryngol Allied Sci 1994;19(4):287–289
7. Cervin A, Wallwork B. Macrolide therapy of chronic rhinosinusitis. Rhinology 2007;45(4):259–267
8. Ramavat AS, Deka RC. Role of low dose macrolide given for long duration in patients with chronic rhinosinusitis. Paper presented at: the 13th Asian Research Symposium in Rhinology; November 20–21, 2008; Bangkok, Thailand
9. Ponikau JU, Sherris DA, Kita H, Kern EB. Intranasal antifungal treatment in 51 patients with chronic rhinosinusitis. J Allergy Clin Immunol 2002;110(6):862–866
10. Ponikau JU, Sherris DA, Weaver A, Kita H. Treatment of chronic rhinosinusitis with intranasal amphotericin B: a randomized, placebo-controlled, double-blind pilot trial. J Allergy Clin Immunol 2005;115(1):125–131
11. Deka RC, Chokkalingam V, Vishnoi RK, Kumar R. Topical amphotericin B and steroid in AFS. Otolaryngol Head Neck Surg 2007;137(2):40
12. Deka RC. Allergic fungal sinusitis. Paper presented at: the 9th Asian Research Symposium on Rhinology (ARSR); November 19–21, 2004; Mumbai, India
13. Deka RC. Topical amphotericin B & corticosteroid spray in controlling allergic fungal sinusitis. Paper presented at: the 26th ISIAN (International Symposium on Infection & Allergy of the Nose); February 1–4, 2007; Kuala Lumpur, Malaysia
14. Deka RC. Allergic fungal rhinosinusitis. Paper presented at: the 12th Asian Research Symposium on Rhinology (ARSR); November 28–29, 2007; Manila, Republic of Philippines
15. Wormald PJ. Uncinectomy and middle meatal antrostomy, including canine fossa puncture. In: Endoscopic sinus surgery anatomy: In three-dimensional reconstruction and surgical technique. New York: Thieme Medical Publishing; 2005: 25–34
16. Albu S, Tomescu E. Small and large middle meatus antrostomies in the treatment of chronic maxillary sinusitis. Otolaryngol Head Neck Surg 2004;131(4):542–547
17. Kirihene RK, Rees G, Wormald PJ. The influence of the size of the maxillary sinus ostium on the nasal and sinus nitric oxide levels. Am J Rhinol 2002;16(5):261–264
18. Nagi MM, Desrosiers MY. Algorithms for management of chronic rhinosinusitis. Otolaryngol Clin N Am 2005; 38(6): 1137–1141

22 Management of Persistent Maxillary Sinusitis: The View from China

Geng Xu, Jianbo Shi, Guanxia Xiong, Kejun Zuo, and Abusaleh Muneif

When performing maxillary sinus surgery in our practice in China, we have found that the following points must be addressed:

1. Whether to open the maxillary sinus ostium
2. The position and scope of the opening
3. The opening pattern
4. Maxillary sinus disease management

Whether to Open the Maxillary Sinus Ostium

The surgeon must determine whether a patient requires opening and enlargement of the natural ostium for the treatment of sinus disease. For the sinus to function in a healthy manner, the drainage pathway must be unobstructed. Ob-

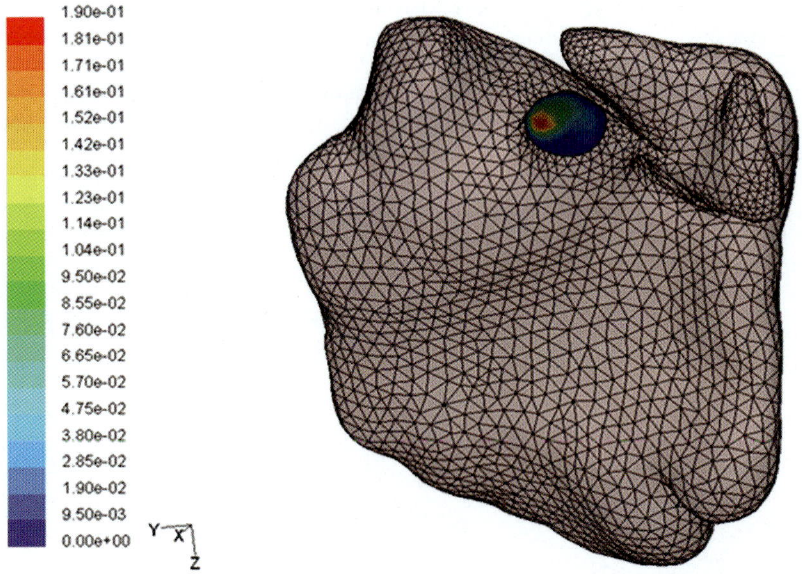

A

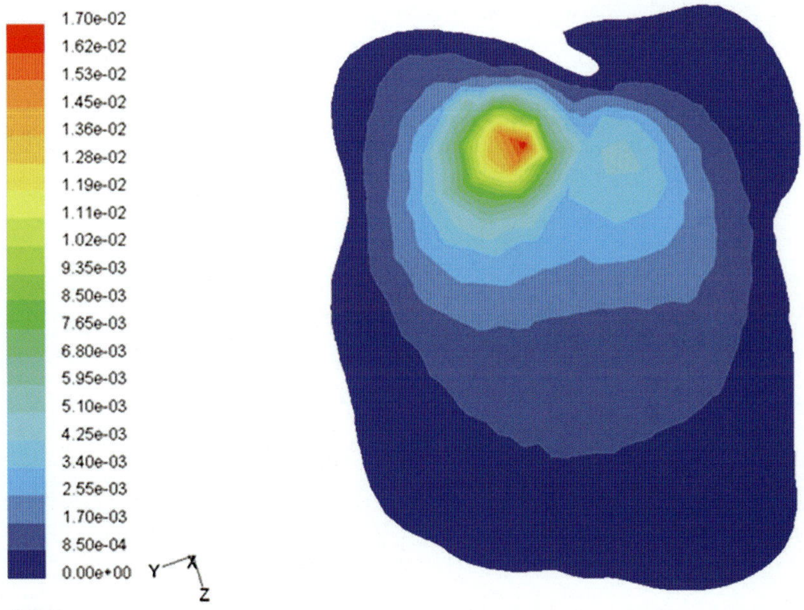

B

Fig. 22.1 (A–D) Computer simulation of nasal cavity and maxillary sinus air current and air exchange. After opening the maxillary sinus ostium, the maxillary sinus air current quantity changes. **(A,B)** Normal unoperated maxillary sinus ostium area. Note that only a small air current appears to enter the maxillary sinus proper (36.15 mL/s).

struction of the sinus ostium results in a barrier to normal sinus ventilation and drainage, with consequent physiologic changes within the maxillary sinus. Changes in the oxygen and carbon dioxide composition, sinus pressure and airflow, pH, and ciliary function have all been documented in the obstructed and diseased sinus.[1] Surgically opening a blocked sinus opening should be done in cases where it may help to reestablish a natural sinus environment.

In our experience, the obstructed maxillary sinus ostia will often clear with medical treatment alone. In cases where inflammation is persistent, sinus outflow obstruction will not clear, polyps or other masses are present, surgery is indicated. However, surgery may change the sinus environment by opening it to the nasal passageway. The size and shape of the surgical opening may impact the characteristics of the sinus mucosa. In the normal nonoperated sinus, there is little exchange with nasal ventilation,[2,3] in part due to the concealed nature of the natural opening by the uncinate process.

When air enters the nasal cavity it does not directly interact with the maxillary sinus. To examine the relationship between nasal cavity ventilation and maxillary sinus aeration, we did a computer simulation of the nasal–paranasal sinus ventilation exchange. We found that in the normal unoperated condition, only a slight amount of air from the nasal cavity enters the maxillary sinus (2.938 mL/s). In the postsurgical maxillary sinus, this relationship changes significantly, and air enters the maxillary sinus at 5.914 mL/s (**Fig. 22.1**).[4] It is possible that this change in sinus anatomy and ventilation is accompanied by a change in the sinus' physiologic environment. Some authors have found that insufficient gas exchange in the maxillary sinus base is associated with an increase in maxillary sinus floor carbon

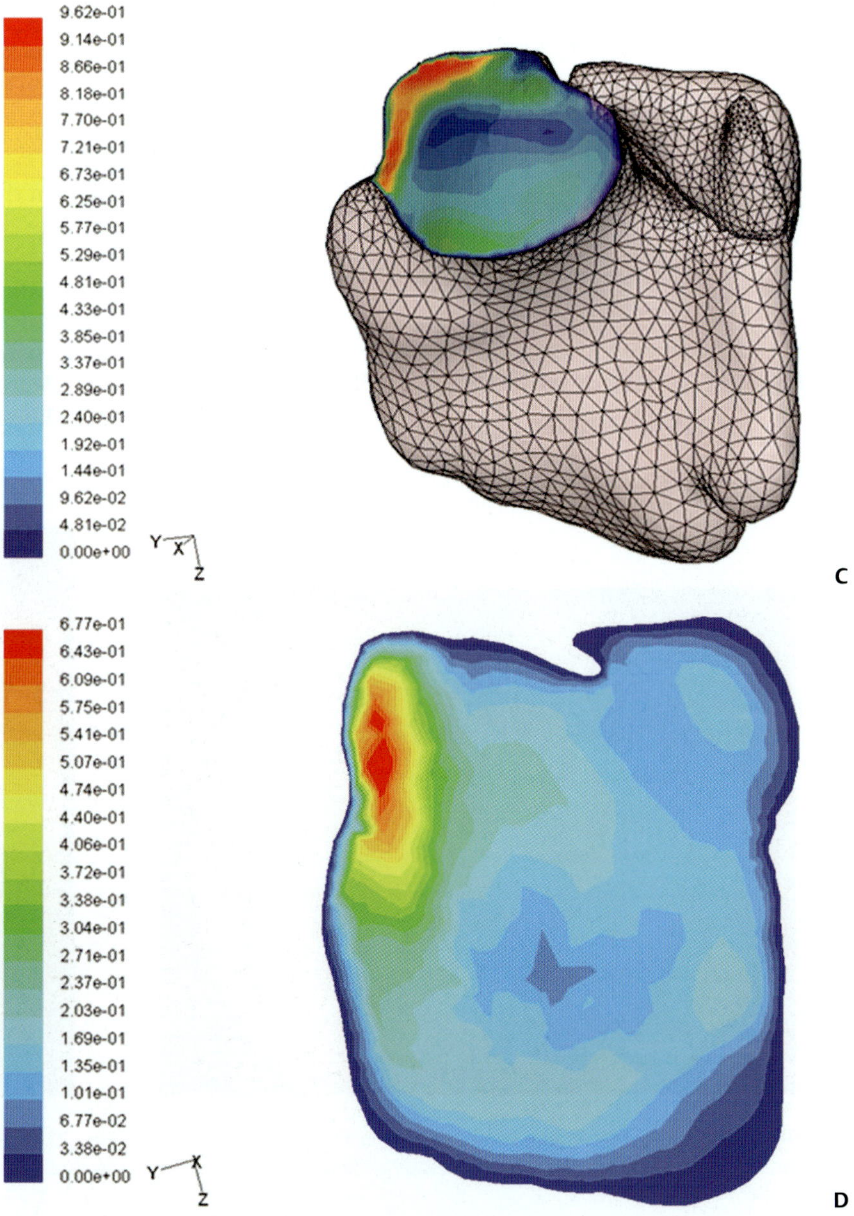

Fig. 22.1 *(continued)* **(C,D)** After enlarging the maxillary sinus ostium, air current into the sinus increases.

dioxide differential pressure, and subsequent partial oxyphil agglomeration.

In the normal condition, bacteria, viruses, and other foreign material that enter the nasal cavity invade the maxillary sinus itself very infrequently. In the postsurgical sinus, this relationship between the nasal cavity and the sinus is changed. Therefore, we advocate minimal surgery to the ostium itself in cases where the ostium can be healed by surgical removal of surrounding obstructive pathology (i.e., nasal polyps). In many cases, we believe opening or enlarging the maxillary sinus os may be unnecessary. We recall Professor Heinz Stammberger's oft-repeated admonition at the First International Course of Functional Endoscopic Sinus Surgery in Vienna in 1992, "Maxillary sinus surgery is a surgery of the nasal cavity external wall." One must recognize that surgical opening and enlargement of the sinus ostium will alter the internal sinus environment.

Maxillary ostium mucous membrane inflammation and hypertrophy can create stenosis or blockage of the sinus outflow pathway. In these situations, the sinus ostium may require a surgical opening or expansion. When this is required, we favor the use of straight pliers to enlarge the ostium by roughly 0.5 to 1.0 cm. In some instances, due to severe mucous membrane polyposis or postoperative scar proliferation the surgical ostium may become obstructed again. When this occurs, we favor the use of further expansion and enlargement of the interior maxillary sinus wall.

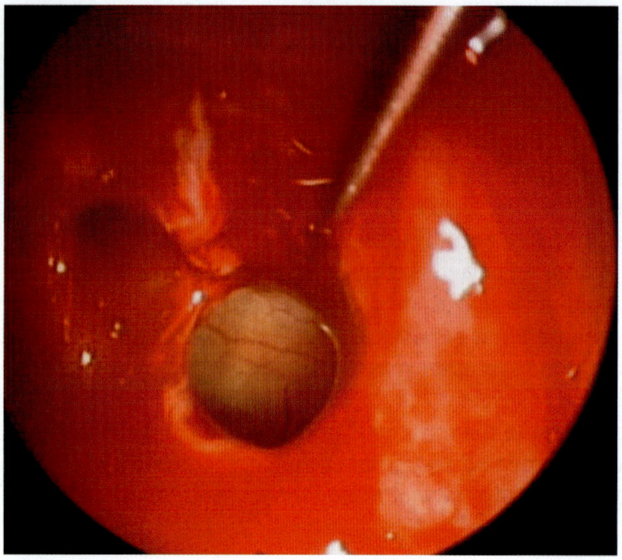

Fig. 22.3 Endoscopic image demonstrating left maxillary sinus ostium opening/expansion.

Location and Size of the Maxillary Sinus Opening

It has been well documented that the natural drainage pathway of the maxillary sinus is toward the natural ostium located in the anteromedial aspect of the sinus. This drainage pathway persists even in the light of surgical openings made elsewhere along the medial sinus wall.[5–8] Research in support of this concept has been performed in China, as well. In one study, an inferior meatal antrostomy was created in patients with maxillary sinus infections. Subsequently, using a 70-degree nasal endoscope for guidance, dye was placed into the sinus through the inferior antrostomy. Drainage of this dye was then observed over a 60-minute period. Of

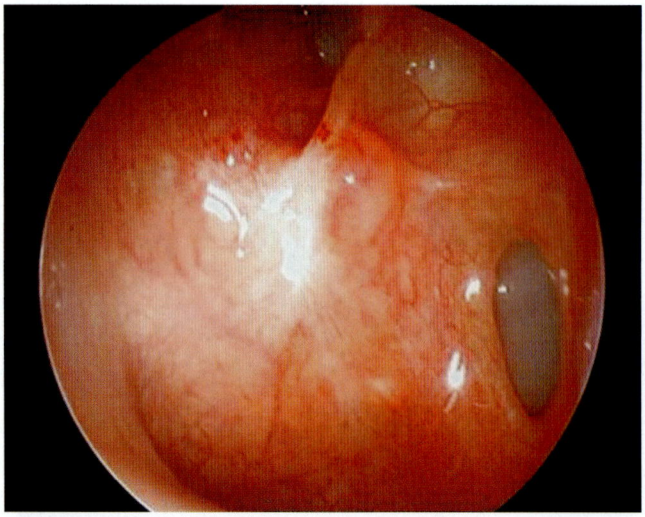

Fig. 22.2 Endoscopic image showing that maxillary sinus empyema cannot be drained from the inferior meatus artificial orifice.

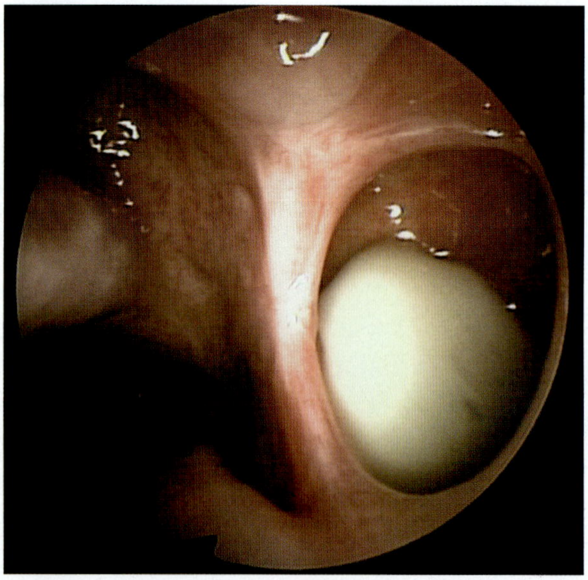

Fig. 22.4 Endoscopic image showing that because of the scars around the maxillary sinus ostium, the sinus empyema cannot drain.

11 patients enrolled in this study, the dye in seven patients discharged through the natural ostium, whereas the dye in four patients discharged through both the ostium and the inferior nasal meatus orifice. In two of the seven patients, persistent empyema prevented drainage through the inferior antrostomy site (**Fig. 22.2**).

The results of this study support the concept of the surgical enlargement of physiologic drainage pathways as opposed to the creation of alternate sites of gravity-dependent drainage. This study reinforces the principle that in cases of maxillary sinus surgery, it is more favorable to enlarge the natural aperture, and not to create a secondary artificial orifice (**Fig. 22.3**). At present, most sinus surgeons in China adhere to this principle and favor enlargement of the natural maxillary ostium over creation of an inferior meatal artificial orifice.

The Maxillary Sinus Ostium Opening Pattern

Improvement of maxillary sinus drainage may require opening or expanding the natural ostium. In some cases, even when the surgical antrostomy is open, the sinus secretions agglomerate and pool in the sinus cavity, resistant to discharge (**Fig. 22.4**).[9] Situations such as this indicate that the maxillary sinus cilium system's route of transmission is blocked despite an apparently open surgical antrostomy.

Several experiments at the Otorhinolaryngology Hospital of the First Affiliated Hospital of Sun Yat-sen University were designed to shed light on the pathophysiology underlying this obstruction to sinus drainage. One-hundred thirty unoperated sinuses were examined, along with 30 postsurgical sinuses. The following observations were made.

- Ninety-seven of 130 (71%) unoperated sinuses had a "dry river bed" type drainage pathway in which mucous from the maxillary sinus was swept by cilia over the inferior edge of maxillary ostium, passed through the "the river bed" area along the medial aspect of the turbinate into the lower middle nasal meatus, and then drained into the nasopharynx (**Fig. 22.5**).
- The maxillary ostium superior, inferior, anterior, and posterior quadrants are covered entirely by cilia. The cilia length and the density do not have significant differences in these quadrants. There is a lack of nonciliated cell or secretory cell's distribution nearby. The cilia direction in all quadrants sweeps mucous toward the inferoposterior area of the ostium.
- Regardless of patient position—upright, seated, or supine—dye which is placed into the maxillary sinus exits via the ostium inferior edge, drains, and enters the middle nasal meatus directly (**Fig. 22.6**). Even when the maxillary sinus is filled with purulent secretion, discharge is still via the inferior edge of the ostium (**Fig. 22.7**).
- In the postsurgical group of 30 participants who had a ring-like expanded maxillary ostium, drainage was along the inferior edge in 4 participants (13.3%), and along the posterior edge and/or superior edge in 17 participants (56.7%) (**Fig. 22.8**). In nine participants (30%), the tracer material accumulated in the maxillary sinus cavity and/or the sinus assumed revolving/circular transmission movement (**Fig. 22.9**).
- In the postsurgical group where the inferior edge mucosa was retained, the sinus mucous in every case

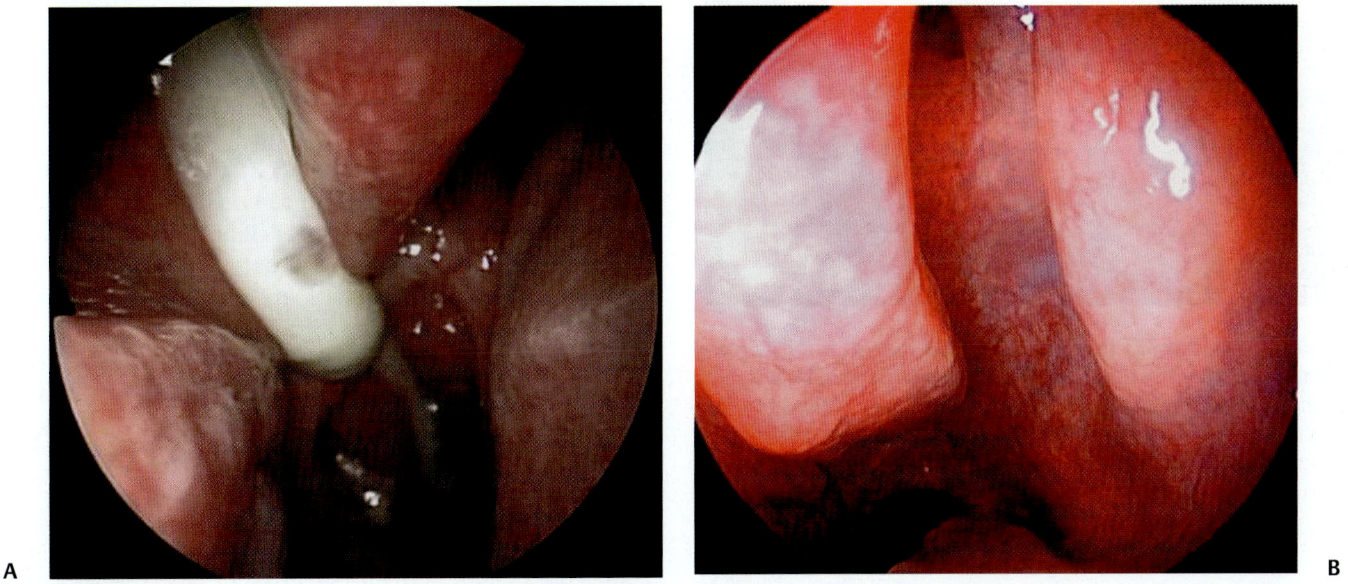

Fig. 22.5 Endoscopic images showing **(A)** the drainage channel of the maxillary sinus ostium inferior quadrant "the river bed type," and **(B)** the drainage channel of the maxillary sinus ostium inferior quadrant "the river bed type," which directly drains into the nasopharynx.

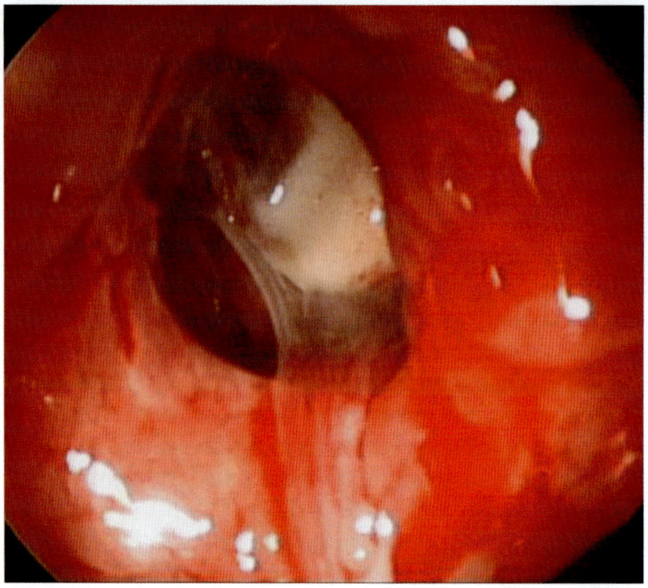

Fig. 22.6 Endoscopic image demonstrating the maxillary sinus filled with purulent secretion, which drains from the inferior edge of the ostium.

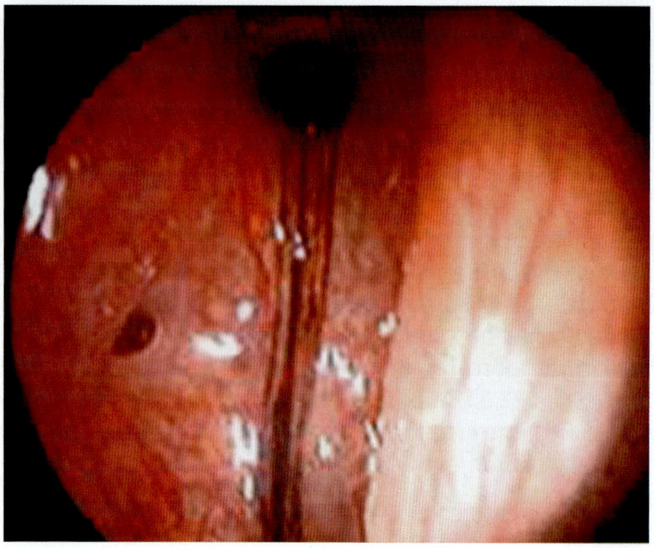

Fig. 22.7 Endoscopic image shows that the maxillary sinus ostium inferior edge is the site for natural sinus drainage via cilia transmission.

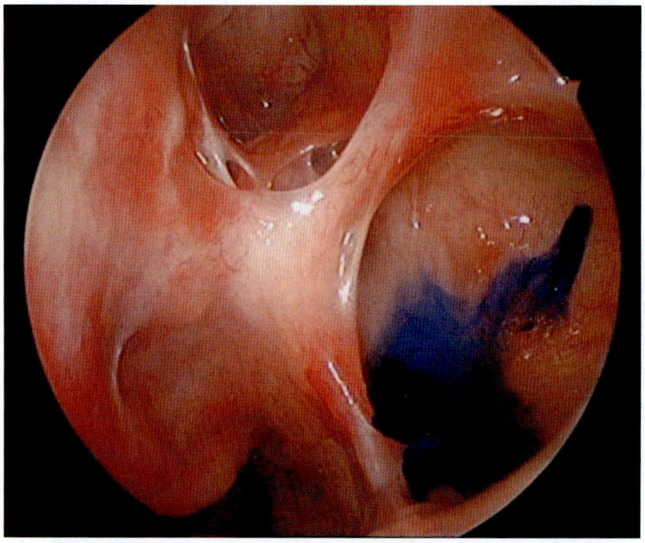

Fig. 22.8 Endoscopic image demonstrates that after a circumferential enlargement of the maxillary sinus ostium, the maxillary sinus displays delayed drainage. Note that the dye placed in the sinus cannot cross the inferior edge of the scar belt. This dye eventually drained out of the maxillary sinus in a superior direction into the ethmoid sinus area.

(100%) (**Fig. 22.10**) entered the middle meatus via the inferior edge of the ostium.

From these clinical observations, the following conclusions were made.

- The maxillary sinus ostium inferior edge is the primary drainage pathway for secretions from the maxillary sinus to enter the middle meatus.
- In the postsurgical sinus in which the inferior edge of the ostium has been retained, maxillary sinus cilia transmission and drainage route do not differ between the postoperative and the nonoperated sinus.
- After a ring-like, circumferential surgical enlargement of the maxillary ostium, the scar ribbon may alter the outflow pathway of maxillary sinus cilium. In this situation, natural drainage patterns are observed in a minority of patients. The majority of patients who undergo circumferential enlargement of their natural ostia experience altered drainage into the middle meatus via the superior or posterior edges. In many of these cases, sinus drainage occurs with difficulty and at an altered rate.
- In functional endoscopic sinus surgery (FESS) if the surgeon has to open and enlarge the maxillary sinus ostium, we recommend enlargement in an anterior or posterior direction. We recommend leaving the inferior edge untouched so that the natural drainage "river bed" patterns may continue in the postsurgical sinus.[9]

A
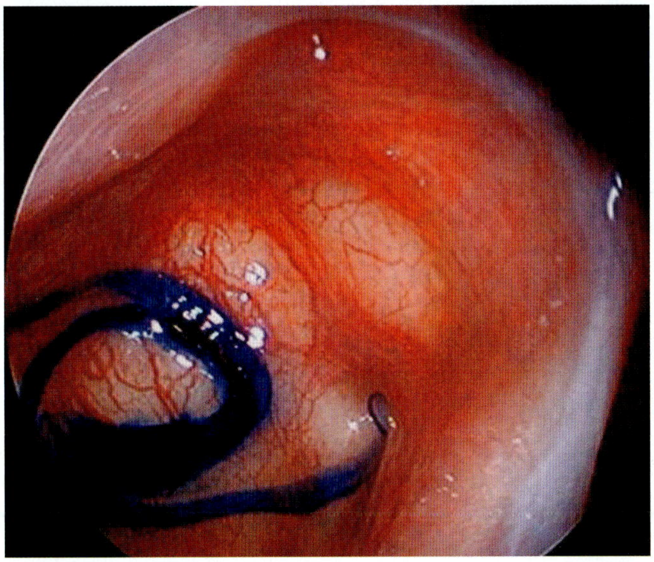
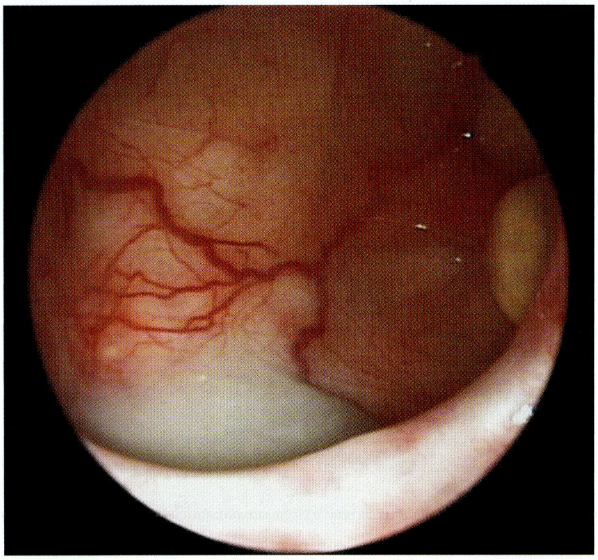
B

Fig. 22.9 Endoscopic images demonstrating that **(A)** after circumferential enlargement of the maxillary sinus ostium, a ring-like scar belt has formed. Note that the dye material cannot cross into the middle meatus, and a rotary, circular drainage pattern has developed. **(B)** In this postsurgical sinus, thick mucopurulent fluid is retained in the sinus and is unable to drain into the nasal cavity due to surgical damage to the inferior edge of the sinus. Small chronic abscesses can also be appreciated residing within the sinus itself.

Maxillary Sinus Disease Management

In cases in which the maxillary sinus disease is secondary to mucous membrane inflammation and hypertrophy without the presence of an obstructive polyp or cyst, enlargement of the sinus ostium is often unnecessary.

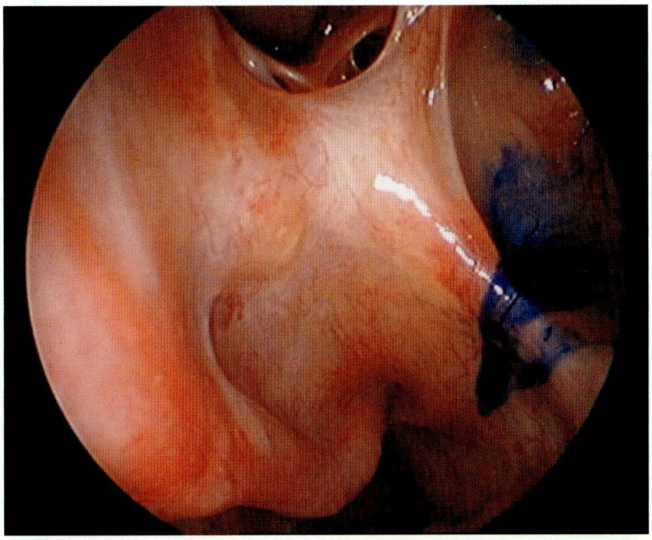

Fig. 22.10 Endoscopic image of a postsurgical sinus in which the inferior edge was preserved: the dye drains over the inferior edge and is transmitted in a natural manner toward the nasopharynx.

In cases where there is an obstruction to sinus drainage, the obstructive mass (e.g., polyp, cyst, etc.) does need to be excised.

It is imperative to try to retain the underlying periosteum in all cases. Powered instrumentation may assist in this goal. In cases where the maxillary sinus mucous membrane has been removed (including the periosteum and basement membrane), there is often a proliferation of poorly functional connective tissue fibers. It is for this reason that every attempt should be made to preserve mucosal lining and periosteum during maxillary sinus surgery.

Pearls

- Surgical opening of the maxillary sinus should include enlargement of the natural ostium.
- In most situations, the enlargement of the maxillary sinus opening should be in a posterior, anterior, and superior direction. Whenever possible, the inferior edge should be left untouched so as not to interfere with natural mucociliary clearance.
- Always try to prevent mucosal stripping, and always try to preserve the sinus periosteum.

References

1. Kennedy DW, Bolger WE, Zinreich SJ. Diseases of the Sinuses. Diagnosis and Management. Ontario: B. C. Derker, Inc.; 2001: 35–45
2. Albu S, Tomescu E. Small and large middle meatus antrostomies in the treatment of chronic maxillary sinusitis. Otolaryngol Head Neck Surg 2004;131(4):542–547
3. Xiong GX, Zhan JM, Jiang HY, et al. Computational fluid dynamics simulation of airflow in the normal nasal cavity and paranasal sinuses. Am J Rhinol 2008;22(5):477–482
4. Xiong G, Zhan J, Zuo K, Li J, Rong L, Xu G. Numerical flow simulation in the post-endoscopic sinus surgery nasal cavity. Med Biol Eng Comput 2008;46(11):1161–1167
5. Terrier G. Rhinosinusal Endoscopy. Diagnosis and Surgery. Milano: Zambon Group; 1991: 167–170
6. Stammberger H, Hawke M. Essentials of Endoscopic Sinus Surgery. St. Louis, MO: Mosby-Year Book, Inc.; 1993: 1–12
7. Waguespack R. Mucociliary clearance patterns following endoscopic sinus surgery. Laryngoscope 1995; 105(7 Pt 2, Suppl 71):1–40
8. Asai K, Haruna SI, Otori N, Yanagi K, Fukami M, Moriyama H. Saccharin test of maxillary sinus mucociliary function after endoscopic sinus surgery. Laryngoscope 2000;110(1):117–122
9. Xu CL, Zuo KJ, Xu G. [Impact of draining mode of enlarged maxillary ostium on mucociliary transportation system]. Zhonghua Er Bi Yan Hou Tou Jing Wai Ke Za Zhi 2008;43(4):259–262

23 Management of Persistent Maxillary Sinusitis: The View from Japan

Keiichi Ichimura

Buoyed by the sentiment that the Japanese economy could "no longer be termed postwar," Japan's gross national product expanded at an average annual rate of 10% between the mid-1950s and the end of the 1960s.[1] Until then, chronic sinusitis (CS) was so common in Japan that it was considered a national affliction. It was treated mainly with surgery, although a considerable number of cases were recalcitrant. The pathophysiology of CS has changed and the infiltrating cells in polyps or sinus mucosa have changed dramatically since then. In 1964, Okuda[2] reported the dominant infiltrating cells in polyps found in Europeans were eosinophils, which were different from those seen in Japanese patients (lymphocytes and neutrophils). Since then, the rate of eosinophil-dominant polyps has increased and has matched the European level of eosinophil infection.

Before 1970, sinusitis developed mainly due to an anatomic abnormality in the lateral nasal wall. Inflammation was located in the maxillary sinus and the dominant infiltrating cells in the sinus mucosa were lymphocytes or neutrophils. However, this type of sinusitis has decreased and is now treated by macrolide treatment and endoscopic sinus surgery (ESS).

After 1970, increased numbers of allergic rhinitis patients with a type-1 allergy developed CS. Insufficient ventilation and drainage due to mucosal swelling in the nose were regarded as a cause. This was often seen in severe cases of allergic rhinitis or in pediatric cases. Concomitant usage of drugs for allergic rhinitis such as receptor antagonists or release inhibitors of chemical mediators is effective for this condition.

The introduction of macrolides as agents for controlling CS in the 1990s dramatically improved outcome. Sinusitis, however, characterized by recalcitrant inflammation of the eosinophil-dominant mucosa became recognized,[3] and this type of inflammation showed poor results even with macrolide treatment. The main locus in the early stage of this type of sinusitis was in the ethmoid cells, although pansinus involvement occurred later. This type of sinusitis was highly associated with bronchial asthma and could be controlled only by steroids. The number of such cases is still increasing and ESS is used in its treatment. The use of macrolides for treatment of these patients could reduce the number of patients undergoing ESS. Yet there are still patients who will require the surgery, especially eosinophil-dominant infiltration cases. Concomitant treatment of CS with pre- and postoperative macrolide treatment and the addition of steroids treatment is now the choice of treatment for this condition. The process of CS seen in Japanese is presented in **Fig. 23.1**.

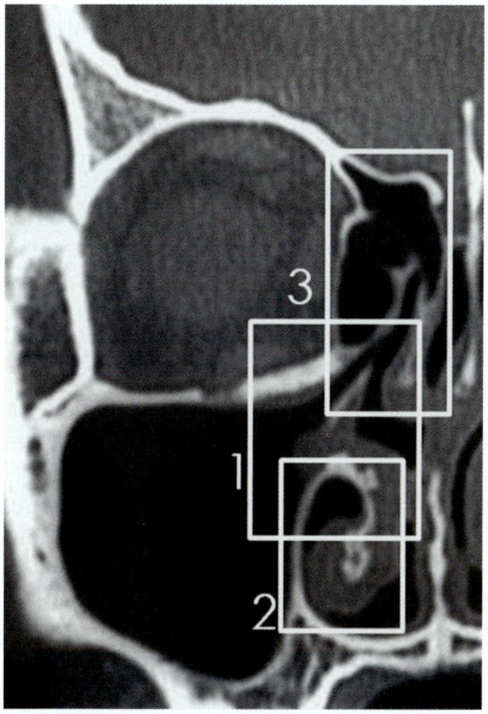

Fig. 23.1 The history of sinusitis treatment in Japan. (1) Before 1970, sinusitis developed mainly because of an anatomic abnormality in lateral nasal wall. Inflammation was located in the maxillary sinus. Neutrophil-dominant infiltration is present at the sinus mucosa. This type of sinusitis is a good indication for macrolide treatment and endoscopic sinus surgery. (2) Sinusitis accompanied by allergic rhinitis increased after 1970. Insufficient ventilation and drainage due to mucosal swelling in the nose seems to be the cause. This type is often accompanied by severe cases of allergic rhinitis and is observed frequently in pediatric cases. Concomitant antiallergic drug usage is effective. (3) Sinusitis caused by recalcitrant inflammation of the eosinophil-dominant mucosa was recognized in the 1990s. The main locus is in the ethmoid cells, followed by pansinus involvement; eosinophil infiltration is dominant. This type of sinusitis is highly associated with bronchial asthma. Poor results are obtained with macrolide therapy.

History of Sinusitis Treatment in Japan

Early in the 17th century, the Japanese feudal government broke off all relations with foreign countries, prohibited foreign travel, and entered an era of isolation. Japan's modernization began in 1867 following the abandonment of the isolation policy. Until then, Japanese patients had been treated with traditional Chinese herbal medicine. For Japan, modernization meant Westernization. In the late 19th century, Japanese doctors, such as Okonogi, Kanasugi, and Kako who had studied otolaryngology in Germany, introduced Western techniques for the treatment of sinusitis. Dr. Okada was the first man to study at overseas universities at the government's expense. After coming back from 4 years' study in Berlin, Munich, and Vienna, he became the first professor of the Department of Otolaryngology, University of Tokyo Hospital in 1898. Dr. Watsuji, the first professor of otolaryngology at the University of Kyoto Hospital, also studied in Berlin. He developed a sinus operation, which is similar to Denker's approach except that the inferior turbinate is left intact. He developed his approach in 1905—the same year as Denker. Thus, in Japan this approach has been named the Watsuji–Denker method. Professor Kubo studied abroad at Killian's clinic in Freiburg before he became a professor at Fukuoka University Hospital. He was the first surgeon to report cases of postoperative maxillary cyst in the world.[4]

In the early 20th century, the prevalence and severity of sinusitis in Japan was high. Because of the lack of effective drugs, most patients underwent surgery for the treatment of sinusitis. The Caldwell–Luc method was used for maxillary sinusitis and Killian's method for frontal sinusitis. However, once the importance of ethmoid cells in controlling CS was established, surgeons soon introduced the ethmoidectomy. Dr. K. Takahashi was the first surgeon to perform an endonasal ethmoidectomy in Japan (1918). Kuwana (1918) and Hirogami (1926) developed an ethmoidectomy through the maxillary sinus via the Caldwell–Luc approach. Dr. Kurosu developed the pansinectomy in 1929, which gave access to the ethmoid, frontal, and sphenoid sinuses through the maxillary sinus, nostril, and facial skin. Professor Nishihata at Keio University Hospital developed a combined sinectomy via the Caldwell–Luc approach and the endonasal approach in 1931. The latter method had been performed widely in Japan until the introduction of ESS in the 1980s. Professor R. Takahashi of Jikei University Hospital had performed an endonasal sinus operation in 1950[5] and tried to popularize the procedure. This method performed without the aid of a scope of any kind, required keen eyes and great surgical skill. This limited its use as a general procedure. The first report of ESS was done by Dr. Kaneko, one of Professor Takahashi's pupils, in 1980.[6] Since then, Professors Ohnishi and Moriyama of the Department of Otolaryngology at Jikei University Hospital have contributed to the teaching of ESS in Japan.

As the cause of CS had not yet been established, effective conservative or medical treatment was not available until the introduction of macrolides. Antibiotics, antiinflammatory enzymes, and antihistamines had been used with limited effect. In the 1960s, the prevalence of sinusitis in children was as high as 30 to 40%. After 1980, it was reduced to 3 to 4%. In addition, the severity of sinusitis was high until 1980. Moderate and severe cases amounted to 40% in those days; it was not until 1995 that the rate was reduced.[7]

The Impact of Sinobronchial Syndrome

Sinobronchial syndrome (SBS) is defined as the coexisting pathologies of CS and nonspecific chronic lower airway inflammation, which includes chronic bronchitis, bronchiectasis, and diffuse panbronchiolitis (DPB). Allergic inflammation, such as bronchial asthma and allergic rhinitis, are not included in this category. Parenchymal lesions, such as pneumonia, are also not included. Typical SBS cases show pansinus lesions in diagnostic imaging and are classified as resistant-to-treatment. The history of SBS dates back to the end of the 19th century.[8] However, it has been within the past 30 years that the cause of this syndrome has been found to be an abnormality of the systemic airway defense mechanism. The incidence of family occurrence is extremely high; it amounts to two-thirds in SBS patients.[9] B54 in the B locus of human leukocyte antigen (HLA) is a characteristic antigen in mongoloids and is highly recognized in SBS patients. The incidence of B54 in Japanese control patients is ≥10% ; in DPB patients it is 50 to 70%.[9] In patients with bronchiectasis or chronic bronchitis, the prevalence is also high, although less than that of DPB. So, a portion of SBS patients may be regarded as having a genetic disease. DPB is sometimes seen in Caucasoids, but is common in Mongoloids. Nevertheless, B54 is not found in DPB patients in Korea, but HLA A11 is highly identified.[10] The disease susceptibility gene may exist between the two HLA loci on chromosome 6.

This genetic theory explains how both nasal and bronchial symptoms occur simultaneously. Yet the bronchiolar region is regarded as "silent zone" in view of symptomatology. Therefore, the difference of reactivity and standby capacity between the upper and lower airway tissues may be attributed to a time lag in manifestation.

DPB was first reported in Japan in 1969. Cases were reported in the English literature in 1983.[11] DPB is a diffuse chronic inflammation of the respiratory bronchiole and their peribronchiolar regions. It is considered a small airway disease because it usually involves terminal bronchiole and more proximal airways. DPB is accompanied by CS without exception. Before the introduction of macrolide therapy, DPB had the following characteristics:

1. Prognosis of the patient was poor; the 5-year survival rate was as low as 63% and the death rate in each year was 10%.[12]
2. The results of a Caldwell–Luc operation for the sinus lesion were not good compared with other types of CS.[13]
3. Complete cure after sinus surgery was rare.
4. The lower airway symptoms did not necessarily improve, even in the patients whose sinus symptoms improved.

The introduction of macrolide therapy along with ESS made SBS a curable condition.

Macrolide Treatment

Japan was the first country to begin macrolide therapy. Macrolide therapy was started as the result of an accidental discovery by Dr. Kudoh. He had treated a 52-year-old male DPB patient with steroids and various antibiotics for 5 years without any effect and the patient discontinued consultation. Two years later in 1980 the patient came to see him with minimal symptoms and his PaO2 had improved from 55 to 85 torr. Dr. Kudoh was surprised at the patient's improved condition and learned that he had consulted Dr. Miyazawa in Matsumoto City (200 km northwest to Tokyo) for 2 years. His prescribed drugs were almost the same as those Dr. Kudoh had prescribed in his earlier treatment, except for the addition of 600 mg a day of erythromycin (EM). Normally we would think that such a low dose would not work. But Dr. Kudoh could not help but believe what he saw and accepted the validity of this regimen. To confirm this treatment, the first open trial of low-dose, long-term EM therapy was started immediately. After 6 months to 3 years of treatment with 600 mg of EM, symptoms and clinical parameters were markedly improved in 18 patients. FEV 1 and PaO2 were significantly increased on average from 1.61 to 2.17 L ($p < 0.01$) and from 65.2 to 75.1 mm Hg ($p < 0.01$), respectively. Small nodular shadows on chest x-ray (CXR) films disappeared in more than 60% of the cases.[14] A subsequent national-level controlled study with placebo was performed in 1990 with significantly better results.[15] In the 1970s before EM treatment, the overall 5-year survival rate was 63% as stated earlier. Between 1980 and 1984, fluoroquinolones were started for treating *Pseudomonas aeruginosa*, but the survival rate was still limited to 72%. After 1985, when EM therapy was introduced, the 5-year survival rate was 91%.[12] As a result, EM treatment became a standard therapy for chronic lower airway inflammatory disease including DPB.

As DPB always accompanies CS, EM therapy for DPB also then affects sinus pathology. Nasal symptoms get better during EM therapy. The first EM trial for CS was done in 1990 among patients with CS-associated DPB. EM showed remarkable effectiveness.[16] The next trial was performed by Kikuchi and others[17] in 26 adult patients with CS regardless of the presence of lower airway inflammatory diseases in 1991. They were treated with 400 to 600 mg of EM per day for an average of 7.9 months. Rhinorrhea was reduced in 60%, postnasal drip in 50%, nasal obstruction in 60%, hyposmia in 11.8%, and a sense of dullness in the head was absent in all the study's patients. Rhinoscopy showed reduced mucosal swelling in 10.5%, lower volume of rhinorrhea in 80%, better quality of rhinorrhea in 70%, and reduced postnasal drip in 85.7%. Clinical efficacy was unrelated with sensitivity of EM for bacteria identified. No significant side effects were noted in any of the patients during this therapy; however, this was not due to EM's antibacterial activity.

The same authors then proceeded to study 130 CS patients, including 21 pediatric patients.[18] EM at 400 to 600 mg per day for adults and at 200 to 300 mg per day for children was administered orally for an average of 5.4 months and at least 3 months. Subjective symptoms—excluding dysosmia—and objective findings—excluding mucosal swelling—were improved after treatment. The results of this EM study were as follows:

1. Adequate clinical effect was obtained with half or less of ordinary dose.
2. The clinical course is slowly, but surely improved with time and reliable effect was obtained at 2 to 3 months.
3. This treatment is more effective in cases of hypersecretion-type CS.
4. The clinical effect in children was somewhat less than that found in adults. (Successive studies have yielded better outcomes in pediatric cases.)[19]
5. Clinical efficacy was unrelated with the presence of lower airway diseases or history of sinus surgery.

A subsequent trial was done with new 14-membered macrolides. Clarithromycin (CAM) and roxithromycin (RXM) also showed effectiveness for CS. The first article describing the use of macrolides in patients with CS appeared in the English literature in 1996. Hashiba and Baba[20] treated 45 adult CS patients with CAM, 400 mg daily for 8 to 12 weeks. Twenty (44%) of these patients had undergone previous sinus surgery. Improvements in symptoms and rhinoscopic findings were directly related to the duration of macrolide therapy. The investigators noted improvement rates of 5%, 48%, 63%, and 71%, respectively, after 2, 4, 8, and 12 weeks of therapy. After 12 weeks of therapy, 64% of patients had reduced viscosity of nasal secretions, 56% had reduced quantity of nasal secretions, 62% had decreased postnasal drip, and 51% had reduced nasal obstruction. Clinical benefit in patients with CS also was observed following long-term administration of roxithromycin, 150 mg daily.[21]

Roxithromycin was tried on polyps associated with chronic rhinosinusitis.[22] Forty adult patients were enrolled and were grouped according to whether they received azelastine or not. Duration of medication was at least 2 months. More than half the cases experienced shrinkage of nasal polyps in various extents in both groups. The rate of polyp disappearance was 16% in each group.

A number of studies have been done to ascertain macrolides mechanism of action, outside their antibacterial effect. As DPB is a typical neutrophil-derived inflammatory condition, some novel actions relating neutrophils were examined. Macrolides inhibit accumulation and activation of neutrophils, suppress expression of adhesion molecules, block production of proinflammatory cytokines, and hamper lymphocyte activation. It has recently been found that even sub-MIC of 14-membered ring macrolides exhibits inhibitory effects on biofilm formation and the expression of virulence factors such as pyocyanine, elastase, and proteases. Macrolides inhibit water secretion by blocking Cl^-- channels via epithelial cells.[23] They also inhibit mucin secretion.[24] The novel actions of macrolides are summarized in **Table 23.1**.

The pathologic mechanism of developing CS is complicated. Where the ostia of the sinuses presents in the middle meatus is called the ostiomeatal complex (OMC). If this part is blocked, ventilator and drainage impairment will occur and the gas composition and pH in the sinuses will change. As a result, bacterial proliferation occurs, and the mucosal lamina propria in the sinuses thickens. The blockade of the ostia is then reinforced, which creates a "vicious circle." Any treatment of CS aims to break this cycle. Antral lavage can do this by clearing accumulated fluids in the sinuses, whereas antibiotics act specifically against bacterial proliferation. Topical management including a topical vasoconstrictor helps to open the ostium; whereas mucolytics improve mucociliary clearance. Macrolides (1) inhibit the accumulation of inflammatory cells, (2) block cytokine production, (3) decrease water and mucin secretion, (4) restore mucociliary clearance, and (5) hamper biofilm formation.

Table 23.1 Novel Actions of Macrolides

1. On host
Inhibit cytokine production
Inhibit active oxygen generation
Inhibit production of chemotactic factors, such as lipopolysaccharide (LPS) and tumor necrosis factor-alpha (TNF-α) from fibroblasts
Suppress the activation of nuclear factor-kappa B and activator protein-1
Accelerate both differentiation and proliferation of monocytes-macrophage system cells
Enhance intrinsic glucocorticoid production
Inhibit chloride channel opening
Suppress mucin production
2. On bacteria
Potentiate serum sensitivity
Suppress expression of virulence factors (pyocyanine, elastase, protease)
Restrain production of biofilm
Inhibit quorum sensing system

There are many different treatment options for CS. Among medical treatments, macrolide treatment produces the most improvement with the exception of steroid treatment. With macrolide treatment, many patients can avoid surgery. Nevertheless, in mild or moderate cases of CS, a combination of drugs has proven to be the most effective treatment. The low-dose long-term administration of macrolide should be used for recalcitrant cases. For the treatment of CS, macrolide therapy should be used for hypersecretion-type CS, a refractory case, and for certain postoperative conditions.

In 1998, the following clinical guidelines for long-term macrolide therapy was announced by the Society for Novel Actions of Macrolides Study Group (**Table 23.2**).[25]

1. What macrolides should be used?
   The 14-membered macrolides (EM, CAM, RXM)
2. What are the appropriate doses to prescribe?
   Half of an ordinary dose is recommended. For adults, daily doses are EM 400 to 600 mg, CAM 200 mg, and RXM 150 mg. For children, daily doses are EM 8 to 12 mg/kg and CAM 4 to 8 mg/kg.
3. How long should they be used?
   For 3 months at first. At 3 months the efficacy of the drug should be evaluated. If ineffective, change to another treatment. It is important to shorten the duration of medication to avoid adverse effects and the development of resistant bacterial strains. Even if effective, medication should be stopped.

Table 23.2 Guidelines for Macrolide Therapy

Fourteen-membered macrolides (EM, CAM, RXM) are recommended.
Half of an ordinary dose is recommended. For adults, daily doses are EM 400–600 mg, CAM 200 mg, RXM 150 mg. For children, EM 8–12 mg/kg, CAM 4–8 mg/kg
Macrolides are used for 3 months at first. At 3 months the efficacy of the drug should be evaluated. If failed, change to another treatment. Even if effective, medication should be stopped at 6 months to prevent adverse effects and the development of resistant bacterial strains.
If symptoms recur, treatment should be restarted. Tachypraxis has not been recognized so far.
In the following conditions, additional treatments may be required: the presence of type 1 allergy or bronchial asthma, obstruction at the OMC, coexistence of polyps, and acute exacerbation. Additional treatments include surgery and steroids.

Abbreviations: EM, erythromycin; CAM, clarithromycin; RXM, roxithromycin; OMC, ostiomeatal complex.

4. If effective, when should the treatment be stopped?
   Even if effective, stop at 6 months.
5. What should be done if the symptoms recur?
   Macrolide treatment should be restarted. Tachypraxis has not been recognized so far.
6. Under what conditions may additional treatment be required?
   The presence of type 1 allergy or bronchial asthma, obstruction at the OMC, coexistence of polyps, and acute exacerbation limit the efficacy of macrolides. In such conditions, additional appropriate treatment, such as surgery or the administration of steroids, may be required.

This guideline was also incorporated with no modification in 2006 in the Japan Rhinologic Society's Practical Guidelines for Sinusitis.[26]

Indications in children are different from those in adults. In pediatric CS, signs and symptoms are unstable and bacterial infection is prominent, whereas the incidence of irreversible mucosal lesions including polyps is low. CS may spontaneously remit during adolescence. Thus, long-term treatment is not the sole option. Indications of pediatric CS are the presence of purulent or mucopurulent nasal discharge and if its duration is longer than one month. Evaluation should be done at 2 months and the term of treatment should be as brief as possible.[27]

Side effects reported were gastrointestinal upset and abnormality of liver function. These adverse effects will occur within 3 months at which point the medication should be stopped. The incidence of an adverse effect was reported as 7.2% with EM, 2.5% with CAM, and 1.9% with RXM.[28] The cessation of treatment due to side effects was 2.8% with EM and 0% with CAM and RXM in Japan. Severe adverse effects have not been recognized so far. Hence, macrolide therapy is considered a safe treatment.

One possible problem posited in macrolide treatment is the increase in the prevalence of resistant strains of bacteria. Mean types of bacteria during macrolide treatment were investigated by Hashiba and others.[29] Twenty-seven patients were included in the study. No numerical change was confirmed during and at the end of the treatment compared with baseline. Maeda et al presented 26 patients with chronic lower airway inflammation who had been administered macrolides for more than 10 years.[30] Adverse effects were observed in only two cases (dysgeusia and raised liver enzyme level); they disappeared soon after cessation and never reappeared in the next administration. Long-term administration of macrolides had no effect on sensitivity of identified bacteria from the sputa to β-lactum antibiotics.

To date, there has been no direct evidence for increased antibiotic-resistant bacteria in the nasal and oral cavity. And to the best of my knowledge, there have been no reports of patients treated with long-term macrolides who experienced life-threatening infectious disease with macrolide-resistant bacteria. Nevertheless, new antiinflammatory macrolides without antimicrobial activity should continue to be developed. EM201 was developed as a metabolic product of EM; it has no antibiotic effect, but still has motilin-like action. From this product, EM 703 was created as a new macrolide derivative, which reinforced antiinflammatory activity but was weak in solubility and stability. Then the EM 900 series compounds (901, 905, 914, and 939) were de-

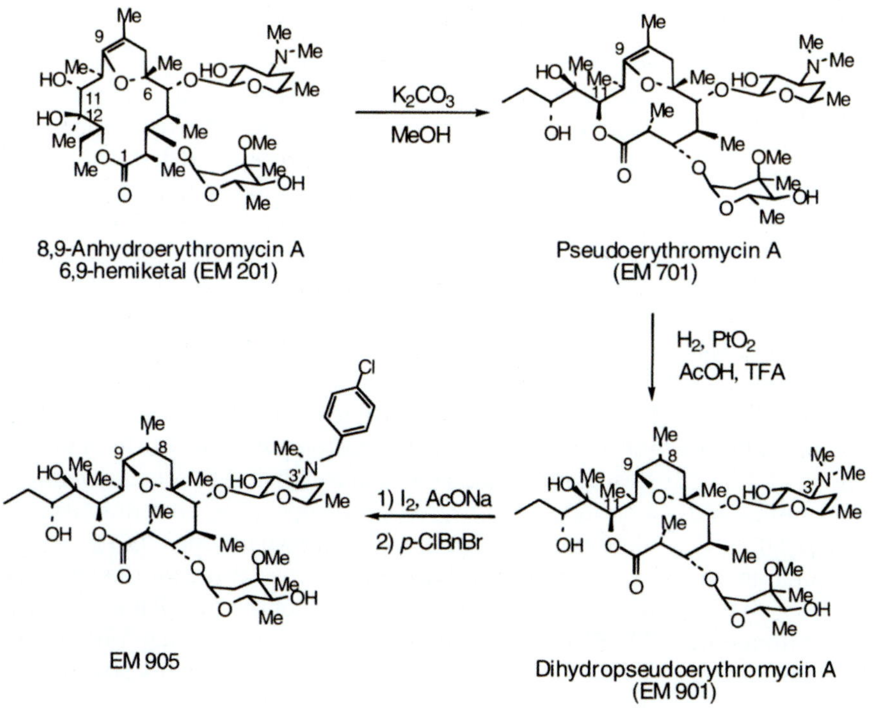

Fig. 23.2 Synthesis of the EM 900 series.

veloped (**Fig. 23.2**). They have no influence on CYP3A4. They are now being investigated in vitro; their induction potency of monocytes on macrophages has been shown to increase 30 times as much as that of EM.[31] Further investigation of this series is required.

As mentioned here earlier, macrolide therapy has reduced the rate of ESS. In cases of extensive mucosal pathology and those of obstructed OMC that are usually resistant to macrolide therapy, removal of polyps is very useful. Macrolide therapy is continued in the postoperative course. Patients who are candidates for surgery are recommended to have macrolides prior to the surgical procedure. Although not published before, minimizing inflammation by macrolides decreased volume of bleeding during surgery. With the introduction of postoperative macrolide therapy, the symptomatic improvement rate after ESS has become 90% compared with 80% obtained before.[32]

Eosinophilic Sinusitis

A histologic study by Iino et al indicated that macrolide treatment is effective in sinusitis with lymphocyte-dominant or neutrophil-infiltrating patterns of submucosal infiltrating cells, but not effective in sinusitis with an eosinophil-dominant pattern.[33] Some cases recur even after the combination treatment of macrolide therapy and ESS. A retrospective analysis of postoperative cases revealed that the cases associated with bronchial asthma or with eosinophil-dominant infiltration in the sinus tissue had poor results.[34] Haruna and Moriyama[35] proposed the term, *eosinophilic sinusitis* to describe the infiltration of activated eosinophil in the sinuses. Diffuse eosinophil-dominant polyposis and eosinophil mucin rhinosinusitis (Ferguson[36]) are terms that describe similar conditions. Eosinophilic sinusitis includes sinusitis combined with nonatopic asthma, aspirin-induced asthma, Churg–Strauss syndrome, allergic fungal sinusitis, and eosinophil-infiltration sinusitis without lower airway lesions.

The clinical characteristics of eosinophilic sinusitis are as follows:

1. Age at onset is ~40.
2. This type of sinusitis is usually involved bilaterally and associated with multiple edematous polyps.
3. Stronger pathologic changes are present around the middle turbinate and less in the inferior turbinate.
4. The majority of patients complain of dysosmia.
5. Accumulation of thick mucus with eosinophil infiltration is observed.
6. This condition is remotely related to allergic rhinitis and shows varied quantities of immunoglobulin E (IgE).
7. Bronchial asthma and aspirin-induced asthma are accompanied by the condition.
8. Eosinophil count in blood and value of eosinophilic cation protein (ECP) in serum and nasal mucosa are increased.
9. The ethmoid sinuses are mainly involved in the early stages followed by pansinus involvement.
10. This disease is resistant to treatment, especially to surgical therapy.
11. The administration of systemic steroids is effective for this condition.

Ishitoya et al[37] proposed the following diagnostic criteria for eosinophilic sinusitis. According to these criteria, eosinophilic sinusitis accounts for 15% of the CS that requires surgery.

1. Computed tomography (CT) findings: ethmoid/maxillary (E/M) score ratio*≧1 and score of ethmoid cells≧3
   *E/M score ratio = (CT score of anterior ethmoid cells + score of posterior ethmoid cells) / (score of maxillary sinus × 2) (after Lund–McKay score)
2. Eosinophil count in blood: ≧6% or 400/μL
3. Eosinophil count* in nasal polyps: ≧350 in the field of view at 400-fold magnification.
   *In a polyp specimen that has been stained with hematoxylin-eosin, five areas where eosinophils are found in a higher percentage are selected and the number of eosinophils is counted at 400-fold magnification and the mean of the value of the top three areas is obtained.
4. The presence of typical clinical findings: dysosmia, nasal obstruction, thick mucous discharge, etc.
5. All asthmatic patients have CS. About 10% of asthmatic patients have aspirin sensitivity. The condition is characterized by raised leukotrene (LT)s in the serum and urine.

Maxillary Sinus Surgery and Postoperative Treatment

For maxillary sinus lesions, a wide opening of the natural ostium (NO) and middle meatus is essential for ensuring reliable working space during surgery. If there are polyps in the middle meatus, they should be removed first. The middle meatus is widened by resection of the uncinate process. For performing uncinectomy we Japanese use a Kurosu elevator (**Fig. 23.3A**) instead of the Freer elevator widely used in Western countries. For easier management of the NO we remove the ethmoidal bulla and open the other anterior ethmoidal cells. If there is no ethmoidal involvement, opening of the (third) basal lamella of the ethmoid is not necessary; however, we usually open it to secure the ventilation route of the maxillary sinus in the postoperative period. In this initial stage, the NO can be seen in over half the patients even with a straight, zero-degree endoscope. (The procedure used to identify and widen the NO is shown in **Video 23.1**).

To enlarge the NO, the knife specialized for the membranous portion of the medial wall of the maxillary sinus (**Fig. 23.3B**) is used followed by retrograde cutting forceps (**Fig. 23.3C**) for forward or vertical enlargement and straight cutting forceps (**Fig. 23.3D**) for backward widening. The posi-

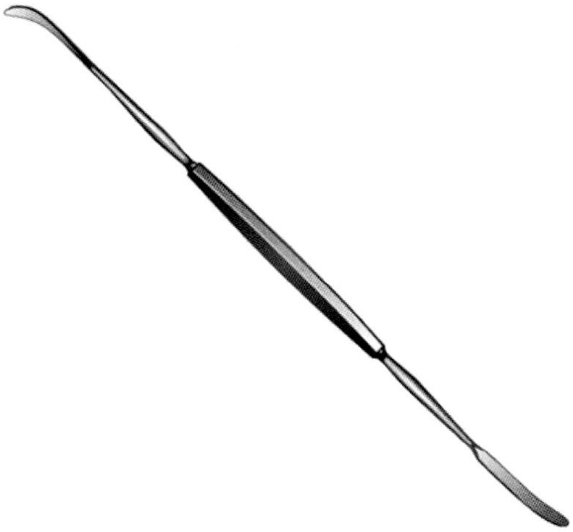
A

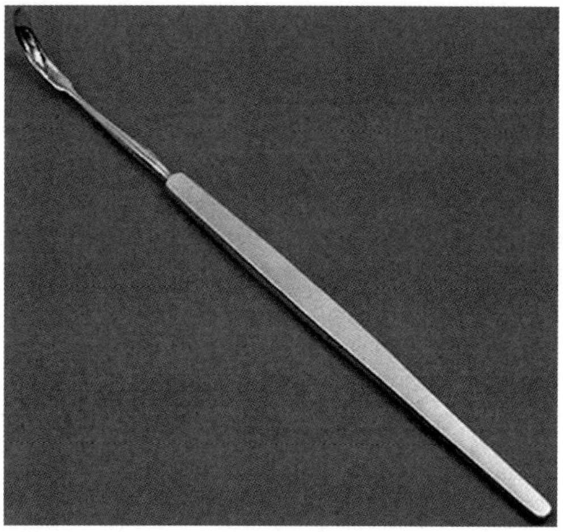
B

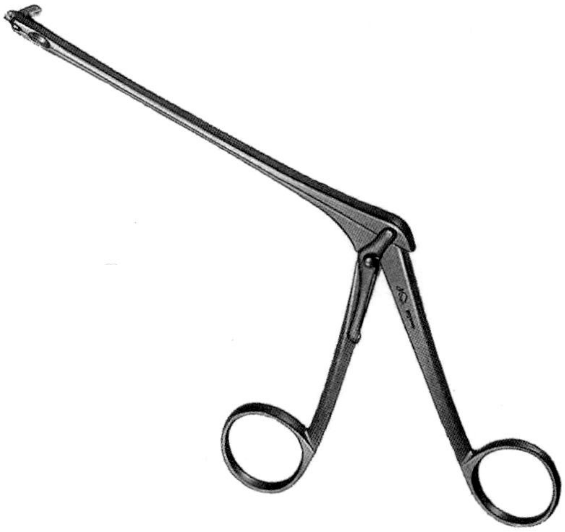
C

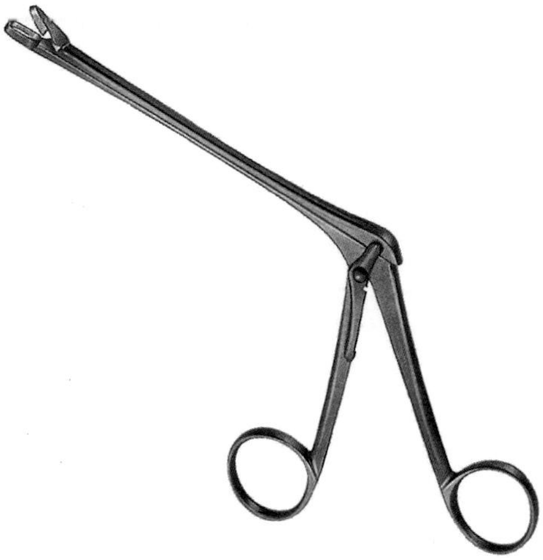
D

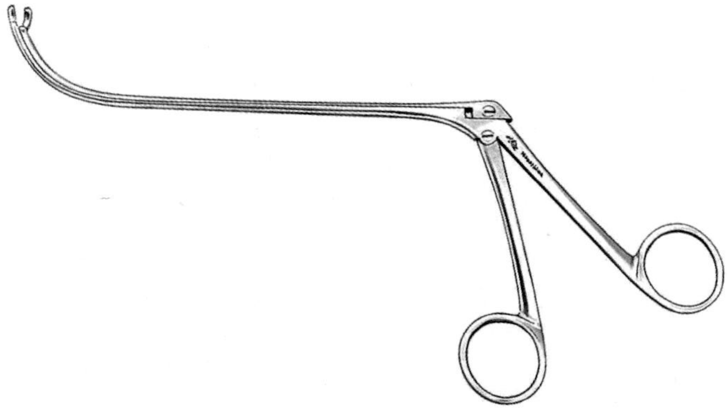
E

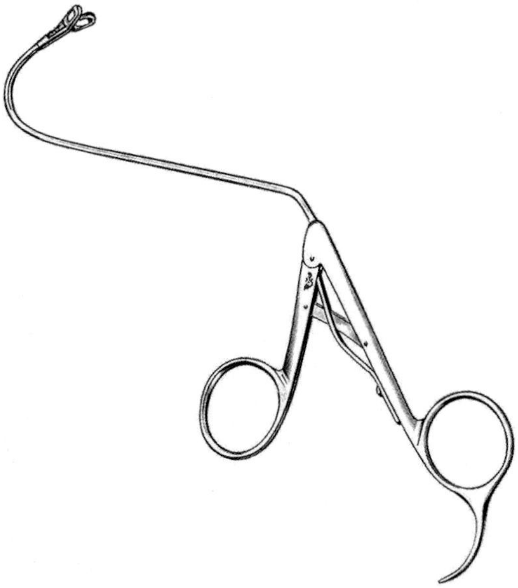
F

Fig. 23.3 (A–F) Instruments for surgery. **(A)** Kurosu elevator. **(B)** Membranous portion knife. **(C)** Ashikawa's retrograde cutting forceps (opening to the right). **(D)** Ashikawa's straight cutting forceps. **(E)** Nishihata's greatly curved spoon forceps. **(F)** Kikawada's spoon forceps (135 bent).

tion of the knife cut is on the membranous portion of the medial wall at a height between both ends of the middle turbinate. The window should have a diameter of not less than 1 cm. Care should be taken not to injure the nasolacrimal duct during a forward enlargement procedure. Removal of the mucosa in the sinus is unnecessary. Instead, the edematous swollen membrane is trimmed with a microdebrider, Nishihata's greatly curved spoon forceps (**Fig. 23.3E**), or a malleable suction tube without exposing bony surface.

The anteroinferior portion of the sinus is the difficult part to handle because it is out of reach of instruments through the middle meatus. If pathology is present there, we have two options. One is to use Kikawada's spoon forceps (135 degrees) (**Fig. 23.3F**), which can put the unreachable within reach and another is to make a hole at the lateral wall of the inferior meatus as anterior as possible. This hole is big enough to pass through suction tubes, slender curved forceps, or a microdebrider. We usually create a hole of 5-mm width. The trimming procedure is continued with forceps, suction tubes, or a microdebrider passed through this control hole. Illumination is provided by a 70-degree endoscope set in the middle meatus. If the alveolar recess of the sinus is well developed, the management of the anteroinferior part is still difficult even with the creation of an inferior meatal hole. In such cases, a small incision is made at the gingivobuccal sulcus and a small hole around 5-mm width is created at the anterior wall of the sinus with a chisel or drill. The trimming is performed through the hole in the same fashion as from the inferior meatal window. If there are tenacious fluid, fungus balls, caseous masses, or foreign bodies, irrigation with saline is effective.

The surgical procedure for eosinophilic sinusitis is almost the same as that for CS. Important reminders are (1) to suction the pooled thick fluid in the sinuses as completely as possible, (2) to avoid adhesion due to the formation of multiple wound surfaces at the olfactory cleft and superior meatus, and (3) to make a single sinonasal cavity by widening ostia of sinuses and removing ethmoid cell walls.

Postoperative treatment is very important. We usually ask patients to visit weekly for the first postoperative month, biweekly the next month, monthly for the next 4 months, and then once evert 3 months until one year of non-eosinophilic sinusitis. Because mild and moderate cases are controlled by macrolide therapy, the patient who undergoes surgery needs intense follow-up and requires treatment during the postoperative period. Mucociliary function is recovered by 3 months after surgery. At each visit, endoscopic observation of the nose and sinuses is mandatory. In the early postoperative stage, excessive fibrin masses and crusts are suctioned and removed gently. Bleeding should be avoided as much as possible so as not to prolong the healing process. Secretions collected in the sinus are flushed with saline. Small polyps, edematous mucosa, and granulations are managed by placing cottons soaked with adrenaline and steroids followed by aerosol therapy. We remove polyps at every visit after the postoperative 3 weeks. Topical steroids and oral low-dose macrolides are applied for 2 months postoperatively. Eosinophilic sinusitis often re-occurs even after the postoperative third month. For this condition, peroral administration of steroids for some days soon after the operation and regular postoperative therapy is applied along with administration of topical steroids and leukotriene receptor antagonists for as long as 3 to 6 months. As for aspirin-sensitive asthma (ASA), the addition of topical cromolyn helps to prevent recurrence after surgery. Oral steroids (prednisolone 20–30 mg/day) are administered for several days to offset the recurrence of polyps.

The postoperative improvement rate was 88% in patients with lymphocyte-dominant sinus mucosa; 69% in patients with eosinophil-dominant mucosa.[34] If patients with histopathologically diagnosed eosinophilic sinusitis were divided into two groups according to whether they had bronchial asthma, the percentage of patients without nasal symptoms after surgery was 38% for the asthma group compared with 89% for the non-asthma group.[38]

Postoperative Maxillary Cyst

Maxillary sinus surgery via the Caldwell–Luc approach has a complication of postoperative maxillary cyst (POMC). The first report on POMC was presented by Professor Kubo as "Postoperative Wangenzyste" in 1927.[3] Before the introduction of ESS, we were busy surgically removing POMCs. Because of the absence of prospective studies, the incidence of POMC is not known. From an imaging study of POMCs, latent asymptomatic cysts have been found in other area in 34% of POMC cases.[39] Although there has been no study on whether these asymptomatic cysts present with symptoms later, Iinuma estimated this rate as 3.4%.[40] In my experience, this figure seems reasonable and can be applied to the incidence of POMC. The most prevalent period of occurrence is 11 to 15 years postoperatively. A POMC is most often found at the anteromedial part of the maxillary sinus. A monocyst is present in more than 50% of cases, followed by double (30%) and triple (10%) cysts.[41] There are several theories on POMC development, but two are considered to be reasonable proposals. The retention cyst theory posits that the remnant sinus mucosa is surrounded by granulation tissue at the postoperative period, and as a result, pathologic closed cavity develops. The invagination theory proposes that the upper and medial wall of the maxillary sinus invaginated to the center of the sinus and the traffic route to the middle meatus became stenotic and formed a closed cavity. Patients with a POMC complain of pressure symptoms according to the localization of the cyst, cheek swelling, cheek pain, nasal obstruction, toothache, gingival swelling, palatal swelling, epiphora, diplopia, and proptosis. There is a short acute exacerbation stage and a long intermittent stage. Bony erosion develops in the acute stage. Even in the intermittent stage, a bony destruction process will develop gradually due to prostaglandin E2 (PGE2) and collagenase in the accumulated fluid. When such pressure symptoms appear, the history of sinus surgery and the scar at the gingivobuccal sulcus indicate the diagnosis of POMC. CT and/or magnetic resonance imaging (MRI) are essential tools for determining the treatment modality. After acute exacerbation with antimicrobials, the endoscopic endonasal opening of the cyst is the current surgical choice. The exceptions are far laterally placed cysts or cysts with an extremely thick bony wall. In creating a large opening at the inferior meatus, identification of the nasolacrimal duct outlet is important to avoid injuring it. (In **Video 23.2**, the author shows how to identify the nasolacrimal duct outlet using dye infusion.)

The introduction of ESS and the resultant decrease in the number of Caldwell–Luc operations reduced the numbers of POMCs. This is a good trend for patients with CS. The chance, however, of surgery for POMC is still quite high. In the case of a dentigerous cyst, the cyst needs total removal because of high recurrence rate after simple cystostomy and the risk of a keratinizing primordial cyst. (The procedure of removing the cyst wall of a dentigerous cyst via the middle meatus and inferior meatus is shown in **Video 23.3**.)

Conclusion

Until 20 years ago, the sinusitis refractory to treatment was sinobronchial syndrome. Introduction of macrolide therapy and ESS was able to control this condition. Recently, eosinophilic sinusitis has become a treatment challenge. Extensive and minute surgery along with elaborate postoperative treatment and the administration of steroids is the treatment protocol at present.

Pearls

- CS can be divided into three types: (1) with lymphocytes or neutrophil dominant infiltration in the mucosa, (2) associated with allergic rhinitis, (3) associated with bronchial asthma or with eosinophil-dominant infiltration in the mucosa.
- Recommended treatment for type 1 is macrolide treatment; in unresponsive cases ESS is recommended.
- Recommended treatment for type 2 is macrolide treatment with antiallergic drugs.
- Recommended treatment for type 3 is ESS with macrolide treatment in the pre- and postoperative period along with a short course of systemic steroids in the postoperative period and at recurrence of polyps.
- Creating a large hole in the membranous portion of the medial wall of the maxillary sinus and ethmoidectomy is a key point in maxillary sinus surgery. Bony surface exposure should be avoided.
- Decreased numbers of postoperative maxillary cysts is due to the abandonment or restriction of the Caldwell–Luc operation.

References

1. Nippon Steel Technical Information Center. Nippon: The land and its people (8th ed). Gakuseisya, Tokyo, 2006.
2. Okuda M, Sato S, Kamata K, et al. The problem of idiosyncrasy and affection of nasal mucous membrane. Jibiinkoka 1964;30:5–13 (Abstract in English)
3. Hamilos DL, Leung DY, Wood R, et al. Evidence for distinct cytokine expression in allergic versus nonallergic chronic sinusitis. J Allergy Clin Immunol 1995;96(4):537–544
4. Kubo I. A buccal cyst occurred after a radical operation of the maxillary sinus. Z F Otol Tokyo 1927;3:896–897 (in Japanese)
5. Takahashi R. Endonasal surgery for chronic ethmoiditis. Syujutu 1950;4:105–116 (in Japanese)
6. Kaneko Y. Endonasal surgery with rigid fiberscope. Nippon Jibiinkoka Gakkai Kaiho 1980;19:61–62 (in Japanese)
7. Yajin K. Pathogenesis and treatment of chronic sinusitis. Hiroshima, Japan: Department of Otolaryngology, Hiroshima University School of Medicine; 2001:28–233 (in Japanese)
8. Lichtwitz L. Über die bedeutung von eiterungen der nebenhöhren der nase als ursache von erkrankungen der tieferen luftwege. Dtsch Med Wochenschr 1895;44:1328–1329
9. Suzaki H, Kudoh S, Sugiyama Y. Sinobronchial syndrome in Japanese people. Am J Rhinol 1990;4:133–139
10. Park MH, Kim YW, Yoon HI, et al. Association of HLA class I antigens with diffuse panbronchiolitis in Korean patients. Am J Respir Crit Care Med 1999;159(2):526–529
11. Homma H, Yamanaka A, Tanimoto S, et al. Diffuse panbronchiolitis. A disease of the transitional zone of the lung. Chest 1983;83(1):63–69
12. Kudoh S, Azuma A, Yamamoto M, Izumi T, Ando M. Improvement of survival in patients with diffuse panbronchiolitis treated with low-dose erythromycin. Am J Respir Crit Care Med 1998;157(6 Pt 1):1829–1832
13. Ichimura K, Mineta H, Mizuta K, et al. The effect of sinus surgery on sinobronchial syndrome. Jibiinkoka 1987;59:733–737 (abstract in English)
14. Kudoh S, Uetake T, Hagiwara K, et al. Clinical effect of low-dose, long-term erythromycin chemotherapy on diffuse panbronchiolitis. Jpn J Thorac Dis 1987;25:632–642 (abstract in English)
15. Kudoh S. Erythromycin and DPB. Ther Res 1990;11:93–96 (in Japanese)
16. Suzaki H, Sugita K, Kudoh S, et al. Why erythromycin is effective for diffuse panbronchiolitis? Its effect for chronic sinusitis associated with diffuse panbronchiolitis. Ther Res 1990;11:29–31 (in Japanese)
17. Kikuchi S, Suzaki H, Aoki A, Ito O, Nomura Y. Clinical effect of long-term low-dose erythromycin therapy for chronic sinusitis. Pract Otol (Kyoto) 1991;84:41–47 (abstract in English)
18. Kikuchi S, Yamasoba T, Suzaki H, et al. Long-term low-dose erythromycin therapy for chronic sinusitis. Pract Otol (Kyoto) 1992;85:1245–1252 (abstract in English)
19. Iino Y. Macrolide therapy for sinusitis in children. Pediatr Otorhinolaryngol Jap 1996;17:39–40 (abstract in English)
20. Hashiba M, Baba S. Efficacy of long-term administration of clarithromycin in the treatment of intractable chronic sinusitis. Acta Otolaryngol 1996;525:73–78
21. Shinkawa A, Miyake H, Sakai M. Clinical evaluation of roxithromycin in chronic sinusitis–long-term treatment. Nippon Jibiinkoka Kansensyo Kenkyukai Kaishi 1993;11:102–106 (abstract in English)

22. Ichimura K, Shimazaki Y, Ishibashi T, Higo R. Effect of new macrolide roxithromycin upon nasal polyps associated with chronic sinusitis. Auris Nasus Larynx 1996;23:48–56
23. Tamaoki J, Isono K, Sakai N, Kanemura T, Konno K. Erythromycin inhibits Cl secretion across canine tracheal epithelial cells. Eur Respir J 1992;5(2):234–238
24. Goswami SK, Kivity S, Marom Z. Erythromycin inhibits respiratory glycoconjugate secretion from human airways in vitro. Am Rev Respir Dis 1990;141(1):72–78
25. Hashiba M, Suzaki H, et al. Guideline of macrolide therapy for chronic sinusitis (proposal). Jpn J Antibiot 1998;51(Suppl A):86–89 (in Japanese)
26. Japan Rhinologic Society. Handbook for Management of Sinusitis. Tokyo: Kanehara Publ; 2006 (in Japanese)
27. Hashiba M. Problems in macrolide treatment of pediatric sinusitis. Jpn J Rhinol 2002;41:109 (in Japanese)
28. Yoshida H. Macrolide treatment–literature review on indication. Jpn J Rhinol 2002;41:100–102 (in Japanese)
29. Hashiba M, Kondo K, Hamashima A, et al. [Effect of macrolide therapy on microbes in nasal cavity and larynx of patients with chronic paranasal sinusitis]. Jpn J Antibiot 2001;54(Suppl C):102–105 (in Japanese)
30. Maeda K, Nakagawa T, Yonekawa S, et al. Clinical study of patients with chronic lower airway infection who have administered macrolide treatment for more than 10 years. Jpn J Antibiot 2008;61(Suppl A):92–94 (in Japanese)
31. Shima H, Sunazuka T, Omura S. Novel macrolide EM900 series with anti-inflammatory action. Jpn J Antibiot 2007;60(Suppl A):39–43 (in Japanese)
32. Moriyama H, Yanagi K, Ohtori N, Fukami M. Evaluation of endoscopic sinus surgery for chronic sinusitis: post-operative erythromycin therapy. Rhinology 1995;33(3):166–170
33. Iino Y, Okura S, Shiga J, Toriyama M, Kudo K. [Histopathological studies on paranasal mucosa from patients treated with erythromycin]. Nippon Jibiinkoka Gakkai Kaiho 1994;97(6):1070–1078 (abstract in English)
34. Yanagi K. Studies regarding chronic sinusitis under endoscopic sinus surgery. Evaluation of endoscopic findings and pathological findings of maxillary sinus. O R L Tokyo 1998;41:15–37 (abstract in English)
35. Haruna S, Otori N, Yanagi K, Moriyama H. Eosinophilic sinusitis. O R L Tokyo 2001;44:195–201 (abstract in English)
36. Ferguson BJ. Eosinophilic mucin rhinosinusitis: a distinct clinicopathological entity. Laryngoscope 2000;110(5 Pt 1):799–813
37. Ishitoya J. Eosinophilic sinusitis. JOHNS 2004;20:1865–1879 (in Japanese)
38. Dejima K, Adachi N, Oshima A, et al. [Outcomes of endoscopic sinus surgery in chronic sinusitis cases complicated/ not complicated by bronchial asthma and eosinophilic infiltration of the sinus mucosa]. Nippon Jibiinkoka Gakkai Kaiho 2008;111(2):58–64 (abstract in English)
39. Iinuma T. X-ray diagnosis of the postoperative cysts of the maxilla. Jibiinkoka 1972;44:959–963 (abstract in English)
40. Iinuma T, Mizutani A, Miyagawa K. New aspect of postoperative maxillary cyst. Supplement. Pract Otol (Kyoto) 1974;67:427–436 (abstract in English)
41. Hirota Y, Iinuma T, Haruyama K, Fukamauhi A, Fugimaki Y. [Postoperative polycystic cysts of the maxillary sinus]. Nippon Jibiinkoka Gakkai Kaiho 1982;85(7):756–765 (abstract in English)

24 Learning from a Difficult Case: Recurrent Maxillary Sinus Inverted Papilloma

Kevin C. Welch and James A. Stankiewicz

As seen throughout this book, diseases of the maxillary sinus range from the simple to the complex and from the benign to the malignant. Likewise, medical and surgical approaches to these conditions vary and reflect both the nature of the disease and the skill set of the surgeon. Therefore, recalcitrant disease of the maxillary sinus often requires innovative treatment paradigms to completely eradicate disease.

Inverted papilloma (IP) is a benign exophytic and polypoid soft tissue neoplasm arising from Schneiderian (ectodermal) mucosa characterized by inward growth of the neoplasm through the mucosa.[1–3] It is also noteworthy for its locally aggressive nature, rate of recurrence, and rate of conversion to squamous cell carcinoma.[1–8]

In the not-so-distant past, resection of IPs was performed through numerous open approaches with long-term rates of recurrence ranging from 20 to 100%[9] and often significant morbidity. More recently, the endoscopic resection of IPs has been described.[4,8–14] In addition to superior illumination and magnification, the endoscopic removal of IP can result in improved outcomes[4] with a greater degree of patient acceptance. Despite the evolution of hand instruments and the introduction of stereotactic navigation, certain areas of the paranasal sinuses continue to present technical challenges due to prohibitive anatomy. The lateral and anterior walls of the maxillary sinus represent two such areas. In many instances, endoscopic resection must be combined with external approaches (e.g., Caldwell–Luc or midfacial degloving procedure) to reach these areas.

The modified endoscopic medial maxillectomy (MEMM) has been described for the resection of sinonasal neoplasia,[15,16] as well as in revision surgery for recalcitrant inflammatory disease.[17] Using this technique, areas of the maxillary sinus previously inaccessible during endoscopic sinus surgery (ESS) may be reached and tumors such as an IP can be effectively removed through this approach. We present a case of a patient with recurrent IP based on the lateral wall of the maxillary sinus and demonstrate how this extended endoscopic procedure can be used successfully to treat tumors in this location.

Case Presentation

History

A 53-year-old male patient with a Krouse stage III inverted papilloma of the left maxillary sinus presented with recurrent disease. Examination revealed a wide maxillary antrostomy with partial resection of the middle turbinate and partial ethmoidectomy. Small foci of implanted IP in the ethmoid and frontal recess and recurrent IP in the posterior and lateral aspects of the maxillary sinus were identified.

With a 0-degree telescope, inspection of the tumor within the maxillary sinus was challenging due to the limitations presented by the anatomy. With the use of a 30-degree telescope, the tumor could be seen more extensively (**Fig. 24.1**); however, the delineation between tumor and normal tissue was challenging due to the limitations presented by the patient's anatomy.

Radiologic Evaluation

Computed tomography (CT) was used to assess the extent of recurrence. Computed tomography in patients with IP is very helpful in determining the site of attachment because

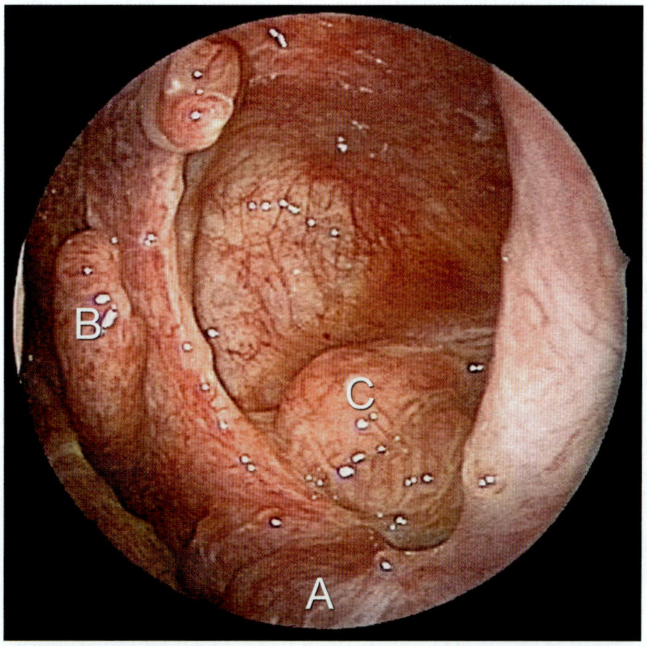

Fig. 24.1 Endoscopic view of the tumor with a 30-degree telescope. A, The inferior turbinate, B, middle turbinate stump, and C, inverted papilloma can be seen. Even with a 30-degree telescope, the complete extent of the tumor cannot be seen.

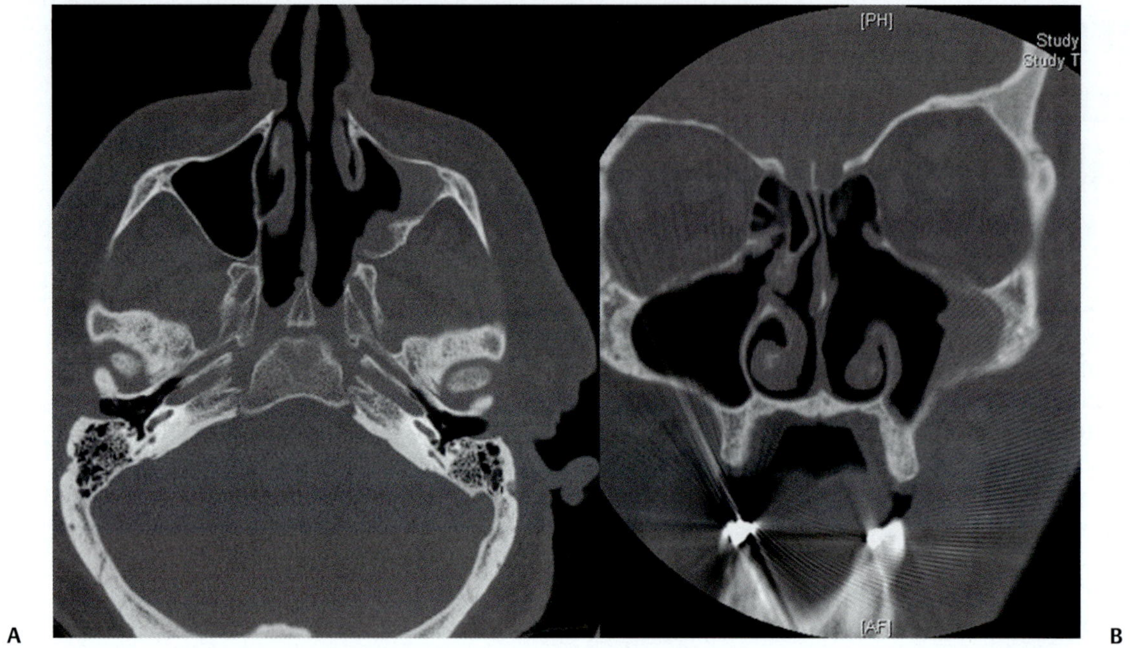

Fig. 24.2 **(A,B)** Computed tomography (axial and coronal) of the patient with recurrent inverted papilloma. **(A)** In the axial image, note the region of soft tissue thickening centered on the lateral aspect of the left maxillary sinus. **(B)** There is an area of thickened bone which represents the likely site of attachment. In the coronal image, the lateral, superior, and inferior extent of the tumor can be seen.

bony thickening has been reported to be associated with the pedicle of the tumor.[18] In this patient, repeat CT imaging revealed a soft tissue mass in the posterior and lateral aspects of the left maxillary sinus and bony thickening along the lateral aspect of the maxillary sinus (**Fig. 24.2**). This correlated with the identified location of recurrence.

Operative Technique

The MEMM is performed under general anesthesia with the use of total intravenous anesthesia (TIVA). The use of TIVA has been shown[19,20] to reduce intraoperative blood loss and is helpful in cases involving extensive surgery when blood loss might be expected to be high. Preoperatively, the nose is decongested topically with 0.5% oxymetazoline, and 4% topical cocaine is used prior to endoscopy. The mucosa of the inferior turbinate and lateral nasal wall is infiltrated with 1% lidocaine with 1:100,000 epinephrine to help achieve hemostasis. Additionally, a transoral pterygopalatine injection can be performed by inserting a 25-gauge needle bent at 2.5 cm into the greater palatine foramen opposite the second molar to provide additional vascular control.

The majority of the resection is done with 4-mm, 30-degree, and 70-degree telescopes. In this case, an antrostomy and partial ethmoidectomy had been previously performed. (In the event that the maxillary sinus had not been previously entered, the uncinate process is resected with a sickle knife or backbiting instrument and the natural os of the maxillary sinus is identified midline along the maxillary line and is widened with through-cutting forceps or the microdebrider.) Once a wide antrostomy is performed, the valve of Hasner is identified in the inferior meatus. The valve is lo-

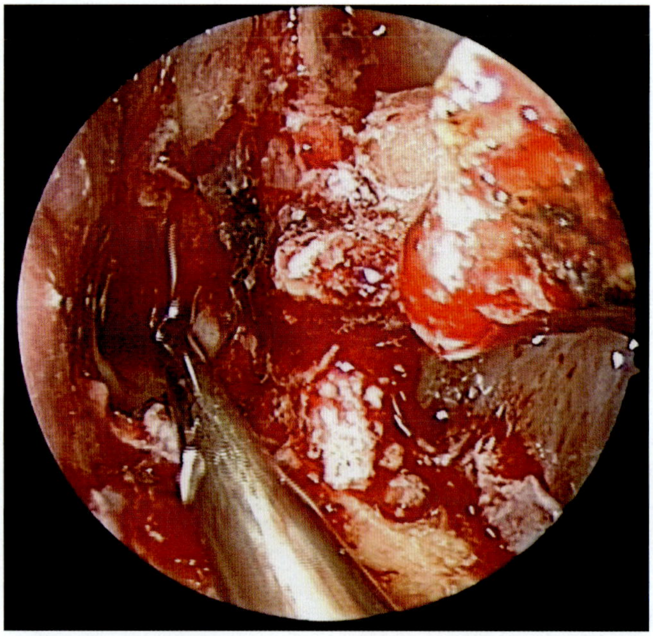

Fig. 24.3 Endoscopic view of the modified endoscopic medial maxillectomy. The inferior turbinate has been removed. The medial maxillary wall has been made flush with the floor of the nasal cavity. Lastly, an inferior meatal window has been made to increase access to the anterior wall of the maxillary sinus.

cated ~30 to 35 mm posterior to the limen nasi and must be identified prior to performing the maxillectomy; otherwise, the surgeon risks injury to the valve and/or lacrimal duct. An inferior turbinectomy is performed next using the endoscopic scissors. The inferior turbinate is incised between the anterior one-third and the posterior two-thirds of the turbinate, just behind the valve of Hasner. Cautery can be used to help with hemostasis, but care must be taken to avoid injury to the mucosal flap of the valve.

The mucosa along the lateral nasal wall is incised, and a mucoperiosteal flap is elevated toward the septum. (This flap is preserved and later draped into the maxillary defect.) A series of through-cutting instruments is used to resect the medial maxillary wall. If needed, a high-speed irrigating drill can be used to remove bone too thick for through-cutting punches. This is performed so that the maxillary sinus opens directly onto the floor of the nasal cavity. Because the valve of Hasner opens superiorly in the inferior meatus, the medial maxillary wall inferior to the valve of Hasner can be resected to provide additional exposure and room for instrumentation; this is performed with a backbiting instrument (**Fig. 24.3**) until the anterior wall of the maxillary sinus is reached near the piriform aperture. The use of navigation software (**Fig. 24.4**) can also be very helpful in confirming the precise anatomic location of the tumor and the exposure created during the approach.

At this point, the exposure is complete (**see Video 24.1**) and the resection of the tumor begins. If the tumor is bulky in nature, it is carefully debulked until the site of attachment is reached. Using the curette and giraffe forceps, margins around the lesion are taken to ensure that preserved mucosa is free of tumor. Using the 70-degree endoscope and curved instruments, the tumor is carefully elevated off the posterior and lateral aspects of the maxillary sinus. In this instance, a malleable curved suction and curette is used to elevate

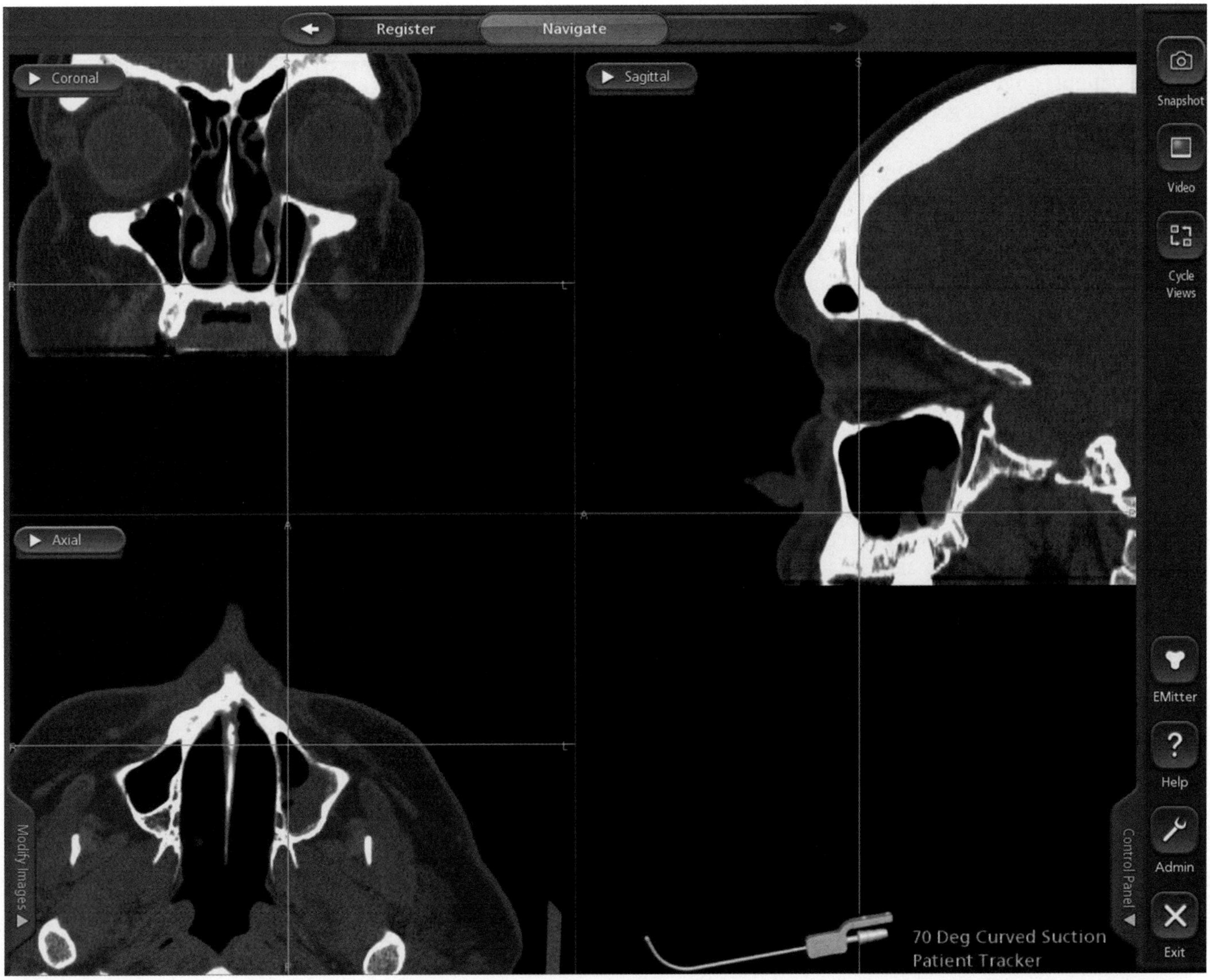

Fig. 24.4 Triplanar images of the patient during surgery. Notice that when the modified endoscopic medial maxillectomy has been performed, angled instruments can be used to access the inferior, lateral, and anterior aspects of the maxillary sinus.

the tumor off the bone. Instruments are passed through the medial maxillectomy as well as through the inferior meatal window to aid in the resection of the lesion. Once resected, the maxillary sinus is inspected thoroughly to evaluate for unaddressed foci of tumor. Stereotactic probes are used to correlate the endoscopic view with the CT images to confirm the completeness of the resection. Cautery is performed throughout the maxillary sinus to help achieve hemostasis and to fulgurate nests of IP. Because nests of IP have been demonstrated to infiltrate the underlying bone at the site of attachment, this bone must be removed.[21] High-speed 15-degree and 70-degree rotating diamond burs are used to thin the bone along the attachment site of the tumor to address these nests (**see Video 24.2**). After a final inspection, the maxillary sinus is filled with a hemostatic agent.

Postoperative Care

The postoperative care of the patient involves serial debridements and long-term surveillance. Given the considerable rates of recurrence,[4,8,15] long-term surveillance is necessary in these patients, and particular attention to the pathology for the presence of any degeneration into squamous cell carcinoma is necessary.

Irrigation with saline solution is proven to be beneficial and provide symptomatic relief to patients undergoing endoscopic sinus surgery.[22–24] Irrigation also helps to manually debride blood clots and crusting.[24] The role of antibiotics in this type of procedure has not been studied in a controlled manner; however, we believe prophylactic treatment with oral antibiotics is useful, especially in the presence of exposed bone where infection may easily occur.

Alternative Procedures

The MEMM presented here represents only one method of approaching and resecting the recurrent IP. As previously mentioned, a medial maxillectomy combined with a Caldwell–Luc procedure would have provided similar access with the benefit of a zero-degree telescope placed through the canine fossa into the antrum. The drawback of this adjuvant approach is the sublabial incision and canine fossa puncture. Other external procedures (midfacial degloving, open maxillectomy, etc.) could have been considered as primary or adjuvant surgical methods. Drawbacks of the external approaches are the incisions created and potential disfigurement and discomfort. Another method described by Harvey et al[25] involves the creation of a septal window to obtain access to the lateral and anterior aspects of the maxillary sinus and simultaneously provide more direct visualization of the attachment site with a zero-degree or 30-degree telescope. The drawback of this approach is the creation of a controlled septal perforation that requires repair at the termination of the case.

Conclusion

Recurrent IP can be a challenge to treat, especially if the tumor is attached to the lateral aspect of the maxillary sinus. However, the MEMM offers adequate exposure when combined with angled instruments and angled telescopes for the resection of difficult to reach tumor attachment sites within the maxillary sinus.

Pearls

- Intraoperative blood pressure and heart rate control, as well as thorough injection, will help minimize blood loss and improve visualization.
- Preserving a nasal floor mucosal flap helps cover exposed bone after the case is completed.
- Visualization with a 70-degree endoscope is performed through the mega-antrostomy while instruments can be passed through the inferior meatal window.
- Use of image guidance can help confirm that all areas of the maxillary sinus are addressed by the surgeon.
- Long-term surveillance is critical so that any recurrence is promptly identified and treated.

References

1. Hyams VJ. Papillomas of the nasal cavity and paranasal sinuses. A clinicopathological study of 315 cases. Ann Otol Rhinol Laryngol 1971;80(2):192–206
2. Lampertico P, Russell WO, MacComb WS. Squamous papilloma of upper respiratory epithelium. Arch Pathol 1963;75:293–302
3. Ringertz N. Pathology of malignant tumors arising in the nasal and paranasal sinus cavities and maxilla. Acta Otolaryngol 1938;27:31–42
4. Busquets JM, Hwang PH. Endoscopic resection of sinonasal inverted papilloma: a meta-analysis. Otolaryngol Head Neck Surg 2006;134(3):476–482
5. Kaufman MR, Brandwein MS, Lawson W. Sinonasal papillomas: clinicopathologic review of 40 patients with inverted and oncocytic schneiderian papillomas. Laryngoscope 2002;112(8 Pt 1):1372–1377
6. Lawson W, Ho BT, Shaari CM, Biller HF. Inverted papilloma: a report of 112 cases. Laryngoscope 1995;105(3 Pt 1):282–288
7. Weissler MC, Montgomery WW, Turner PA, Montgomery SK, Joseph MP. Inverted papilloma. Ann Otol Rhinol Laryngol 1986;95(3 Pt 1):215–221
8. Wolfe SG, Schlosser RJ, Bolger WE, Lanza DC, Kennedy DW. Endoscopic and endoscope-assisted resections of inverted sinonasal papillomas. Otolaryngol Head Neck Surg 2004;131(3):174–179

9. Sham CL, Woo JK, van Hasselt CA. Endoscopic resection of inverted papilloma of the nose and paranasal sinuses. J Laryngol Otol 1998; 112(8):758–764
10. Schlosser RJ, Mason JC, Gross CW. Aggressive endoscopic resection of inverted papilloma: an update. Otolaryngol Head Neck Surg 2001;125(1):49–53
11. Sukenik MA, Casiano R. Endoscopic medial maxillectomy for inverted papillomas of the paranasal sinuses: value of the intraoperative endoscopic examination. Laryngoscope 2000;110(1):39–42
12. Wormald PJ, Ooi E, van Hasselt CA, Nair S. Endoscopic removal of sinonasal inverted papilloma including endoscopic medial maxillectomy. Laryngoscope 2003;113(5):867–873
13. Zhang G, Rodriguez X, Hussain A, Desrosiers M. Outcomes of the extended endoscopic approach for management of inverted papilloma. J Otolaryngol 2007;36(2):83–87
14. Stankiewicz JA, Girgis SJ. Endoscopic surgical treatment of nasal and paranasal sinus inverted papilloma. Otolaryngol Head Neck Surg 1993;109(6):988–995
15. Lawson W, Kaufman MR, Biller HF. Treatment outcomes in the management of inverted papilloma: an analysis of 160 cases. Laryngoscope 2003;113(9):1548–1556
16. Lund VJ. Optimum management of inverted papilloma. J Laryngol Otol 2000;114(3):194–197
17. Woodworth BA, Bhargave GA, Palmer JN, et al. Clinical outcomes of endoscopic and endoscopic-assisted resection of inverted papillomas: a 15-year experience. Am J Rhinol 2007;21(5):591–600
18. Sham CL, King AD, van Hasselt A, Tong MC. The roles and limitations of computed tomography in the preoperative assessment of sinonasal inverted papillomas. Am J Rhinol 2008;22(2):144–150
19. Eberhart LH, Folz BJ, Wulf H, Geldner G. Intravenous anesthesia provides optimal surgical conditions during microscopic and endoscopic sinus surgery. Laryngoscope 2003;113(8):1369–1373
20. Wormald PJ, van Renen G, Perks J, Jones JA, Langton-Hewer CD. The effect of the total intravenous anesthesia compared with inhalational anesthesia on the surgical field during endoscopic sinus surgery. Am J Rhinol 2005;19(5):514–520
21. Chiu AG, Jackman AH, Antunes MB, Feldman MD, Palmer JN. Radiographic and histologic analysis of the bone underlying inverted papillomas. Laryngoscope 2006;116(9):1617–1620
22. Hauptman G, Ryan MW. The effect of saline solutions on nasal patency and mucociliary clearance in rhinosinusitis patients. Otolaryngol Head Neck Surg 2007;137(5):815–821
23. Talbot AR, Herr TM, Parsons DS. Mucociliary clearance and buffered hypertonic saline solution. Laryngoscope 1997;107(4):500–503
24. Tomooka LT, Murphy C, Davidson TM. Clinical study and literature review of nasal irrigation. Laryngoscope 2000;110(7):1189–1193
25. Harvey RJ, Sheehan PO, Debnath NI, Schlosser RJ. Transseptal approach for extended endoscopic resections of the maxilla and infratemporal fossa. Am J Rhinol Allergy 2009;23(4):426–432

25 Learning from a Difficult Case: Accessing the Anterolateral Maxillary Sinus

Richard J. Harvey

Aggressive exposure is not necessary for inflammatory disease. There are 90- and 120-degree microdebriders (Medtronic, Jacksonville, FL) to access the maxillary sinus via a wide antrostomy. The maxillary trephine technique can provide access without these angled instruments[1] and a modified medial maxillectomy (MMM) can be performed for those with chronically dysfunctional sinus mucosa not being effectively treated via antrostomy alone.[2,3] For tumor resection, exposure needs to be greater. Traditional surgical approaches include midface degloving and transfacial options. Transfacial approaches are hindered by the subsequent scar, alar retraction, and potential functional deformity to eye closure. Without significant bone removal, open access suffers from an increasingly narrow surgical corridor as the dissection proceeds posteriorly. Endoscopic approaches have the advantage of a wide field, near-vision dissection, while maintaining a narrow surgical approach. Visualization can be superior with an endoscopic approach compared with the microsurgical access.[4] The removal of juvenile nasopharyngeal angiofibroma (JNA) and inverted papilloma (IP) are the case examples for successful endoscopic tumor removal. The literature is now filled with reports of low recurrence rates for these lesions when managed with an entirely endoscopic approach, even for extensive lesions.[5–8]

For lateral pathology, however, the use of angled endoscopes and instruments becomes necessary. This is especially true for more anterior and laterally based lesions (**Fig. 25.1**). The use of angled scopes greatly enhances the visualization, but angled instruments do not always afford the equivalent dissection technique compared with zero-degree surgery. As endoscopic techniques begin to encompass more extensive benign disease and even malignancy, more accurate dissection is required to improve our removal of pathology, control bleeding, and minimize morbidity.[9] Working with curved instruments, angled endoscopes, and a single nostril often leaves the surgeon with curette only and "scraping" techniques for tumor removal.

For the removal of large JNA, a posterior septectomy is often performed to improve access and the working field. Similarly, a superior septal window is used for extended surgery of the frontal sinus and recess. The subsequent functional impairment of either a posterior or superior septal window is minimal for most patients. Crusting, bleeding, support, and airflow changes do not appear to be a common cause of morbidity. An anterior septectomy is not feasible as the anterior septum plays an important role in the support of the external nose, forms part of the the nasal valve, and will often cause airflow changes with resultant crusting, whistling, and bleeding.[10] The use of large pedicled septal flaps from skull base reconstruction[9,11] has changed our approach for more anterior and lateral pathology. We use an anterior transseptal approach, created by the elevation of large septal flaps, a cartilaginous septal window, and reconstruction at the end of the procedure.

The concept of a transseptal approach is not entirely novel. Wormald et al have discussed the concept of nonopposing septal incisions to provide additional retraction and access to JNA.[8] However, it has been our experience with large pedicled septal flaps[9,12,13] in skull base surgery that has allowed an evolution in the way we manage extensive anterolateral sinonasal lesions. Additional anatomic studies have shown that even a large MMM or total medial maxillectomy (TMM) does not provide adequate access for many patients.[14]

Some pathologies have significant anterior attachments; for others, a transseptal approach is made in a stepwise fashion after defining the tumor origin. We utilize the following algorithm when accessing more anterolaterally based disease: transnasal direct, middle meatal antrostomy (MMA), modified medial maxillectomy (MMM),[2] total medial maxil-

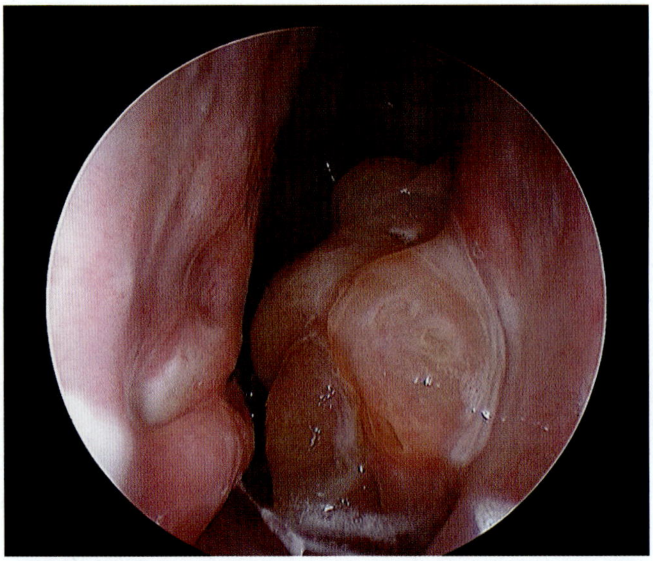

Fig. 25.1 Endoscopic view of recurrent left inverted papilloma protruding into the left nasal cavity.

lectomy[15] (TMM; with removal of the lower lacrimal apparatus), and a combined transseptal MMM/TMM.

Case Presentation

History

A very active 72-year-old man with a Krouse stage 3 inverted papilloma of the left maxillary sinus presents with progressive nasal obstruction and postnasal mucoid discharge. He has had two previous endoscopic procedures then a further open lateral rhinotomy to remove the disease. It has now been 10 years since his first surgery, 2 years since his last procedure, and 18 months since last review.

He has had a previous septoplasty, left middle turbinectomy, wide antrostomy, subtotal resection of his inferior turbinate, and a partial ethmoidectomy. Endoscopic examination easily identifies the tumor (**Fig. 25.1**) and the orbital floor and medial wall are not involved in the disease.

Surgery was indicated for this patient because he had progressive symptoms, was otherwise fit with no comorbidities, and there was the potential for malignant change. Atypia, dysplasia, carcinoma-in-situ, and squamous cell carcinoma can all occur in papilloma. Malignant change within the inverted type of papilloma has been well documented.[16] Krouse originally described a 9.1% rate of squamous cell carcinoma in his cohort.[17] This has been supported by a recent meta-analysis of a published case series, which reported a synchronous carcinoma rate of 7.1% and a metachronous rate of 11%.[18] It was widely speculated that atypical and dysplastic change was precancerous,[17] but this is not supported by the literature. Degree of atypia, mitotic index, and recurrence appear to have little correlation with carcinoma transformation.[19,20] Carcinoma-in-situ should be closely followed as these cases may represent precancerous change or undetected carcinoma from sampling errors.[18]

Radiologic Evaluation

Computed tomography (CT) forms the basis for the assessment. The site of the tumor can be seen by a corresponding area of osteitis[21,22] in the zygomatic recess of the left maxilla (**Fig. 25.2**). The previous anterior maxillary wall defect is also present (**Fig. 25.3**). The potential for tumor to have migrated in the premaxillary soft tissue should be recognized here. Similar seeding into extrasinus tissue, including the face, can occur through a lateral rhinotomy approach (**Fig. 25.4**). Considering the multiple previous procedures and open surgery, magnetic resonance imaging (MRI) was performed that confirmed tumor was confined to the maxillary sinus.

Operative Technique

Endoscopic transseptal surgery is performed under general controlled hypotensive anesthesia. Total intravenous anesthesia is associated with better mucosal hemostasis.[23,24] Cotton pledgets containing adrenaline 1:1000 are placed in the nasal cavity over the areas of surgical access for 10 minutes before the surgical procedure. The septum is infiltrated with 1% lidocaine with adrenaline 1:100.000.

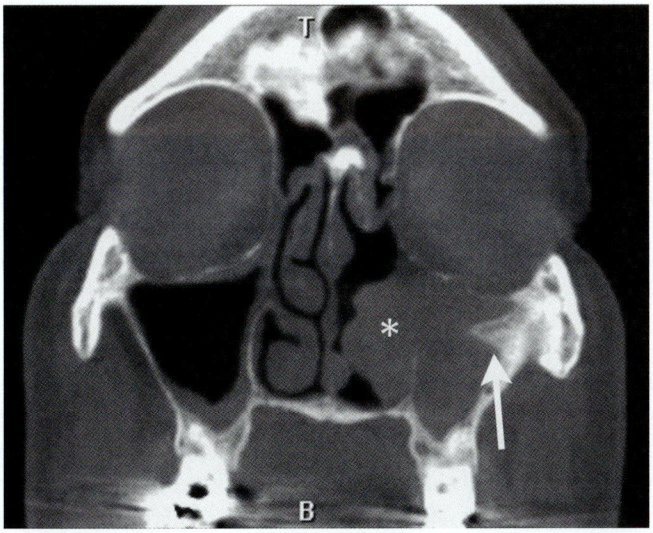

Fig. 25.2 Computed tomography evaluation: The recurrent left inverted papilloma protruding into the left nasal cavity can be seen (*). An area of osteitis and neo-osteogenesis is a landmark for the origin of the tumor (*arrow*).

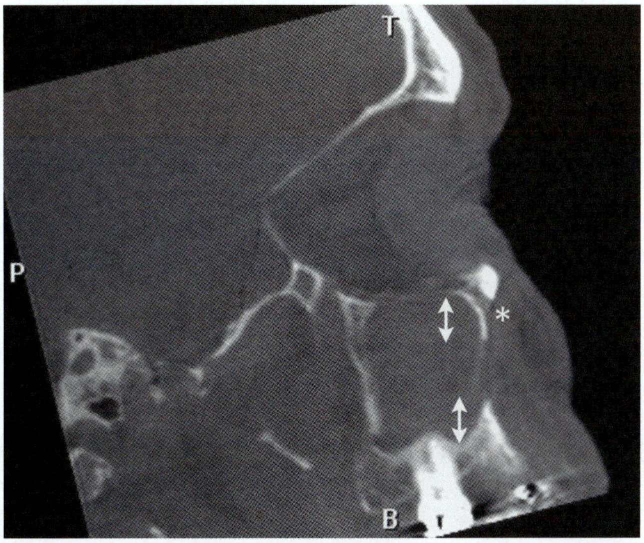

Fig. 25.3 Computed tomography evaluation: The exit of the infraorbital nerve can be seen (*). The previous anterior open approach has fallen well short of exposing the area to be addressed (*double-ended arrows*).

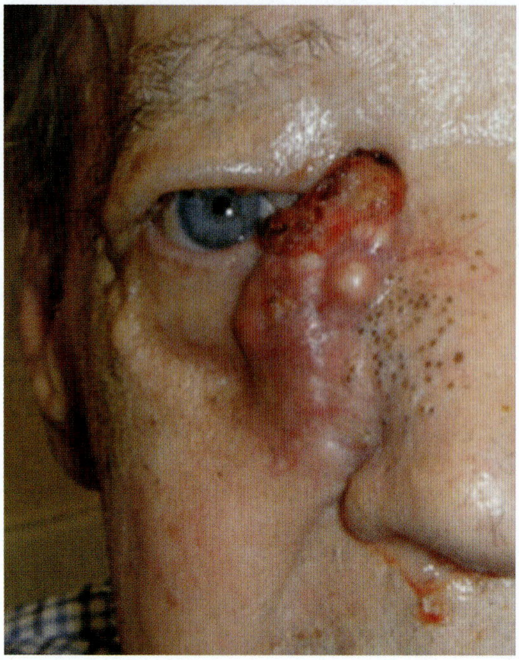

Fig. 25.4 Violation of natural barriers to spread: skin, dural, and periorbital can lead to tumor seeding and difficult to manage disease. Although squamous cell carcinoma conversion was suspected, this papilloma was benign on multiple biopsies.

For some patients it is possible to predict the insertion site by a corresponding area of osteitis.[21,22] Early planning in the need for a transseptal approach makes surgery more straightforward. But for many, the exact attachment of their sinonasal tumor is not evident until the time of surgery. The resection often follows a stepwise MMA, MMM, TMM, and then transseptal access, as the origin is elucidated.

The decision to go to a transseptal approach should come early in the operation. Make this judgment on preoperative imaging and operative location of tumor attachment. Dissection will proceed very quickly via a transseptal approach compared with working with 70-degree scopes and angled instruments.

The contralateral septal mucosa is generally chosen to raise the main mucoperiosteal/perichondrial flap. This ensures that it can be conveniently tucked away between the contralateral middle turbinate and posterior septum to avoid accidental injury during instrumentation on the operative side. The nasal floor incision begins far lateral in the inferior meatus. The superior incision is made as high as possible near the nasal dorsum. Both are brought forward to join a hemitransfixion incision. This mucoperichondrial/periosteal flap is pedicled posteriorly on the septal branch of the sphenopalatine artery. There is some foreshortening of the flap after elevation and the additional width is important for adequate reconstruction. A window of septal cartilage is removed beginning at the head of the inferior turbinate. The area usually comprises a 1.5 × 2 cm area that then allows both endoscope and instrument to work comfortably through the septum. The ipsilateral mucosa over this area is raised as an inverted "U" flap with a random blood supply based inferiorly from the nasal floor (**see Video 25.1**, which demonstrates the development and closure of a septal window).

After MMM, 2-mm Kerrison rongeurs are used via the transseptal route to remove the remaining medial wall down to the nasal floor. Attention is then turned to removing the medial wall anteriorly. It is possible to resect the wall underneath the Hasner valve for access. But experience has found that this leads to inadequate exposure of the anterior wall. The lower lacrimal apparatus is resected and reconstructed at the end of the case. We drill away the bone at the attachment of most benign tumors as tumor pseudopods are often extended into the nearby bone.[25]

There is usually little active bleeding at the completion of tumor removal. The clean mucosal edges and rough diamond drilled bone offer good hemostasis (**Fig. 25.5**). A dissolvable hemostatic dressing (Surgiflo; Johnson & Johnson Medical, North Yorkshire, UK) is used to fill the cavity. Prior to closure, the lacrimal duct is exposed for a length of 6 to 8 mm. This membranous duct is then marsupialized. A formal dacryocystorhinostomy can be performed, but we have found this unnecessary in the majority of cases. Dissolvable sutures are used to reconstitute the septum. We do not replace the septal cartilage. It is usually removed piecemeal and is far less than that often removed during septoplasty. Thin Silastic (Dow Corning, Midland, MI/Barry, UK) sheets are placed on either side. They should be sized to include coverage of the nasal floor. One or two 3/0 Prolene (Ethicon, Somerville, NJ) transseptal sutures are used to secure the silastic sheets (**see Video 25.2**, which demonstrates the approach and resection for this patient).

Postoperative Care

Patients are discharged on the same day or morning after depending on analgesic control. Oral antibiotics are used for 2 weeks and usually consist of amoxicillin and clavulanic acid (GlaxoSmithKline, Mississauga, Ontario, Canada) and clavulanic acid combination twice a day. Nasal irrigation begins at 24 to 36 hours postsurgery. This is performed with a high volume squeeze bottle (NeilMed Sinus Rinse; NailMed Pharmaceuticals, Inc., Santa Rosa, CA) twice a day only. Silastic sheets are removed 2 to 3 weeks postoperatively (**see Video 25.3**). Exposed cartilage and bone appears to heal extremely well under the Silastic and avoids crusting. They are thin and so allow patients to breathe and irrigate with minimal interference. For inverted papilloma, a collation of literature reports recurrence rates of 12.8% for endoscopic resection, 17.0% for lateral rhinotomy, and 34.2% for other limited resections.[18] Selection bias may exist for some of the published reports, but the Krouse Staging System used to provide a comparison basis is well accepted in the literature (**Table 25.1**).

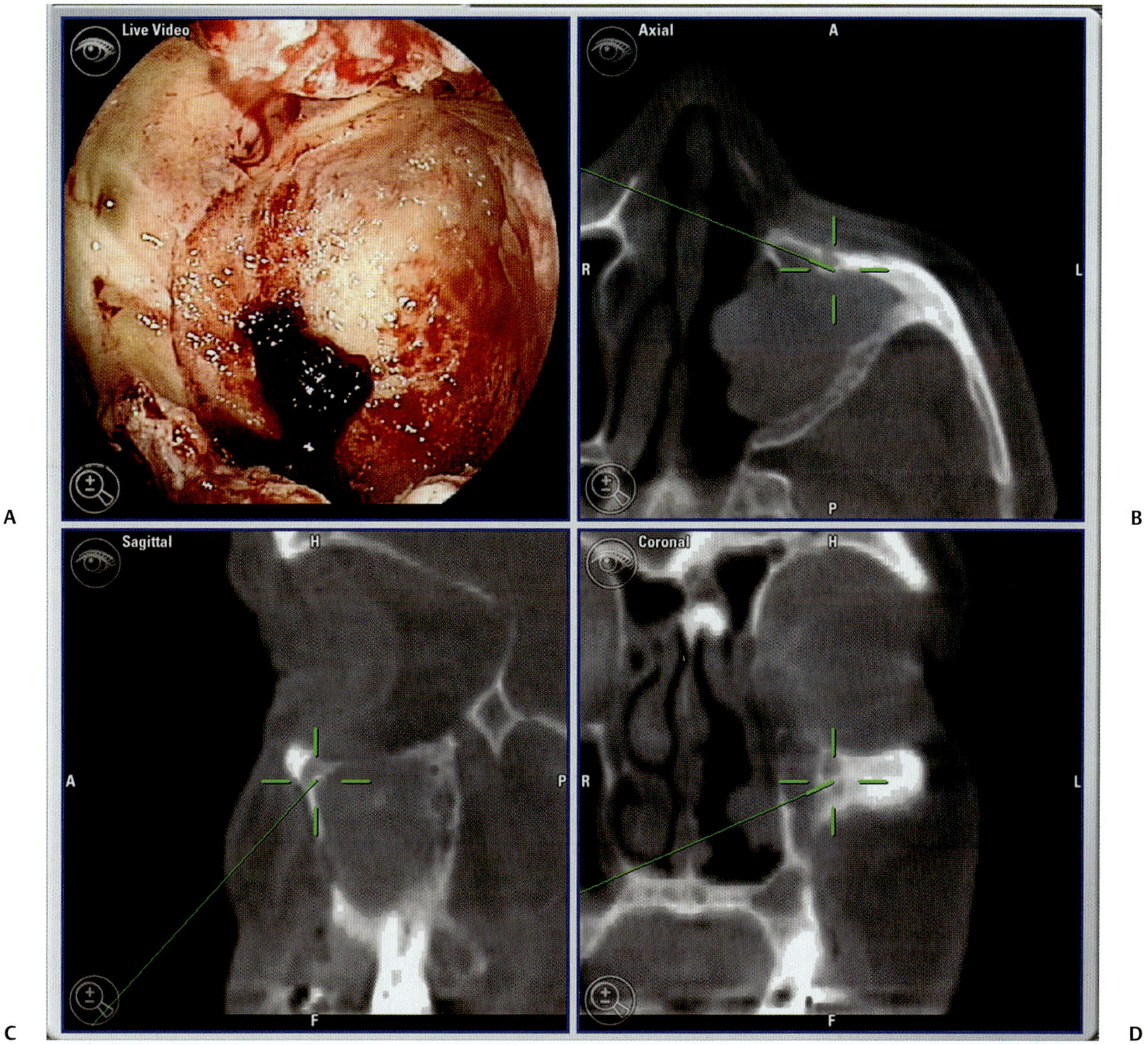

Fig. 25.5 (A–D) Intraoperative images from image guidance system (IGS; not necessary for this type of surgery), but demonstrates well the area of resection and the angle of approach. Here the IGS probe is on the internal exit point of the infraorbital nerve.

Other Approaches

Other approaches exist to access the anterolateral maxillary sinus. Endoscopic maxillotomy has been described and can provide similar access.[26] This procedure involves the removal of the medial buttress via osteotomies (**see Video 25.4**). The lacrimal apparatus is disrupted as with a TMM. The anterior superior alveolar nerve, the canine root, and potential loss of lateral support of the alar cartilage to the piriform aperture can all occur with this approach. Performed endoscopically, the resultant alar retraction and collapse is limited

Table 25.1 Krouse Staging for Inverted Papilloma

T1	Tumor isolated to one area of the nasal cavity without extension to the paranasal sinuses
T2	Tumor involves medial wall of the maxillary sinus, ethmoid sinuses, and/or ostiomeatal complex.
T3	Tumor involves the superior, inferior, posterior, anterior, or lateral walls of the maxillary sinus; frontal sinus; or sphenoid sinus.
T4	Tumor with extra-sinonasal extent or malignancy

compared with similar lateral rhinotomy approaches, but can still occur. The maxillary trephine has been popularized by Wormald and can provide either additional instrument or endoscopic access through the anterior maxilla.[26] This is an excellent adjunct to a lateral infratemporal fossa or lateral maxillary lesion. However, for those pathologies involving the anterior wall itself, the trephine does not improve surgical access and will come through tumor in its approach.

Conclusion

Most maxillary sinus masses can be successfully managed via direct single or simple bilateral transnasal access. However, when pathology arises anterior and lateral to the inferior orbital nerve, the transseptal approach greatly enhances the endoscopic surgeon's ability to completely remove disease. Direct, straight ahead, endoscopic dissection is possible for even these most anterolateral lesions. The morbidity from anterior septal reconstruction must be weighed against the need for access and complete tumor removal. The transseptal approach affords access to areas previously thought inaccessible with an endoscopic technique.

Pearls

- Converting to a transseptal access early affords quicker subsequent dissection.
- Oversize the contralateral septal flap. Do not hesitate to start at the squamous-mucosal junction.
- Silastic splints are essential as they prevent fibrinous adhesions and protect the flaps.
- Secondary bone pain is common at 5 to 7 days after aggressive drilling in the maxillary sinus. Nonsteroidal antiinflammatory drugs (NSAIDs) are effective analgesia rather than opioids.
- Do not fear the lower lacrimal system. Remove the inferior nasolacrimal system to remove disease. Robust superior reconstruction is possible.
- The extent of exposure and its subsequent morbidity should be dictated by the disease.
- Simple nonopposing incisions seem appealing and maybe appropriate for a rectractor, but as a working channel it is awkward, does not easily accommodate both instruments, results in traumatized mucosa, and blood has a tendency to run down the endoscope.

References

1. Singhal D, Douglas R, Robinson S, Wormald PJ. The incidence of complications using new landmarks and a modified technique of canine fossa puncture. Am J Rhinol 2007;21(3):316–319
2. Woodworth BA, Parker RO, Schlosser RJ. Modified endoscopic medial maxillectomy for chronic maxillary sinusitis. Am J Rhinol 2006;20(3):317–319
3. Cho D-Y, Hwang PH. Results of endoscopic maxillary mega-antrostomy in recalcitrant maxillary sinusitis. Am J Rhinol 2008;22(6):658–662
4. Catapano D, Sloffer CA, Frank G, Pasquini E, D'Angelo VA, Lanzino G. Comparison between the microscope and endoscope in the direct endonasal extended transsphenoidal approach: anatomical study. J Neurosurg 2006;104(3):419–425
5. Robinson S, Patel N, Wormald PJ. Endoscopic management of benign tumors extending into the infratemporal fossa: a two-surgeon transnasal approach. Laryngoscope 2005;115(10):1818–1822
6. Rice DH. Endonasal approaches for sinonasal and nasopharyngeal tumors. Otolaryngol Clin North Am 2001;34(6):1087–1093, vii
7. Wormald PJ, Van Hasselt A. Endoscopic removal of juvenile angiofibromas. Otolaryngol Head Neck Surg 2003;129(6):684–691
8. Douglas R, Wormald PJ. Endoscopic surgery for juvenile nasopharyngeal angiofibroma: where are the limits? Curr Opin Otolaryngol Head Neck Surg 2006;14(1):1–5
9. Stamm AC, Vellutini E, Harvey RJ, Nogeira JF Jr, Herman DR. Endoscopic transnasal craniotomy and the resection of craniopharyngioma. Laryngoscope 2008;118(7):1142–1148
10. Lanier B, Kai G, Marple B, Wall GM. Pathophysiology and progression of nasal septal perforation. Ann Allergy Asthma Immunol 2007;99(6):473–479, quiz 480–481, 521
11. Harvey RJ, Nogueira JF, Schlosser RJ, Patel SJ, Vellutini E, Stamm AC. Closure of large skull base defects after endoscopic transnasal craniotomy. J Neurosurg 2009;111(2):371–379
12. Hadad G, Bassagasteguy L, Carrau RL, et al. A novel reconstructive technique after endoscopic expanded endonasal approaches: vascular pedicle nasoseptal flap. Laryngoscope 2006;116(10):1882–1886
13. Harvey RJ, Sheehan PO, Debnath NI, Schlosser RJ. Transseptal approach for extended endoscopic resections of the maxilla and infratemporal fossa. Am J Rhinol Allergy 2009;23(4):426–432
14. Wormald PJ, Ooi E, van Hasselt CA, Nair S. Endoscopic removal of sinonasal inverted papilloma including endoscopic medial maxillectomy. Laryngoscope 2003;113(5):867–873
15. Snyder RN, Perzin KH. Papillomatosis of nasal cavity and paranasal sinuses (inverted papilloma, squamous papilloma). A clinicopathologic study. Cancer 1972;30(3):668–690
16. Krouse JH. Endoscopic treatment of inverted papilloma: safety and efficacy. Am J Otolaryngol 2001;22(2):87–99
17. Mirza S, Bradley PJ, Acharya A, Stacey M, Jones NS. Sinonasal inverted papillomas: recurrence, and synchronous and metachronous malignancy. J Laryngol Otol 2007;121(9):857–864
18. Christensen WN, Smith RR. Schneiderian papillomas: a clinicopathologic study of 67 cases. Hum Pathol 1986;17(4):393–400
19. Weissler MC, Montgomery WW, Turner PA, Montgomery SK, Joseph MP. Inverted papilloma. Ann Otol Rhinol Laryngol 1986;95(3 Pt 1):215–221
20. Yousuf K, Wright ED. Site of attachment of inverted papilloma predicted by CT findings of osteitis. Am J Rhinol 2007;21(1):32–36
21. Lee DK, Chung SK, Dhong HJ, Kim HY, Kim HJ, Bok KH. Focal hyperostosis on CT of sinonasal inverted papilloma as a predictor of tumor origin. AJNR Am J Neuroradiol 2007;28(4):618–621
22. Eberhart LH, Folz BJ, Wulf H, Geldner G. Intravenous anesthesia provides optimal surgical conditions during microscopic and endoscopic sinus surgery. Laryngoscope 2003;113(8):1369–1373

23. Wormald PJ, van Renen G, Perks J, Jones JA, Langton-Hewer CD. The effect of the total intravenous anesthesia compared with inhalational anesthesia on the surgical field during endoscopic sinus surgery. Am J Rhinol 2005;19(5):514–520
24. Chiu AG, Jackman AH, Antunes MB, Feldman MD, Palmer JN. Radiographic and histologic analysis of the bone underlying inverted papillomas. Laryngoscope 2006;116(9):1617–1620
25. James D, Crockard HA. Surgical access to the base of skull and upper cervical spine by extended maxillotomy. Neurosurgery 1991;29(3):411–416
26. Singhal D, Douglas R, Robinson S, Wormald PJ. The incidence of complications using new landmarks and a modified technique of canine fossa puncture. Am J Rhinol 2007;21(3):316–319

26 Learning from a Difficult Case: Inverted Papilloma Involving the Anterior Wall of the Maxillary Sinus

Christos C. Georgalas and Wytske J. Fokkens

Although an inverted papilloma (IP) is the most common benign neoplasia of the paranasal sinuses, its features have always been controversial. It was thought that it frequently undergoes malignant transformation, that it invades the orbit and the brain, and that it recurs many years after its excision. We know now that this is not true. The initial reports of up to 53% risk of malignant transformation referred (in a significant portion of the cases) to missed ab initio malignant tumors. A retrospective review of 123 cases of IP at the Institute of Laryngology and Otology at Gray's Inn Road Hospital in London[1] showed elegantly how reports of malignant change have decreased at the same time as reports of synchronous malignancy have risen. A review of 2297 cases of documented synchronous and metachronous tumors revealed that the real risk of malignant transformation of IP is ~3%, but the risk of an IP harboring a carcinoma is more than double (7–8%).[2]

Similarly, 21 cases of an IP invading the brain have been reported in the literature:[3] 10 of which had SCC, and 9 of the 11 remaining patients had recurrent disease. The cases involving the orbit are rare enough to merit publishing as case reports.[4] In terms of timing of recurrence, we now understand that recurrences are mostly cases of residual disease, with 80% of them presenting within 2 years from resection.

■ Management

The management advocated for IP in the seventies was simple intranasal excision, which perhaps unsurprisingly was associated with recurrence rates of up to 71%.[5] A decade later, the application of the principles of oncologic head and neck surgery led to more extensive surgery (lateral rhinotomy/medial maxillectomy) being performed—and the recurrence rates plummeted to less than 20%.[6] The introduction of the endoscope led to the first attempts at endoscopic removal.[7] As more surgeons published their results, it became feasible in 2006 to undertake a meta-analyses of their outcomes.[8,9] These meta-analyses looked at 292/353 and 714/1060 cases of endoscopic and open techniques, respectively, and both reached broadly similar results, namely, that the endoscopic approach is associated with better outcomes and lower recurrence compared with the external approach: 12 versus 17% or 12 versus 20%, respectively. However, caution is indicated in interpreting these findings: They were based on simple observational studies which (in the case of the second meta-analysis) lacked nonrandomized or even historical controls. It is also not clear how adequately synchronous tumors were excluded, how many of those treated had recurrent tumors, how thorough was the follow-up, and more importantly, how was selection bias dealt with. At the dawn of the endoscopic excision, the smallest tumors would (logically) have been chosen for endoscopic management. Although these meta-analyses reveal that endoscopic excision has become the current standard, they also make clear that there is a need to standardize excision, follow-up, exclusion of synchronous tumors, and apply staging.[10]

■ Our Technique

We feel that a discussion of endoscopic versus external excision can be potentially misleading. The use of an endoscope, per se, tells us about the "endoscopic approach" as much (or as little) as the use of a scalpel tells us about an external approach. What is important is what is removed and how it is removed rather than how it is visualized while being removed. We favor a targeted/step approach, tailoring the excision to the extent of the disease.

The IP is endoscopically evaluated and the possibility of creating free margins is checked. The attachment of the IP is determined. The most limited approach possible is chosen. When the IP is attached to the orbital roof or the superior part of the lateral or posterior wall of the maxillary sinus, removal by a normal infundibulotomy is usually possible. Attachments to the lower part of the lateral or posterior wall can sometimes be removed by making a big antrostomy or an extra access through the inferior meatus or the anterior wall. If the attachment is very broad or located at the medial wall of the maxilla, a more radical approach is often indicated with complete removal of the medial wall (medial maxillectomy). The inferior turbinate, is removed when involved by disease or for visualization, as part of medial maxillectomy, whereas the middle turbinate is removed only when involved by the IP.

Based on this rationale, we routinely plan surgery after assessing both the computed tomography (CT) and the magnetic resonance imaging (MRI) scans. We specifically look for signs of osteitis, to help us identify the area of attachment to the sinus wall.[11] We are prepared to change plans intraoperatively, always aiming to achieve a removal on healthy margins, and ideally en bloc. To attain this, we

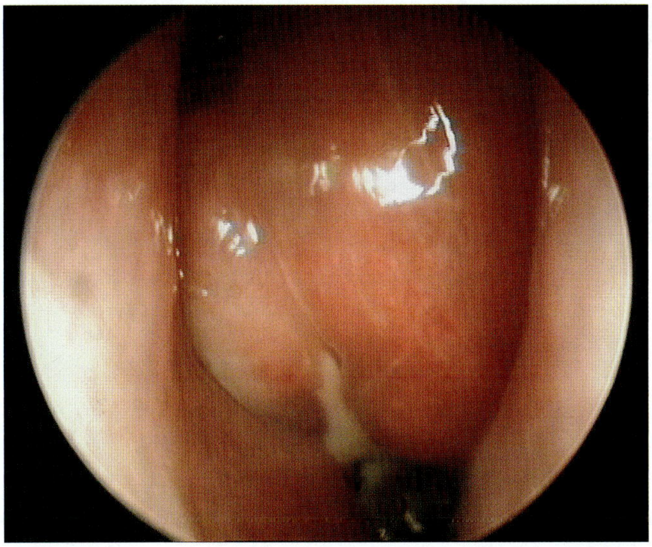

Fig. 26.1 Preoperative endoscopic photograph of the tumor in the nasal cavity.

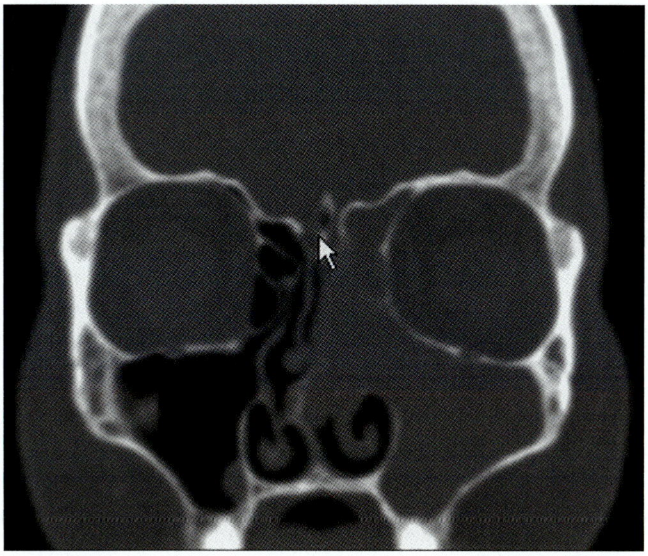

Fig. 26.2 Computed tomography scan of the sinuses: note the osteitis sign.

actively search intraoperatively for the site of attachment of the IP and remove it with a 1-cm cuff of healthy mucosa around it. After the IP removal, the areas of mucosa adjacent to the IP attachment are burned with diathermy and/or the underlying bone is drilled with a diamond burr, to remove microscopic extensions of the IP.

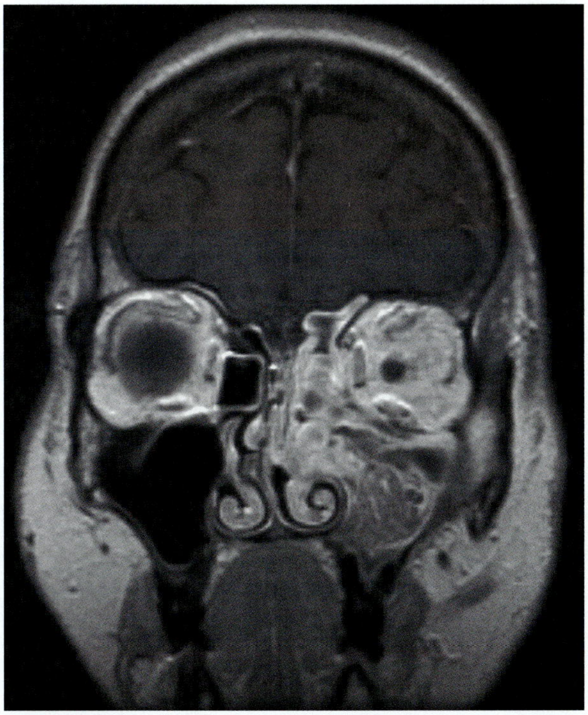

Fig. 26.3 Magnetic resonance imaging of the sinuses.

The Case

A 65-year-old woman presented in our clinic with progressive left-sided nasal obstruction. On rigid endoscopy, a large fleshy polyp was visualized extending through the middle meatus, deflecting medially the middle turbinate and partly obstructing the nasal cavity (**Fig. 26.1**).

A biopsy confirmed the clinical diagnosis of an inverted papilloma. The CT and MRI scans are shown in **Figs. 26.2** and **26.3**. On the basis of the scans and the histologic report, a medial maxillectomy, anterior and posterior ethmoidectomy was planned.

We start by applying topical cocaine powder in cotton buds soaked in 1 mg/mL epinephrine. Initially, we assess the extent of the tumor specifically trying to identify the location and extent of attachment. If we decide that the medial wall has to go because of the broad attachment to the medial wall and floor of the maxillary sinus, we subsequently proceed with a medial maxillectomy (**see Video 26.1**). In this case, we start by incising the mucosa with a 45-degree disposable keratome knife and subsequently reflect the mucosa over the projected osteotomy sites. A 3-mm chisel is used for both osteotomies, always first anterior to the nasolacrimal duct then under the inferior turbinate. The medial wall of the maxillary sinus is subsequently reflected medially and the nasolacrimal duct identified and cleanly resected with sharp scissors. If necessary, the maxillectomy opening is further enlarged anteriorly and inferiorly with a 15-degree diamond burr and a Kerrison punch, aiming always to completely visualize the anterior wall of maxillary sinus. At this stage, the whole attachment of the papilloma in the maxillary sinus should be clearly visualized. We find that malleable suction elevators are very helpful for removing a 10-mm cuff of normal mucosa around the papilloma attachment. Subsequently, the papilloma is followed in the ethmoids, from the lamina papyracea to the middle turbinate, all the way to the sphenoid ostium. The frontal recess is visualized via a Draf 2a. The sphenopalatine artery is ligated and the papilloma is removed en bloc. The bony maxillary wall where the papilloma was attached is drilled using a 70-degree diamond drill and the cavity inspected with a 70-degree endoscope. We sent all the specimens (including that in the debrider trap) for histology, to avoid missing a synchronous malignant tumor.

Discussion

A complete removal of inverted papilloma is vital, if one is to avoid recurrence and the need for subsequent operations. As shown in this case, we feel that it is frequently possible to perform an en bloc resection and remove completely the tumor using a targeted approach. In the case of maxillary sinus tumors involving the anterior maxillary wall, adequate visualization and subsequently complete removal can be accomplished via a medial maxillectomy (endoscopic Denker), in our opinion in most cases without the need for canine fossa trephination. However, the use of a 30- and 45-degree endoscope and curved drills and shavers is imperative, as is assessment of the whole specimen in the pathology laboratory.

Pearls

- Always assess the papilloma with both CT and MRI. The bony detail included in the CT is important to recognize the presence of intrasinus septa, Haller cells, and the relative depth of the orbit and the nasolacrimal duct; MRI (especially T2-weighted MRI with intravenous contrast) can differentiate between tumor and retained secretions.
- It is increasingly recognized that the papilloma attachment can be predicted with some degree of accuracy from signs of osteitis: always try to assess the CT for such signs.
- Hypotensive anesthesia and adequate local vasoconstriction are useful for a bloodless field and adequate visualization during the operation.
- Try to remove en bloc the medial maxillary wall and the papilloma. Use a 3-mm chisel to perform the inferior and anterior/medial osteotomies on the maxillary sinus wall.
- Always aim to clearly visualize and cleanly cut the nasolacrimal duct. In our opinion, there is no indication for the routine use of nasolacrimal duct stents.
- A 70-degree diamond drill and curved suction diathermy are important to completely remove any remnants of the papilloma as well as its attachments in the maxillary sinus walls.
- Remember to send the whole specimen (including any parts of the specimen within the debrider trap) for histology. Although the chance of malignant transformation of a papilloma is minimal, the chances of a synchronous malignant tumor are not insignificant.

References

1. Woodson GE, Robbins KT, Michaels L. Inverted papilloma. Considerations in treatment. Arch Otolaryngol 1985;111(12):806–811
2. Mirza S, Bradley PJ, Acharya A, Stacey M, Jones NS. Sinonasal inverted papillomas: recurrence, and synchronous and metachronous malignancy. J Laryngol Otol 2007;121(9):857–864
3. Vural E, Suen JY, Hanna E. Intracranial extension of inverted papilloma: An unusual and potentially fatal complication. Head Neck 1999;21(8):703–706
4. Bajaj MS, Pushker N. Inverted papilloma invading the orbit. Orbit 2002;21(2):155–159
5. Trible WM, Lekagul S. Inverting papilloma of the nose and paranasal sinuses: report of 30 cases. Laryngoscope 1971;81(5):663–668
6. Myers EN, Schramm VL Jr, Barnes EL Jr. Management of inverted papilloma of the nose and paranasal sinuses. Laryngoscope 1981;91(12): 2071–2084
7. Waitz G, Wigand ME. Results of endoscopic sinus surgery for the treatment of inverted papillomas. Laryngoscope 1992;102(8):917–922
8. Karkos PD, Fyrmpas G, Carrie SC, Swift AC. Endoscopic versus open surgical interventions for inverted nasal papilloma: a systematic review. Clin Otolaryngol 2006;31(6):499–503
9. Busquets JM, Hwang PH. Endoscopic resection of sinonasal inverted papilloma: a meta-analysis. Otolaryngol Head Neck Surg 2006;134(3):476–482
10. Krouse JH. Development of a staging system for inverted papilloma. Laryngoscope 2000;110(6):965–968
11. Yousuf K, Wright ED. Site of attachment of inverted papilloma predicted by CT findings of osteitis. Am J Rhinol 2007;21(1):32–36

27 Learning from Two Difficult Cases: Transmaxillary Approaches to the Pterygopalatine Space

Hwa J. Son and Rakesh K. Chandra

Prior to advances in instrumentation for endoscopic sinus surgery, access to the middle cranial skull base behind the maxillary sinus was difficult, often involving facial incisions and/or neurosurgical access. Disease processes ranging from cerebrospinal fluid (CSF) leak, infections, and various neoplasms are occasionally found in anatomic spaces behind the posterior wall of the maxillary sinus, including the pterygopalatine space (PPS) and the lateral sphenoid recess (LSR), a pneumatization of the sphenoid sinus lumen into the pterygoid root.

Traditional approaches to the retromaxillary spaces include midfacial degloving or lateral rhinotomy with medial maxillectomy, Caldwell–Luc, and subtemporal craniotomy. Endoscopic transmaxillary approaches with image guidance provide a superior visualization while being less invasive and more aesthetically favorable. The special anatomic relationship of the PPS and the LSR allow endoscopic approaches to these regions through the posterior wall of maxillary sinus and indications for endoscopic techniques continue to broaden. This chapter will illustrate surgical techniques of transmaxillary approaches to the PPS as adaptations of those previously described for the LSR.

■ Anatomy

The posterior wall of the maxillary bone articulates medially with the palatine bone. The PPS is a small space bounded anteriorly by these structures and posterosuperiorly by the sphenoid. The PPS has free connections to the orbit, palate, skull base, infratemporal fossa, and nasal cavity, thus providing a path of least resistance to various disease processes.

The sphenopalatine foramen, found between sphenoid and palatine bone, contains the sphenopalatine artery, which is the main blood supply to the posterior nasal cavity. The inferior orbital fissure, at the junction of sphenoid and maxillary bone, opens to the orbital floor and transmits the distal branch of the maxillary nerve as the infraorbital nerve. Transmaxillary approaches offer access to the extradural skull base up to the foramen rotundum (containing the maxillary nerve) and pterygoid canal (containing the Vidian nerve). The pyramidal process of the palatine bone makes up the floor with its greater and lesser palatine foramina as the communications of the PPS inferiorly (**Table 27.1**).[1]

Occasionally, pneumatization of the lateral portion of the sphenoid bone, either the greater wing or the pterygoid process, occurs forming an LSR. This is observed in up to 25 to 48% of patients[2] and is extensively pneumatized in 8% of cases. In this case, the roof of the sphenoid sinus lies directly beneath the middle cranial fossa and temporal lobe. Defects in the skull base in the LSR or the infratemporal fossa can be accessed via transmaxillary approaches as well.

■ Pathology That May Be Encountered in the Pterygopalatine Space

Juvenile nasopharyngeal angiofibroma (JNA) is the most common lesion in the PPS. It is thought to originate from the aperture of sphenopalatine foramen. Although a benign neoplasm, it is a locally invasive and a high vascular tumor. Radiologically, the pathognomonic sign is the Holman–Miller

Table 27.1 Pterygopalatine Space (PPS) Anatomy and Its Contents

Foramina/Fissures	Location within PPS	Contents
Inferior orbital fissure	Anterosuperior wall (roof)	Infraorbital nerve
Pterygomaxillary fissure	Lateral wall	Internal maxillary artery
Sphenopalatine foramen	Medial wall	Sphenopalatine artery
Greater palatine foramen	Floor	Greater palatine nerve/artery
Lesser palatine foramen	Floor	Lesser palatine nerve/artery
Pterygoid canal	Posterior wall	Vidian nerve
Foramen rotundum	Posterior wall	Maxillary nerve

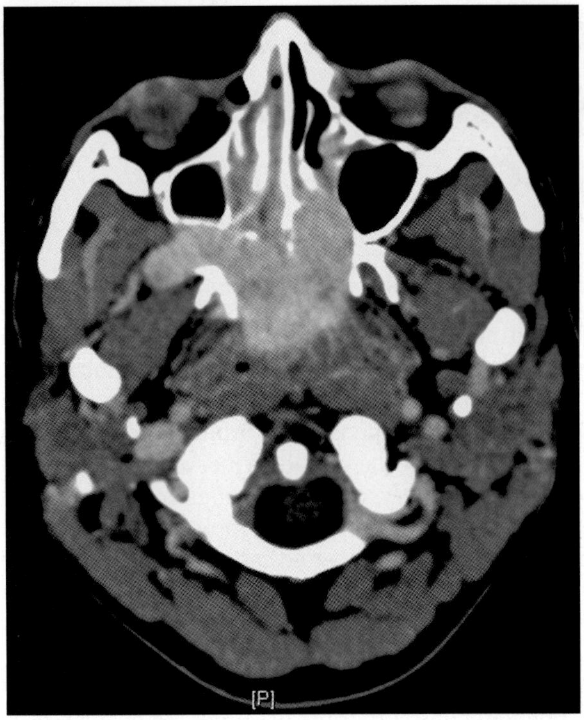

Fig. 27.1 Computed tomography scan of sinus, axial cut showing right-sided juvenile nasopharyngeal angiofibroma in the pterygopalatine space, displacing the posterior wall of the maxillary sinus anteriorly.

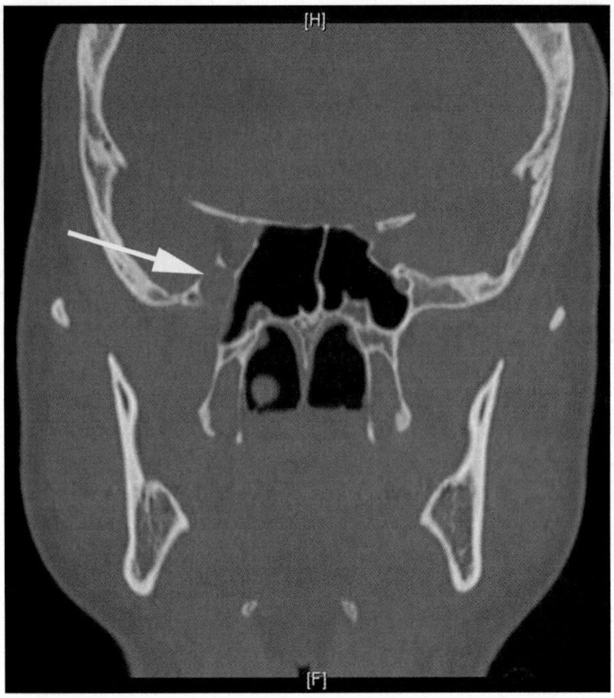

Fig. 27.2 Computed tomography scan of sinus, coronal cut showing right-sided schwannoma widening foramen rotundum (*arrow*).

sign, where there is an anterior displacement of the posterior wall of maxillary sinus wall due to mass (**Fig. 27.1**). Angiography is performed to evaluate for the feeding vessel, the most common vessel being the branches of internal maxillary artery. For smaller tumors, an endoscopic approach is ideal.[3,4] Schwannoma is another lesion that can involve the maxillary division of the trigeminal nerve in the PPS. It is a slowly growing tumor and they can expand through thin parts of bone and widen the natural ostium (**Fig. 27.2**). Traditionally, these tumors in the PPS were removed through lateral rhinotomy or facial degloving approach. In a benign mass where en bloc resection is not necessary, endoscopic surgery is well suited.[5] Other pathologies such as mucocele, invasive fungal infection, lymphoma, and inverting papilloma can extend to the PPS as well. Biopsies can be performed to confirm diagnoses of such conditions, and formal surgical resection may be indicated.

Rarely, the temporal lobe can herniate into the PPS or LSR through a congenital or traumatic skull base defect, causing CSF rhinorrhea, recurrent meningitis, and possibly seizures. Traditionally, several invasive measures were used such as anterior subtemporal craniotomy or facial degloving. Bolger et al popularized the transpterygoid approach to the LSR and described this in detail through cadaver studies.[6] Bolger and Osenbach reported six patients treated for encephalocele of the LSR endoscopically with up to 25-month follow-up, without recurrence or significant complications.[7] Transmaxillary access to the PPS is an adaptation of these

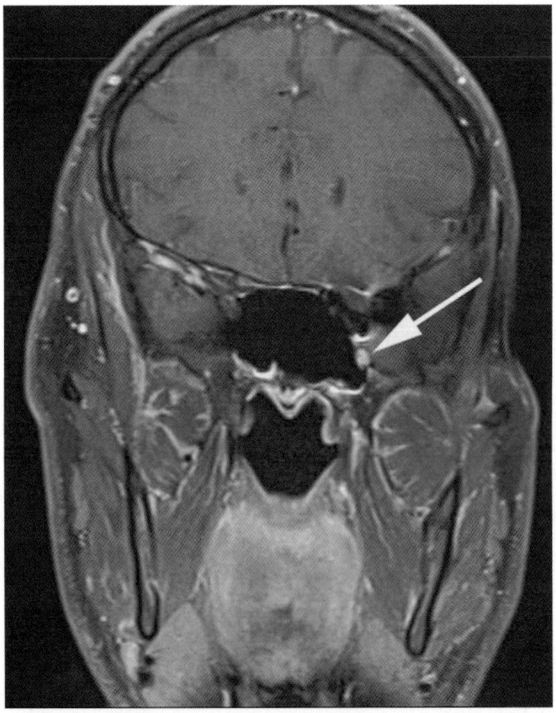

Fig. 27.3 Magnetic resonance image of the neck, coronal cut showing left enlargement V2 nerve, in recurrent adenoid cystic carcinoma of lacrimal gland with perineural invasion (*arrow*).

approaches to the LSR, involving removal of the ascending process of the palatine bone and posterior maxillary sinus wall via a wide antrostomy.

Occasionally, tumors spread beyond the bony confines of the PPS via the previously described foraminal portals. A classic example of this is reflected by perineural invasion by adenoid cystic carcinoma, which can track intracranially along nerves of the cavernous sinus wall. The palatine branch of the maxillary nerve innervates the mucosa of the hard palate, which contains many minor salivary glands and can also harbor neoplasm. As tumors pass through foramina, they enlarge these bony openings, creating a characteristic appearance on imaging studies (**Fig. 27.3**).[8]

Surgical Technique

The two cases presented (**see Videos 27.1 and 27.2**) illustrate the transmaxillary approach to the pterygopalatine space. Case 1 describes a patient with a history of lacrimal adenocarcinoma previously treated with orbital exoneration, chemotherapy, and radiation. He presented with lip numbness, and MRI suggested perineural recurrence along the second division of the trigeminal nerve. After consultation with the multispecialty tumor board, excisional biopsy was advocated. This was performed via a transmaxillary approach to the pterygopalatine space through a wide maxillary antrostomy, takedown of the palatine process and posterior maxillary wall, and identification of the neural foramen and canal in the posterior-superior compartment of the space. Case 2 presents a patient with cerebrospinal fluid rhinorrhea whose preoperative imaging revealed a large meningocele arising from the left temporal region, filling the pterygoid space posterior to the pterygoid plate, splaying the pterygoid plates. This was accessed via a transmaxillary approach to the pterygopalatine space through a wide maxillary antrostomy, takedown of the palatine process and posterior maxillary wall, and identification of the attenuated bone of the pterygoid root. Opening of the latter layer of bone exposed the meningocele sac, which was resected and decompressed. The defect was closed with a fascia lata flap and bulk from the flap was also utilized to obliterate dead space in the pterygoid and pterygopalatine spaces.

When approaching the pterygopalatine fossa, depending on the pathology, it may be prudent to anticipate the need for transfusion, given proximity to the internal maxillary arterial system and pterygoid plexus of veins. Preoperative angiography and embolization is necessary in certain cases such as JNA. Neurosurgical consultation is a significant consideration, particularly in the setting of encephalocele or CSF leak. MRI and CT should both be obtained and image-guided surgical navigation is useful intraoperatively.

The usual preparations for the endoscopic sinus surgery are undertaken. Nasal cavities are topically vasoconstricted and anesthetized with pledgets soaked with 4% cocaine and oxymetazoline. Needle injection with 1% lidocaine with 1:100,000 epinephrine is applied to the axilla of the middle turbinate and the region of the sphenopalatine foramen. Intraoral injection of the greater palatine foramen can also be employed.

Zero-degree telescopic visualization is utilized throughout the initial stages of the dissection. First, uncinectomy is done, and middle meatal antrostomy is performed through the natural ostium. This is enlarged posteriorly into the region of the posterior fontanel using through-cut forceps as well as a microdebrider. A wide antrostomy is the first key to the procedure. For extended lesions, anterior and posterior ethmoidectomy may be required with identification of the skull base in the posterior ethmoid. Then sphenoidotomy is begun by identifying the root of the superior turbinate, followed by resection of the lower third of the turbinate body to expose the rostrum. The natural ostium will be posterior and just medial to the resected portion of the turbinate body. The sphenoid is entered using a curette and the ostomy is enlarged using a combination of Kerrison forceps, as well as through-cut forceps and/or the microdebrider. The sphenoidotomy is lowered toward the floor of the sinus. During this maneuver, it is often necessary to control the posterior septal branch of the sphenopalatine artery, which courses along the rostrum inferior to the sphenoid os.

The mucosa is then elevated in a submucoperiosteal plane, from the posterior wall of the maxillary sinus. Next, using the 4-mm diamond choanal atresia burr, the ascending process of the palatine bone, as well as the bone from the posterior wall of the maxillary sinus is removed, thus opening the anteromedial walls of the PPS. The sphenoidotomy is enlarged laterally and brought into communication with the soft tissue of the sphenopalatine foramen and medial pterygopalatine space. Using a combination of the drill, and Blakesley and Kerrison forceps, the opening into the posterior wall of the maxillary sinus is further enlarged laterally to expose the soft tissue in the pterygopalatine space. Angled telescopes (30- and 45-degree) are useful in this process, but occasionally, it is necessary to perform a Caldwell–Luc antrostomy to augment lateral access from an anterior trajectory. One should recall the pathologic process can significantly thin the posterior wall. Branches from the internal maxillary artery in the pterygopalatine space should be identified and bleeding controlled using electrocautery and/or surgical clips. Dissection using endoscopic microscissors through the pterygopalatine space fat can be performed to tease vascular branches away from the area of pathology, which can be confirmed with stereotactic correlation.

Dissection should proceed from inferomedial to superolateral until the foramen rotundum is encountered. The nerve within the foramen rotundum can be identified. Using an elevator, dissection can proceed in a subperiosteal plane along the uppermost aspect of the pterygoid root. If further dissection is necessary, the diamond drill can be utilized to remove bone along the medial hemisphere of the foramen rotundum, allowing dissection of the nerve along the body of the lateral sphenoid wall to the point of the cavernous sinus. Adequate biopsy specimen or resection of mass concludes the procedure.

Additional visualization in the region of the internal maxillary arterial branches should confirm hemostasis in this location. A small amount of absorbable hemostat can be placed over cauterized areas or venous plexi. In patients with defects of the floor of the middle cranial fossa, grafts are utilized to reconstruct the defect, support the temporal lobe, and obliterate the dead-space in the PPS. The displaced mucosa of posterior maxillary wall is then redraped; in cases where a CSF leak or cranial base defect was repaired, it is necessary to bolster the closure with a pack or Foley balloon within the maxillary sinus.

Conclusion

The literature describes multiple alternatives for the management of lesions behind the posterior maxillary sinus wall, including JNA, schwannoma, carcinoma with perineural invasion, and CSF leak with meningocele.[9,10] Here we illustrated how management of these pathologies can be successfully and safely accomplished through an endoscopic maxillary antrostomy. In our experience, the use of image guidance and meticulous exposure are critical to the procedure.

Pearls

To accomplish the meticulous exposure, the following are needed:
- Wide antrostomy
- Identification of the orbital process of the palatine bone
- Control of internal maxillary arterial branches
- Use of a drill, when necessary, to address dense bone of the pterygoid root
- Consideration of a Caldwell–Luc if enhanced lateral exposure is required

References

1. Moore KL, Dalley AF. Clinically Oriented Anatomy. 5th ed. Baltimore: Lippincott Williams & Wilkins; 2006
2. Etter L. Atlas of Roentgen Anatomy of the Skull. Springfield, IL: Charles C. Thomas; 1955
3. Borghei P, Baradaranfar MH, Borghei SH, Sokhandon F. Transnasal endoscopic resection of juvenile nasopharyngeal angiofibroma without preoperative embolization. Ear Nose Throat J 2006;85(11):740–743, 746
4. Wormald P. Endoscopic Sinus Surgery: Anatomy, Three-Dimensional Reconstruction, and Surgical Technique. New York: Thieme Medical Publishing; 2005
5. Pasquini E, Sciarretta V, Farneti G, Ippolito A, Mazzatenta D, Frank G. Endoscopic endonasal approach for the treatment of benign schwannoma of the sinonasal tract and pterygopalatine fossa. Am J Rhinol 2002;16(2):113–118
6. Bolger WE, Osenbach R. Endoscopic transpterygoid approach to the lateral sphenoid recess. Ear Nose Throat J 1999;78:36–46
7. Bolger WE. Endoscopic transpterygoid approach to the lateral sphenoid recess: surgical approach and clinical experience. Otolaryngol Head Neck Surg 2005;133(1):20–26
8. Som PM, Curtin HD. Head and Neck Imaging. St. Louis, MO: Mosby; 2003
9. Lane AP, Bolger WE. Endoscopic transmaxillary biopsy of pterygopalatine space masses: a preliminary report. Am J Rhinol 2002;16(2):109–112
10. DelGaudio JM. Endoscopic transnasal approach to the pterygopalatine fossa. Arch Otolaryngol Head Neck Surg 2003;129(4):441–446

28 Three Difficult Cases in the Management of Maxillary Sinus Disease

Maria L. Wittkopf and James A. Duncavage

The maxillary sinus, as we have seen in this book, is without a doubt the most difficult sinus to cure medically or surgically. The endoscopic sinus surgeon can perform a flawless endoscopic antrostomy and yet fail to improve the diseased state of the sinus. Similarly, the endoscopic sinus surgeon can revise a scarred maxillary antrostomy and fail to improve the ability of the sinus to drain properly. Finally, the revision endoscopic sinus surgeon can remove the diseased lining in a failed maxillary antrostomy case and still find that the postoperative maxillary sinus is in no way improved than its preoperative state.

Our intent in this concluding chapter is to present three cases of maxillary sinusitis, in which the patients have failed to improve their symptoms following attempted surgical treatment. The authors of previous chapters have elucidated how to perform a maxillary antrostomy successfully. They have also illustrated how to identify and correct technical reasons for failure. In this chapter, we would like to discuss the most difficult cases that we have encountered in the previous 23 years at Vanderbilt University Medical Center (Nashville, TN). The following discussion assumes that the patient has undergone a previous maxillary antrostomy, which has failed, but that no abnormalities in the surgical technique for the antrostomy have been found.

Before presenting you with the three cases, we will outline the treatment philosophy that has been used to evaluate and treat our maxillary sinus patients:

- The first treatment point is to adequately manage the patient medically, once maxillary sinusitis has been diagnosed via computed tomography (CT) scan or directly by nasal endoscopy. In my practice, adequate management includes the use of systemic steroids for a minimum of 10 days and oral antibiotics for a minimum of 3 weeks. All attempts are made to obtain a culture endoscopically, from the middle meatus or directly from the maxillary sinus.
- A second point concerns the management of biofilms. In the case of an isolated maxillary sinus infection, irrigation via the maxillary antrostomy site is utilized to break up and flush out the infected materials. All irrigations are cultured. If *Staphylococcus* is isolated on culture, mupirocin is instilled directly into the maxillary sinus and the patient is placed on culture-directed antibiotics. Further treatments of the biofilms are initiated by weekly office visits to irrigate and instill mupirocin.
- If bacteria are isolated on culture that is not amenable to oral antibiotics, either due to allergy or to the lack of a suitable oral antibiotic, an infectious disease consult is obtained. Once the plan for intravenous (IV) antibiotics is initiated, plans are made either to see the patient weekly for biofilm treatment, or to see the patient at 3 weeks to evaluate the effectiveness of the IV antibiotic. If at 3 weeks there is observable improvement, then the patient proceeds on to a complete course of IV treatment, usually lasting 6 weeks.

In our experience, one of two results will occur with the treatments outlined above. The patient will improve and become healthy, or the sinus will not improve and the patient will relapse. The usual case is that the sinus will relapse quickly after the weekly treatments or after the cessation of the IV antibiotics.

The patients in our three cases were all treated in the manner just described. When the maxillary sinus fails to improve, our diagnosis is failure of the ciliated respiratory epithelium to regenerate. Given that the maxillary sinus must drain against gravity, an intact ciliary clearance mechanism must be present and functional. The data we have used to guide our management of the failed cilia are based on our experience with the use of Caldwell–Luc surgery to manage this group of patients. Our review of this group of maxillary sinus patients found a 93% success rate to manage the maxillary sinus after removal of the maxillary sinus lining via a Caldwell–Luc approach.[1]

■ Case 1

The first case is a 67-year-old man with a chief complaint of chronic nasal crusting and nasal drainage. He had a history of two previous sinus surgeries and was on Coumadin following an aortic valve replacement. Nasal endoscopy revealed metaplastic changes in both maxillary sinuses. In addition, the nasal cavities were filled with crust and purulent material. A CT scan of the sinuses revealed bilateral maxillary sinus opacification. A culture with sensitivities was obtained from both maxillary sinuses.

The patient was then treated with numerous culture-directed antibiotics without improvement. The recommended plan of treatment was a bilateral Caldwell-Luc operation. The clinical findings at the time of surgery revealed avascular bone along the medial wall of the left maxillary sinus and purulent debris within both maxillary sinuses. The sinus mucosa was also found to be edematous. Microscopically, the left maxillary sinus lining was found to be polypoid and edematous with markedly inflamed respiratory mucosa and submucosa with severe chronic inflammation and mild acute inflammation. There were areas of necrotic inflammatory debris, fragmented fungal hyphal forms, and benign reactive bone. On the right side, the mucosa was likewise found to be polypoid and the submucosa also revealed severe chronic and mild acute inflammation, along with fragments of benign bone, but no definite fungal organisms. Part of the pathology report stated that "the mucosa exhibits relatively prominent plasmacytic and lymphocytic infiltrates. A few areas of ulceration and acute inflammation are present."

The follow-up at one month noted no signs of infection in either maxillary sinus. The patient returned at 2 months with complaints of globus sensation and postnasal drip. The endoscopic findings were crusting in the bilateral maxillary sinuses. Topical Pulmicort (AstraZeneca, Pharmaceuticals, LP, London, UK) was instituted. The patient returned 2 months later with complaint of hoarseness and nasal crusting. A culture was taken, the Pulmicort was stopped, and Bactroban (GlaxoSmithKline, Mississauga, Ontario, Canada) was started topically. The culture was positive for *Klebsiella*. Appropriate antibiotic management was initiated.

The patient returned 3 months later. His complaint at that time was persistent postnasal drip. Physical exam revealed scarring of the bilateral maxillary sinuses. A CT scan of the sinuses was obtained. It noted significant opacification within the bilateral maxillary sinuses. Given the CT findings, exploratory surgery was recommended with a possibility of bilateral Caldwell–Luc approaches.

One month later the patient was taken to the operating room. The surgical findings were a small area of loculated purulence within the right maxillary sinus and no purulence within the left maxillary sinus (**Fig. 28.1**). The postoperative visit at one week found the patient well healed and much improved. He was continued on Flonase (GlaxoSmithKline, Mississauga, Ontario, Canada) and Bactroban topically. The patient was followed regularly and was taken back to the operating room about a year later for continued chronic maxillary sinusitis unresponsive to medical management. He underwent bilateral revision endoscopic maxillary antrostomies with tissue removal and bilateral maxillary sinoscopies. Intraoperative findings at that time included loculated areas of purulence involving the right maxillary and no loculated areas on the left, but scarring of the antrostomies bilaterally. He returned to the operating room about 4 months later for nasal endoscopy given the persistent opacification of the bilateral maxillary sinuses. The findings at that time included scarring of left and right maxillary openings and his maxillary sinuses were filled with scar tissue. No pockets of purulent material were noted. The patient continues his use of Flonase and Bactroban topically. He continues to be followed regularly in our clinic and has had no new problems.

This case illustrates the following important points:

1. The maxillary sinus respiratory lining can become irreversibly damaged as exemplified by the first pathology report. The treatment of the diseased lining in these cases may require its removal.
2. Once the diseased lining is removed, the assessment of the status of the sinus may be limited on endoscopic exam. The use of the CT scan may also be limited due to

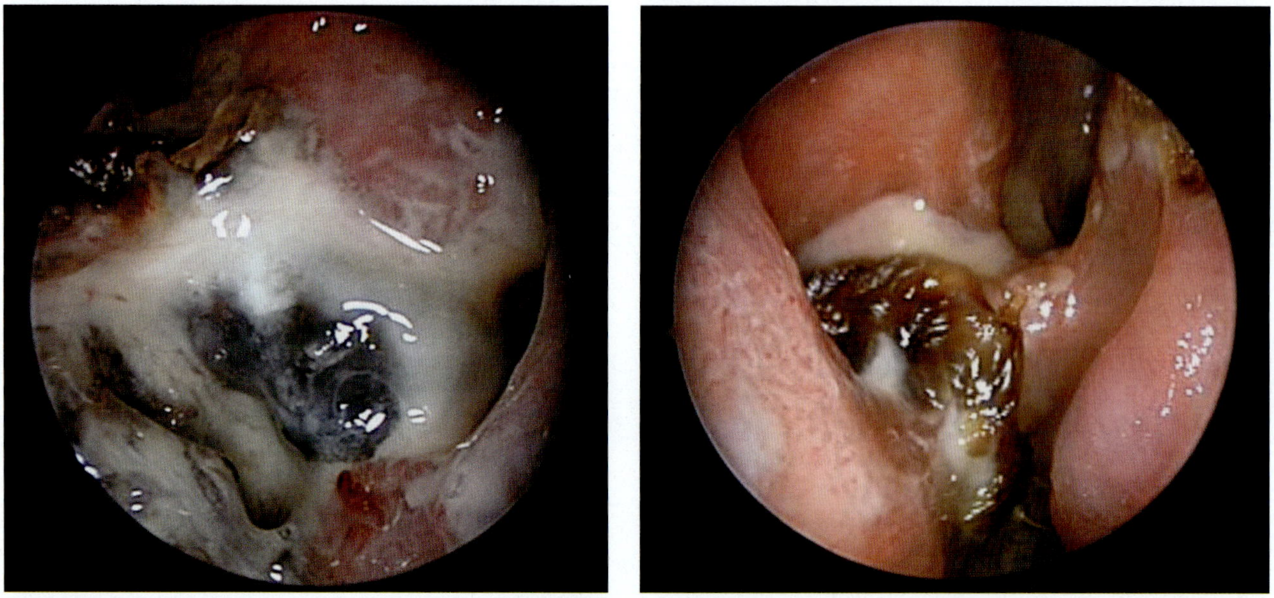

A B

Fig. 28.1 (A,B) Intraoperative findings looking into the patient's left maxillary sinus with a 30-degree endoscope.

the development of scarring that can obliterate the interior of the maxillary sinus. The inability to assess the sinus in the office may require a second look in the operating room.

3. The need to get pre- and postoperative CT scans.

Case 2

The second case is a 43-year-old woman who presented with recurrent episodes of maxillary sinusitis causing foul-smelling nasal drainage. She had undergone a previous endoscopic sinus surgery with bilateral maxillary antrostomies in January of 1999, and a septoplasty in 1988. The endoscopic exam revealed scarring at both maxillary antrostomies. Cultures were obtained in clinic, but were nondiagnostic. A sinus CT scan was read as bilateral maxillary mucopurulent thickening, as well as opacification in the frontal sinuses and left ethmoid cells. The patient was taken to the operating room on December 31, 2001, and underwent correction of the scarring at both maxillary antrostomies. Scar tissue was found between the natural maxillary ostium and the surgical ostium. Pathologically, the specimen was unremarkable, only revealing chronic inflammation.

The patient continued to have recurrent episodes of maxillary sinusitis, which were culture-positive for *Staphylococcus*. She underwent numerous treatments with antibiotics and endoscopic debridement of the bilateral maxillary sinuses. Her maxillary sinus cultures began to grow *Serratia* along with *Staphylococcus*. After failure of numerous antibiotics, bilateral Caldwell–Luc operations were performed on March 16, 2006. Crusting, edema, and purulent debris were found in both maxillary sinuses. The pathology report found respiratory-lined mucosa with marked edema, acute and chronic inflammation, and occasional eosinophils (~5 per high-powered field). The culture was positive for *Serratia*.

The patient eventually improved over the course of one year. She then relapsed with recurrent maxillary sinus infection, which was culture-positive for *Pseudomonas*. Oral antibiotics and debridements failed to control the infection. The infectious disease team was consulted and the patient was started on 6 weeks of IV antibiotics with weekly debridements. The medical management failed to control the maxillary sinusitis and the symptoms of malodorous nasal drainage. A second Caldwell–Luc procedure was performed on the left maxillary sinus on September 15, 2008. The findings were very hyperplastic, edematous membrane with an abscess pocket in the medial inferior aspect of the sinus. *Pseudomonas* was found on culture. The pathology report found respiratory mucosa with granulation tissue and chronic inflammation, but no increase in eosinophils (**see Video 28.1**).

The patient's postoperative clinical course was remarkable for persistent pseudomonal maxillary sinusitis. Immunologic and genetic testing revealed that her immunoglobulin levels were within normal limits (immunoglobulin G [IGG] level was 1131 mg/dL with reference range of 694–1618, IGA level was 202 mg/dL with reference range of 68–378, and IGE level was 44 IU/mL with reference range of 0–99). Cystic fibrosis testing revealed that the patient was a carrier of the ΔF508 mutation, detected in one allele (Poly dT tract in intron 8–5/9). Her seat chloride test was 32 mEq/L. (Reference range: less than 40 mEq/L sweat chloride = normal; 40–60 mEq/L sweat chloride = borderline; greater than 60 mEq/L sweat chloride = abnormal.)

Case 3

The third patient is a 76-year-old man who presented with a chief complaint of odor from his nose along with crusting and nasal congestion. His history was remarkable for three previous sinus surgeries, and type II diabetes. Nasal endoscopy revealed marked mucosal edema involving both maxillary sinuses with a question of scarring at both natural maxillary sinus openings. There was a large amount of nasal crusting. A CT scan found circumferential moderate mucosal thickening within the bilateral maxillary sinuses. A culture was taken from the maxillary sinuses and reported light growth of upper respiratory bacteria. He was started on ciprofloxacin and scheduled for surgery for possible Caldwell–Luc procedures.

The patient was taken to the operating room approximately one month later and found to have purulence in the maxillary sinuses with discrete abscesses within the maxillary sinus cavities, loculated purulence in the posterior ethmoid sinuses, and purulence in the right sphenoid. The patient underwent removal of scarring at both maxillary sinus openings and removal of diseased maxillary mucosa via a sinoscopy approach. A culture taken during surgery found a light growth of coagulase-positive *Staphylococcus*. The pathology report found respiratory mucosa with chronic inflammation and up to 20 eosinophils per high-power field.

Postoperatively, the patient did not show improvement in his maxillary sinus disease. Approximately 2 months later, he underwent bilateral Caldwell–Luc procedures. The surgical findings were massive edema and purulence pus within the maxillary sinuses. Intraoperative culture was again positive for heavy growth of coagulase-positive *Staphylococcus*. The pathology report found edematous respiratory mucosa and submucosa with extensive lymphoplasmacytic inflammation. An unofficial hematology consult revealed that the report findings were consistent with chronic inflammation. Since the last operative intervention, the patient has had weekly maxillary sinus debridements and is using a saline nasal wash. The crusting and odor have diminished and although they are still present, they no longer affect the patient's quality of life. The maxillary sinus lining continues to be swollen and inflamed. A sweat chloride was performed and found to be 53 mEq/L. (Reference range: less than 40 mEq/L sweat chloride = normal; 40–60 mEq/L sweat chloride = borderline.) The patient is scheduled for genetic testing to determine if he has a variant of cystic fibrosis.

The two patients discussed in Cases 2 and 3 have required multiple medical and surgical treatments of their maxillary sinus disease as a result of unhealthy maxillary sinus mucosa. They both show evidence of a symptomatic carrier state for the cystic fibrosis (CF) gene. The patient in Case 2 has been shown to be a carrier for ΔF508 mutation, which is the most common CF mutation worldwide, although she had a sweat chloride test within normal limits. Conversely, the patient discussed in Case 3 had a borderline sweat chloride test, although thus far genetic testing has not revealed him to carry a known CF mutation. Furthermore, this patient's pathology report noted up to 20 eosinophils per high-power field, a known marker for inflammation. Studies have shown that chronic rhinosinusitis (CRS) patients with hypereosinophilia have a worse prognosis when compared with controls.[2] Treatment paradigms for hypereosinophilic CRS have shifted to involve control of the inflammation and away from antimicrobial and surgical treatments.[3]

Cystic fibrosis has been known to be associated with CRS, but the story does not stop there.[4] The majority of patients with CF suffer from CRS and 20% of patients will eventually require surgical treatment of their sinuses.[5] More recent data suggest that there is a higher prevalence of CRS in carriers for the CF gene as compared with the general population. More specifically, 36% of CF carriers were noted to have signs and symptoms of CF as compared with 13 to 14% in the general population.[6] The patient discussed in Case 2 is known to be a carrier for the CF gene. Furthermore, the bacteriology of the maxillary sinusitis in this patient is characteristic for that found in airway infections of CF. *Staphylococcus aureus* and *Pseudomonas aeruginosa* have long been considered of primary importance with respect to virulence.[7] This would explain the propensity for developing CRS in the patient in Case 2 as well as the difficulty in managing her maxillary sinus disease.

The difficulty in establishing the existence of a CF mutation in the patient discussed in Case 3, in the setting of difficult to treat sinus disease and intermediate sweat chloride test, is not surprising when one bears in mind that there are more than 1600 CF mutations.[8] Mild cystic fibrosis without pulmonary symptoms has also been previously described with some CF mutations. There are many cases reported in the literature of patients with adult-onset or atypical presentations of CF.[9–11] This may delay confirmation of the diagnosis in a patient with a borderline sweat chloride test as studies have shown that a borderline sweat chloride test can be associated with a CF phenotype or it can exist in patients who do not exhibit the CF phenotype.[12] Some authors advocate looking for CF and ciliary dyskinesia mutations in all patients displaying signs and symptoms of atypical or severe and persistent CRS.[13] A borderline sweat chloride test can therefore be thought of as predictor of CF, but not the basis for a definitive diagnosis.

Conclusion

Maxillary sinusitis and sinusitis in general have become common clinical entities affecting ~15% of adults.[14] Patent ostia, mucus of the proper viscosity, and actively beating cilia are necessary to protect against infection of the paranasal sinuses. Sinusitis that does not respond to appropriate medical therapy is often treated surgically.[15] Underlying disease processes that affect the upper airway such as asthma, cystic fibrosis, ciliary dyskinesia, and allergic rhinitis complicate the treatment of maxillary sinusitis, both medically and surgically.[16,17] Some authors have suggested that patients with chronically diseased maxillary sinuses and poor mucociliary clearance from long-standing inflammation or scarring from previous surgery, may benefit from an endoscopic maxillary mega-antrostomy and avoid persistent sinus mucosa stripping.[18] Others have suggested that endoscopic revision of the maxillary sinus yields comparable outcomes to a repeat Caldwell–Luc procedure in patients with a history of previous failed Caldwell–Luc surgery, and thus, endoscopic revision surgery is a viable alternative for surgical rehabilitation of the post-Caldwell–Luc maxillary sinus.[19] The authors believe that even though endoscopic sinus surgery techniques have proven to be safe and effective in the vast majority of patients requiring surgical management, the Caldwell-Luc procedure is safe and effective as described, and should remain in the repertoire of surgeons managing the maxillary sinus.[20]

We have presented three cases from our experience, which illustrate the difficulty that can be encountered in treating maxillary sinus disease despite careful medical and surgical management. Whether the maxillary sinus mucosa is irreversibly damaged during a prior procedure, as the first case exemplifies, or whether the lining is diseased as a result of a genetic predisposition, as illustrated in the last two cases, a difficult problem is posed to the treating physician and sinus surgeon. When treating these patients, one must keep in mind that the focus of management, both medical and surgical, should be on maintaining the health of the sinus mucosa, which ensures good ciliary function and patent sinus ostia, thus achieving adequate mucociliary flow.

Pearls

- Always take an endoscopic-directed culture of the maxillary sinus.
- Always do an endoscopic debridement during antibiotic therapy to break up the biofilm
- Weekly endoscopic debridements may be necessary.
- Use of systemic steroids may be helpful.
- Endoscopic surgical exploration may be indicated to determine the nature and extent of disease.
- Always send tissue to the laboratory when in the operating room.
- In cases of persistent sinusitis, consider immune workup and infectious disease consultations.
- In cases of persistent sinusitis, consider sweat chloride/genetic testing.

References

1. Cutler JL, Duncavage JA, Matheny K, Cross JL, Miman MC, Oh CK. Results of Caldwell-Luc after failed endoscopic middle meatus antrostomy in patients with chronic sinusitis. Laryngoscope 2003;113(12):2148–2150
2. Zadeh MH, Banthia V, Anand VK, Huang C. Significance of eosinophilia in chronic rhinosinusitis. Am J Rhinol 2002;16(6):313–317
3. Amrol D, Murray JJ. Alternative medical treatment strategies for chronic hyperplastic eosinophilic sinusitis. Curr Opin Otolaryngol Head Neck Surg 2005;13(1):55–59
4. Wang X, Moylan B, Leopold DA, et al. Mutation in the gene responsible for cystic fibrosis and predisposition to chronic rhinosinusitis in the general population. JAMA 2000;284(14):1814–1819
5. Ramsey B, Richardson MA. Impact of sinusitis in cystic fibrosis. J Allergy Clin Immunol 1992; 90(3 Pt 2, 3Pt 2)547–552
6. Wang X, Kim J, McWilliams R, Cutting GR. Increased prevalence of chronic rhinosinusitis in carriers of a cystic fibrosis mutation. Arch Otolaryngol Head Neck Surg 2005;131(3):237–240
7. Gilligan PH. Microbiology of airway disease in patients with cystic fibrosis. Clin Microbiol Rev 1991;4(1):35–51
8. http://www.genet.sickkids.on.ca/cftr
9. Bargaglia E, Margolliccib M, Luddib A, Rottolia P, Bartalinib G. Unusual phenotype of cystic fibrosis patient, compound-heterozygous for 2789+5G-A/DF508 mutations. Respir Med CME 2008;1:85–86
10. Paranjape SM, Zeitlin PL. Atypical cystic fibrosis and CFTR-related diseases. Clin Rev Allergy Immunol 2008;35(3):116–123
11. Boyle MP. Nonclassic cystic fibrosis and CFTR-related diseases. Curr Opin Pulm Med 2003;9(6):498–503
12. Goubau C, Wilschanski M, Skalická V, et al. Phenotypic characterisation of patients with intermediate sweat chloride values: towards validation of the European diagnostic algorithm for cystic fibrosis. Thorax 2009;64(8):683–691
13. Coste A, Girodon E, Louis S, et al. Atypical sinusitis in adults must lead to looking for cystic fibrosis and primary ciliary dyskinesia. Laryngoscope 2004;114(5):839–843
14. www.cdc.gov
15. Slavin RG. Sinusitis in adults. J Allergy Clin Immunol 1988;81(5 Pt 2): 1028–1032
16. Kim JE, Kountakis SE. The prevalence of Samter's triad in patients undergoing functional endoscopic sinus surgery. Ear Nose Throat J 2007;86(7):396–399
17. Ryan MW. Diseases associated with chronic rhinosinusitis: what is the significance? Curr Opin Otolaryngol Head Neck Surg 2008;16(3):231–236
18. Cho DY, Hwang PH. Results of endoscopic maxillary mega-antrostomy in recalcitrant maxillary sinusitis. Am J Rhinol 2008;22(6):658–662
19. Han JK, Smith TL, Loehrl TA, Fong KJ, Hwang PH. Surgical revision of the post-Caldwell-Luc maxillary sinus. Am J Rhinol 2005;19(5):478–482
20. Matheny KE, Duncavage JA. Contemporary indications for the Caldwell-Luc procedure. Curr Opin Otolaryngol Head Neck Surg 2003;11(1):23–26

Index

Note: Page numbers followed by *f* and *t* indicate figures and tables, respectively

F

G